Manual ot
Clinical
Psychopharmacology

Seventh Edition

Manual of
Clinical
Psychopharmacology

Seventh Edition

Alan F. Schatzberg, M.D.

Kenneth T. Norris, Jr., Professor and Chairman,
Department of Psychiatry and Behavioral Sciences,
Stanford University School of Medicine, Stanford, California

Jonathan O. Cole, M.D.

Professor of Psychiatry, Harvard Medical School, Boston;
Senior Consultant, McLean Hospital, Belmont;
Psychiatric Training Consultant, St. Elizabeth's Medical Center,
Brighton, Massachusetts

Charles DeBattista, D.M.H., M.D.

Professor of Psychiatry and Behavioral Sciences;
Director, Depression Clinic and Research Program;
Director, Medical Student Education in Psychiatry,
Department of Psychiatry and Behavioral Sciences,
Stanford University School of Medicine, Stanford, California

Washington, DC
London, England

To buy 25–99 copies of this or any other APPI title at a 20% discount, please contact APPI Customer Service at appi@psych.org or 800-368-5777. To purchase 100 or more copies of the same title, please e-mail bulksales@psych.org for a price quote.

Copyright © 2010 Alan F. Schatzberg, M.D., Jonathan O. Cole, M.D., and
  Charles DeBattista, D.M.H., M.D.
ALL RIGHTS RESERVED

Manufactured in the United States of America on acid-free paper
14   13   12   11   10   5   4   3   2   1
Seventh Edition

American Psychiatric Publishing, Inc.
1000 Wilson Boulevard
Arlington, VA 22209-3901
www.appi.org

Library of Congress Cataloging-in-Publication Data
Schatzberg, Alan F.
  Manual of clinical psychopharmacology / Alan F. Schatzberg, Jonathan O. Cole,
Charles DeBattista.—7th ed.
    p. ; cm.
  Includes bibliographical references and index.
  ISBN 978-1-58562-377-8 (pbk. : alk. paper)
  1. Psychopharmacology—Handbooks, manuals, etc. 2. Psychotropic drugs—
Handbooks, manuals, etc. I. Cole, Jonathan O. II. DeBattista, Charles. III. Title.
  [DNLM: 1. Psychopharmacology. 2. Mental Disorders—drug therapy.
3. Psychotropic Drugs—pharmacology. QV 77 S312m 2010]
  RM315.S37 2007
  616.89′18—dc22

                                                              2007004385

British Library Cataloguing in Publication Data
A CIP record is available from the British Library.

Contents

List of Tables

List of Figures

Preface

This is the seventh edition of our *Manual of Clinical Psychopharmacology*, whose first edition appeared in 1986. As with that original edition and all subsequent editions, our intention has been to provide a readable, up-to-date guide to clinical psychopharmacology. Reader response generally has indicated the manual has met the original goal. However, the ever-expanding number of available agents with widening indications has led to understandably larger editions of the manual. Still, we have attempted to maintain a collegial, reader-friendly style. In this regard, we have added summary tables with key information on classes of psychotropics to serve as quick-reference guides. We have also reorganized and expanded all the chapters over the past few editions to reflect changes in current treatments. Because the field changes so rapidly, we are now increasing the frequency of new editions of the manual.

The manual reflects our most up-to-date thinking about specific agents—efficacy, dosing, side effects, and so forth. Material is largely evidence based, with an intermingling of our personal experiences. These experiences are offered as guides for the reader's own practice. We encourage the reader to cross-check recommendations (particularly doses) with other standard references and texts, particularly the latest edition of the *Physicians' Desk Reference*.

There are so many people to thank in writing this type of book. Our families have been patient and understanding of our need to spend time on this project. Charles DeBattista joined us in writing the third edition and has played an increasingly vital role in the writing of each successive edition.

Sadly, Jonathan Cole died in mid-2009. The field has lost one of the original pioneers in psychopharmacology, a man of great intelligence and humanism. We dedicate this edition to his memory.

Robert Chew made numerous editorial suggestions that were of great help. The editorial staff at American Psychiatric Publishing, Inc. (APPI)—John McDuffie, Bessie Jones, Greg Kuny, Tammy Cordova, Susan Westrate, and Judy Castagna—deserve a great deal of credit for their support, critical reading, and technical know-how. The APPI leadership—Bob Hales and Ron McMillen—have unwavering confidence in us as authors, and we are eternally grateful to them. We are also appreciative of our colleagues and trainees at McLean Hospital and Stanford University. Our experiences have been enriched by their insights. Last, we are indebted to the many patients we have treated over the past decades. They have taught us much about drug treatment.

We hope the reader will find this seventh edition of the manual even more informative and helpful than the first six, and we look forward to your feedback as we plan for future editions.

Alan F. Schatzberg, M.D.

Jonathan O. Cole, M.D. (posthumous)

Charles DeBattista, D.M.H., M.D.

December 2009

Disclosure of Competing Interests

Jonathan O. Cole, M.D.—No competing interests to disclose.

Charles DeBattista, D.M.H., M.D.—*Grant support:* Abbott, AstraZeneca, Cephalon, CNS Response, Corcept, Cyberonics, Eli Lilly, GlaxoSmithKline, NARSAD, National Institute of Mental Health, Neuronetics, Novartis, Pfizer, Pritzker Foundation, Wyeth; *Speaker/Consultant:* Bristol-Myers Squibb, Cephalon, Corcept, Cyberonics, Eli Lilly, GlaxoSmithKline, Pfizer, Wyeth; *Stock:* Corcept.

Alan F. Schatzberg, M.D.—*Consultant:* Abbott, BrainCells, Bristol-Myers Squibb, Corcept, Eli Lilly, Forest, GlaxoSmithKline, Merck, Neuronetics, Novartis, Pathway Diagnostics, Pfizer, Quintiles, Wyeth; *Equity:* BrainCells, CeNeRx, Corcept (co-founder), Forest, Merck, Neurocrine, Pfizer, PharmaNeuroBoost, Somaxon; *Intellectual property:* Named inventor on pharmacogenetic use patents on prediction of antidepressant response and on glucocorticoid antagonists in psychotic major depression.

1

General Principles of Psychopharmacological Treatment

Psychiatry has experienced a rapid metamorphosis since the 1970s in its methods of treatment. The move from a largely psychoanalytic orientation toward a more biological stance radically changed not only its basic approaches to patients but also the professional identities of psychiatrists. For most older psychiatrists, the transformation in the 1980s and 1990s was not easy. At first, keeping up with ever-expanding information on biological theories, new laboratory tests, computerization, new medications, and new additional uses for old medications was in itself a full-time occupation—one that often allowed little time or energy for integrating current information into daily practice. Moreover, the proliferation of biological and psychopharmacological information occurred so rapidly that the task of integrating biological and psychotherapeutic approaches became ever more difficult. By now, however, the most arduous parts of the transition are over for most practitioners, and over the past two or more decades a cadre of psychiatrists, well versed in psychopharmacology, has been trained.

Some academics and practitioners have argued that psychopharmacological approaches have become the essence of psychiatry, whereas for many years others insisted that these drugs merely masked underlying diseases, worked against conflict resolution, interfered with therapy, and so forth. Our impression has been that most practitioners today have developed more balanced, practical approaches, combining elements of both psychotherapy and psychopharmacology. In an odd way, academic psychiatry, with its sometimes hypertrophied and polarized approaches, lagged behind clinical practice. Indeed, we believe intuitively that psychiatry as a medical subspecialty is incorporating aspects of psychosocial, psychobiological, and psychopharmacological theories to form a truly new psychiatry.

One major reason for this is that although psychotropic drugs exert profound and beneficial effects on cognition, mood, and behavior, they often do not change the underlying disease process, which is frequently highly sensitive to intrapsychic, interpersonal, and psychosocial stressors. As a rule, beneficial outcomes can be achieved only by simultaneously reducing symptoms and promoting the capacity of the individual to adapt to the exigencies of his or her life. Strikingly, some practitioners of internal medicine have embraced psychosocial principles to help treat illnesses such as hypertension, rheumatoid arthritis, and juvenile diabetes. Similarly, psychiatrists who embrace psychopharmacology as the be-all and end-all will probably find themselves in the same position as internists who feel that prescribing thiazides is a simple solution to hypertensive illness. Conversely, practitioners of psychoanalysis should not expect that approach to cure or significantly reduce vegetative symptoms in endogenously depressed patients. Rather, they need to realize the potential benefits of alternative treatments—particularly psychotropic medication.

For practitioners who did not have extensive experience, the transition to a more pharmacological practice was not without difficulties. A favorable clinical outcome after prescribing a psychotropic drug does reinforce confidence in psychopharmacological approaches. Practically speaking, since favorable outcomes can often be effected more quickly with a psychopharmacological approach than with psychotherapy, confidence in psychopharmacology could be achieved more readily. The selective serotonin reuptake inhibitors (SSRIs), with their ease of use and wide therapeutic effects, helped practitioners become effective pharmacological treaters.

Although this book is primarily a guide to psychopharmacology, it should not lead the reader to conclude that understanding how to select and prescribe psychotropic medications obviates the basic need to comprehensively evaluate and understand psychiatric patients. Our primary purpose is to provide the reader-practitioner with basic and practical information regarding the many classes of psychiatric medications. This book is written as a practical, usable clinical guide to the selection and prescription of appropriate drug therapies for individual patients, drawing on our own clinical experience as well as on the scientific literature. It is not a series of meticulously documented review papers; therefore, statements in the text are sometimes not individually referenced. However, each chapter is followed by a list of selected relevant articles and books for readers who want to go beyond the material presented here. Starting with the fourth edition, in response to some readers' suggestions, we did increase the number of references, both cited in the text and listed in the bibliographies of individual chapters. We also added new sections and provided summary tables to act as quicker reference sources. We have continued to make modifications through this current edition, and we hope the reader will find this edition as—if not even more—useful than previous editions.

General Advice

Today, younger psychiatrists have generally been more formally trained in psychopharmacology than were many older colleagues. For less experienced practitioners of psychopharmacology, a number of practical steps can help in developing skills and achieving favorable outcomes. Generally speaking, we recommend that practitioners concentrate first on one or two drugs per drug class—SSRIs, typical and atypical antipsychotics, mood stabilizers, and so forth—and become fully familiar with how to use them (e.g., dosage, side effects). One's armamentarium of medication can then be widened over time and through further experience.

The physician should have available some key resource materials, such as textbooks on psychopharmacology and the *Physicians' Desk Reference* (PDR). (Some helpful titles are found in Appendix B at the end of this manual.) These materials can be supplemented with pharmacology newsletters, which provide useful current information. For the "modern agers," downloading a product like Epocrates onto your computer or phone is very handy and provides one essentially with an electronic PDR.

Moreover, practitioners should be familiar with a number of books directed at the lay audience that can help supplement information provided to patients (see Appendix B at the end of this manual).

It is also a good idea to identify local psychopharmacological consultants who can provide second opinions when needed—for example, if patients fail to respond or if they experience severe side effects.

Practice Guidelines

Since the early 1990s, practice gudelines have been developed by professional societies as well as academic leaders. Such guidelines can be helpful, since they are generally based on evidence in the literature. Unfortunately, there are limitations imposed by overreliance on these guidelines. First, guidelines may quickly become out of date with the reporting of evidence or new indications or new treatments. Second, available evidence in the published literature may be for agents that are not the most effective for treating patients with more atypical or comorbid conditions. Third, evidence often breaks down when the practitioner encounters a lack of response to the initial therapy, leaving him or her to fall back once again on clinical experience or judgment. Fourth, recommendations can often be based on the consensus opinions of experts. These opinions are helpful but are not necessarily accurate. Last, guidelines may be most helpful for nonspecialist practitioners and less helpful for more experienced treaters of patients with refractory conditions. In the end, there is still a need for considerable art in the practice of medicine.

Legal, Ethical, and Economic Issues

It seems prudent to discuss briefly a number of legal, ethical, and economic issues that arise in psychopharmacology. Because a comprehensive discussion of all these is beyond the scope of this manual, the reader is referred elsewhere for specific information (see Appendix B). An excellent review of work in this area, by Hoop et al. (2009), is available.

Informed consent has become an increasingly important issue in medicine. Standard medical practice has long called for informing patients of the benefits versus the risks of various surgical and medical procedures. In the past decade, greater attention has been paid to the question of informed consent; for psychiatry, however, several key problems quickly arise. For one, psychiatrists must wrestle with the problem of evaluating the patient's capacity either to understand fully the benefits and risks of the medication prescribed or to interpret the provided information in a reflective and beneficial way. Obviously, this issue is particularly pressing with psychotic patients, and legal guardianship may be required at times to effect adequate informed consent. Fortunately, these patients represent a minority of the average practitioner's patient population.

Paranoid but competent patients present practical problems that are best overcome by creating a solid working relationship. Such patients are less commonly encountered than are highly anxious, obsessive, or agitated patients, who are prone to a phobic approach to medication. The practitioner at first glance may view informed consent in such cases as an insurmountable obstacle. Practically speaking, however, such patients will be anxious even if the practitioner does not inform them of side effects. Indeed, disclosing the facts often relieves their anxiety. It also connotes a respect for the severity of their illness and the need to assume some risks mutually.

Should the physician inform the patient of every side effect listed in the PDR or merely highlight the most common ones? Some courts have judged that physicians may be liable if they do not tell the patient of every side effect. Practically speaking, most clinicians do not do so—for several reasons, including the time involved and concern for unduly frightening the patient. The latter is particularly relevant when one reflects on the fact that package-insert information lists virtually all side effects ever reported in drug trials, even if they were not due to the drug, plus side effects observed only or mainly with similar drugs. Still, we are impressed that patients not only have ready access to copies of the PDR, a product like Epocrates, and consumer guides to medications but also commonly use them. In a sense, these practices begin to obviate the physician's apparent problem. Physicians need to enter into an open dialogue with all patients regarding the benefits and side effects of medication, even (or particularly) patients who are self-taught. Patients who read the PDR need to be informed of the relative probability of the occurrence of one or another side effect. For example, patients should be made to realize that a dry mouth as the result of a tricyclic antidepressant (TCA) is to be expected, but that agranulocytosis or anaphylaxis is extremely rare. Our experience is that patients are reassured by the physician's belief (and hope) that these side effects will not be encountered. Today, package inserts often include tables comparing side effects in patients treated with a given drug with those observed with a placebo. This places the issues in a much better perspective. Some physicians routinely give patients written materials (often a separate sheet for each medication) that spell out the medication's relative risks. This works well, but only if the practitioner feels comfortable with this approach and it becomes truly routine in his or her practice.

For many years until the introduction of atypical antipsychotics, a particularly difficult problem revolved around the informed consent regarding the risk of developing tardive dyskinesia, an unfortunate side effect generally due to long-term treatment with the more typical antipsychotic medications (see Chapter 4: "Antipsychotic Drugs"). Tardive dyskinesia is less of a real risk in psychiatric practice today. It was shown to affect some 14% of patients receiving maintenance therapy with standard neuroleptic medication for 3 or more years, and it may have been more common in patients with affective disorders than in those with schizophrenia. Thus, practitioners had to be particularly conservative in administering neuroleptics to patients who did not demonstrate frequent or chronic psychotic episodes. However, because chronic psychotic disorders do unfortunately exist, even prudent practice with first-line antipsychotics could not eliminate the risk of tardive dyskinesia. Newer antipsychotics offer greater promise for reducing the risk of this problem, although the risk has not been completely eliminated.

What should the physician tell the patient about tardive dyskinesia, and when? Here, a variety of approaches have been developed. One is to inform the patient and/or the family of the risk of tardive dyskinesia before prescribing typical neuroleptics. This may be too anxiety provoking and impractical, particularly for acutely psychotic patients, because tardive dyskinesia is generally a long-term side effect and there is a pressing need to help the patient quickly. Another approach is to broach the subject of the risk of tardive dyskinesia after approximately 4–6 weeks of treatment with a typical antipsychotic, before embarking on long-term or maintenance therapy. This seems more prudent to us. The risk with atypical antipsychotics is low.

Should one obtain written verification of informed consent? Here, too, different approaches have emerged. Some institutions and practitioners have adopted formal, written informed consent. Others have followed traditional verbal informed-consent procedures and have placed written documentation of the interchange in the patient's record. Still others have routinely provided the patient with additional written information (beyond that provided in the PDR) regarding the risks of tardive dyskinesia or other side effects but have not asked the patient to provide written informed consent. Each of these approaches has its advantages and its proponents. Currently, we recommend that 1) practitioners and institutions adopt some formal, documented disclosure of the risk of tardive dyskinesia with typical neuroleptics, 2) they combine this with conservative administration of typical neuroleptics (in terms of both time and dosage), and 3) they and the patient cooperate in monitoring the patient for the emergence of dyskinetic movements. Much of this issue is less relevant today, since initiation of long-term therapy with typical antipsychotics is relatively uncommon in this country.

With the release of clozapine, psychiatrists needed to seriously consider adopting a standard documented informed-consent procedure for this potentially lethal but therapeutically unique drug. Patients who are incompetent to give informed consent should have a guardian who provides the consent. Clozapine-like agents, such as olanzapine, without the apparent risks for agranulocytosis have largely obviated the problem, but there are still patients with refractory conditions who require clozapine therapy.

Although the atypical antipsychotics are safer in some ways than were first-generation agents, weight gain, insulin resistance (metabolic syndrome), and diabetes are major worries with some of these agents, particularly olanzapine and clozapine. Diabetic ketoacidosis is a rare but serious side effect that has garnered a great deal of attention. More common, however, is the weight gain seen with several of the newer compounds, with a possible loss of insulin sensitivity. Patients who begin taking these agents should be monitored closely for both weight gain and insulin resistance. Patients should be warned about such side effects if the agent is thought to have an increased risk (e.g., clozapine, olanzapine). As indicated in Chapter 4 ("Antipsychotic Drugs"), the offending agent may need to be discontinued.

Since the early 1990s, physicians have been increasingly faced with the dilemma of prescribing standard drugs for indications that have not been approved by the U.S. Food and Drug Administration (FDA) or at doses that are higher than those recommended in the PDR. In some instances when this practice is followed, drugs can be misprescribed, and this can obviously be dangerous. In many other instances, considerable clinical or research data that have emerged point to potentially great benefits to many patients, but package-insert information may not have been changed because of economic or regulatory factors. For example, imipramine had for many years been commonly prescribed to both outpatients and inpatients at a dosage of 300 mg/day. Still, the package insert stated that outpatients should not receive more than 225 mg/day. In part, this reflected the fact that approved dosage regimens were determined on the basis of data generated many years previous, when a greater proportion of seriously depressed patients had been treated as inpatients and before plasma levels were applied (see Chapter 3: "Antidepressants"). The package insert was never changed. Additional studies designed to document further the efficacy and safety of higher dosages would be too costly for drug manufacturers, who can no longer hope to recoup the costs of such study because the patents for the drug have long since expired. One pharmaceutical manufacturer several years ago applied for and was granted FDA approval to raise the maximum daily dose of its nortriptyline compound (Pamelor) from 100 to 150 mg/day. A manufacturer of an identical nortriptyline compound, Aventyl, did not apply, and that product called for only a 100-mg maximum daily dose. Thus, we had on the U.S. market two identical nortriptylines with different maximum daily doses. Aventyl is now off the U.S. market.

Examples of so-called nonapproved uses in previous editions of this manual included the use of imipramine and phenelzine in treating agoraphobia or panic disorder and, for many years, the use of carbamazepine in treating manic-depressive illness. Over the years, many other of such uses emerged, including valproic acid for maintenance therapy in bipolar disorder, SSRIs in treating body dysmorphic disorder and related disorders, and bupropion in treating attention-deficit disorder. A reasonable body of data supports the effectiveness of these drugs for these indications, but market conditions and regulatory guidelines may result in some, or even all, of these drugs' not being granted official new indications.

One generally nonapproved indication for SSRIs has been in adolescent depression. The FDA had warned that efficacy data for this class and for venlafaxine are limited and that these agents carry a risk for increasing suicidal behavior. Fluoxetine appears to be an exception on both counts and is now approved for children and adolescents ages 8–18 years. We thus recommend initially using fluoxetine in adolescents with depression. Should patients not respond, alternatives can be considered, and if an alternative agent is used, the practitioner should provide clear documentation. The risks and benefits of these agents need to be discussed with young patients and their parents whenever possible. Since the FDA instituted a black box warning about the potential risk of using antidepressants in adolescents and children, prescription rates by pediatricians have dropped by approximately 20% (Nemeroff et al. 2007). Suicide rates among the young may be rising. A report by Gibbons et al. (2006) points to a significant rise in suicide rates in younger male adolescents (about age 15 years) in the Netherlands after institution of the warning. These data indicate that discussion of side effects without discussing potential benefits can have unfortunate results.

Is the practitioner at legal risk in prescribing drugs for nonapproved indications? Generally, the American Medical Association and the FDA have taken the position that the use of any marketed drug for nonapproved indications or at higher dosages for individual patients is within the purview of the clinician. PDR is not an official textbook of medical practice, but rather a compendium of drug information for marketing purposes. It sets limitations on what pharmaceutical companies can claim for their products. Malpractice is based on failure to practice within community norms. Still, many clinicians will not easily accept the risk of being sued—even if such a suit may have little merit—by a patient who experiences an untoward reaction to a standard drug used for a nonapproved indication or to a dose of a drug that is higher than the recommended maximum dose.

What are the solutions? Until various forces (both patients and physicians) come to the fore to effect a change in the system for widening indications or for redefining maximum doses, each clinician must decide whether to assume the risk. However, although clinicians may attempt a conservative approach, they will at some point encounter patients who will require alternative treatments. One possible aid is to acquire outside consultation from more expert psychopharmacologists or from other practitioners in the community. Another is to explain the scope of the problem to patients, providing them with available published reports on positive benefits and documenting these actions in their records. Some physicians will ask for written documentation that the patient has been informed. In the end, there are no simple solutions, and the physician will at some point be faced with this problem.

Another issue faces psychiatrists who treat patients with treatment-resistant conditions. Many antidepressant and antipsychotic drugs are available in Canada or in European countries. Before clomipramine received FDA approval in 1989, Canadian drugstores were mailing the drug regularly to the United States after receiving a prescription and a check from the patient. With the growth of pressure from patients with AIDS, the FDA and the U.S. Customs Service appeared to view favorably (or at least passively) the importation of a 3-month supply of drugs not available in the United States for the treatment of an individual patient. Well-established drugs such as mianserin, older monoamine oxidase inhibitors (iproniazid, nialamide), and newer drugs such as moclobemide and tianeptine are available in Canada and Europe, and psychiatrists or patients may be able to obtain them through pharmacies, colleagues, friends, or relatives there.

Many patients received Canadian clomipramine for years without our ever hearing of a malpractice suit. Nevertheless, the possibility existed. State laws have varied as to whether such use is or was appropriate. Psychiatrists who want to treat patients with imported drugs not approved in the United States should consider the risks to themselves as well as to their patients. We recommend having the patient sign an informed-consent document if a foreign medication is to be used. Information on the issue can be obtained from the FDA Web site (www.fda.gov).

King (1998) discusses these issues and outlines the procedures for obtaining FDA and investigational new drug application approval, primarily for investigational agents.

One important facet of psychopharmacological practice is to document various steps in treatment: diagnosis, drug dose regimen, other medications, informed consent, and so forth. Practical tips have been articulated in a paper by Lamb (2001).

A somewhat related issue has emerged over the past few years with the Internet. Some patients have ordered medications online, often from abroad, and we have suspected that many of the preparations are not legitimate. One recent patient entirely lost her positive response to aripiprazole augmentation after she had reordered over the Web. The preparation from India did not produce any effect. She recaptured the benefit when she went back to taking the U.S. proprietary preparation.

Managed care has had a tremendous impact on psychiatric practice. Building on the initial success of psychopharmacology, it has in a sense reshaped psychiatric practice—primarily along pharmacological lines. By providing limited benefits, it has forced psychiatrists to emphasize drug treatment. This has been a somewhat shortsighted approach, resulting in many patients' receiving limited care. Moreover, the limited sessions and the avoidance of hospitalization lead at times to unrealistic expectations by patients and their families and inordinate pressure on providers. Although psychopharmacological approaches imply ease of care for a large caseload of patients, providers must keep in mind that responses to treatment are gradual at best and that any short-term successes must be followed by the continuation and maintenance phases of treatment.

Cost containment has led many health plans to prefer generic compounds over proprietary drugs. We are frequently asked about the advisability of prescribing generic compounds. For many years, the FDA has required only that a manufacturer demonstrate that a given dose of a compound will produce blood levels within 20%–30% of those produced by the proprietary form. Obviously, for some medications (e.g., TCAs) this standard can prove problematic. Lower blood levels of a TCA may result in the patient's not achieving therapeutic levels when treated with traditional doses. Moreover, switching to an equivalent dose of a generic compound in patients who have responded to a given dosage of a standard antidepressant may result in loss of therapeutic effect. Differences between generic and proprietary forms can go in both directions. Use of the generic form could lead to higher, potentially toxic blood levels. In August 2001, fluoxetine became available in a generic formulation. Fluoxetine produces relatively high concentrations in blood and brain, and generic forms did not prove to be problematic. Similarly, we have not heard of problems with generic paroxetine. A few years ago, this issue came to the fore again with the concern that some generic cardiac medications may not have offered efficacy equal to that seen with the brand product. In our last edition, we noted it is conceivable that, in the future, efficacy will need to be demonstrated for generic formulations, and, indeed, there were recent problems with a generic formulation of bupropion.

Almost 20 years ago, the FDA had ordered that a number of generic benzodiazepine compounds be removed from the market because they had fallen below minimum standards. Thus, quality control of the manufacturing of generic compounds may not necessarily meet acceptable standards. However, there may be significant variability between different batches of the same proprietary drug as well, and large pharmaceutical companies have had other problems with the manufacturing of proprietary compounds. In recent years, generic compounds in general have appeared closer in equivalency to their proprietary counterparts.

In early editions, we had recommended that physicians start their patients on proprietary compounds (particularly in the case of TCAs) and adjust dosages until therapeutic benefit was achieved and side effects were limited. Generic compounds could then be used for maintenance therapy. Blood levels for the specific medication, if available, could be obtained while the patient was still being treated with the proprietary compound—before switching to the generic—and rechecked while the patient was taking the equivalent dose of the generic if the patient lost therapeutic benefit or experienced side effects. Over the years we have come to feel less staunchly about this, in part because a good deal of practice today is with generic medication and the TCA class is used much less commonly. Also, we do not have good data on therapeutic blood levels of the second-generation compounds, and blood levels are less readily available. Still, as noted above, issues can on occasion arise.

Another consequence of cost containment is health plans' insistence that patients obtain 3-month supplies of medications, generally during maintenance therapy. Obviously, for patients with a history of abuse of medications or suicidal behavior or with medications with narrow safety margins, this requirement can prove problematic. We recommend using good clinical sense in deciding how many pills or capsules to prescribe. Frequently, local pharmacies will work with physicians and patients to come to a clinically and economically sound compromise (e.g., agreeing to hold supplies in patients' names but dispensing in 1- to 2-week quantities). However, this practice is a problem with mail-order drugs that are made available through health insurance plans. Again, newer medications tend to have wide safety margins, and the problem has to a large extent been obviated.

There has been recent controversy about the propriety of states and municipal governments condoning the large-scale importation of pharmaceuticals approved in the United States from Canada and other countries. The FDA has opposed this attempt to reduce costs in part because the origin, safety, and efficacy of medications imported from Canada cannot be verified (for further infomation, see the FDA Web site: www.fda.gov/importeddrugs). At the time of writing, this issue is unresolved.

In this book, we provide practical information regarding many different psychotropic drugs. Information regarding dosages is for adult patients (ages 18–60 years) unless otherwise noted. We have included information derived from our reading of the psychiatric literature as well as from our own clinical practice. We attempt to indicate, whenever possible, the uses that officially have not been approved by the FDA for marketing purposes, but we also attempt to provide readers with sufficient data to aid them in deciding whether or how they may want to prescribe specific drugs. In so doing, we are not endorsing the use of these specific drugs but are realistically attempting to place a drug in its proper perspective. We believe real-world psychiatric practice dictates that we give the practitioner information based either on the scientific literature or on common clinical use, even though a drug's indications may not yet have been changed or—perhaps because of economic reasons—may never be changed. Information about specific agents should be checked against the PDR and package inserts to ensure accuracy before prescribing for specific patients.

Bibliography

Applebaum PS: Legal and ethical aspects of psychopharmacologic practice, in Clinical Psychopharmacology, 2nd Edition. Edited by Bernstein JC. Boston, MA, Wright PSG, 1984

Erickson SH, Bergman JJ, Schneeweiss R, et al: The use of drugs for unlabeled indications. JAMA 243:1543–1546, 1980

FDA does not approve uses of drugs (editorial). JAMA 252:1054–1055, 1984

Gibbons RD: Efficacy and safety of antidepressants for depression and suicide risk in youth and adults: results of new analyses. Neuropsychopharmacology 31 (suppl 1): S50, 2006

Gutheil TG: Liability issues and malpractice prevention, in Handbook of Clinical Psychopharmacology. Edited by Tupin JP, Shader RI, Harnett DS. Northvale, NJ, Jason Aronson, 1988, pp 439–453

Hoop JG, Layde JB, Weiss LR: Ethical considerations in psychopharmacological treatment and research, in The American Psychiatric Publishing Textbook of Psychopharmacology, 4th Edition. Edited by Schatzberg AF, Nemeroff CB. Washington, DC, American Psychiatric Publishing, 2009, pp 1477–1495

King SM: Legal and risk management concerns relating to the use of non-FDA approved drugs in the practice of psychiatry. Rx for Risk 6(2):1–7, 1998

Lamb K: Risk management and medication prescribing/administering. Rx for Risk 9(1):1–3, 2001

Nemeroff CB, Kalali A, Keller MB, et al: Impact of publicity concerning pediatric suicidality data on physician practice patterns in the United States. Arch Gen Psychiatry 64:466–472, 2007

Nonapproved uses of FDA-approved drugs. JAMA 211:1705, 1970

Slovenko R: Update on legal issues associated with tardive dyskinesia. J Clin Psychiatry 61 (suppl 4):45–57, 2000

Use of approved drugs for unlabeled indications. FDA Drug Bulletin, April 1982 [entire issue]

Use of drugs for unapproved indications: your legal responsibility. FDA Drug Bulletin, October 1972 [entire issue]

2

Diagnosis and Classification

Since the late 1970s, psychiatry has paid greater attention to rigorous diagnosis and classification, as evidenced by the 1980 publication of the then forward-thinking DSM-III (American Psychiatric Association 1980). Unlike earlier editions, DSM-III provided detailed diagnostic criteria and descriptive diagnoses. Subsequent editions, including DSM-III-R (American Psychiatric Association 1987) and DSM-IV (American Psychiatric Association 1994) (the text revision of which, DSM-IV-TR, was published in 2000; American Psychiatric Association 2000), refined these diagnostic criteria and made changes primarily on the basis of new empirical data and the results of field trials. Much of the attention to more rigorous nosology had been sparked by advances in the biology and treatment of various psychiatric disorders, making precise diagnosis ever more important. For example, the response to lithium carbonate of many patients diagnosed as having bipolar (manic-depressive) illness fostered diligent efforts to discriminate between manic-depressive illness and schizophrenia, which resulted in a change of diagnosis for many patients and alterations in their treatment.

Approaches to psychopharmacological treatment are often based on trying to match a given treatment or a combination of treatments with a specific diagnosis. Although this approach represents the ideal, it is effective only in approximately 60% of patients because

- Many patients have a disorder not easily classified into one particular syndrome.
- Many patients have comorbid disorders.
- Some patients with a seemingly classic disorder may not respond to a traditional drug.
- Various drugs (e.g., anticonvulsants) have increasingly been shown to exert wider actions than their drug class eponym suggests. (When first used in bipolar disorder, anticonvulsants were not approved for the syndrome. Controlled clinical trials did eventually lead to U.S. Food and Drug Administration [FDA] approval for valproate, lamotrigine, and carbamazepine in treating this disorder.) Today, except for clozapine, second-generation antipsychotics are approved in the treatment of acute mania. However, only olanzapine, aripiprazole, and quetiapine have indications in the maintenance treatment of bipolar disorder.

Thus, the clinician for many years had to combine the "ideal" paradigm with a more flexible approach—one in which the clinician attempted to match a given treatment with various clusters of symptoms rather than with an overall syndrome. The danger of this approach, however, is that if carried too far, it can result in overly innovative treatment or even unhealthy polypharmacy. Obviously, the clinician must attempt to develop a general strategy for matching a range of specific treatments to patients with particular diagnoses or symptoms. It is best to do the following:

1. Ascertain whether patients meet symptom criteria for a disorder (e.g., major depression with or without melancholia);
2. Determine the class of drug (e.g., tricyclic antidepressants [TCAs] or selective serotonin reuptake inhibitors [SSRIs]) or treatment that is commonly thought to be effective in treating that disorder; and
3. Prescribe classic representatives of the given drug class (e.g., imipramine or citalopram); this can be followed by a shift to less traditional medications or to combinations of medications if initial trials do not prove effective.

Such an approach is sound overall; however, clinicians must be aware that diagnostic classifications have inherent limitations that can make diagnoses misleading. For example, many patients who had been diagnosed with DSM-III major depression did not respond to antidepressant drugs, and they often required some form of psychotherapy (e.g., interpersonal psychotherapy or cognitive therapy). In part, this was due to the limited number and type of symptoms required for a disorder to be diagnosed as major depression. Indeed, although major depression is commonly mistaken as representing an endogenous type of depressive illness, in fact—historically and practically speaking—endogenous depression, which is classically believed to respond to TCAs, is only a subtype of major depression. DSM-III-R and DSM-IV (and DSM-IV-TR) criteria for major depression are somewhat tighter than they were in DSM-III—a change that obviated the problem to some degree.

As discussed below, the development of DSM-V is already well under way, with an anticipated release date of 2013. It is expected that DSM-V will to some extent use dimensional characterization to better describe patients' disorders. This could aid in better treatment selection for an individual patient.

Although comprehensive discussion of psychiatric classification is beyond the scope of this manual, it is still useful to review the current (DSM-IV) system and the prevalence rates for major categories of adult psychiatric disorders and to highlight which types of psychopharmacological agents often prove most beneficial in each category. Prevalence rates provided in this chapter are based primarily on reports from the Epidemiologic Catchment Area (ECA) study and the National Comorbidity Survey (NCS).

Mood Disorders

Mood disorders, by definition, are pathological affective states. In DSM-III-R, these disorders were divided into bipolar and depressive disorders, which were then further subdivided into distinct entities. In addition, the severity of the disorder and the degree of psychosocial precipitants and seasonal pattern were specified. In DSM-IV (and DSM-IV-TR), this classification was largely retained (Table 2–1). Revisions included the elimination of organic mood disorder and the addition of bipolar II disorder, an atypical depression qualifier, substance abuse–related mood disorder, and mood disorder due to a medical condition.

Bipolar Disorders

Bipolar disorders are subdivided into bipolar I disorder (mixed, manic, or depressed), bipolar II disorder, cyclothymic disorder, and bipolar disorder not

Table 2–1.   DSM-IV-TR mood disorders

Depressive disorders
  Major depressive disorder
    Single, recurrent
    Melancholic, psychotic, atypical, seasonal
  Dysthymic disorder
    Early, late onset
  Depression not otherwise specified
Bipolar disorders
  Bipolar I
    Manic, mixed, depressed
  Bipolar II
    Hypomanic, depressed
  Cyclothymic disorder
  Bipolar disorder not otherwise specified
Other mood disorders
  Mood disorder due to a general medical condition
  Substance-induced mood disorder
  Mood disorder not otherwise specified

otherwise specified. To be diagnosed with bipolar disorder (manic-depressive illness), the patient must currently meet criteria for hypomania or mania or must have had a prior episode that met the criteria for either of these syndromes. The current episode is further categorized according to whether the patient is manic, depressed, or experiencing a mixed-affect state.

DSM-IV criteria for mania include a distinct period of persistently elevated or irritable mood sufficient to cause harm or to result in hospitalization. At least three of seven symptoms need to be included (four if only irritability is present): increase in goal-directed activity, increased speaking, flight of ideas, inflated self-esteem, decreased need for sleep, distractibility, and overinvolvement in high-risk activities (e.g., spending sprees, reckless driving). As in DSM-III, the current criteria indicate that symptoms must persist at least 7 days, or for any duration if the symptoms require hospitalization. However, if the symptoms last for fewer than 7 and more than 4 days and do not severely affect functioning or require hospitalization, the episode meets the criteria for hypomania, and bipolar II disorder is diagnosed. Any previous episode that met the criteria for mania would make the diagnosis bipolar I disorder, regardless of whether the current episode is hypomanic. The 6-month and lifetime prevalence rates of mania in the general population were approximately 0.5% and 0.8%, respectively, in the ECA study data and were slightly higher in the NCS.

The classic psychopharmacological treatment approach for overall mood stabilization of these disorders has involved lithium carbonate or lithium citrate. Carbamazepine, oxcarbazepine, valproic acid, some benzodiazepines, and atypical antipsychotics have also been shown to have mood-stabilizing effects, most prominently in acute mania (see Chapter 5: "Mood Stabilizers"). Treatment of acute hypomania or mania includes the mood-stabilizing drugs noted above as well as antipsychotics and sedative-hypnotics for sleep. Treatment of bipolar depression often requires combining lithium or valproate with treatments used for major depression (see subsection "Depressive Disorders" in this chapter). The combination of olanzapine and fluoxetine was approved for bipolar depression. Lamotrigine has been approved for the prevention of depressive episodes. At one time, mixed states were more responsive to anticonvulsants than to lithium, but this is no longer clear.

The major strides made toward a wider redefinition of bipolar manic states have undoubtedly resulted in more patients receiving mood stabilizers. The potential benefit to many patients in this broadening of diagnoses must be weighed against a procrustean tendency to overdiagnose the disorder in order to justify lithium or other thymoleptic treatment. Not uncommonly, clinicians see patients who have a chronic disorder that was once termed schizophrenia but has been rediagnosed as either a bipolar manic-depressive illness or a schizoaffective illness. Likewise, the affective instability and impulsivity of borderline personality disorder are sometimes mistaken for symptoms of bipolar II disorder. Unfortunately, many such patients do not respond to mood stabilizers; this points to certain inherent limitations in overbroadening this category.

Cyclothymic disorder is a more chronic and less severe illness than bipolar disorder. For the criteria for this disorder to be met, a 2-year course with repeated episodes of mild mood cycles is required. Patients with cyclothymic disorder may develop superimposed bipolar I or II disorder. Many investigators claim that lithium carbonate is of benefit to some patients with cyclothymic disorder.

Depressive Disorders

Major depressive episode is by definition a unipolar disorder if the patient does not have a history of hypomania or mania (i.e., a bipolar disorder). Six-month and lifetime prevalence rates for major depressive episode in the ECA study were 3% and 6%, respectively, and women are twice as commonly affected as men. The 12-month and lifetime prevalence rates for major depression in the NCS were much higher: 10.3% and 17.1%, respectively.

Criteria for a major depressive episode consist of a variety of signs and symptoms, including appetite disturbance, sleep disturbance, psychomotor retardation or agitation, suicidality, decreased interest in life, and guilt. Obviously, some of these symptoms are those that European and American investigators have used to describe endogenous depression. However, a patient may meet criteria for a major depressive episode without demonstrating much in the way of endogenous depression symptoms. In DSM-III-R, only four symptoms were required to meet the diagnosis of major depressive episode; DSM-IV (and DSM-IV-TR) requires five symptoms. However, in both systems, only a 2-week duration of symptoms is needed in order for the criteria to be fulfilled. Major depression has been shown to respond to many different types of antidepressants, including the TCAs, SSRIs, serotonin-norepinephrine reuptake inhibitors (SNRIs), monoamine oxidase inhibitors (MAOIs), and other available agents.

A subtype of major depression (melancholic features) more closely resembles endogenous depression. In DSM-IV (and DSM-IV-TR), the criteria for this subtype have been modified from DSM-III and DSM-III-R criteria. The current diagnosis requires anhedonia or lack of pleasure from enjoyable stimuli. In addition, three of the following six symptoms must be present: diurnal variation, marked psychomotor retardation or agitation, early-morning awakening, significant anorexia or weight loss, excessive or inappropriate guilt, and distinct quality of the depressed mood. Biological abnormalities such as dexamethasone nonsuppression and hyperadrenocorticism are thought to be more common in major depression with melancholia than in less severe forms of depression, but these abnormalities are not included in the current criteria. It is still not clear whether major depression with melancholic features fully approximates endogenous depression. The criteria include brief time periods similar to those for major depression but, at present, do not include earlier criteria for good past response to biological therapies. The disorder responds to all of the antidepressants, although recently there has been considerable debate as to whether the SSRIs are less effective than the TCAs in the treatment of melancholia. Further research will, it is hoped, lead to even better phenomenological definition of this disorder.

DSM-IV (and DSM-IV-TR) includes a specifier to indicate a subtype of major depression that has been described for many years in the psychiatric literature: *atypical depression*. This disorder, unlike melancholia, is characterized by significant reactivity of mood to pleasurable stimuli, in addition to at least two of four other symptoms: significant weight gain or increase in appetite, excessive sleeping, sensitivity to interpersonal rejection, and heaviness in the limbs. This subtype appears to be less responsive to TCAs but more responsive to MAOIs and possibly to SSRIs.

Another specifier included in DSM-IV (and DSM-IV-TR) is *postpartum onset*. Women have increased vulnerability to a variety of mood disorders, including depression and mania, in the postpartum period. The new specifier may be used when mood symptoms develop within 4 weeks of giving birth.

DSM-IV (and DSM-IV-TR) also includes *mixed anxiety-depressive disorder* in Appendix B as a disorder for further study. The criteria for this disorder include persistent or recurrent dysphoric mood for at least 1 month, with symptoms including worry, irritability, fatigue, sleep disturbance, and difficulty concentrating. Some data suggest that the SSRIs and other antidepressants may be useful for this condition. Recent data suggest that this is a relatively rare disorder.

Finally, a very important subtype of major depressive episode—*major depressive episode with psychotic features*—by definition involves delusional thinking, evidenced by guilty or nihilistic delusions, hallucinations, and even communicative incompetence. This subtype represents 15%–19% of all major depressions. Typically, patients who have depression with psychotic features are much less responsive to monotherapy with antidepressants. They typically require the addition of an antipsychotic or of electroconvulsive therapy. Recent data suggest that glucocorticoid antagonists may be effective in the treatment of this disorder (DeBattista et al. 2006; Flores et al. 2006). (Two of us [A.F.S. and C.D.] do have a conflict of interest with a company attempting to develop these agents for this use; see "Disclosure of Competing Interests" at the beginning of this manual.)

Table 2–2. DSM-IV-TR schizophrenia spectrum disorders

Schizophrenia
  Paranoid
  Disorganized
  Undifferentiated
  Catatonic
  Residual
Schizophreniform
Schizoaffective

Dysthymic disorder is a more chronic condition, and its symptoms by definition are not severe enough to meet the criteria for major depression. In DSM-III, the criteria for dysthymic disorder were broad, and a number of the symptom criteria (e.g., anxiety, irritability, and obsessionality) were not specifically those of depression. The current nomenclature requires two of the following six depressive symptoms: appetite disturbance, sleep disturbance, fatigue, decreased self-esteem, decreased concentration or indecisiveness, and hopelessness. DSM-IV dropped the distinction between primary and secondary dysthymic disorder because of lack of evidence for the validity of this distinction. Lifetime prevalence rates for dysthymic disorder were approximately 3% in the ECA study and 6.4% in the NCS. SSRIs are useful in treating this disorder. Older evidence suggested that dysthymic disorder preferentially responded to MAOIs over TCAs. The data on the utility of antidepressants for dysthymic disorder, historically, were sketchy, but studies on the SSRIs have clarified this issue.

Schizophrenia and Other Schizophrenia Spectrum Disorders

Schizophrenia and other schizophrenia spectrum disorders, in contrast to disorders of mood, are primarily disorders of cognition and thinking. These syndromes are heterogeneous, having multiple subtypes (as described in DSM-IV-TR, pp. 313–317) (Table 2–2). Of particular importance in these conditions are delusions (often persecutory or bizarre in nature), prominent and persistent hallucinations (primarily auditory), disorganized speech, disorganized or catatonic behavior, and negative symptoms such as flat affect and avolition.

The course of the illness is chronic (at least 6 months) and often deteriorating, and the patient commonly shows social isolation and withdrawal. Six-month and lifetime prevalence rates of schizophrenic disorders in the ECA study were 0.8% and 1.3%, respectively.

Primary treatments are the atypical antipsychotics (e.g., olanzapine, risperidone, quetiapine), as well as the first-generation, neuroleptic antipsychotics, which include phenothiazines, butyrophenones, and thioxanthenes. Acute management may include the addition of valproate to the atypical antipsychotic agent. Some investigators have also reported limited benefit with lithium. The efficacy of TCAs and SSRIs for some anergic, depressed patients with schizophrenia has also been demonstrated—interestingly, with a relatively low incidence of worsening of psychosis.

Schizophreniform and schizoaffective disorders are also subsumed under the category of schizophrenia spectrum disorders. Schizophreniform disorder differs from schizophrenia only in the duration of illness—lasting from 4 weeks to 6 months. This is a rarer disorder, with 6-month and lifetime prevalence rates of 0.1%. Acute treatment for this condition generally involves antipsychotic agents. The term *schizoaffective disorder* is used to describe patients with chronic symptoms of schizophrenia who also meet the criteria for mania, hypomania, or depression in the course of their illness. In schizoaffective disorder, the psychotic symptoms are not limited to the concurrent affective episodes. For example, some patients with an episodic mood disorder and a significant thought disorder as seen in schizophrenia would receive this diagnosis. Furthermore, patients with residual evidence of psychosis when their mood disorder is in remission may also receive this diagnosis. Such patients often receive the most complex drug regimen in a valiant effort to control a mix of affective, schizophrenic, and even anxiety symptoms.

Anxiety Disorders

The DSM-III classification of anxiety disorders was radically different from its predecessor, DSM-II (American Psychiatric Association 1968), and the more recent editions and revisions have elaborated further on this approach. Anxiety in DSM-III was divided into two main categories: phobias and anxiety

Table 2–3.   DSM-IV-TR anxiety disorders

Panic disorder without agoraphobia
Panic disorder with agoraphobia
Agoraphobia without history of panic disorder
Specific phobia
Social phobia
Obsessive-compulsive disorder
Posttraumatic stress disorder
Acute stress disorder
Generalized anxiety disorder
Anxiety disorder due to a general medical condition
Substance-induced anxiety disorder
Anxiety disorder not otherwise specified

states. Since then, the broad distinction between anxiety states and phobias has been dropped. In DSM-IV (and DSM-IV-TR), the anxiety disorders are divided into 12 subtypes (Table 2–3). They include panic disorder (with and without agoraphobia), specific phobia (formerly called simple phobia, such as phobia of heights or of snakes), agoraphobia (fear of being in places where escape options are limited), generalized anxiety disorder (GAD), obsessive-compulsive disorder (OCD), and anxiety disorder due to a general medical condition or related to substance abuse. In addition, DSM-IV (and DSM-IV-TR) anxiety disorders include posttraumatic stress disorder (PTSD) and incorporate a new, related diagnosis: acute stress disorder. This diagnosis was added to describe a reaction to a traumatic stressor occurring within 1 month of the stressor and lasting 2 days to 4 weeks.

Whereas considerable progress in classifying anxiety is reflected in the recent editions and revisions of DSM, a great deal of confusion and debate still remains. This is particularly evident in the lingering questions of how to subdivide the group of disorders included under agoraphobia, agoraphobia with panic attacks, panic disorder, social phobia, and GAD.

The specific phobias include encapsulated fears and avoidance of specific stimuli (e.g., heights, animals, closed spaces). Animal phobias are almost exclusively found in females and generally begin in childhood. The 6-month and lifetime prevalence rates of simple phobias are extremely high: approximately

8% and 13%, respectively, in both the ECA study and the NCS. These conditions are generally treated with behavior therapy.

Social phobias involve intense and undue fears and avoidance of interpersonal interactions, urinating in public bathrooms, and other events. They occur in both sexes and begin in late adolescence and early adulthood. Social phobia in adolescence may be a prodrome of major depression in adulthood. MAOIs, SSRIs, and SNRIs are effective in treating patients with this disorder.

Agoraphobia—the fear of being in places where escape may be difficult or embarrassing (e.g., supermarkets or shopping malls)—attracted considerable attention in the 1980s, particularly reflected by the numerous psychopharmacological and psychotherapeutic studies on DSM-III-defined agoraphobia with panic attacks. As indicated, panic disorder may occur with or without agoraphobia. When frank panic attacks are not present, a diagnosis of agoraphobia without panic is made. Patients with this presentation may experience partial panic attacks (*limited symptom attacks*). Some investigators have argued that agoraphobia does not occur without significant limited-symptom or panic attacks; however, analysis of ECA study data indicates that agoraphobia without frank panic attacks is far more common than was once thought. Agoraphobia is far more common in women than in men, and the mean age at onset is the late 20s. The lifetime prevalence rate of agoraphobia is approximately 4%. The disorder can be disabling because patients may markedly constrict their daily activities. The phobic aspects may be treated via behavior therapy or psychotherapy. Acute symptomatic relief may be best effected with benzodiazepines.

The criteria for panic disorder in DSM-IV (and DSM-IV-TR) are somewhat broader than they were in DSM-III-R. Panic disorder is characterized by recurrent, unexpected panic—acute, almost incapacitating anxiety—followed by persistent fear (lasting at least 1 month) of having another attack. (This criterion contrasts with the DSM-III-R criterion requiring four attacks in 4 weeks.) The attacks are characterized by at least 4 of 13 symptoms, including dyspnea, chest discomfort, palpitations, lightheadedness, sense of dread, hot and cold flashes, sweating, and faintness. If the symptoms are associated with agoraphobia, a diagnosis of panic disorder with agoraphobia is made. The 6-month and lifetime prevalence rates of panic disorder in the ECA study were found to be approximately 0.8% and 1.1%, respectively, whereas the lifetime prevalence in the NCS was 3.5%. Women have panic disorder about twice as commonly as men.

Panic disorder with and without agoraphobia may be responsive to a variety of agents, including many TCAs, MAOIs, SSRIs, SNRIs, reboxetine (not available in the United States), alprazolam, and clonazepam. There is some indication that agoraphobia also may be responsive to these agents even if panic symptoms are not evident.

In DSM-III, GAD is characterized by persistent anxiety of at least 1-month duration. The more recent editions and revisions of DSM reflect that GAD is chronic, lasting at least 6 months. DSM-IV simplified the 18-symptom checklist in DSM-III-R by clustering symptoms in six areas: fatigue, motor tension (shakiness, tension, trembling), irritability, difficulty concentrating, sleep disturbance (usually initial insomnia), and restlessness. DSM-IV, in its criteria for panic, severely limited the use of this diagnosis by designating patients with one panic attack followed by GAD symptoms as having panic disorder. Earlier studies pointed to prevalence rates ranging between 2% and 6%. In the NCS and the ECA study, 1-year prevalence of GAD as defined by DSM-III-R criteria was estimated to be 3%, and lifetime prevalence was estimated to be about 5%.

Various drug classes may be effective in treating GAD; these include benzodiazepines, buspirone, barbiturates, antihistamines, phenothiazines, and meprobamate. However, of these medications, benzodiazepines have been overwhelmingly the most commonly prescribed. The TCAs have also been shown to be effective in treating this disorder, as has trazodone. Other antidepressants, including the SSRIs and venlafaxine, have also proved effective in the treatment of GAD and now have FDA-approved indications. Pregabalin has been reported to be effective in several double-blind studies but has, of this writing, not received an indication from the FDA for treatment of GAD.

OCD is characterized by obsessions and compulsions producing significant distress. DSM-IV (and DSM-IV-TR) attempts to clarify the distinction between obsessions and compulsions. By DSM-III-R criteria, a counting ritual could be either an obsession or a compulsion; however, in DSM-IV, an obsession is an idea, thought, or impulse that is experienced as being intrusive or inappropriate and that provokes anxiety. A compulsion, on the other hand, is a repetitive behavior or mental image that serves the function of avoiding or relieving anxiety. Thus, in DSM-IV (and DSM-IV-TR), most counting rituals are compulsions, even though they are repetitive thoughts, as opposed to actions. In Europe, OCD is commonly regarded as a mood rather than an anxiety disorder. The disorder is more common in women than in men, and 6-month and lifetime prevalence rates were 1.5% and 2.5%, respectively, in the ECA study. Often, patients with pronounced obsessive-compulsive symptoms are, on closer inspection, found to meet the criteria for major depression. Many studies have found that clomipramine, a TCA with pronounced serotonin reuptake–blocking properties, is effective, and it is FDA approved for this condition. The SSRIs have also been demonstrated to be effective for this condition, and fluoxetine, fluvoxamine, sertraline, and paroxetine have received FDA approval for the treatment of OCD. Other TCAs and MAOIs have been found, in limited studies, to be much less effective.

Disorders such as trichotillomania, kleptomania, and body dysmorphic disorders appear to be closely related to OCD. Trichotillomania is characterized by a recurrent pulling out of one's hair. The hair pulling has a compulsive quality in that it is ego-dystonic but relieves tension. Likewise, kleptomania is characterized by compulsive stealing without an agenda of monetary gain. However, trichotillomania and kleptomania are listed as impulse-control disorders in DSM-IV (and DSM-IV-TR) and not anxiety disorders or variants of OCD. Body dysmorphic disorder is listed under somatoform disorders. Interestingly, the SSRIs have proved to be very useful in treating most patients with trichotillomania and in some patients with kleptomania or body dysmorphic disorder.

PTSD has come under increased attention since the Vietnam War. The disorder is characterized by the existence of a recognizable stressor that is likely to evoke distress in most individuals. Previous trauma is reexperienced via recurrent recollections or dreams of the event or a sudden sense that the event is recurring. Often patients with this disorder demonstrate decreased responsiveness to or involvement with the external world. Common symptoms include startle responses, memory or concentration problems, sleep disturbance, guilt about surviving, avoidance of stimuli that mimic or simulate the event, and recrudescence of symptoms upon exposure to such stimuli. Although the disorder has achieved wide popular interest because of the political aspects of the Vietnam War, similar disorders, such as traumatic war neurosis in World War II pilots, have long been reported in the literature. The prevalence of the disorder has been reported to be 1%. In civilian PTSD, rape and car accidents are common stressors.

Psychopharmacological treatment for PTSD was for many years not well studied. A number of earlier studies suggested that phenelzine (an MAOI) and imipramine could reduce specific symptoms but had limited overall effect. Likewise, carbamazepine was shown to have some utility for treating the reexperiencing of traumatic events that characterizes the disorder. Adrenergic receptor agents such as propranolol and clonidine have been used to decrease the autonomic hyperarousal of PTSD. The SSRIs paroxetine and sertraline are effective in the treatment of PTSD, and they have received FDA approval for the disorder. Other SSRIs and SNRIs are likely to be effective as well.

DSM-IV (and DSM-IV-TR) includes the new diagnosis *acute stress disorder*. This term describes the acute reaction to a traumatic stressor in the period immediately after the stressful event. The disorder is characterized by the same trauma that may precipitate PTSD, but the diagnosis focuses on anxiety symptoms that occur within 1 month of an extreme stressor. The diagnosis requires three of five symptoms: emotional numbing, derealization, depersonalization, amnesia, and being in a daze. It is expected that the development of an acute stress disorder may predict a typically more chronic disorder such as PTSD. At this time, there are no reliable studies on the pharmacological treatment of acute stress disorder. However, it is expected that antianxiety agents such as benzodiazepines may come to play a key role in the treatment of this disorder.

Somatoform Disorders

Somatoform disorders represent a class of disorders involving physical complaints that are without objective medical basis. The five major illnesses in this group are somatization disorder, conversion disorder, pain disorder, hypochondriasis, and body dysmorphic disorder. The prevalence rate of this group of disorders was approximately 0.1% in the ECA study, and the disorders were predominantly found in women. Somatoform pain disorder has been reported to respond to antidepressant therapy. The other disorders have not been shown to be particularly responsive to older psychopharmacological therapies, but some cases of hypochondriasis and body dysmorphic disorder have been effectively treated with SSRIs. Of interest is the observation that the SNRIs venlafaxine and duloxetine are both effective in diabetic neuropathic pain. Duloxetine has received FDA approval for use in that disorder, as has pregabalin, an analog of gabapentin. Duloxetine also appears to reduce pain in patients with major depression. Several studies, in both clinic and community samples, now point to chronic pain being commonly comorbid with major depression (Ohayon and Schatzberg 2003).

Personality Disorders

In DSM-IV (and DSM-IV-TR), personality disorder diagnoses are made on Axis II. Generally, these disorders have not been found to respond robustly to psychopharmacological treatment; however, medication may reduce certain symptoms. Three personality disorders are of particular note for this manual: borderline personality disorder, paranoid personality disorder, and antisocial personality disorder. Borderline personality disorder, which has attracted great interest and study in recent years, is characterized by impulsivity, unstable and intense interpersonal relationships, inappropriate and intense anger, identity disturbances, affective instability, self-destructive physical acts, and a chronic sense of emptiness. DSM-IV also added stress-induced paranoid ideation or dissociative symptoms. Patients with this disorder (or variants of the disorder) may respond to mood-stabilizing agents (initially for emotionally unstable character), phenelzine (for hysteroid dysphoria), and low doses of antipsychotics. More recently, SSRIs have proved of significant utility in treating the dysphoria, aggression, and impulsivity common in borderline personality disorder, and valproate has been shown to be effective in decreasing aggressive outbursts.

Paranoid personality disorder is characterized by pervasive, unwarranted suspiciousness, hypersensitivity, and restricted affectivity. By definition, the paranoia is not due to schizophrenia or paranoid disorder. Although the somatic treatment of paranoid personality has not been well studied, trials of atypical antipsychotics or lithium carbonate may prove useful in this disorder.

Antisocial personality disorder is characterized by chronic antisocial behavior, with onset before age 15. This personality disorder is characterized by repeated unlawful acts and lying, impulsivity, irresponsibility, disregard of the safety of others, and lack of remorse over misdeeds. DSM-IV also added the requirement of evidence of a conduct disorder before the age of 15. This disorder is three times more common in men than in women. Six-month and lifetime ECA study prevalence rates for the disorder are approximately 0.8% and 2.5%, respectively. Pharmacotherapy has not proved particularly helpful in the treatment of this disorder. However, mood-stabilizing agents have been somewhat useful in treating impulsive, repetitive violent outbursts in some patients.

Psychoactive Substance Use Disorders

Two major classes of substance abuse or dependence (alcohol and drugs) were emphasized in DSM-III. In DSM-III-R and DSM-IV, criteria were provided for abuse of and dependence on psychoactive substances in general. *Abuse* reflects pathological use of a substance or impairment in social and occupational performance secondary to substance use. *Dependence* includes a psychological need for continuing a substance as well as abuse of, tolerance of, or characteristic symptoms on withdrawal from the particular substance.

The prevalence of substance use disorders is, unfortunately, high in the United States. Six-month and lifetime prevalence rates for alcohol dependence/abuse were approximately 5% and 13%, respectively, in the ECA study, and these rates are similar to those in the NCS. Alcohol abuse/dependence is five times more common in men than in women. Drug abuse/dependence is somewhat less common: 6-month and lifetime prevalence rates are 2% and 6%, respectively. Drug abuse/dependence is only slightly more common in men than in women.

In disorders involving substance use or abuse, pharmacological treatment is generally aimed at ameliorating symptoms of withdrawal or at promoting abstinence, either by producing physical discomfort in the face of intoxication (e.g., disulfiram for alcohol abuse) or by blocking drug-induced euphoria (e.g., methadone or naltrexone). Acamprosate has been approved for promoting abstinence in alcoholic patients postwithdrawal. When the substance has been abused in the context of another disorder (such as major depression), treatment of the underlying disorder (e.g., with an SSRI) is warranted.

Child and Adolescent Disorders

Two disorders that in DSM-IV (and DSM-IV-TR) are categorized as disorders with onset in childhood or adolescence deserve mention. Bulimia, characterized by intense eating binges, occurs in both adolescents and adults and has been thought by some investigators to be related to depression or affective disease. Although there is some debate as to the nature of the possible relationship, it is clear that many patients with bulimia respond to treatment with antidepressants, including TCAs and SSRIs. Some bulimic patients also respond to behavior therapy. The other syndrome—attention-deficit/hyperactivity disorder (ADHD)—is characterized by hyperactivity and poor attention span. Classically, ADHD has its onset in childhood, but an adult form almost certainly exists (usually in patients who were hyperactive as children). Patients with this disorder respond well to stimulants and may also respond to TCAs and perhaps to bupropion or venlafaxine as well. Atomoxetine has been approved for use in children and adults with the disorder (Michelson et al. 2001). The drug is a potent norepinephrine reuptake blocker with little effect on serotonin or dopamine.

FDA Approval of Symptom Reduction Strategies

For many years, the FDA's position was to approve specific medications for specific disorders (e.g., fluoxetine for major depression or OCD). Recently, the FDA has begun to approve indications for symptom reduction in multiple disorders. For example, intramuscular olanzapine has been approved for acute relief of agitation, and various atypical antipsychotics are being studied for the relief of psychosis or behavioral disinhibition in Alzheimer's disease. It is likely we will have a host of adjunctive medications approved for components of multiple disorders.

DSM-V and Pharmacogenetics

DSM-V will attempt to incorporate data from recent studies on biology (e.g., genetics) into a new nomenclature. There will be efforts to deal more reasonably with the common comorbidities seen in practice. Dimensions will be developed to capture key characteristics such as psychosis, cognitive dysfunction, severity, anxiety, and depression. A recent report by Regier et al. (2009) highlights the approach being used. It is likely that DSM-V will be in field trials when this edition of our manual appears, with promulgation of DSM-V not occurring until 2013.

Genetics is likely to help with both classification and treatment. The Human Genome Project has provided us with a great deal of data on our own genetic building blocks. This information will, it is hoped, provide us with allelic variations of genes related to specific syndromes or symptoms. Such data will ultimately help clarify the relationship of many disorders that often occur comorbidly, such as childhood ADHD and bipolar disorder, GAD and major depression, and schizophrenia and bipolar disorder. It is not unlikely that genetic information, particularly that regarding symptoms, could lead to a new classification system with newly defined syndromes based on a combination of biological, genetic, and clinical data.

Pharmacogenetics could ultimately play a role not only in reclassifying psychiatric disorders but also in defining optimal treatment algorithms. If a specific allelic variation predicted a response to a specific treatment, our next manual could conceivably have a series of recommendations regarding using a specific drug for a patient with a disorder (e.g., major depression) who also has a particular allelic variation. A number of groups have reported that the long allelic form of the serotonin transporter predicts more robust responses to SSRIs. We and others have reported that individuals with short-form homozygotes for the serotonin transporter demonstrate poor responses or significant side effects while taking SSRIs (Murphy et al. 2004; Serretti et al. 2006). Our group has also reported that in depressed geriatric patients, the *APOE4* allele predicted response to mirtazapine (Murphy et al. 2003a), and the 102TC SNP for the serotonin 5-HT$_{2A}$ receptor predicted intolerance to paroxetine (Murphy et al. 2003b). Thus, it is possible that in the near future drug selection will be determined in part by laboratory testing. (For discussion of possible conflicts, see "Disclosure of Competing Interests" at the beginning of this manual.)

Summary

Accurate diagnosis and classification provide clues for developing psychopharmacological strategies. However, the clinician should not expect to find complete correlations between the types of patients encountered in practice and the classic prototypes in the literature. This caveat may prove particularly important when the clinician follows a patient over many years. In such a case, a flexible approach needs to be developed—one that includes routine and regular reassessment of the patient's condition and consideration of the need for changes in medication. These issues are discussed in more detail in subsequent chapters of this manual.

Bibliography

American Psychiatric Association: Diagnostic and Statistical Manual of Mental Disorders, 2nd Edition. Washington, DC, American Psychiatric Association, 1968

American Psychiatric Association: Diagnostic and Statistical Manual of Mental Disorders, 3rd Edition. Washington, DC, American Psychiatric Association, 1980

American Psychiatric Association: Diagnostic and Statistical Manual of Mental Disorders, 3rd Edition, Revised. Washington, DC, American Psychiatric Association, 1987

American Psychiatric Association: Diagnostic and Statistical Manual of Mental Disorders, 4th Edition. Washington, DC, American Psychiatric Association, 1994

American Psychiatric Association: Diagnostic and Statistical Manual of Mental Disorders, 4th Edition, Text Revision. Washington, DC, American Psychiatric Association, 2000

Bauer MS, Dunner DL: Validity of seasonal pattern as a modifier for recurrent mood disorders for DSM-IV. Compr Psychiatry 34:159–170, 1993

Bourdon KH, Boyd JH, Rae DS, et al: Gender differences in phobias: results of the ECA community survey. J Anxiety Disord 2:227–241, 1988

Boyd JH, Burke JD, Gruenberg E: Exclusion criteria of DSM-III: a study of co-occurrence of hierarchy-free syndromes. Arch Gen Psychiatry 41:983–989, 1984

DeBattista C, Belanoff J, Glass S, et al: Mifepristone versus placebo in the treatment of psychosis in patients with psychotic major depression. Biol Psychiatry 60:1343–1349, 2006

Fink M: Catatonia in DSM-IV (editorial). Biol Psychiatry 36:431–433, 1994

Flores BH, Kenna H, Keller J, et al: Clinical and biological effects of mifepristone treatment for psychotic depression. Neuropsychopharmacology 31:628–636, 2006

Frances A, Mack AH, First MB, et al: DSM-IV meets philosophy. Journal of Medical Philosophy 19:207–218, 1994

Gelenberg AJ, Lydiard RB, Rudolph RL, et al: Efficacy of venlafaxine extended-release capsules in nondepressed outpatients with generalized anxiety disorder: a 6-month randomized controlled trial. JAMA 283:3082–3088, 2000

Kessler RC, McGonagle KA, Zhao S, et al: Lifetime and 12-month prevalence of DSM-III-R psychiatric disorders in the United States: results from the National Comorbidity Survey. Arch Gen Psychiatry 51:8–19, 1994

Liebowitz MR: Mixed anxiety and depression: should it be included in DSM-IV? J Clin Psychiatry 54:4–7 [discussion 17–20], 1993

Marks I, Lader M: Anxiety states (anxiety neurosis): a review. J Nerv Ment Dis 156:3–18, 1973

Michelson D, Wernicke J, Heiligenstein J, et al: LY 139603 (tomoxetine) a new, nondopaminergic intervention for ADHD. Poster presented at the 41st annual meeting of the National Institute of Mental Health New Drug Clinical Drug Evaluation Unit, Phoenix, AZ, May 2001, Poster Session II-55

Murphy GM, Kremer C, Rodrigues HE, et al: The apolipoprotein E epsilon 4 allele and antidepressant efficacy in cognitively intact elderly depressed patients. Biol Psychiatry 54:665–673, 2003a

Murphy GM, Kremer C, Rodrigues HE, et al: Pharmacogenetics of antidepressant medication intolerance. Am J Psychiatry 160:1830–1835, 2003b

Murphy GM Jr, Hollander SB, Rodrigues HE, et al: Effects of the serotonin transporter gene promoter polymorphism on mirtazapine and paroxetine efficacy and adverse events in geriatric major depression. Arch Gen Psychiatry 61:1163–1169, 2004

Myers JK, Weissman MM, Tischler GL, et al: Six-month prevalence of psychiatric disorders in three communities. Arch Gen Psychiatry 41:959–967, 1984

Nathan PE: DSM-IV: empirical, accessible, not yet ideal (editorial). J Clin Psychol 50:103–110, 1994

Ohayon M, Schatzberg AF: Using chronic pain to predict depressed morbidity in the general population. Arch Gen Psychiatry 60:39–47, 2003

Pope HG Jr, Lipinski JF: Diagnosis in schizophrenia and manic-depressive illness: a reassessment of the specificity of "schizophrenic" symptoms in the light of current research. Arch Gen Psychiatry 35:811–828, 1978

Regier DA, Boyd JH, Burke JD Jr, et al: One-month prevalence of mental disorders in the United States. Arch Gen Psychiatry 45:977–986, 1988

Regier DA, Narrow WE, Kuhl EA, et al: The conceptual development of DSM-V. Am J Psychiatry 166:645–650, 2009

Robins LN, Helzer JE, Weissman MM, et al: Lifetime prevalence of specific psychiatric disorders in three sites. Arch Gen Psychiatry 41:949–958, 1984

Rush AJ, Weissenburger JE: Melancholic symptom features and DSM-IV. Am J Psychiatry 151:489–498, 1994

Sadler JZ, Hulgus YF, Agich GJ: On values in recent American psychiatric classification. Journal of Medical Philosophy 19:261–277, 1994

Schatzberg AF: Classification of affective disorders, in The Brain, Biochemistry, and Behavior (Proceedings of the Sixth Arnold O. Beckman Conference in Clinical Chemistry). Edited by Habig RL. Washington, DC, American Association for Clinical Chemistry, 1984, pp 29–46

Schatzberg AF, Rothschild AJ: Psychotic (delusional) major depression: should it be included as a distinct syndrome in DSM-IV? Am J Psychiatry 149:733–745, 1992 [also see comments]

Schatzberg AF, Kremer C, Rodrigues H, et al: Mirtazapine vs paroxetine in elderly depressed patients. Poster presented at the 41st annual meeting of the National Institute of Mental Health New Drug Clinical Drug Evaluation Unit, 2001, Poster Session I-62

Serretti A, Cusin C, Rausch JL et al: Pooling pharmacogenetic studies on the serotonin transporter: a mega-analysis. Psychiatry Res 145:61–65, 2006

Sheehan DV, Sheehan KH: The classification of anxiety and hysterical states, I: historical review and empirical delineation. J Clin Psychopharmacol 2:235–244, 1982a

Sheehan DV, Sheehan KH: The classification of anxiety and hysterical states, II: towards a more heuristic classification. J Clin Psychopharmacol 2:386–393, 1982b

Smeraldi E, Zanardi R, Benedetti F, et al: Polymorphism within the promoter of the serotonin transporter gene and antidepressant efficacy of fluvoxamine. Mol Psychiatry 3:508–511, 1998

Stein MB, Fyer AJ, Davidson JR, et al: Fluvoxamine treatment of social phobia (social anxiety disorder): a double-blind, placebo-controlled study. Am J Psychiatry 156:756–760, 1999

Woody G, Schuckit M, Weinrieb R, et al: A review of the substance use disorders section of the DSM-IV. Psychiatr Clin North Am 16:21–32, 1993

3

Antidepressants

According to the Centers for Disease Control and Prevention 2007 annual report "Health, United States," antidepressants are the most commonly prescribed agents in all of medicine (National Center for Health Statistics 2007). The wisdom of such a widespread use of this class of medications is debated in the literature and the popular press. However, what is not debatable is that clinicians have felt increasingly comfortable in prescribing these medications. The growing popularity of antidepressants rests on a number of factors, including their efficacy in the treatment of depression, broad spectrum of activity, relative safety, and ease of use. Factors such as marketing also have played a role in the widespread adoption of antidepressants in clinical practice.

The utility of antidepressants in the treatment of major depression has been established in a half century of randomized clinical trials. Relative to placebo, antidepressants appear to generally be effective in reducing the different symptom domains of major depression, effecting a 50% improvement in overall symptoms from baseline, achieving higher rates of remission of symptoms, and preventing relapse in patients with recurrent major depression. Advantages over placebo are most evident in more severe forms of depression. The placebo response rate has grown steadily in clinical trials, and many trials are no longer adequately powered to show a difference from placebo. As a result, only about half the antidepressant trials in the FDA database show separation from placebo.

Some investigators have come to the conclusion that when negative trials, including unpublished studies, are included in meta-analyses evaluating the efficacy of antidepressants, the advantages of antidepressants are small and may not outweigh the potential disadvantages. This conclusion is probably incorrect. First of all placebo in depression trials is not simply the administration of a sugar pill in a vacuum. In clinical depression trials, there are many nonspecific effects that would be difficult to replicate outside the research setting. These include extensive contact over weeks or months with highly devoted research personnel and physicians. The placebo might be administered in an inpatient setting with all the attendant therapeutic effects a hospitalization might provide. The increase in placebo response rates also means that many studies may be underpowered to show a difference now, in contrast to years ago. Underpowering of sample sizes in depression trials contributes to more trials failing to show a separation from placebo. Finally, studies that have demonstrated only minor benefits of antidepressants over placebo have tended to focus on change from baseline scores on a standardized rating scale such as the Hamilton Depression Rating Scale (HDRS). Antidepressants are known to have benefits to patients that might not be adequately captured by evaluating mean differences in scores on a depression scale. We know that antidepressants may impact a whole variety of symptoms that are not adequately captured on a scale such as the HDRS, including pain, different dimensions of anxiety, work productivity, and cognition. These nondepression effects of antidepressants are very important in determining patient well-being but are not fully assessed by evaluating symptom dimensions of antidepressant effects.

The popularity of antidepressants stems in no small part from the broad spectrum of uses these agents possess. In addition to their use in the treatment of major depression, antidepressants emerged in the 1990s as a viable treatment for most anxiety disorders. Many of the selective serotonin reuptake inhibitors (SSRIs) and serotonin-norepinephrine reuptake inhibitors (SNRIs) have received FDA indications for treatment of generalized anxiety disorder (GAD). Compared with other treatments for GAD, such as benzodiazepines, the antidepressants appear to be at least as effective, although slower acting.

However, the antidepressants lack the risk of dependence more common to the benzodiazepines. The SSRIs have also been approved for the treatment of panic disorder, posttraumatic stress disorder (PTSD), social anxiety disorder, and obsessive-compulsive disorder (OCD) and are now first-line treatments for these conditions. The efficacy of the antidepressants in treating anxiety disorders such social anxiety is often greater than that seen in the treatment of major depression.

While the treatment of major depression and anxiety disorders constitutes the major uses of antidepressants, these medications treat a variety of psychiatric conditions. Antidepressants are approved to treat bulimia and premenstrual dysphoric disorder (fluoxetine, sertraline). Off-label uses have included the treatment of negative symptoms of schizophrenia, agitation in dementia, impulse-control disorders, and borderline personality.

Approved psychiatric uses of antidepressants include treatment of pain conditions such as neuropathic pain and fibromyalgia (duloxetine) and smoking cessation (bupropion) and enuresis (imipramine). Off-label uses have included use in the treatment of vasomotor symptoms of menopause, migraine prophylaxis, and treatment of premature ejaculation.

The popularity of newer antidepressants such as the SSRIs, SNRIs, bupropion, and mirtazapine, relative to the older tricyclic antidepressants (TCAs) and monoamine oxidase inhibitors (MAOIs) also arises from their relative ease of use and safety. Most of the newer antidepressants are administered once daily, and the starting dose is often the therapeutic dose. While all antidepressants have side effects that limit their use, newer agents tend to be considerably better tolerated than either the TCAs or the MAOIs. In addition, most newer antidepressants are relatively safe in overdose, whereas an overdose of a TCA or MAOI is commonly lethal.

Most of the newer antidepressants and all of the older antidepressants are now quite inexpensive since going off patent and becoming available in generic form. In fact, as of this writing, a 90-day supply of most antidepressants costs $10 at one major pharmacy chain. Only the most recently available agents (escitalopram, duloxetine, and desvenlafaxine) do not have generic equivalents as of this writing.

Limitations of the antidepressants include side effects, slow onset of action, and lack of efficacy in many patients. Novel agents are under investigation currently that may address some of the shortcomings of currently available antidepressants. For example agomelatine, a melatonin 1 (MT_1) and melatonin 2 (MT_2) receptor agonist and 5-HT_{2C} antagonist, may have fewer sexual side effects and promote restful sleep in ways that current agents may not. Triple reuptake inhibitors, such as tesofensine, that block the reuptake of dopamine as well as serotonin and norepinephrine, appear to promote weight loss and may act more rapidly than available agents. Antiglucocorticoid agents might act quickly and be effective in treating some patients not treatable with current medications. However, novel agents with nonmonoaminergic mechanisms have fared poorly in randomized controlled clinical trials, and it is unclear whether any of these more novel agents will be demonstrated to have the efficacy and tolerability to allow them to join the many antidepressants currently available.

History

The modern antidepressants were discovered serendipitously. In the early 1950s, investigators noted that tuberculosis patients showed prolonged elevation of mood when treated with iproniazid (Marsilid), an MAOI thought to be an antituberculosis agent. Iproniazid proved ineffective for tuberculosis, but its impact on mood led to some of the earliest double-blind studies in psychopharmacology, demonstrating that MAOIs were effective antidepressant agents. The biological and pharmacological observations that MAOIs were antidepressants and that monoamine oxidase degraded norepinephrine and serotonin (5-HT) became cornerstones of the so-called biogenic amine theories of depression.

Iproniazid was taken off the U.S. market some time ago because of fear that it causes hepatic necrosis. For many years the use of other MAOIs declined, partly because of the introduction of TCAs and partly because of the occurrence in patients of significant hypertensive crises.

The TCAs were also discovered serendipitously. The first reports on TCA efficacy in depression came from Professor Kuhn (1958) in Switzerland, who astutely noted that a three-ringed compound, imipramine, which was being investigated as a treatment for schizophrenia, appeared to elevate mood even though it did not relieve psychosis. The drug was similar in structure to the phenothiazines, but a simple substitution of nitrogen for sulfur in the central ring appeared to confer unique antidepressant properties.

Two antidepressants with a four-ringed structure, maprotiline and amoxapine, have pharmacological effects similar to those of the more traditional TCAs. These effects are not unexpected, because the development of many of the earlier antidepressant compounds was based on the similarity of their activity in certain animal models to that of prototypical TCAs—a similarity that led some to call them "me-too drugs." However, there are both subtle and pronounced differences among many of the so-called me-too drugs. For example, amoxapine is a potent $5\text{-}HT_2/5\text{-}HT_3$ antagonist. Another four-ringed antidepressant, mirtazapine, has a very different profile than that of the TCAs. Mirtazapine appears to increase norepinephrine release by blocking presynaptic α_2 receptors. This release also appears to, in turn, stimulate serotonin release. Like many TCAs, mirtazapine is very antihistaminic but lacks the antimuscarinic effects seen in the TCAs.

The success of traditional antidepressants in treating depression led to a search in the pharmaceutical industry for compounds that would have the efficacy of the TCAs without many of the adverse effects, such as cardiotoxicity. In 1972, a research team composed of Bryan Malloy, Dave Wong, and Ray Fuller synthesized an agent at Eli Lilly labeled LY86032 that possessed these properties. This compound was altered somewhat to produce fluoxetine hydrochloride (Prozac). After an initial release in Belgium and South Africa, fluoxetine was released to the U.S. market in 1988. The first serotonergic agent, trazodone, had been released in 1981, but it did not have nearly the impact of fluoxetine. No other drug in the history of psychiatry has received as much attention, both positive and negative, as has fluoxetine. In any case, fluoxetine offered an alternative to traditional agents because it retained the efficacy of traditional antidepressants but did not have many of their side effects. In addition, fluoxetine appeared safe in overdose. As a result, fluoxetine and related antidepressants have supplanted the TCAs as the first-line agents in the treatment of major depression. Sales for fluoxetine alone topped $2 billion in 2000 in the United States. (Fluoxetine went off patent in mid-2001.) This success prompted other pharmaceutical companies to investigate agents that selectively enhance 5-HT function, and several other new agents were later released.

The search for selective medications has also led to the introduction of new classes of antidepressants. Venlafaxine, which is a selective SNRI, appears to possess much of the efficacy of TCAs without the overdose risks and the myriad side effects of the TCAs. Its metabolite desvenlafaxine appears to be a more balanced serotonin-norepinephrine drug than its parent. Duloxetine is the most noradrenergic of the available SNRIs. Selegiline, a selective monoamine oxidase B (MAO-B) agent at low oral doses, circumvents some of the problems of traditional MAOIs when given transdermally or, for that matter, sublingually. Selective and reversible inhibitors of monoamine oxidase A (RIMAs) represent another attempt to render difficult-to-tolerate MAOIs in a more manageable form.

Despite the tremendous success of the newer classes of antidepressants in enhancing safety and tolerability, there has been no appreciable success in improving the efficacy and the latency of onset of the antidepressants. As with the traditional agents, no more than 50%–65% of patients with major depression will respond to any given trial with a newer antidepressant, and no agent has been able to reduce reliably the 1–2 months or longer it appears to take for the drugs to show maximum benefits. Reducing the latency of antidepressant effects and enhancing efficacy are both important goals of future research efforts.

General Principles of Antidepressant Use

Although the antidepressants vary considerably in their mechanisms of action, toxicity, dosing, and potential for drug interactions, some clinical decisions apply to the use of all antidepressants. These include the criteria for choosing an antidepressant, deciding what dose is adequate, and determining the optimal duration of treatment.

Choosing an Antidepressant

As the number of antidepressants available has steadily increased, choosing an agent has become somewhat more difficult. Although side-effect profile is generally mentioned as the primary factor in choosing an antidepressant, optimally matching an antidepressant to a specific patient is as much art as science. Patient parameters, including subtype of depression, age, sex, and medical status, are matched with drug parameters such as side effects, safety, and cost.

The general wisdom is that all antidepressants on the market are equally efficacious in the treatment of depression. This is unlikely. Depression is much too heterogeneous to suggest that agents with diverse actions all work equally well for all types of depression.

The notion that antidepressants are equally efficacious is based on the fact that it has not been possible to show that any antidepressant is reliably more than 50%–70% effective in a given clinical trial. In contrast, placebos tend to be about 30% effective in outpatient trials. Efficacy is usually defined as a 50% improvement on a standard depression rating scale such as the HDRS. When remission, rather than more general improvement, is the criterion for efficacy, differences between antidepressants may begin to emerge. Even a 5% difference between classes of antidepressants in the ability to achieve remission would be clinically meaningful. However, adequately powering a study to show such a difference would take a sample size of several thousand subjects. The funding to do such a trial is prohibitive. Thus, a meta-analysis of similar studies is often employed to increase power and detect smaller differences. There had been some speculation that antidepressants with more complex neurotransmitter effects, such as the TCAs, venlafaxine, duloxetine, mirtazapine, and MAOIs, may achieve more complete remissions than SSRIs, and this hypothesis has been investigated. Some, such as the meta-analysis by Thase et al. (2001), indicated that venlafaxine was significantly more likely to effect a remission than were the SSRIs with which it was compared. However, this area is controversial. The FDA had chided Wyeth for using the Thase study in their marketing, pointing out that venlafaxine superiority may only be inferred against fluoxetine. Indeed, more recent meta-analyses by Nemeroff et al. (2003) and Weinmann et al. (2008) failed to show a clear advantage of venlafaxine over SSRIs overall. One major problem is that the original venlafaxine studies were not designed to compare maximum doses over time or to treat to remission.

In a review of randomized clinical trials by Montgomery and colleagues (2007), the authors concluded that there is evidence of probable superiority of some antidepressants over others. This review found that three antidepressants—clomipramine, venlafaxine, and escitalopram—tended to show superiority in efficacy in comparison studies. The review relied more on direct comparisons than meta-analyses to come to this conclusion. Indeed, many psychiatrists would concur that clomipramine, venlafaxine, and escitalopram may offer efficacy advantages over other agents. However, the advantages are relatively modest and may be outweighed by disadvantages for many patients, including side effects and cost.

When subtypes of depression such as atypical, melancholic, and psychotic depressions are evaluated, differences between antidepressant classes appear.

Atypical depressions, which are characterized by mood reactivity along with reverse vegetative symptoms such as increased sleep and appetite, have long been shown to respond better to MAOIs than to TCAs. Since atypical depression may also respond well to SSRIs and bupropion, these agents still would be first-line agents in the treatment of this subtype. However, it may be quite reasonable to consider an MAOI for a patient with treatment-resistant depression with atypical features. The availability of transdermal selegiline, with its favorable side-effect profile and lack of dietary restrictions, should probably now be the first MAOI that is considered in either atypical or treatment-resistant depression.

There continues to be a debate as to whether melancholic or psychotic depression responds better to TCAs or SNRIs than to SSRIs. Although most studies of antidepressant efficacy in these subtypes have involved TCAs, prospective, head-to-head comparisons have never been done, and the literature remains inconclusive. Melancholic depression clearly appears to respond to TCAs, and it may be more reasonable to start with venlafaxine or mirtazapine, which are TCA-like in their dual actions, than with an SSRI. Likewise, psychotic depression has responded to electroconvulsive therapy (ECT); amoxapine, which is a tetracyclic agent; or the combination of a TCA and an antipsychotic. There are some recent controlled data showing that the combination of fluoxetine and olanzapine is also effective, and this would be the recommended first-line strategy because of safety and ease of use.

The age of the patient is an important consideration in antidepressant choice. In geriatric patients, toxicity is more likely because of the number of concurrent medications they are taking, increased fat-to-muscle ratios, and reduced hepatic function and renal clearance. Among the SSRIs, escitalopram, citalopram, and sertraline appear to be among the best tolerated and the least likely to have serious pharmacokinetic interactions. Likewise, venlafaxine and mirtazapine have a low risk of interactions in geriatric patients. However, there has been some concern about the safety of venlafaxine in frail nursing home patients (Oslin et al. 2003). TCAs and MAOIs tend to be more poorly tolerated in geriatric patients and would be second- or third-line agents in this population, although some geriatricians still emphasize nortriptyline for elderly melancholic patients, and isocarboxazid was well tolerated in geriatric studies done some years ago.

Gender is also an important factor in tolerability and efficacy of a given antidepressant class. Substantial evidence suggests that men may respond to and tolerate the TCAs better than do women. Conversely, premenopausal women appear to do better with serotonergic agents than do men. Thus, men may be better treated with venlafaxine, duloxetine, or a TCA, and women may be better treated with an SSRI or a 5-HT$_2$ antagonist. Although clinicians would generally be advised not to start with a TCA because of safety concerns, it may be better to start male patients with a more noradrenergic agent than with an SSRI. Again, head-to head comparison studies are needed before clearer recommendations can be made, and this area is still controversial.

The medical status of the patient is an important consideration in choosing an antidepressant. Patients with pain conditions may do better with duloxetine, venlafaxine, or a TCA than with other agents. There is some evidence that the SNRIs and TCAs may be effective in treating both depression and some types of pain conditions. Patients with a history of a seizure disorder, stroke, or head trauma are more safely treated with an SSRI or venlafaxine than with a TCA or bupropion. Likewise, patients with a history of arrhythmia or coronary artery disease are more safely treated with serotonergic agents than with TCAs or MAOIs. Caution should be used in prescribing nefazodone for AIDS patients who are taking protease inhibitors, since it may increase toxicity of the protease inhibitors through pharmacokinetic interactions.

The primary drug parameters in choosing an antidepressant are side effects and safety. Most SSRIs are generically available and quite inexpensive. Older agents such as the TCAs and MAOIs usually require more visits and monitoring, and this may offset the low expense of the drugs. The SSRIs are relatively safe in overdose and better tolerated than the TCAs and MAOIs for most patients. The SNRI venlafaxine may also be less safe in overdose than are the SSRIs but safer than the TCAs. From safety alone, it is difficult to justify using a TCA or an MAOI as a first treatment option. Most of the SSRIs are given once per day, and the starting dose is sometimes the therapeutic dose. Thus, the SSRIs are also among the easiest agents to use. Recently, NICE, the British advisory group, noted that overdoses with venlafaxine were more likely to be lethal than overdoses with SSRIs. For a while, it advised against first-line use of the drug and recommended routine ECG monitoring but eventually changed its position. The FDA had not agreed.

Side effects differ considerably from class to class. Among the more important long-term side effects that influence compliance are weight gain and sexual dysfunction. The TCAs, MAOIs, and mirtazapine are probably the most problematic agents for weight gain, whereas fluoxetine and bupropion may be the least problematic. Sexual dysfunction is common to most antidepressants, especially the MAOIs, clomipramine, and the SSRIs. A number of agents are less likely to cause sexual side effects; these include nefazodone, bupropion, and mirtazapine. In addition, novel antidepressants such as agomelatine and transdermal selegiline also appear to have low risk for sexual side effects. It has been suggested that more noradrenergic SNRIs, such as duloxetine, may also have lower rates of sexual side effects than do the SSRIs, but no comparison has yet been completed.

Another common approach to choosing an antidepressant is to target specific symptoms of a depressive episode. For example, a patient with depression characterized by insomnia might benefit from a sedating agent such as mirtazapine or a tertiary-amine tricyclic. Patients with significant anxiety tend to be treated with an SSRI or SNRI. Patients with insomnia or anxiety may also be treated with the combination of an SSRI or SNRI and a hypnotic or benzodiazepine. Alternatively, many clinicians will choose a more stimulating antidepressant such as bupropion or transdermal selegiline in treating patients who are experiencing hypersomnia and fatigue. Patients with significant cognitive deficits or executive functioning problems might be treated with a noradrenergic agent such as bupropion or duloxetine (Raskin et al. 2007). This targeted approach to the treatment of depression is intuitively sound but not necessarily supported by empirical data.

In many areas of medicine, laboratory studies help guide the clinician in choosing a medication for a specific condition. For example, a bacterial culture helps the selection of a specific antibiotic or sensitivity in internal medicine, and genotyping is increasingly guiding treatment in gyn-oncology. At this time, psychiatry lacks a biological assay that might help us choose a specific treatment. There are very preliminary data to suggest that a number of approaches might help clinicians in making antidepressant choices in the future. For example, functional magnetic resonance imaging and positron emission tomography have shown some promise in early detection of whether an antidepressant might be effective or not by imaging early changes in limbic mood-generating areas and connectivity to cortical regions. Quantitative electroencephalography (QEEG) has shown benefit in some studies of prediciting subsequent response to a specific antidepressant by changes in prefrontal brain wave activity in the first week. Other small and very preliminary studies have found that QEEG might predict specific classes of agents a patient is most likely to respond to based on comparisons with a referenced database of responders. Genomics may also play an important role in determining the best choice of an antidepressant. Polymorphisms in the promoter region of the serotonin transporter (5HTTPRL), for example, have shown some predictive ability to determine who is more likely to respond to serotonergic versus noradrenergic antidepressants or who is more likely to experience SSRI-induced side effects. Likewise, commercially available cytochrome P450 (CYP) 2D6 AmpliChip genetic assay should theoretically help with determining tolerability and dosing in a given individual, although the data on this potential benefit are mixed. There are some data to suggest that the AmpliChip might predict side effects of TCAs but not SSRIs (Murphy et al. 2003). It seems likely that, in the coming decades, genomics, functional imaging, and tools like QEEG may provide additional data on which to make a clinical decicion about the choice of an antidepressant, and this would be most welcome. Until then, clinical judgment remains the only viable option in terms of antidepressant choice.

Dosage and Administration

The optimal dose of an antidepressant is the smallest efficacious dose that has the least side effects. The decision about how much to push the dose of an antidepressant always comes down to balancing efficacy and side effects. If, with a given dose of antidepressant, there are no signs of improving symptoms after 4 weeks, the chances are very small that that dose will ever be effective (Quitkin et al. 1996). Likewise, older patients with depression who fail to achieve at least 30% improvement by week 4 have only a 17% chance of achieving a remission by week 12 (Sackeim et al. 2005). On the other hand, partial response in the first 4 weeks predicts more complete response over the next 8 weeks, even if the dose is held constant. If a given dose is tolerated and not producing partial benefits at 4 weeks, the dose should be increased rather than the medication switched. Generally, increasing the dose every 2 weeks gives some opportunity for the clinician to assess the benefits and side effects of a given dose. If the increase in dose is tolerated and less than complete remission is observed, the dose should be gradually increased to the maximum recommended dose.

Duration of Treatment

Although standard antidepressant trials in the 1960s and 1970s were often 4 weeks, 6- to 12-week trials are the current standard. It is difficult to assess the efficacy of an antidepressant in less than 4 weeks. Furthermore, it is unlikely that 4 weeks will be adequate to assess higher doses in a tolerant patient. Quitkin et al. (1984), in reviewing a large series of depressed patients who were treated with traditional TCAs, concluded that relatively few patients demonstrated significant improvement after only 2 weeks of therapy and that many required as long as 6 weeks to respond. Years ago, our group (Schatzberg et al. 1981) reported that patients with slow response to maprotiline and those with rapid response could be identified biologically by their pretreatment urinary levels of 3-methoxy-4-hydroxyphenylglycol (MHPG), which are indicative of norepinephrine function. Patients with low MHPG levels demonstrated rapid responses (in less than 14 days), and those with very high MHPG levels needed 4–6 weeks of treatment. More recent reviews by Nierenberg et al. (1995, 2000) have also suggested that failure to improve while taking a given dose of fluoxetine for 4 weeks predicts failure to respond at 8 and 12 weeks.

All patients who respond to a given dose of an antidepressant should be maintained at that dose for at least 6–12 months. The continuation of all antidepressants studied to date appears to substantially reduce the risk of relapse. In a major National Institute of Mental Health collaborative study (Prien et al. 1984), imipramine was generally more effective than placebo or lithium in preventing relapse of major depression over a 2-year maintenance period. In contrast to that study, two earlier major studies, one in the United States and the other in the United Kingdom, found lithium to be as effective as TCAs in preventing relapses in patients with unipolar depression. In the U.S. study by Prien et al. (1984), the overall relapse rate in the unipolar group was relatively high (64%; 49% in the imipramine group), and the authors argued for the need to develop newer, alternative strategies, perhaps with drugs other than TCAs. (For further discussion of maintenance therapy in affective disorders, see Chapter 4: "Antipsychotic Drugs.") In the first edition of this manual, we indicated that after receiving maintenance therapy for some 3–4 months at the doses at which they responded, many patients can be maintained at lower doses (½ to ¾ that of the original dose) for the remaining months. However, the results of Frank et al. (1990) suggest that full doses are needed for successful maintenance therapy. These investigators found that 80% of patients with recurrent depression were free from relapse or recurrence for 3 years when full doses of imipramine (average of 200 mg/day) were maintained. We second the recommendations of Frank and colleagues that patients be maintained at their therapeutic dosage levels unless pronounced side effects are present. More recent studies examining the maintenance efficacy of venlafaxine demonstrated that patients are about twice as likely to stay well during treatment over the course of 2 years as patients randomly assigned to a placebo during this period. In the maintenance venlafaxine study, patients continued on their acute dose unless side effects required a dosage decrease (Kornstein 2008). Since depression recurs in some 87% of patients within 15 years of the index episode, long-term maintenance therapy should certainly be considered for anyone who has had three or more serious depressive episodes or two episodes in the past 5 years.

However, emerging data on the neurobiology of depression put into question whether it is always wise to wait until the second or third episode to consider long-term or lifetime maintenance treatment. Some studies have now suggested that depression could be associated with a progressive loss of volume in the hippocampus and perhaps other brain areas, including anterior cingulate and medial orbital frontal cortex. Furthermore, these changes may progress as a function of duration of depressive illness and the number of recurrences a patient experiences (Maletic et al. 2007). These morphological changes may be difficult to overcome or could perhaps become permanent. In addition, the cumulative alterations in brain morphology are consistent with the progressive nature of depression in many patients. Subsequent recurrence may be more resistant to treatment, more chronic, more severe, and less related to external stresses. Recurrences may also be associated with an accumulation of cognitive deficits, especially memory loss, that is consistent with the observation of progressive loss in the hippocampus (Gorwood et al. 2008). In fact, Gorwood and colleagues (2008) estimated a permanent loss of 2%–3% in memory performance for each of the first four episodes of depression a patient experiences. Thus, it may be advisable for some patients to consider long-term maintenance treatment even after one initial serious depressive episode.

Long-term treatment with antidepressants can represent a challenge for the patient in adhering to the prescribed regimen. Most patients are not enamored by the idea of continuing to take antidepressants for long periods of time. Stigma, side effects, cost, and inconvenience all contribute to nonadherence to maintenance antidepressant treatment. Several interventions can increase compliance. It is helpful to educate the patient and family about the course of depressive illness, the length of time it takes for antidepressants to work, and the need to continue treatment when the patient is feeling better. We increasingly educate patients about the potential for depression-associated progressive brain changes and long-term cognitive deficits that have been increasingly reported in the literature. Reviewing potential side effects is also helpful. Asking for feedback and answering any questions the patient may have allows the clinician to check the patient's understanding of the prescribed treatment. Instructing the patient to not change the dosage or discontinue the medication without consulting his or her physician is often helpful as well.

Selective Serotonin Reuptake Inhibitors

Although the TCAs were the dominant class of antidepressants worldwide for more than 30 years, the SSRIs overtook them in popularity in just a decade. Currently, this class includes fluoxetine, paroxetine, sertraline, fluvoxamine, citalopram, and escitalopram (Figure 3–1). Fluvoxamine does not have an FDA-approved indication for the treatment of depression but received an approval for social anxiety in 2008 in addition to its long-standing indication for OCD. In addition, fluvoxamine is marketed in many countries as an antidepressant. Unlike the TCAs or any other group of prescribed psychotropic agents, the SSRIs, particularly fluoxetine, have had tremendous exposure in the scientific literature.

These drugs have been both vilified and praised in the lay press, but the popularity of the SSRIs among patients and physicians has remained quite consistent. The enormous popularity of these agents is due in no small part to their favorable safety and side-effect profile relative to the MAOIs and the TCAs. The SSRIs have also proved to have a broad spectrum of activity in a variety of psychiatric disorders, and they have an additional advantage in that it is easier to attain the optimal therapeutic dose. In addition, all the SSRIs except escitalopram are now generic and quite inexpensive. In 2008, a major pharmacy chain was selling most of the SSRIs for about 3–4 dollars for a month's supply. Some long-acting formulations such as weekly fluoxetine, paroxetine CR, and fluvoxamine CR remain on patent and are more expensive. However, not all patients tolerate or respond to the SSRIs, and, as suggested earlier (see "Choosing an Antidepressant" subsection earlier in this chapter), they may not

Selective serotonin reuptake inhibitors (SSRIs): overview

Efficacy	First-line treatment in MDD (FDA approved for all except fluvoxamine), dysthymia PD (FDA approved for fluoxetine, paroxetine, and sertraline) OCD (FDA approved for all except citalopram and escitalopram) Social anxiety disorder (FDA approved for sertraline, fluvoxamine, and paroxetine) PTSD (FDA approved for sertraline and paroxetine) Bulimia (FDA approved for fluoxetine) GAD (FDA approved for paroxetine and escitalopram) PMDD (FDA approved for fluoxetine [Sarafem only], paroxetine [controlled release only], and sertraline)
Side effects	GI side effects (nausea, diarrhea, heartburn) Sexual dysfunction ($\downarrow$ libido, delayed orgasm) Headache Insomnia/somnolence
Safety in overdose	Generally safe in overdose to 30–90 days' supply; manage with vital sign support, lavage Seizures/status epilepticus (rare)
Dosage and administration	Citalopram, paroxetine, fluoxetine: qd dosing, starting at 10–20 mg, increasing to a maximum of 40 mg (citalopram), 50 mg (paroxetine), and 80 mg (fluoxetine). Escitalopram: qd dosing, starting at 10 mg, increasing to 20 mg after minimum of 1 week. Sertraline: starts at 25–50 mg and is increased, as needed, to 200 mg maximum.
	Full benefits in 4–8 weeks
Discontinuation	Paroxetine, fluvoxamine, sertraline: discontinuation associated with parasthesias, nausea, headaches, flulike symptoms 1–7 days after sudden discontinuation
Drug interactions	MAOI (**contraindicated**): serotonin syndrome $\uparrow$ TCA levels (paroxetine, fluoxetine) $\uparrow$ Carbamazepine, phenobarbital, phenytoin levels $\uparrow$ Haloperidol, clozapine levels (fluvoxamine) $\uparrow$ Theophylline levels (fluvoxamine) $\uparrow$ Encainide, flecainide levels (**avoid**)

Note. FDA = U.S. Food and Drug Administration; GAD = generalized anxiety disorder; GI = gastrointestinal; MAOI = monoamine oxidase inhibitor; MDD = major depressive disorder; OCD = obsessive-compulsive disorder; PD = panic disorder; PMDD = premenstrual dysphoric disorder; PTSD = posttraumatic stress disorder; TCA = tricyclic antidepressant.

Figure 3–1. Chemical structures of selective serotonin reuptake inhibitors (SSRIs).

be as effective as other antidepressants for some types of depression and some specific symptoms, such as pain.

Pharmacological Effects

As the name of this class of antidepressants indicates, the SSRIs selectively block the reuptake of 5-HT through their inhibiting effects on the Na^+/K^+ adenosine triphosphatase (ATPase)–dependent serotonin transporter (SERT) in presynaptic neurons. Compared with a standard TCA such as amitriptyline, which has about an equal tendency to block neuronal reuptake of 5-HT and norepinephrine, fluoxetine is 200 times more selective in blocking the reuptake of 5-HT than of norepinephrine. Fluoxetine is approximately 4 times as potent a 5-HT reuptake inhibitor in vitro as is amitriptyline, and paroxetine is approximately 80 times as potent an inhibitor as amitriptyline. Of the five currently available SSRIs, paroxetine and citalopram appear to be the most potent 5-HT uptake blockers.

However, selectivity is a relative term. Although the SSRIs are more selective than, say, the TCAs, all the SSRIs impact other neurotransmitter systems, at least modestly. For example, there is in vitro evidence that paroxetine at high dosages (>40 mg/day) may be as much, if not more, of a norepinephrine reuptake blocker as is venlafaxine. Sertraline also appears to block the reuptake of dopamine and may be more potent in this regard than bupropion. Likewise, paroxetine may have as strong of an anticholinergic effect as desipramine.

The reuptake-blocking properties of the SSRIs enhance general serotonergic tone in at least two distinct steps. Initially, the SSRIs contribute to a significant increase in the availability of 5-HT in the synaptic cleft. However, it is unlikely that this effect has any bearing on antidepressant efficacy, because the SSRIs share the delayed onset of action typical of all antidepressants. With recurrent administration of the drugs, however, there is a reduction in the sensitivity of the somatodendritic and terminal 5-HT_{1A} autoreceptors, and the time course of this effect is associated more closely with antidepressant response. In addition, blockade of SERT by chronic administration of SSRIs is associated with an increase in neurotrophin expression. SSRIs enhance transcription of neurotrophic factors, including brain-derived neurotrophic factor (BDNF). The increase in antidepressant-induced BDNF is associated with an increase in synaptogenesis, neurogenesis, and neuronal resilience. These increases appear to be an important consequence of long-term administration of SSRIs and other effective antidepressant classes.

Unlike the TCAs, the SSRIs have relatively little affinity for histaminic (H_1, H_2), muscarinic, or α_1-adrenergic receptors. Although sertraline may have 25% of the in vitro affinity for α_1-adrenergic receptors that imipramine has, this finding is of little clinical relevance. On the other hand, paroxetine has weak but somewhat clinically meaningful antimuscarinic activity. The anticholinergic affinity for paroxetine is roughly equivalent to that for desipramine. In general, however, the selective nature of the SSRIs results in the very favorable side-effect profile and the large therapeutic index possessed by these drugs.

The SSRIs are extensively metabolized by hepatic enzymes, especially the cytochrome P450 2D6 enzyme (Table 3–1). Sertraline is also metabolized via the cytochrome P450 3A3/4 enzyme. Only fluoxetine and sertraline have pharmacologically active metabolites (Table 3–2). Fluoxetine is demethylated to norfluoxetine, and sertraline is metabolized to N-desmethylsertraline and a hydroxyketone. As a result, the functional half-lives of fluoxetine and sertraline are considerably longer than those of paroxetine and fluvoxamine. Fluoxetine has a half-life of about 34 hours; the half-life of norfluoxetine is at least 1 week. Sertraline has a half-life of about 26 hours, and the half-lives of its metabolites tend to range from 48 to 72 hours. Both paroxetine and fluvoxamine have half-lives that average under 20 hours, whereas citalopram has a half-life of around 35 hours. With repeated administration of the drugs, the half-lives of all of the SSRIs, but particularly paroxetine and fluoxetine, increase substantially, because the drugs appear to inhibit their own metabolism. Thus, the functional half-lives of fluoxetine and norfluoxetine, with continued use, are closer to 2–3 weeks. Plasma level monitoring of the SSRIs has not proved clinically useful. The variability of SSRI plasma levels among individuals is so great that it has been nearly impossible to correlate efficacy or toxicity with plasma levels.

Indications

The SSRIs are indicated primarily for the treatment of major depression, and numerous studies have supported this use. A large number of double-blind, placebo-controlled studies have established that the SSRIs are useful in the treatment of mild to moderate major depression in outpatients (Rickels and Schweizer 1990). Some studies also suggest that the SSRIs are also efficacious in the treatment of more severe depression. In fact, Montgomery and colleagues (2007) concluded that evidence supporting escitalopram in severe depression may be stronger than evidence for other antidepressants. The SSRIs

Table 3–1. Inhibition of cytochrome P450 enzymes by antidepressants

Enzyme	Drugs metabolized	Antidepressant inhibitors
2D6	TCAs (hydroxylation) bupropion venlafaxine thioridazine 1C antiarrhythmics β-blockers paroxetine risperidone codeine haloperidol clozapine benztropine perphenazine	fluoxetine (norfluoxetine) sertraline (desmethylsertraline) paroxetine fluvoxamine and citalopram (weakest)
1A2	caffeine theophylline phenacetin TCAs (demethylation) clozapine diazepam	fluvoxamine
3A3/4	alprazolam triazolam TCAs (demethylation) terfenadine astemizole carbamazepine erythromycin dexamethasone citalopram escitalopram cyclosporine	fluoxetine sertraline fluvoxamine nefazodone
2C19	TCAs (demethylation) warfarin tolbutamide phenytoin diazepam	fluoxetine fluvoxamine sertraline

Note. TCA = tricyclic antidepressant.

Table 3–2. Pharmacokinetics of selective serotonin reuptake inhibitors (SSRIs)

SSRI	Half-life (hours)	Metabolite and its half-life	Peak plasma level (hours)	% Protein bound
fluoxetine	24–72	norfluoxetine, 7–14 days	6–8	94
sertraline	25	N-desmethylsertraline, 2–3 days	6–8	95
paroxetine	<20	NA	2–8	99
fluvoxamine	15	NA	2–8	77
citalopram	35	NA	4–6	91
escitalopram	32	S-demethylcitalopram	5	56

Note. NA = not applicable.

are effective in atypical depression, in combination with standard antipsychotics in the treatment of psychotic depression, and in the maintenance therapy of recurrent depression in trials lasting 1 year. In addition, SSRIs are also useful in the treatment of chronic major depression with dysthymia. Some clinicians have come to regard these agents as the treatments of choice for these disorders.

However, there is ongoing debate about the role of the SSRIs in more serious forms of depression, including melancholia. Large meta-analyses and randomized controlled trials have failed to show a significant difference in efficacy between SSRIs and TCAs or SNRIs in the treatment of severe depression (Beilski et al. 2004; Hirschfeld 1999). Still, relatively few studies of SSRIs have involved more severely depressed inpatients, and some of the studies that did involve such patients did not directly compare the SSRIs with older agents such as the TCAs. Some studies that made these direct comparisons suggested that paroxetine was inferior to clomipramine in inducing remission in melancholic inpatients (Danish University Antidepressant Group 1990) and that fluoxetine was much less effective than nortriptyline in treating melancholic elderly cardiac patients who were hospitalized for depression (Roose et al. 1994). These studies defined response not as a reduction in overall severity but rather as remission. Other studies have failed to find any difference in efficacy between the TCAs and SSRIs in more severely depressed inpatients. This debate about the efficacy of the SSRIs in more severe depression is likely to continue.

The available data suggest that the SSRIs may not be quite as effective in treating some seriously depressed elderly inpatients but that they do have a more favorable side-effect profile than either the TCAs or SNRIs.

The second indication for the SSRIs is the treatment of OCD. The utility of clomipramine (a serotonergic TCA) in the treatment of OCD was first noted in 1968. Since that time it has become clear that other serotonergic agents are also useful in the treatment of this historically difficult-to-treat disorder (Chouinard et al. 1990; Tollefson et al. 1994). Fluvoxamine, fluoxetine, sertraline, and paroxetine all have an FDA indication for the treatment of OCD, but all the SSRIs have demonstrated efficacy in treating the disorder. SSRI doses for the treatment of OCD are usually higher than those required for the treatment of depression, and the latency to response is usually longer.

A third indication for the SSRIs, and a fairly well studied one, is the treatment of eating disorders, particularly bulimia nervosa. Fluoxetine has been shown to have a positive effect on the binge-purge cycle in some bulimic patients (Fluoxetine Bulimia Nervosa Collaborative Study Group 1992). The SSRIs may also ameliorate the carbohydrate craving and mood disturbance associated with bulimia nervosa and obesity. Fluoxetine and sertraline have been shown to have a modest effect on weight and food intake in obese patients. Unfortunately, most patients who lose weight in the course of therapy with an SSRI gain it back over time. There are few data on the use of the SSRIs to treat classic anorexia nervosa, but one report suggested that fluoxetine may be useful for this condition (Kaye et al. 1991). The largest controlled study to date of fluoxetine in the prevention of relapse in anorexic patients failed to show any benefit for fluoxetine in preventing relapse relative to placebo (Walsh et al. 2006). However, this study involved adults with a more chronic form of the illness, and there may be subsets of anorexic patients who appear to do better while taking an SSRI.

Finally, there appears to be a role for the SSRIs in the treatment of most other anxiety disorders, including panic disorder, social anxiety disorder, GAD, and PTSD. Although patients with panic disorder may be sensitive to the activating effects of some SSRIs, most are able to tolerate a slow titration of dosage upward. For example, some reports indicate that although some patients do not tolerate an initial dosage of 20 mg/day of fluoxetine, many patients are able to benefit if the starting dosage is 5 mg/day (Schneier et al. 1990).

The SSRIs, including citalopram and fluvoxamine, all appear, on the basis of published data, to be effective in treating panic disorder. Paroxetine, sertraline, and fluoxetine have received an FDA-approved indication for the treatment of panic disorder.

In 1999, paroxetine received an FDA-approved indication for treating social anxiety disorder, and preliminary data support the use of other SSRIs in the treatment of this disorder. A number of double-blind studies indicate that paroxetine at dosages of 20–50 mg/day is more effective than placebo in alleviating symptoms, including undue fear and avoidance of interpersonal interaction. Further, paroxetine appears to reduce the significant disability associated with more severe forms of this disorder (Stein et al. 1998). Fluvoxamine also received, in 2008, approval for the treatment of social anxiety disorder. Other SSRIs, including escitalopram, have positive controlled trials in the treatment of social anxiety but have not received approval for this indication. In general, the SSRIs appear at least as efficacious in the treatment of social anxiety as they are in the treatment of major depression. However, while social anxiety disorder is among the more common anxiety disorders, it is also less commonly diagnosed and treated than other anxiety disorders.

Posttraumatic stress disorder is associated with a variety of comorbid conditions, especially depression and substance abuse. SSRIs have been used since the late 1980s to treat some of the symptoms of PTSD, including depression, insomnia, hyperarousal, and agitation. There is substantial evidence that fluoxetine, paroxetine, and sertraline help alleviate these symptoms and may even impact comorbid substance use. In 1999, sertraline became the first drug to be approved by the FDA for the treatment of PTSD. Many PTSD patients treated with sertraline appear to require doses above 100 mg/day of sertraline for maximum effects. With paroxetine, a dosage of 20 mg/day appears to be about as effective as 40 mg/day in treating PTSD.

The SSRIs should help with GAD, and paroxetine and escitalopram have received FDA approval for this indication. Paroxetine, at dosages of 20–50 mg/day, was effective in reducing anxiety by 60% on the Hamilton Anxiety Rating Scale. Large-scale studies of escitalopram have also shown benefit in the treatment of generalized anxiety.

Premenstrual dysphoric disorder (PMDD) is a very disruptive monthly occurrence for about 3% of the female population. In 1995, in the first large study of fluoxetine in the treatment of PMDD (Steiner et al. 1995), 20- and

60-mg doses were more effective than placebo for treating symptoms over six consecutive menstrual cycles. The effect was seen as early as the first cycle after initiation of the medication. Since then, a number of studies have supported the use of SSRIs, especially fluoxetine and sertraline, in treating this disorder. Both of these drugs have also been used as intermittent treatment in the luteal phase of the cycle and appear to be effective (Jermain et al. 1999). In 1999, fluoxetine (Sarafem) became the first medication approved for the treatment of PMDD.

The list of disorders in which the serotonergic system plays a part is long, and the potential role for the SSRIs is continually expanding. The SSRIs appear to be useful in treating the anger or impulsive aggression associated with some personality disorders (Kavoussi et al. 1994; Rinn et al. 2002) and perhaps certain pain disorders such as diabetic neuropathy and fibromyalgia (Wolfe et al. 1994), although here the mixed norepinephrine-serotonin reuptake blockers appear to be far more effective.

Side Effects

As noted previously, the SSRIs tend to be safer and better tolerated than their predecessors. There have been many overdoses in clinical practice with the SSRIs, but these have rarely been eventful. In fact, a review of 234 fluoxetine overdose attempts, with doses up to 1,500 mg, failed to reveal any fatalities, and more than half the patients were completely asymptomatic (Borys et al. 1992). Nothing more than supportive care was required for any patient. Moderate overdoses (5–30 times the total daily dose) are rarely serious. Nonetheless, fatal overdoses with SSRIs have occurred. One analysis suggests that as many as 14/1,000 overdoses with SSRIs might be fatal (McKenzie and McFarland 2007). However, many of these overdoses are complicated by the ingestion of additional substances. Still, a rate of 0.14 % of SSRI overdoses associated with fatality is a fraction of the rate of lethal TCA overdoses and also lower than the fatal overdoses seen with venlafaxine. The usual cause of death appears to be complications of seizures or status epilepticus and typically involves ingesting thousands of milligrams (Barbey and Roose 1998).

In early clinical studies, approximately twice as many patients were likely to drop out because of adverse effects of TCAs as because of adverse effects of SSRIs. The SSRIs are largely devoid of the anticholinergic side effects that plague the TCAs. Furthermore, orthostatic hypotension does not typically occur with SSRI use. In general, the SSRIs also appear to be better tolerated than are the MAOIs, and SNRIs as well. That is not to say that all people tolerate the SSRIs better than they do other classes of antidepressants. Some patients who cannot tolerate an SSRI's sexual side effects, for example, might do well with some SNRIs, bupropion, or even transdermal selegiline.

The most common reasons patients discontinue the SSRIs early in treatment are gastrointestinal (GI) side effects. These include nausea, diarrhea, cramping, heartburn, and other symptoms of GI distress. The gut is lined with 5-HT receptors, including 5-HT$_3$, which appear to be responsible for SSRI-induced GI distress. Whereas the earliest reports suggested that approximately 20%–30% of patients treated with fluoxetine developed GI side effects, the incidence in clinical practice has been much lower. In early studies, the dosage was often started at 20 mg/day but reached 60 mg/day by the end of the first week. In clinical practice, the starting dosage of 20 mg/day is maintained for 3 weeks, and nausea is both less common and less severe. Furthermore, the GI side effects tend to diminish over the first 2–4 weeks of treatment.

Several strategies may be useful in reducing SSRI-induced GI distress. The first is a slow titration of the medication. Starting at half, or less than half, of the usual starting dose and moving the dose up slowly in sensitive patients allows adaptation to occur. Another strategy is instructing patients to take their medication with meals. A full stomach appears to mitigate some GI distress. Other 5-HT$_3$ antagonists, such as dolasetron (Anzemet) and ondansetron (Zofran), are also clearly helpful but are too expensive to use routinely. Mirtazapine (Remeron) is a fairly potent 5-HT$_2$ and 5-HT$_3$ antagonist and has been used in combination with SSRIs. In fact, oncologists and anesthesiologists are increasingly using mirtazapine as a less expensive alternative to the traditional 5-HT$_3$ antagonists for treating postoperative and chemotherapy-induced nausea (Kast and Foley 2007).

Another group of side effects commonly encountered with SSRIs is related to central nervous system (CNS) activation. At least 10%–20% of patients receiving SSRI therapy complain of insomnia, jitteriness, and agitation in the course of treatment. These side effects are not particularly surprising, given the selective, but not specific, effect of SSRIs on CNS serotonergic transmission. That is, the SSRIs affect diffuse serotonergic pathways, and some of these pathways contribute to CNS arousal. For this reason, fluoxetine, which has a reputation for activating properties, should be taken in the morning, when it is less likely to interfere with sleep. Likewise, if patients develop insomnia with other SSRIs, it is often effective to have the patients take the dose earlier in the day. Occasionally, patients require modest doses of a benzodiazepine (e.g., clonazepam 0.5 mg bid, lorazepam 0.5 mg bid, alprazolam 0.25 mg bid) early in the course of therapy to help with agitation and sleep. Trazodone is another commonly used agent shown to be helpful at doses of 50–100 mg at bedtime for SSRI-induced insomnia. A number of case reports also suggest that trazodone may augment response in the SSRIs.

Conversely, some patients may become sedated on SSRIs. This effect is seen mostly with paroxetine. When sedation occurs, taking the dose at about 8:00 P.M. is useful for matching the peak blood level with the optimal time of sedation (about 2:00 A.M.). Some patients taking other SSRIs experience the emergence of a numbed or anergic feeling in the context of a euthymic mood. Donald Klein has recommended low dosages of bromocriptine (2.5 mg qd or bid) or stimulants to counteract this effect. Modafinil (Provigil) has been applied to counteract antidepressant-induced hypersomnia. Modafinil is a stimulant with low abuse potential and is FDA approved for the treatment of narcolepsy and idiopathic hypersomnia. We have found that doses of 100–200 mg in the morning are helpful in alleviating treatment-emergent somnolence (DeBattista et al. 2003). In addition, modafinil may have a role in helping other dimensions of depression, including fatigue and cognition.

In recent years, it has become clear that treatment-emergent sexual dysfunction is a much bigger problem with SSRI treatment than was previously recognized. Premarketing studies suggested that the incidence of sexual dysfunction—including delayed ejaculation, anorgasmia, impotence, and diminished libido—was less than 4%. However, more recent reports suggested that the incidence may be closer to 30%–40% for all of the SSRIs. Although accommodation to sexual side effects does occur in some patients, such improvement may take months or even years. Holding the dose of shorter-acting SSRIs, such as paroxetine and sertraline, for 24 hours prior to anticipated sexual activity has been anecdotally reported to be helpful in some 50% of patients. The long half-life of fluoxetine makes this approach ineffective.

A number of interventions to counteract treatment-emergent sexual dysfunction have been described (Table 3–3), but most have not been well studied. Virtually all the reported benefits of adjunctive agents for treatment-emergent

Table 3–3. Adjunctive agents for selective serotonin reuptake inhibitor (SSRI)–induced sexual dysfunction

Adjunctive agent	Dosage	Studies
buspirone	20–60 mg/day	Landen et al. 1999; Norden 1994
bupropion	75–150 mg/day	Ashton and Rosen 1998; Labbate and Pollack 1994; DeBattista et al. 2005
sildenafil	50–100 mg prn	Ashton and Bennett 1999; Gupta et al. 1999; Nurnberg et al. 1999a, 1999b, 2008; Fava et al. 2006a
tadalafil	10–20 mg	Seagraves et al. 2007
vardenafil	10–20 mg	Rosen et al. 2006
Ginkgo biloba	60–240 mg/day	Wheatley 2004
amantadine	100–300 mg/day	Balon 1996; Shrivastava et al. 1995
cyproheptadine	4–12 mg prn	Aizenberg et al. 1995; Keller Ashton et al. 1997
yohimbine	5.4 mg tid	Jacobsen 1992; Price and Grunhaus 1990

sexual side effects are based on case reports or open-label studies. A few controlled studies have been completed, but their findings are not conclusive. In one of the few double-blind studies of sexual dysfunction antidotes to be published, buspirone, a partial agonist of the 5-HT_{1A} receptor, was shown to be useful in treating SSRI-induced sexual dysfunction in some patients at dosages of 20–60 mg/day (Landen et al. 1999). However, another double-blind study of buspirone in the treatment of SSRI-induced sexual side effects did not find buspirone to be useful in this regard (Michelson et al. 2000). Mirtazapine was also ineffective in a controlled trial, although olanzapine, a $5\text{-HT}_2/D_2$ antagonist, was significantly more effective than placebo (Michelson et al. 2002). Switching to bupropion (Walker et al. 1993) or adding bupropion at dosages of 75–150 mg/day to the SSRI regimen (Ashton and Rosen 1998; Hirschfeld 1999; Labbate and Pollack 1994) has proved useful in some cases. We completed a double-blind study of bupropion as an add-on therapy and found it helpful for mood but not for sexual performance at a fixed dosage of 150 mg/day (DeBattista et al. 2005). Bupropion was found to be only marginally effective at increasing sexual arousal; however, a dose of 300 mg or more may be needed to improve sexual function. Clayton and colleagues (2004) found that bupropion at a dosage of 150 mg bid improved desire and interest in sexual activity on some measures after 4 weeks. The use of sildenafil (Viagra) has been reported to be significantly more effective than placebo in men with SSRI-induced sexual dysfunction (Nurnberg et al. 2001; Fava et al. 2006a). The reported utility of sildenafil in countering SSRI-induced sexual side effects is somewhat counterintuitive, since the most common sexual side effects of SSRIs are decreased libido and delayed orgasm rather than erectile problems. However, sildenafil has been reported to increase overall sexual satisfaction in both men and women. In a controlled study in women, we observed sildenafil (50–100 mg/day) to be significantly more effective than placebo in improving global measures of sexual function in patients with purported antidepressant-induced sexual side effects (Nurnberg et al. 2008). Similar agents such as vardenafil also appear to be effective in antidepressant-associated sexual dysfunction, at least in men (Rosen et al. 2006). Cyproheptadine at dosages of 4–12 mg/day may reverse some of the dysfunction. Unfortunately, cyproheptadine may also reverse the antidepressant or antiobsessive effects of the SSRIs and is quite sedating. The α-adrenergic agonist yohimbine helps some patients (Jacobsen 1992) but was ineffective in a controlled trial (Michelson et al. 2002). Unfortunately, yohimbine can be quite anxiogenic for some patients, and this effect tends to be counterproductive. Similarly, some case reports have suggested that dopaminergic agents such as amantadine, amphetamine, and bromocriptine may be helpful for some patients. The ancient herb *Ginkgo biloba* has been anecdotally reported to help some patients with SSRI-induced sexual dysfunction. However, beneficial effects may require a higher dosage (e.g., 240 mg/day) for weeks, and such dosages have sometimes been associated with GI side effects, increased bleeding, and confusion in elderly patients. As is often the case, more carefully controlled studies have failed to show a benefit of *Ginkgo biloba* in treating antidepressant-induced sexual dysfunction (Wheatley 2004). Given the lack of evidence supporting ginkgo and the potential for some side effects, we do not encourage patients to try it.

A number of other adverse effects are associated with the SSRIs, but these occur less consistently. Headaches may occur early in the course of therapy with some patients. On the other hand, the SSRIs have shown some utility in the prophylaxis of migraine when used long-term. Autonomic symptoms such as excessive perspiration and dry mouth are frequently reported. Excessive perspiration is very problematic for some patients. Anecdotal approaches to the treatment of SSRI-induced perspiration, such as the use of β-blockers and anticholinergic agents, are largely untested. α_2-Adrenergic agents may be helpful here. Tremor may develop in a dose-related pattern and is often responsive to propranolol in modest dosages (10 mg tid). Dry mouth is seen in some 20% of patients treated with paroxetine, reflecting the mild anticholinergic effects of this medication.

The question of whether weight gain is associated with chronic use of SSRIs has become a focus of interest. In general, it has been difficult to reliably correlate significant weight gain with SSRI treatment. After a year of treatment, most of the SSRIs are associated with either no weight gain or modest weight increases. Among the SSRIs, paroxetine may be somewhat more associated with weight gain and fluoxetine somewhat less.

Teicher et al. (1990) reported the emergence of intense preoccupation with suicide in six patients early in fluoxetine treatment. This phenomenon may also occur with other antidepressants. Subsequent studies and analyses of data sets have failed to find any greater proclivity for suicide with fluoxetine than with other antidepressants (Beasley et al. 1991). In addition, there has been no association of fluoxetine with suicidality in bulimia (Wheadon et al. 1992) or OCD (Beasley et al. 1992). This suggests that the phenomenon of treatment-emergent suicidal thoughts may be an artifact of the patient's underlying depression rather than the result of the medication. However, fluoxetine is associated with agitation or perhaps akathisia-like side effects, and it is conceivable that some depressed patients may become more suicidal when these effects occur (Rothschild and Locke 1991). Rothschild and Locke (1991) reintroduced fluoxetine in three patients who had previously attempted suicide while taking fluoxetine. They reported that all three patients developed severe akathisia with the reintroduction. In two of the three cases, the suicidal distress was relieved by propranolol. Thus, switching to a less activating antidepressant or using a benzodiazepine such as clonazepam or lorazepam or a β-blocker concurrently with the SSRI may be advisable in cases of treatment-emergent suicidal ideation. Some patients who experience this phenomenon while taking a TCA may not experience it with fluoxetine.

The second author (J.O.C.) was involved in the Teicher et al. (1990) report on obsessive suicidal thoughts associated with fluoxetine and believed he would see in rare cases patients who experience this phenomenon. Fisher et al. (1992), in a prescription-based survey, found that 0.5% of patients who had recently filled a fluoxetine prescription called an 800 number to report a new suicidal drive; no patients who had filled trazodone prescriptions reported such adverse effects. The rare incidence of treatment-emergent suicidal thoughts is not a justification for avoidance of SSRIs. The controversial FDA review of antidepessants and suicidality in children found an increased risk of about 3% with the antidepressants and 1.5% with placebo. This resulted in a black box warning regarding the risks of all antidepressants used in adolescents and children. However, this increased risk must be balanced with the improvement in suicidal ideation that occurs in many more patients while they are taking antidepressants.

Studies subsequent to the black box warning that have examined the risk of suicidal behavior with antidepressant use have generally failed to find an association (Hammad et al. 2006a, 2006b; Kaizar et al. 2006; Simon et al. 2006; Sondergard et al. 2006a, 2006b). Of note was the study by Simon et al. (2006), in which risk of suicide attempts was highest in the month before initiation of therapy. Likewise, an analysis of suicide rates in real-life samples estimated that, compared with treatment without antidepressants, treatment with an antidepressant markedly diminished the risk of completed suicides, regardless of age, gender, or parasuicide history (Cougnard et al. 2008). The recent FDA-initiated study of 100,000 patients in an FDA clinical trial database revealed a 2% risk of emergent suicidal-like behavior in subjects 18–25 years of age versus 1% in subjects receiving placebo. Older patients appeared to not show such increased risk, and elderly subjects showed a significant decrease. However, as with adults, there may be small subsets of patients at greater risk for suicidal behavior (e.g., young adults) while taking antidepressants. These could include patients with latent bipolar disorder, patients who experience agitation while taking an antidepressant, and patients who become energized enough while taking an antidepressant to act on suicidal impulses before their mood has substantially improved.

We continue to recommend that these drugs be used in both children/adolescents and adults, but with appropriate warning and monitoring. In view of the clustering of adverse reports with paroxetine in children, it does seem wise to use another agent before trying paroxetine in children.

Overdose

The popularity of the SSRIs rests in part on their safety in overdose (Barbey and Roose 1998). Thousand of overdoses have occurred in the past 20 years, but very few fatalities have resulted from overdosing on an SSRI alone. In 2003 there were 55,977 reported SSRI overdoses in the United States. There were 106 fatalities in this group, and many of the fatalities were complicated by ingestion of other substances (McKenzie et al. 2007). Fluoxetine, the first SSRI in the United States and the most commonly used, has the most fatalities associated with its overdose. Moderate overdoses (at up to 30 times the common daily dose) tend to be associated with minor symptoms. The most common symptoms of large overdoses include vomiting, nausea, tremor, and sedation. At very high doses (more than 75 times the common daily dose), more serious adverse events, cardiovascular events, seizures, and altered or decreased consciousness have been reported.

The most common causes of death in an SSRI overdose are typically complications of status epilepticus and cardiovascular events such as arrhythmias.

Most fatalities have involved the co-ingestion of other drugs, particularly alcohol or drugs dependent on the cytochrome P450 2D6 system, such as the TCAs (Dalfen and Stewart 2001).

In general, lavage and supportive care in the emergency room are all that is required in the vast majority of SSRI overdoses. In severe overdoses or those involving other drugs, cardiac monitoring or interventions for seizure control may be required.

Drug Interactions

The risk of serious drug interactions is fairly limited with SSRIs. However, several types of drug interactions may occur. The most serious of these is the interaction with the MAOIs. Several fatalities have been reported from serotonin syndrome when SSRIs were used in close proximity to MAOIs, even if the drugs were not used concurrently. In two of these cases, fluoxetine had been stopped but an MAOI had been started promptly thereafter. Therefore, an adequate washout must occur after the SSRIs are discontinued before an MAOI is initiated (see "Discontinuation" subsection). Serotonin syndrome has proved difficult to treat. The most important interventions in treating this syndrome are stopping the offending agents and initiating medical support, including lowering of body temperature, if needed. Beyond that, cyproheptadine at a dosage of 16 mg/day may be helpful in less severe cases in which myoclonic jerking is present. Dantrolene may also be helpful (see Chapter 10: "Emergency Department Treatment").

Another type of potential drug interaction occurs as a result of the tendency of the SSRIs to competitively inhibit enzymes of the cytochrome P450 system (Table 3–1). The inhibition of the 2D6 enzyme by the SSRIs is perhaps the best understood. Many drugs are metabolized by this enzyme, including the TCAs, type 1C antiarrhythmic agents, some β-blockers, benztropine, and many antipsychotic medications. Most of the SSRIs are capable of inhibiting the 2D6 enzyme, leading to increased plasma levels of other agents. For example, fluoxetine may be associated with up to an eightfold increase in TCA plasma levels when the two drugs are used concurrently. On a molar basis, fluoxetine, paroxetine, and sertraline are fairly equal in their proclivity to competitively inhibit the 2D6 enzyme, whereas citalopram (and escitalopram) and fluvoxamine do not significantly inhibit this enzyme. Sheldon Preskorn at the University of Kansas reported that 20 mg of fluoxetine raises desipramine levels several times higher than does 50 mg of sertraline. However, other studies indicate that higher dosages of sertraline (e.g., 150 mg/day) can produce significant increases in desipramine levels. Fluvoxamine is about 10 times less potent a competitive inhibitor of the 2D6 enzyme than the other SSRIs, yet it was associated with a twofold increase in amitriptyline levels in two patients and a sevenfold increase in clomipramine levels in a third patient (Bertschy et al. 1991). Fluvoxamine has also been associated anecdotally with significantly increasing clozapine levels, probably through its inhibition of the cytochrome P450 1A2 enzyme. Thus, caution should be exercised when combining any of the SSRIs with drugs predominantly dependent on the 2D6 enzyme, because the risk of toxicity from the concurrent drug will be enhanced. For example, it is prudent to monitor TCA serum levels and electrocardiograms (ECGs) when any of the TCAs are used in combination with an SSRI. However, in a geriatric study, Murphy et al. (2003) failed to find a relationship between specific cytochrome P450 2D6 alleles and the risk of dropping out due to adverse events, even though patients were taking a variety of medical drugs that were known substrates for the 2D6 enzyme.

Although the 2D6 enzyme is the best characterized of the cytochrome P450 enzymes, there are at least five others, and the SSRIs may be associated with the competitive inhibition of some of them as noted above. Fluvoxamine is known to inhibit the 1A2 enzyme, which is responsible for the metabolism of theophylline, caffeine, certain benzodiazepines, and haloperidol. It would therefore be prudent to use lower doses of theophylline when treating asthmatic patients with fluvoxamine. In addition, fluoxetine and fluvoxamine are capable of inhibiting the 3A3/4 enzyme, which degrades such common drugs as triazolo compounds, including alprazolam, triazolam, and trazodone. Increased drowsiness has been reported in patients treated concurrently with SSRIs and alprazolam, but no serious reactions have been reported. However, lower doses of the concomitant drugs may be required. At one point, H_2 blockers were thought to be particularly problematic vis-à-vis untoward interactions, but this has not been borne out.

Among the SSRIs, citalopram and escitalopram currently exhibit the least potential for pharmacokinetic interactions. Citalopram and escitalopram are weak inhibitors of not only cytochrome P450 2D6 but also 3A3/4, 1A2, and 2C19. With venlafaxine, citalopram shares a low risk of drug interactions, which has made it popular in the treatment of geriatric patients.

Dosage and Administration

Among the factors that have contributed to the enormous popularity of the SSRIs is that the starting dose of the drug is frequently the optimal dose as well (Table 3–4). Given the already lengthy latency of onset of antidepressant action, the SSRIs typically do not require a prolonged titration period in which to achieve a therapeutic dose, as is common with the TCAs and the MAOIs.

Fluoxetine is usually initiated at 20 mg/day, and the maximum recommended dosage is 60 mg/day. A review of the efficacy data from double-blind studies of the use of fluoxetine in the treatment of major depression revealed that fluoxetine produced maximal benefits at 20–40 mg/day, with lesser benefit noted at 60 mg/day. In fact, 60 mg/day appeared to be less effective and to have more side effects than did 20–40 mg/day. Because 20 mg was often effective and the drug has a long half-life, the manufacturer finalized the recommended initial dosing at 20 mg/day for 3 weeks, with subsequent increases to 40–80 mg/day if indicated. Patients with significant psychomotor retardation often seem to require at least 40 mg/day. In other patients, 10 mg/day may be effective. The drug is currently available in 10-mg, 20-mg, and 40-mg capsules, as well as in 10- and 20-mg tablets and in a suspension. Dosages as low as

Table 3–4. Selective serotonin reuptake inhibitors (SSRIs) and other available antidepressants: names, formulations and strengths, and dosages

Generic name	Brand name	Formulations[a] and strengths	Usual therapeutic dosage (mg/day)[b]
SSRIs			
citalopram	Celexa	Tablets: 10, 20, 40 mg Oral solution: 10 mg/5 mL (240-mL bottle)	20–40
escitalopram	Lexapro	Tablets: 5, 10, 20 mg Oral solution: 5 mg/5 mL (240-mL bottle)	
fluoxetine	Prozac	Capsules: 10, 20, 40 mg Capsule (weekly): 90 mg Oral solution: 20 mg/5 mL (120-mL bottle) Tablets: 10, 20 mg	20–60
fluvoxamine	Luvox Luvox CR	Tablets: 25, 50, 100 mg Tablets: 100, 150 mg	100–200
paroxetine	Paxil Paxil-CR (controlled-release)	Tablets: 10, 20, 30, 40 mg Oral suspension: 10 mg/5 mL (250-mL bottle) Tablets: 12.5, 25, 37.5 mg	20–50
sertraline	Zoloft	Tablets: 25, 50, 100 mg Oral concentrate: 20 mg/mL (60-mL bottle)	50–200
5-HT$_2$ antagonists			
nefazodone	Generic only	Tablets: 50, 100, 150, 200, 250 mg	300–500
trazodone	Desyrel and generic	Tablets: 50, 100, 150,[c] 300[c] mg	150–300

Table 3–4. Selective serotonin reuptake inhibitors (SSRIs) and other available antidepressants: names, formulations and strengths, and dosages *(continued)*

Generic name	Brand name	Formulations[a] and strengths	Usual therapeutic dosage (mg/day)[b]
Other			
bupropion	Wellbutrin and generic	Tablets: 75, 100 mg	200–450
	Wellbutrin SR (sustained-release)	Tablets: 100, 150, 200 mg	
	Wellbutrin XL (extended-release)	Tablets: 150, 300 mg	
mirtazapine	Remeron	Tablets: 7.5, 15, 30, 45 mg	15–45
		Soltabs: 15, 30, 45 mg	
venlafaxine	Effexor	Tablets: 25, 37.5, 50, 75, 100 mg	75–375
	Effexor-XR (sustained-release)	Capsules: 37.5, 75, 150 mg	
desvenlafaxine	Pristiq	Tablets (extended release): 50, 100 mg	50–100
duloxetine	Cymbalta	Capsules: 20, 30, 60 mg	60–120

Note.   5-HT$_2$ = serotonin$_2$ receptor.
[a]Not available in an injectable form.
[b]Dosage ranges are approximate. Many patients will respond at relatively low dosages (even dosages below those in ranges given above); others may require higher dosages.
[c]Trazodone also available in 150- and 300-mg divided-dose formulations.

2 mg/day can be obtained with the suspension, and this is particularly useful in patients who cannot initially tolerate higher dosages. Patients who have failed to respond to a lower dosage (20 mg) may subsequently improve if the dosage is increased to 40–60 mg/day (Fava et al. 1994).

A number of years ago a 90-mg, once-weekly form of fluoxetine was introduced. This form was designed to be an alternative to daily treatment with fluoxetine at 20 mg/day and is meant for use in the maintenance phase of treatment only. There are patients who prefer taking one capsule weekly rather than daily. Taking one capsule every 3 days appears roughly equivalent to 40 mg/day. Some patients take two capsules per week on the same day to achieve the equivalent of 40 mg/day. (It is unclear, though, whether taking two 90-mg capsules equals 40 mg/day.) However, staggering the dose every 3 days decreases side effects. Dosing the weekly form of fluoxetine every 3 days appears to be well tolerated.

Dosing of paroxetine is much like that of fluoxetine, with an initial dosage of 20 mg/day. The immediate-release form of the drug is currently available in 10-mg, 20-mg, 30-mg, and 40-mg tablets. The tablets are scored, and patients intolerant of a full tablet can have the dose reduced to a half-tablet for 2–3 weeks. If no response is seen, the dosage may then be increased each week by 10–20 mg/day until a maximum dosage of 50 mg/day is achieved. Data suggest that patients with more serious depressions require higher dosages (30–50 mg/day). Controlled-release (CR) paroxetine is currently available in 12.5-mg, 25-mg, and 37.5-mg tablets, which are equivalent to the 10-mg, 20-mg, and 30-mg immediate-release tablets, respectively. (At one point since the last edition, the CR formulation was taken off the market because of quality control issues during the manufacturing.)

Citalopram is dosed at 20–60 mg/day. The new version of citalopram, escitalopram (Lexapro), is more potent and is generally dosed at 10–20 mg/day. The side effects of escitalopram at 20 mg/day roughly equal those seen with citalopram at 40 mg/day.

The dosage range for sertraline is somewhat wider than that for fluoxetine, paroxetine, and citalopram. In addition, a more linear dose-response curve separates sertraline from the other SSRIs, which have a relatively flat dose-response curve. Therapy is usually initiated at 50 mg/day, although, as with the other SSRIs, a lower starting dosage is sometimes required. The 50-mg dose may be continued for 2 weeks, and if no response is seen, the dosage may then be increased weekly by 50 mg/day until a maximum dosage of 200 mg/day is achieved. Sertraline is available in 25-mg, 50-mg, and 100-mg tablets as well as a concentrate. The different tablet strengths are priced similarly. Thus, it is typically more economical to prescribe the scored 100-mg tablets and instruct patients to break them in half to achieve a dosage of 50 mg/day.

Fluvoxamine has a wider dosage range. It is usually initiated at 50–100 mg/day. Because of fluvoxamine's short half-life, dosages higher than 100 mg/day require divided doses in order to optimize drug availability. In premarketing studies, most patients with major depression required dosages in the range of 100 to 200 mg/day. However, some patients required a dosage as high as 300 mg/day. The recommended starting dosage for fluvoxamine CR is 100 mg/day taken at bedtime. As with the immediate-release form, the maximum dosage for fluvoxamine CR is 300 mg/day, but this formulation can be taken once a day.

Discontinuation

Discontinuation symptoms may be less common with the SSRIs than with the TCAs. However, a number of case reports and double-blind studies do indicate that a discontinuation syndrome may occur with the sudden discontinuation of some SSRIs, especially the shorter-acting agents paroxetine, sertraline, and fluvoxamine.

The most common presentation of an SSRI discontinuation syndrome is a flulike condition with malaise, nausea, and headaches occurring within 2–7 days of stopping an SSRI. Paresthesias, dizziness, agitation, and rebound depression have also been reported when the drugs are suddenly discontinued. The mechanism underlying these symptoms is unclear. Because of paroxetine's greater effect at the serotonin transporter, shorter half-life, and anticholinergic properties, discontinuation symptoms may be more common with this agent than with the other SSRIs. Fluoxetine's very long half-life and citalopram's medium half-life may diminish the risk of discontinuation symptoms with these drugs. Of the SSRIs, fluoxetine may be stopped abruptly without much risk of difficulty. However, for the shorter-acting SSRIs, it may be prudent to taper the drugs over several weeks, particularly if the patient required a prolonged titration upward as a result of adverse effects. Tapering by 25% of the dose per week for doses greater than 30 mg of paroxetine, 100 mg of sertraline, and 150 mg of fluvoxamine is quite reasonable if it is practical to do so. In trials of 4 weeks or less, faster taper schedules can be tried, and most patients will not require a taper.

If discontinuation symptoms occur, the first step may be to increase the dose to the previous dose and taper more gradually. Often, resuming the previous dose will resolve the discontinuation symptoms within 48 hours. Occasionally, clinicians have substituted a longer-acting agent such as fluoxetine for a shorter-acting agent such as paroxetine in patients with substantial discontinuation symptoms. However, there are no good data on the safety or efficacy of this approach.

In starting an MAOI after discontinuing an SSRI, a safe washout period depends on the half-life of the drug and its metabolites. For fluoxetine, the manufacturer has recommended waiting 5 weeks when changing from fluoxetine to an MAOI. This period is five times the half-life of the active metabolite of fluoxetine, norfluoxetine. It is conceivable that a shorter period (e.g., 3 weeks) may suffice, but no data are available. The other SSRIs are shorter acting than fluoxetine, and a 2-week washout appears adequate. When going from an MAOI to an SSRI, a period of 2 weeks of no MAOI is recommended before starting the SSRI.

A common question in clinical practice is, Does it make sense to switch from one SSRI to another if one is not working? Although the practice of switching from one SSRI to another is common, very few prospective, controlled data are available to support the practice. Clearly, however, patients who are intolerant of one SSRI may achieve benefit by being switched to another. Brown and Harrison (1995) reported that patients may respond to sertraline after not responding to fluoxetine. The largest study to date to examine the question of switching to another SSRI after failing the first is STAR*D (Rush et al. 2006). In that study, 727 patients who failed to achieve remission while taking citalopram were switched to either sertraline, venlafaxine, or bupropion. The remission and response rates when patients were switched to sertraline were about the same as those for when patients were switched to venlafaxine or bupropion. While this open study design may contribute to one-comparison agents tending to consistently look similar in outcome, the study does support that switching within the class of SSRIs may be as good as switching outside the class. Thase and colleagues (1997) found that patients who had a poor response to an initial trial of sertraline often achieved a good response when switched to fluoxetine. As many as 50% of patients who do not respond to one

SSRI may respond to another. However, melancholic inpatients who do not respond to an adequate trial of an SSRI appear to have a much lower chance of responding to another SSRI. Along the same lines, Sacchetti et al. (1994) found that patients with recurrent major depression were far more likely to respond to the same SSRI they had responded to in a previous episode than they were to respond to a different SSRI. For example, if a patient had responded to fluoxetine in the index depressive episode, he or she had about a 90% chance of responding to fluoxetine in a subsequent episode but only a 50% chance of responding to fluvoxamine. It is unclear from the report whether patients were blinded to the challenge. It is evident that many patients in clinical practice who start off taking one SSRI will end up taking another agent. In a retrospective review, at least 25% of patients treated with one SSRI subsequently ended up taking another SSRI (Nurnberg et al. 1999c). The authors concluded that the SSRIs were not interchangeable, since patients who discontinue one SSRI because of either lack of efficacy or lack of tolerability may do well with another agent. Likewise, in another study, 91% of patients who were intolerant to fluoxetine tolerated sertraline (Brown and Harrison 1995).

Serotonin-Norepinephrine Reuptake Inhibitors (Venlafaxine, Desvenlafaxine, Duloxetine, and Milnacipran)

Venlafaxine (Effexor) (Figure 3–2) is a phenylethylamine that was released to the U.S. market in 1994. In 1998, it became available in an extended-release form (Effexor XR), which is taken once a day. Along with its FDA indication for the treatment of depression, Effexor XR became the first antidepressant approved for the treatment of GAD and has also been approved for the treatment of social anxiety disorder.

In the past several years, venlafaxine has been growing in popularity as a drug with an efficacy and mechanism of action that may be similar to those of TCA drugs without the safety or side-effect liability of the TCAs. Its major metabolite, desmethylvenlafaxine, became available in 2008 for the treatment of major depression. Desvenlafaxine is a more potent reuptake inhibitor of norepinephrine than venlafaxine but is less potent an inhibitor than duloxetine.

Figure 3–2. Chemical structures of the serotonin-norepinephrine reuptake inhibitors (venlafaxine, desvenlafaxine, duloxetine, and milnacipran).

Duloxetine (Cymbalta) was released in 2004 after a long delay. Like ven-lafaxine and desvenlafaxine, it has little affinity for other neurotransmitter receptors such as muscarinic or histaminic. However, it is a relatively more po-tent norepinephrine reuptake inhibitor (NRI) than is venlafaxine. Whether this increased potency translates into improved efficacy is unclear. Initially, we see duloxetine as an antidepressant that will be a first-line agent in depressed patients who have comorbidities such as pain or stress incontinence. Duloxet-ine also makes sense as a first-line agent for patients with serious depressions, including those with melancholic and psychotic subtypes. We suspect it will have an important role to play in treating resistant depression. Over time, the SNRIs have become first-line agents for less severe depression as well.

A fourth SNRI, milnacipran (Savella), was approved in 2009 in the United States for the treatment of fibromyalgia. Many randomized trials have been completed, mostly overseas, in the treatment of major depression, with mixed results.

Pharmacological Effects

In contrast to the SSRIs, the potent 5-HT-blocking effects of venlafaxine are complemented by mild norepinephrine transporter (NET) inhibition. Typi-cally, dosages of venlafaxine above 150 mg/day are needed to see a clinically significant effect on norepinephrine. In contrast, duloxetine is a potent 5-HT and norepinephrine reuptake inhibitor, while desvenlafaxine is a stronger in-hibitor of NET than is venlafaxine but a less potent inhibitor of NET than is duloxetine.

Several other pharmacological properties distinguish the SNRIs. For ex-ample, the SNRIs promote a rapid downregulation of β-adrenergic receptor–coupled cAMP (cyclic adenosine monophosphate). This effect may correlate with an earlier onset of action for the SNRIs, as some premarketing studies have suggested. In addition, venlafaxine and desvenlafaxine are more weakly bound to protein (27%) than are other antidepressants; this weaker binding may decrease the likelihood of displacing tightly bound drugs, such as war-farin and phenytoin. Also, both venlafaxine and desvenlafaxine share with cit-alopram and escitalopram a very low potential for pharmacokinetic drug interactions because they are not potent inhibitors of any cytochrome P450 hepatic enzymes. However, whereas venlafaxine is a substrate for CYP2D6, desvenlafaxine is not. Therefore, desvenlafaxine's metabolism is not affected by drugs that are inhibitors (e.g., fluoxetine) or inducers (carbamazepine) of CYP2D6. In fact, desvenlafaxine does not undergo much hepatic metabolism at all. Relative to other antidepressants, hepatic metabolism of desvenlafaxine is among the most limited. Likewise, milnacipran undergoes very little hepatic metabolism. Milnacipran is mostly excreted unchanged in the urine.

Indications

The SNRIs have proved useful in the treatment of both outpatients with major depression and inpatients with melancholia. Given the ongoing debate about the utility of the SSRIs for more seriously depressed inpatients, the SNRIs appear to provide a safe and effective alternative to the TCAs in treating melancholic patients. In one study, venlafaxine appeared to be markedly more effective than fluoxetine in the treatment of melancholic inpatients (Clerc et al. 1994). Similar studies have suggested that duloxetine may be more effective than SSRIs in achieving remission, but other studies have not demonstrated this finding (Khan et al. 2007).

Like venlafaxine, duloxetine appears to be an effective antidepressant. Several but not all double-blind studies have now demonstrated the utility of duloxetine, particularly at achieving remission of depressive symptoms relative to placebo. In a 9-week trial, duloxetine 60 mg administered once daily was compared with placebo in treating patients with major depression. By the end of 9 weeks, 44% of 123 duloxetine-treated patients had achieved remission, compared with only 16% of the 122 patients receiving placebo (Detke et al. 2002). In a second trial, 173 patients were randomized to treatment with duloxetine up to 120 mg/day, fluoxetine 20 mg/day, or placebo for 8 weeks. Duloxetine appeared to be more likely to achieve response and remission than either fluoxetine or placebo (Goldstein et al. 2002).

Desvenlafaxine is only indicated in the treatment of major depression. Its efficacy in the treatment of major depression appears comparable to other SNRIs. Dosages of 50 mg/day to 400 mg/day have been studied and found to be effective in the treatment of major depressive disorder (MDD). However, the higher dosages were not more effective than lower dosages but were associated with more adverse events. Thus, 50 mg/day is the standard dosage of desvenlafaxine (Lohoff and Rickels 2008).

A second FDA indication for Effexor XR and duloxetine is for the treatment of GAD. All five controlled trials of Effexor XR in the treatment of GAD reported to date have shown superiority to placebo and sometimes to comparison drugs such as buspirone (Davidson et al. 1999; Diaz-Martinez et al. 1998). Some studies indicated that relatively low dosages of Effexor XR (75–150 mg/day) are useful in the treatment of GAD, and most patients obtain some benefit within 2 weeks, with additional improvement often seen over the next 6 weeks of treatment. Studies out to 6 months have reported significantly greater efficacy for Effexor XR over placebo, with many patients continuing to improve beyond their acute responses (Gelenberg et al. 2000). Venlafaxine is approved for the treatment of social anxiety (Altamura et al. 1999; Lenderking et al. 1999). Likewise, venlafaxine has some demonstrated efficacy in the treatment of PTSD, including PTSD that has failed to respond to an SSRI (Hamner and Frueh 1998).

Venlafaxine was also approved for the treatment of social anxiety disorder in 2003. As with the SSRIs, the effects of venlafaxine on social anxiety may be at least as large as its effects in depression and GAD.

Duloxetine's efficacy in the treatment of GAD looks similar to that of venlafaxine. Three pivotal trials in GAD involving about 800 patients indicated that duloxetine-treated GAD patients were significantly more likely to show an improvement, response, and remission on the Hamilton Anxiety Scale than were patients receiving placebo. Duloxetine was effective at dosages of 60–120 mg/day, but higher dosages were not necessarily more effective than lower dosages (Rynn et al. 2008).

Since the mechanism of action of the SNRIs is similar to that of the TCAs, the SNRIs also have utility in treating some pain conditions. Venlafaxine has been studied in the treatment of neuropathic pain, fibromyalgia, and other chronic pain conditions (Davis and Smith 1999; Kiayias et al. 2000; Pernia et al. 2000). Venlafaxine appears to be about as useful as the TCAs and superior to the SSRIs for chronic pain. Dosages over 150 mg/day are often required. Duloxetine also appears to be useful in the treatment of some somatic and pain symptoms. In a study by Detke and colleagues (2002), duloxetine-treated patients had not only an improvement in their depression but a significant reduction in shoulder pain, back pain, and pain that interfered with daily activities. It is likely that, as with the TCAs, the improvement in pain was independent of the improvement in depression. Indeed, studies of duloxetine in the treatment of diabetic neuropathy have shown clear benefit, and duloxetine was approved for the treatment of neuropathy shortly after it was approved for the treatment of depression.

In 2008, duloxetine was also the second drug (after pregabalin) approved for the treatment of fibromyalgia. Two pivotal trials involving about 900 patients demonstrated that duloxetine at dosages of 60 mg/day or 120 mg/day reduced overall pain on the brief pain inventory at 3 months in both studies. In one of the studies, sustained benefit in pain was also seen with 6 months of duloxetine treatment of fibromyalgia (Russell et al. 2008). Lilly, the manufacturer of duloxetine, is expected to seek approval for the drug in an expanded indication for chronic pain in 2009 based on two trials of duloxetine in the treatment of knee pain associated with osteoarthritis and one study in the treatment of chronic back pain. Milnacipran has been used for chronic pain conditions in Europe for some years and received a fibromyalgia indication in the United States in January 2009. Controlled trials with milnacipran show a fairly consistent benefit on the pain component of fibromyalgia but also associated features such as sleep and cognition. The manufacturer of desvenlafaxine is also expected to seek indications for various pain conditions. Early studies have suggested a role of desvenlafaxine in the treatment of neuropathic pain. Not surprisingly, venlafaxine has also shown benefit in pain conditions, including neuropathic pain associated with diabetes in controlled trials. However, because of patent life issues, Wyeth is not seeking a pain indication for venlafaxine, and desvenlafaxine trials have reportedly failed in pain disorders.

The SNRIs have been studied for use in other disorders. For example, a number of studies suggest that venlafaxine may be effective in both childhood and adult attention-deficit/hyperactivity disorder (ADHD) at dosages of 150–300 mg/day. Like other antidepressants that appear useful in ADHD, including desipramine and bupropion, venlafaxine lacks disadvantages of drugs such as methylphenidate that have some potential for abuse and require Drug Enforcement Administration triplicate forms.

Another condition duloxetine may be valuable in treating is stress urinary incontinence. In fact, duloxetine is approved outside the United States for treating stress urinary incontinence. In a large trial involving 533 women, duloxetine at dosages of 20–80 mg/day was superior to placebo in reducing the frequency of incontinence episodes. Patients treated with duloxetine had up to a 64% decrease in incontinence episodes, while patients receiving placebo had

a 41% decrease in such episodes (Norton et al. 2002). The differences from placebo were even greater in patients who had a high baseline frequency of incontinence episodes.

Desvenlafaxine appears to be effective in the treatment of vasomotor symptoms associated with menopause. At dosages of 100 mg/day and 150 mg/day,
desvenlafaxine reduced the number and intensity of hot flashes associated
with menopause in 454 women (Archer et al. 2009), although here, too, there
are failed trials. Earlier work with venlafaxine also suggested benefit in the
treatment of vasomotor symptoms.

Side Effects

The SNRIs share many of the side effects of the SSRIs. For example, GI side effects are common with the SNRIs. In fact, the SNRIs may have a somewhat
greater propensity for causing nausea than do some of the SSRIs. As with the
SSRIs, adaptation to this side effect occurs rapidly, in the first 2–3 weeks of
therapy. Some studies suggest that the rate of sexual side effects seen with duloxetine may be lower than the rate seen with SSRIs. However, these have tended not to apply to specific rating instruments. Any potent serotonin reuptake
inhibitor can cause sexual side effects, and all three SNRIs are potently serotonergic. Nonetheless, it is possible the noradrenergic effects of duloxetine may
mitigate the serotonergic sexual side effects. Venlafaxine and desvenlafaxine,
which are less noradrenergic, may have a greater tendency for sexual side effects,
but no comparison studies have yet been done to examine this issue.

One side effect of the SNRIs that differs from those of the SSRIs is treatment-emergent hypertension. This noradrenergically mediated side effect occurs in about 5% of patients at dosages of venlafaxine (immediate release) less
than 200 mg/day and in 13% of patients at dosages greater than 300 mg/day in
venlafaxine-treated patients. The increase in blood pressure is usually modest,
with an an average increase in diastolic blood pressure of about 5–7 mm Hg
with venlafaxine at high doses and about 2 mm Hg with duloxetine. Desvenlafaxine also shows a dose-related increase in blood pressure, with 0.5% of patients showing a sustained increase in diastolic blood pressure of >90 mm Hg
and 10 points above baseline, compared with about 2.3% of patients treated at
400 mg/day showing this elevation. Duloxetine may also increase blood pressure, but perhaps less so than the other SNRIs. One possible explanation for the
lower rates of hypertension in use of duloxetine may be its greater protein

binding relative to desvenlafaxine and venlafaxine. Nonetheless, it is important to monitor blood pressure, particularly in the first 2 months of treatment at higher doses of the SNRIs. We have seen some patients with a rise in diastolic blood pressure of 20–30 mm Hg while taking an SNRI. If hypertension occurs, reducing the dose is often helpful. If it is not feasible to do so, clinicians should consider adding a β-blocker or an α-blocker. The impression is that hypertension has been less problematic with the extended-release formulation, perhaps reflecting lower total daily doses or lack of peak effects.

A related noradrenergic side effect of SNRIs is an increase in heart rate. The average increase with the SNRIs is around 1-4 bpm (beats per minute), but higher doses are clearly associated with greater increases than lower doses. Some patients, particularly elderly patients with a history of tachyarrhythmias, should be monitored more carefully. An SSRI might be a better choice in these patients.

Hepatotoxicity has been reported with duloxetine in patients with preexisting liver disease, and duloxetine has a hepatic warning in the package insert. Inclusion of the warning was based on a finding of 77 cases of treatment-emergent hepatic events in more than 8,000 treated patients versus 34 cases of treatment-emergent hepatoxicity in more than 6,000 patients with placebo control. The overall rate of hepatic events, such as an increase in liver enzymes to three times above the upper limits of normal, is about 0.008%, a rate similar to that seen in SSRIs and many other drugs. It makes clinical sense to monitor liver function in any patient with preexisting liver disease treated with a drug that undergoes extensive hepatic metabolism. It appears that milnacipran also has some association with elevations in liver function test values, particularly in patients with preexisting liver disease. Thus, it carries the same warning as does duloxetine.

The more potent noradrenergic effects of duloxetine, milnacipran, and, to a lesser extent, desvenlafaxine also result in a variety of anticholinergic-like side effects, including dry mouth, constipation, and urinary retention. Elderly males might be particularly susceptible to retaining urine and should be monitored.

Overdose

Fatal overdoses with venlafaxine, as with the SSRIs, are exceedingly rare but are occasionally reported. As with the SSRIs, moderate overdoses of less than

30 times the daily dose tend to be more associated with GI upset than with other symptoms. Gastric lavage is often helpful in these cases of moderate overdose. More substantial overdoses involving 10 g or more have sometimes resulted in seizures (Bhattacharjee et al. 2001; Gittelman and Kirby 1993; Mainie et al. 2001) and a serotonin syndrome (Spiller et al. 1994). In the United Kingdom, there has been considerable concern about the safety margin of venlafaxine in overdoses (Buckley and McManus 2002). Recently, a warning about risk for lethality in overdose was added to venlafaxine's package insert; the mechanism is unclear. To date, there have been no reported fatal overdoses of duloxetine. Doses up to 1,200 mg have been treated with lavage and supportive care. Likewise, desvenlafaxine has not been associated with fatalities in overdoses to 5,200 mg in the clinical trials. However, in postmarketing surveillance, desvenlafaxine overdoses in combination with other drugs have been sometimes associated with arrhythmias, serotonin syndrome, rhabdomyolysis, and other life-threatening events. Since these were not single-drug overdoses, it is unclear how much desvenlafaxine contributed to the toxicity. Given the additional concern about venlafaxine overdoses relative to SSRIs, it may be prudent also to be more careful about the use of desvenlafaxine in suicidal patients.

Drug Interactions

The SNRIs can precipitate a serotonin syndrome when combined with the MAOIs, and this combination is therefore contraindicated. Similarly, 2 weeks should elapse after stopping an MAOI before starting an SNRI. Because venlafaxine has a short half-life (5 hours for venlafaxine and 11 hours for O-desmethylvenlafaxine), a 1-week washout is sufficient before starting an MAOI.

Venlafaxine and duloxetine are weak inhibitors of cytochrome 2D6. Like citalopram and escitalopram, the SNRIs do not appear to be potent inhibitors of other hepatic enzymes. However, both duloxetine and venlafaxine are metabolized by the 2D6 enzyme and, to some extent, the 1A2 enzyme as well. Therefore, cimetidine, paroxetine, or other drugs that inhibit the metabolism of 2D6 could result in a more pronounced increase in blood pressure or other side effects. Venlafaxine can increase haloperidol blood levels, but this is not mediated by an effect on the 1A2 or 2D6 enzymes. Rather, it may be an effect on excretion.

Desvenlafaxine is neither a substrate nor an inhibitor of CYP2D6. Thus, it is less likely to be a problem than other SNRIs in either an individual who is a genetically slow or rapid metabolizer of CYP2D6 or someone who is also taking a CYP2D6 inhibitor or inducer.

Like desvenlafaxine, milnacipran undergoes minimal CYP450 metabolism, and the majority of the drug is excreted unchanged. It is even less tightly bound to protein (13%) than either desvenlafaxine or venlafaxine. The risk of pharmacokinetic drug interactions appears small with milnacipran.

Dosage and Administration

The manufacturer recommends that the extended-release formulation of venlafaxine (Effexor XR) be initiated at 37.5 mg. Thereafter, doses can be increased by 37.5 mg every 3 days or 75 mg per week until a dosage of 150 mg/day is reached. Beyond that, increases should be at a rate of 75 mg per week. Although the manufacturer suggests that elderly patients do not require a lower starting dosage, many geriatric psychiatrists have found that a starting dosage of 37.5 mg/day is better tolerated. Increase of dosage should be gradual. For the extended-release formulation of venlafaxine, the maximum recommended dosage is 225 mg/day; for the immediate-release form, it is 375 mg/day. We recommend using the extended-release formulation. Most depressed outpatients appear to respond to dosages in the range of 75 to 225 mg/day. Therefore, if no response is seen at the starting dosage for 2 weeks, the dosage may be titrated upward in 37.5-mg increments every 3 days or so, as tolerated. In premarketing studies, the dosage was sometimes increased rapidly to the maximum dosage in the first week of treatment. This rapid titration was sometimes associated with a more rapid onset of action, but it also was poorly tolerated in many cases. Venlafaxine does have a linear dose-response curve, and higher dosages are associated with greater response (as well as more prominent side effects). Inpatients with melancholic depression and patients with depression that was refractory to other treatments often require dosages closer to the maximum dosage of 375 mg/day (for the immediate-release form) administered in divided doses. On occasion we have used even higher dosages (450–600 mg/day) without problem.

We have tried a variety of doses of duloxetine in clinical trials. In general, starting the duloxetine at 20 mg or 30 mg in the morning with food is a reasonable approach. After 3–7 days, we increase the dosage to 60 mg/day. Some patients have less nausea at 30 mg bid, but most patients can manage 60 mg taken once daily. It is reasonable to keep the dosage at 60 mg/day for 4 weeks before going up to 90 mg/day and then 120 mg/day in divided doses. However, dosages above 60 mg/day are not necessarily more effective than 60 mg/day.

A recent trial compared venlafaxine (immediate release) and duloxetine in the treatment of major depression. Starting dosages were 75 mg/day of venlafaxine and 60 mg/day of duloxetine. Duloxetine was associated with twice as high a rate of dropout due to side effects as venlafaxine. These data suggest that 30 mg of duloxetine is more like 75 mg of venlafaxine from a tolerability standpoint.

The starting dosage of desvenlafaxine is 50 mg/day. The registration trials did not demonstrate that higher doses of desvenlafaxine were more efficacious than lower doses. However, the registration trials were not designed or powered to show a difference between different doses. Thus, in a patient who has not responded to 50 mg of desvenlafaxine for 4 weeks, it is not unreasonable to increase the dose to 100 mg. Dosages up to 400 mg/day have been studied. These higher dosages are clearly associated with greater side effects but not necessarily greater efficacy. Therefore, for most patients, the recommended dosage is 50–100 mg/day.

Most of the studies examining the utility of milnacipran in the treatment of depression have started at 50 mg. Nausea has been a problem at these doses. For fibromyalgia, the starting dosage is 12.5 mg/day, with increases to 25 mg/day by day 3 and 50 mg/day by day 7. The target dosage is 100–200 mg/day for fibromyalgia These dosages have also generally been the the ones used in antidepressant trials as well.

Discontinuation

The relatively short half-life and low protein binding of venlafaxine, desvenlafaxine, and milnacipran may predispose patients to an increased risk of discontinuation symptoms when the drug is stopped suddenly. At least half of patients taking desvenlafaxine (and one-third of patients receiving placebo) experience discontinuation symptoms when the medication is stopped suddenly, even at 50 mg/day. Significant dizziness has been reported with rapid discontinuation of venlafaxine, as have paresthesias and the typical SSRI withdrawal symptoms. Therefore, the manufacturer advises tapering the dose for any patient who has been taking the drug for longer than 7 days.

For patients taking venlafaxine for more than 2 weeks, a gradual taper over at least a 2-week period is advised, and some patients may require a 4-week taper or longer. Decreasing the dosage by 37.5 mg every 3 days or 75 mg per week circumvents withdrawal symptoms in many patients. Since the lowest dose of desvenlafaxine is 50 mg, advising the patient to take the drug every other day for 1 week might be beneficial. Milnacipran may be decreased by 25 mg per week but may require tapering by 12.5-mg increments below 50 mg/day. Switching to sertraline (Luckhaus and Jacob 2001) or supplementing the antiemetic ondansetron (Raby 1998) may also help. In the double-blind studies of duloxetine, rapid discontinuation was associated with expected symptoms. However, duloxetine's longer half-life and higher protein binding may be associated with a lower frequency of discontinuation symptoms compared with venlafaxine. Duloxetine may be safely tapered in most patients by decreasing the total dose by 30 mg per week.

5-HT$_2$ Receptor Antagonists (Trazodone and Nefazodone)

Another class of antidepressants act as 5-HT$_2$ antagonists (Figure 3–3; Table 3–5) and have a number of other direct effects on 5-HT receptors that distinguish these agents from the SSRIs. The class currently includes the phenylpiperazine nefazodone and the triazolopyride trazodone. Trazodone was synthesized in Italy in the mid-1960s and eventually released to the U.S. market in 1981. It represented the first 5-HT-specific agent in the United States. Nefazodone was synthesized in the 1980s by Bristol-Myers Squibb (BMS) with the specific intent of improving the side-effect profile of trazodone. Nefazodone became available in the United States in 1995. In December 2001, the FDA issued a "black box" warning about the risk of hepatoxicity associated with nefazodone. In late 2003, BMS withdrew Serzone from markets in the United States and Canada, but nefazodone is still available generically.

Pharmacological Effects

The pharmacology of the 5-HT$_2$ antagonists is somewhat more complex than the name implies, and questions still remain. The principal effect of both trazo-

Nefazodone

Trazodone

Figure 3–3.   Chemical structures of serotonin$_2$ (5-HT$_2$) antagonists.

done and nefazodone appears to be antagonism of the postsynaptic 5-HT$_{2A}$ and 5-HT$_{2C}$ receptors. Nefazodone is the more potent antagonist. This antagonism causes a paradoxical downregulation of 5-HT$_2$ sites, which may explain the antidepressant effects of such 5-HT$_2$ antagonism. The 5-HT$_2$ receptor is also linked with other receptors, including the 5-HT$_{1A}$ receptor, which is thought to be important in depression, anxiety, and violent behavior. There is growing evidence that both nefazodone and trazodone stimulate the 5-HT$_{1A}$ site, possibly through antagonizing the 5-HT$_2$ receptor. In addition to their effects as 5-HT$_2$ antagonists, both trazodone and nefazodone block the reuptake of 5-HT to some extent. Although the inhibition of the 5-HT transporter with these two drugs is weak in comparison to that of the SSRIs, it may be clinically significant.

Finally, *m*-chlorophenylpiperazine (m-CPP), a major active metabolite of both nefazodone and trazodone, is a potent direct agonist of 5-HT, mostly at the 5-HT$_{2C}$ receptor, which may contribute both to the efficacy of the drugs and to their side effects.

Table 3–5. The serotonin$_2$ (5-HT$_2$) antagonists

Drug	Starting dosage (mg/day)	Maximum dosage (mg/day)
trazodone (Desyrel)	50–100	600
nefazodone (Serzone)	50–100	600

Indications

The primary indication for both trazodone and nefazodone is major depression. There are more than two dozen double-blind, placebo-controlled studies of trazodone and at least eight double-blind studies of nefazodone that establish the efficacy of these drugs in the treatment of major depression. Most of these studies suggest that trazodone and nefazodone are as effective as comparison drugs, primarily the TCAs, in the treatment of major depression. However, many of the controlled studies have involved outpatients with mild to moderate major depression, and there have been persistent questions about the efficacy of trazodone in the treatment of more severely depressed patients. Some investigators have suggested that trazodone is not particularly helpful for retarded depressions. However, a review of efficacy studies (Schatzberg 1987) found that there appeared to be no difference between TCAs and trazodone in the treatment of depressed inpatients and of those with more classic endogenous features. Interestingly, the studies that reported the poorest results with trazodone used aggressive dosing, with dosages that reached a total of 300–450 mg in the first week of treatment. Thus, trazodone may be effective and is better tolerated at lower rather than higher doses, particularly at first. At least one study has also concluded that nefazodone is effective in the treatment of more severely depressed inpatients (Ansseau et al. 1994).

Both trazodone and nefazodone appear to be effective anxiolytic agents. The antianxiety effects of the drugs are often evident earlier than the antidepressant effects. A comparison of low-dose trazodone with chlordiazepoxide for general anxiety suggested that the two agents had equal efficacy (Schwartz and Blendl 1974). Likewise, one study suggested that trazodone compared favorably to imipramine and diazepam in the treatment of GAD (Rickels et al. 1993). In depressed patients, anxiolytic effects of nefazodone were noted at dosages less than 250 mg/day (Fontaine et al. 1994), but trazodone, an antidepressant, has shown significant utility as a hypnotic at doses of 25–100 mg at night. Because trazodone is quite sedating and does not have an addiction potential, it offers a safe alternative to the benzodiazepines. Likewise, trazodone has been used successfully to treat SSRI- and MAOI-induced insomnia.

Next to depression, the best-studied disorder treated with nefazodone is PTSD. Currently, nefazodone is among the more common agents prescribed in treating PTSD because of the sleep disturbance, agitation, and comorbid problems of substance abuse and depression. At least six open-label studies of nefazodone in the treatment of PTSD suggested that the drug can help ameliorate nightmares and hyperarousal and decrease anger (Hidalgo et al. 1999). Dosages ranging from 300 to 600 mg/day appear to be efficacious, and large controlled trials are under way to determine their efficacy.

Nefazodone does not share trazodone's utility as a hypnotic, because the former is generally less sedating. However, preliminary data (Armitage et al. 1994) suggested that nefazodone, unlike many psychotropics, may enhance rapid eye movement (REM) sleep and therefore may increase restful sleep in some patients.

Case reports suggest a number of other potential roles for nefazodone. Nefazodone has been reported to be useful in the treatment of social phobia, panic disorder, and PMDD and as an adjunctive agent in the treatment of negative symptoms of schizophrenia.

Side Effects

Although the 5-HT$_2$ antagonists are 5-HT-specific agents, they differ from the SSRIs in mechanism of action and thus in side-effect profile as well (Table 3–6). One common side effect of all currently available serotonergic antidepressants is GI upset. The incidence of nausea with trazodone and nefazodone is less than that found with the SSRIs. However, it was still the leading cause for discontinuation of nefazodone in prerelease trials. Higher doses of trazodone, particularly when taken on an empty stomach, may also be correlated with nausea. As with the SSRIs, the GI side effects of these drugs are lessened by taking them with food.

As reported, neither trazodone nor nefazodone has particularly strong anticholinergic effects. They can, however, produce dry mouth because of their α_1-adrenergic receptor blockade. (Salivation is controlled by both the acetylcholinergic and the noradrenergic systems.) The α_1-adrenergic blockade may

Table 3–6. Common or troublesome side effects of trazodone and nefazodone

Gastrointestinal
 Nausea
 Dyspepsia
 Liver failure (nefazodone—rare)
Adrenergic blockade
 Orthostasis (trazodone >> nefazodone)
 Dizziness
Neurological
 Headaches
 Visual trails (nefazodone > trazodone)
CNS depression
 Sedation (trazodone >> nefazodone)
CNS activation
 Restlessness (nefazodone > trazodone)
Sexual
 Priapism (trazodone)

Note. >> = much greater than; CNS = central nervous system.

also result in significant orthostasis with trazodone, especially in elderly persons. Dizziness and even frank syncope may occur in patients taking large doses of trazodone on an empty stomach, as well as in some elderly patients taking nefazodone. It is therefore useful to monitor blood pressures for orthostasis with vulnerable patients and to encourage proper hydration. Support stockings may also be helpful. The incidence of orthostasis with nefazodone is thought to be lower than with trazodone. However, orthostasis has been reported with higher doses of nefazodone and in vulnerable patients. Trazodone also differs from nefazodone in the amount of sedation it produces. As described, trazodone is very sedating and is useful as a hypnotic at modest doses. Nefazodone may produce daytime somnolence, but this usually occurs at higher doses. Shifting the bulk of the dose to bedtime will mitigate this problem.

CNS activation is generally reported not to be a problem with either drug. However, patients who are deficient in the cytochrome P450 2D6 enzyme or who are taking SSRIs may experience activation secondary to the effects of the metabolite m-CPP, which is cleared by this enzyme. We have also seen some patients develop dysphoric activation on nefazodone, even without recent exposure to the SSRIs. Therefore, starting nefazodone at lower doses appears prudent.

More than 200 cases of priapism have been reported in males treated with trazodone. Although rare, priapism—with an incidence of 1 per 6,000 patients—is very problematic. Risk of trazodone-associated priapism is thought to be higher in younger males with prolonged erections in the morning upon awakening or who can have frequent erections over a relatively short period (several hours). Some patients may require surgical intervention. The acute treatment involves injection of an α-adrenergic receptor agonist (e.g., epinephrine) into the penis. If not treated promptly, priapism may result in permanent impotence. Male patients should thus be warned to stop the drug immediately if they experience any symptoms suggestive of priapism (occasional erections are not problematic) and to seek emergency room treatment if the erection persists longer than 1 hour. At least one case of clitoral priapism has also been reported (Pescatori et al. 1993).

Since priapism is mediated via adrenergic pathways, nefazodone is thought to present less of a problem than trazodone in this regard. There have been no reports of nefazodone-induced priapism, but there have been isolated reports of prolonged erections in men and reports of increased nocturnal penile tumescence. A case of clitoral engorgement, but not priapism, with nefazodone has also been reported.

Sexual side effects generally appear to be rare with nefazodone. In fact, it is difficult to demonstrate that the rate of sexual dysfunction with nefazodone treatment is any higher than with placebo treatment. Feiger and colleagues (1996) found that sertraline and nefazodone were comparable in antidepressant efficacy. However, sertraline had negative effects on sexual function, whereas nefazodone had none.

Visual side effects may also occur in up to 12% of patients taking nefazodone. These side effects often take the form of an afterimage during tracking of moving objects. Interestingly, the afterimage during tracking may be a serotonin-enhancing effect, because other agonists, such as lysergic acid diethylamide (LSD), also produce this effect. Patients should be told that the visual side effects generally improve with time.

In 1999, there was an isolated report at one center of three patients being treated with nefazodone who sustained liver failure. The patients were all women between the ages of 16 and 57 who were treated with 200–400 mg of nefazodone for a period averaging several months (Aranda-Michel et al. 1999). All patients showed significant hepatocellular damage, and two of the three underwent liver transplants. The third recovered without transplantation. In at least one of the patients, a concomitant medication could have contributed to hepatotoxicity. Since that first report, a number of other cases have emerged that led the FDA to advise BMS that they must include a black box warning in the package insert that alerts the public about the risk of severe liver toxicity. The risk is estimated at about 1/250,000 for every patient-year of treatment with nefazodone. In other words, if a quarter million patients were taking nefazodone for a year, one patient would be expected to develop potentially severe liver damage. While these odds are very small, this is about three to four times the background rate for severe liver damage, and use of nefazodone dropped dramatically with the black box warning. BMS voluntarily removed Serzone from the market, but nefazodone is still available generically. Many antidepressants, including TCAs, have rarely and idiosyncratically been associated with fulminant hepatic failure. There do not appear to be clear demographic variables that predict hepatic toxicity from a given antidepressant. However, in any patient with a history of hepatic difficulties, it is prudent to obtain baseline liver enzymes and monitor these periodically. Nefazodone should not be prescribed in any patient with a history of liver disease. We are frequently asked whether a patient who has done well while taking nefazodone should continue the medication. We have not routinely taken patients who have responded to the drug off the medication. If there is a reasonable alternative to nefazodone, it should be considered. If alternatives have been unsuccessful or poorly tolerated, it may be particularly reasonable to continue the nefazodone while informing the patient of the known risk. Patients should also be educated about symptoms of liver illness, including jaundice, anorexia, GI disturbance, and malaise, and the drug should be discontinued if there are any symptoms suggesting toxicity.

Overdose

Trazodone and nefazodone appear to have a wide safety margin in cases of overdose. Doses as high as 10 g of trazodone have been taken without untoward incidents. The lethal dose in animals averages 500 mg/kg.

Although the risk of fatal overdoses with nefazodone or trazodone is very small, a number of reports suggest that the combination of trazodone and other CNS depressants, such as alcohol, can be lethal when taken in overdose.

The usual cause of death is respiratory depression. Although a trazodone overdose alone can result in a seizure or respiratory arrest, the lethal dose in animals approaches half of body weight, or about 500 mg/kg. Nefazodone has been taken in overdoses of up to 12 g, or 20 times the maximum daily dose, without serious effects.

Drug Interactions

The 5-HT$_2$ antagonists are fairly safe in terms of drug interactions. Trazodone may potentiate the effects of other CNS depressants and lead to excessive sedation. Similarly, the postural hypotension associated with trazodone is exacerbated by concurrent antihypertensive agents, and such combinations should be monitored with frequent checks of orthostatic blood pressure. Because both the 5-HT$_2$ antagonist drugs have proserotonergic effects, there is a theoretical risk of precipitating a serotonin syndrome with the MAOIs, particularly at higher doses. However, neither trazodone nor nefazodone is a potent catecholamine reuptake inhibitor (although nefazodone has some reuptake inhibition); therefore, the risk of hypertensive crises with concurrent use of 5-HT$_2$ antagonists and MAOIs is low.

Nefazodone is a potent inhibitor of the cytochrome P450 enzyme 3A3/4. As stated previously, this enzyme is responsible for the metabolism of such common drugs as the triazolobenzodiazepines alprazolam and triazolam, ketoconazole, erythromycin, and carbamazepine. The combination of nefazodone and anti-arrhythmics, pimozide, or ziprasidone may enhance cardiac toxicity. Concurrent use of nefazodone with these agents may raise serum levels, and clinicians should exercise caution in combining these drugs.

Occasionally, switching from the SSRIs to 5-HT$_2$-antagonist drugs, particularly nefazodone, may be problematic. One of the metabolites of nefazodone is m-CPP, which is metabolized via the cytochrome P450 2D6 enzyme. Increased serum levels of m-CPP have been associated with dysphoric agitation. Thus, simultaneous use of an SSRI and nefazodone, either current or recent (before the washout period has ended), may be poorly tolerated in some patients. Fluoxetine can contribute to elevated levels of m-CPP for 4–5 weeks after it is discontinued, and the other SSRIs may have this effect for 1–2 weeks after they are discontinued. Therefore, it would be useful, ideally, to have a washout period between stopping an SSRI and starting nefazodone. However, an alternative strategy is to allow no washout period but start with smaller dosages of nefazodone (50–100 mg/day) and titrate upward more gradually after discontinuing the SSRI.

Dosage and Administration

The manufacturer recommends starting trazodone at 150 mg/day and then increasing the dosage up to 600 mg/day (Table 3–5). Our experience has been that the drug is quite sedating, and we begin patients at 50 mg/day and increase the dosage to 150 mg/day by day 7. Thereafter, each week, we increase the daily dosage by 50–75 mg, up to 300 mg/day. In our experience, patients respond at a modal dosage of 150–300 mg/day.

Because of trazodone's short half-life, the optimal dosing for the treatment of depression is in two or three divided doses a day. The bulk of the dose may be taken at bedtime to mitigate daytime somnolence.

Some investigators have proposed that trazodone has a therapeutic window; as with nortriptyline, too-high plasma levels are associated with poor responses. Our experience suggests this may be so, and several studies have supported a correlation between plasma levels and efficacy (Monteleone and Gnocchi 1990; Spar 1987). Steady-state trazodone plasma levels above 650 ng/mL may be ideal for antidepressant response. However, more study is needed to determine whether it is worthwhile to obtain trazodone plasma levels routinely.

The manufacturer's recommended starting dosage of nefazodone is 100 mg bid. However, we recommend starting at 50 mg bid or lower and increasing the dose by 50 mg every 4 days to reach 200 mg/day. Thereafter, each week, the daily dosage may be increased by 100 mg until a therapeutic dose is achieved. Minimal therapeutic antidepressant dosage is 300 mg/day, and most patients will require at least 400 mg/day. Thus, it is reasonable to titrate the dosage to 400 mg/day and then maintain this dosage for 3–4 weeks. If a response is not observed, the dosage may then be further increased to a maximum of 600 mg/day. The initial dosage in elderly patients should be 50 mg/day. Some patients may feel too sedated or activated at 100 mg bid, but they are often able to tolerate an initial dosage of 50 mg bid. Therefore, we have recently come to start all patients routinely at 50–100 mg/day. The manufacturer recommends bid dosing, but some practitioners prescribe the drug to be administered nightly, and this appears particularly feasible once patients have been on a steady dosage for a few weeks. A slow-release formulation is being developed that would allow once-a-day dosing. However, at the time of this writing, a once-a-day formulation is not available.

Discontinuation

Discontinuation syndromes appear uncommon for both trazodone and nefazodone but have been reported. Some case reports suggested that the rapid discontinuation of trazodone may occasionally lead to withdrawal symptoms, particularly rebound insomnia (Otani et al. 1994). As with the SSRIs, there have been reports of paresthesias and dizziness associated with the sudden discontinuation of nefazodone (Benazzi 1998; Kotlyar et al. 1999; Lauber 1999). Therefore, it is generally prudent to taper these medications rather than to stop them suddenly. The total daily dose of nefazodone and trazodone can be decreased by 50–100 mg each week.

Combined Noradrenergic-Dopaminergic Antidepressant (Bupropion)

Bupropion (Wellbutrin) is a unicyclic antidepressant (Figure 3–4) that was to be released in 1986, but its release was delayed pending an evaluation of its risk of inducing seizures. It was not released until mid-1989, when it became clear that the increased seizure risk was dose related and tended to occur in specific populations. In 1998, bupropion became available in a sustained-release formulation (Wellbutrin SR) that allows twice-a-day administration and also appears to decrease the risk of seizures to about that associated with SSRIs. In 2003, bupropion became available in an extended-release formulation (Wellbutrin XL) for once-a-day dosing. All formulations are now off patent and available generically.

Pharmacological Effects

Bupropion is not a 5-HT reuptake blocker and does not inhibit monoamine oxidase. Its biochemical mode of action is not completely understood. It was hypothesized to act via dopamine reuptake blockade; however, its dopamine-potentiating effects in animals appear to occur at very high dosages and blood levels, well beyond those routinely used in humans. The dopamine reuptake–blocking properties of bupropion are an order of magnitude less than those of

Bupropion

Figure 3–4. Chemical structure of bupropion.

sertraline. Activation of the nucleus accumbens, a common consequence of enhanced dopaminergic transmission, is easier to demonstrate in animal studies of bupropion than in human functional imaging studies. Nonetheless, the dopaminergic effects may be important, because the plasma levels of homovanillic acid, the primary metabolite of dopamine, decrease in patients who respond to bupropion but not in patients who do not respond (Golden et al. 1988).

In recent years, the noradrenergic effects of bupropion have become increasingly evident. The major active metabolite of bupropion, hydroxybupropion, does appear to block the reuptake of norepinephrine in rats. Earlier studies, involving mice, failed to show an effect on norepinephrine, but this species metabolizes the drug differently. Indirect evidence for an effect on noradrenergic activity also comes from data showing that the drug decreases 24-hour excretion of norepinephrine metabolites.

Indications

Bupropion appears to be effective in many types of depression. It has demonstrated utility in outpatients with mild to moderate depression as well as in inpatients with more severe depression. The drug appears to be safe in depressed cardiac patients. There have been reports that the drug is less likely to produce mania or rapid cycling, but episodes of mania on bupropion do occur. Conversely, bupropion has been reported not to induce rapid cycling in patients with bipolar disorder. Since head-to-head comparisons of bupropion and other antidepressants are lacking in the treatment of bipolar depression, it is difficult to fully assess bupropion's proclivity for inducing mania relative to that of other agents. Still, for the treatment of bipolar depression, bupropion is a reasonable first-line agent in addition to mood stabilizers.

The second FDA indication for bupropion is in smoking cessation. Two controlled clinical trials indicate that the sustained-release formulation of bupropion (which is also marketed under the trade name Zyban) administered at 300 mg/day aids in smoking cessation (Goldstein 1998). More than 3,000 patients were studied in a clinical trial of the sustained-release formulation of bupropion in the treatment of smoking cessation. As with the treatment of depression, the benefits of sustained-release bupropion are not immediate and take several weeks or longer to be evident. After 7 weeks of treatment, more than twice as many patients on bupropion 300 mg/day (36%) were abstinent from nicotine as patients administered placebo (17%). At 26-week follow-up, only 19% of bupropion-treated patients and 11% of placebo-administered patients remained abstinent from smoking. These results mirror those commonly seen in smoking cessation studies with nicotine preparations. In a recent trial, we reported that bupropion was no better than placebo in achieving smoking abstinence in adolescents. However, bupropion appeared to significantly decrease nicotine use (Killen et al. 2004). The drug is being studied for appetite suppression.

The most recent indication for bupropion is in the treatment of seasonal affective disorder (SAD). SAD has historically been treated with phototherapy, antidepressants, and mood stabilizers. However, there had been no FDA-approved therapy for this disorder until the approval of bupropion XL. Studies indicate that by starting treatment of bupropion while patients are well, the drug appeared to prevent relapse and time to onset of new depressive symptoms when compared with placebo (Modell et al. 2005). Since some patients with SAD may have illness that falls in the bipolar spectrum, we have found that a mood stabilizer such as lamotrigine or lithium can also be helpful, although there are few empirical data for the use of a mood stabilizer.

Another fairly common use of bupropion is in the treatment of ADHD. Bupropion appears to be effective in the treatment of ADHD in both adults and children (Cantwell 1998). Since bupropion is metabolized to a number of amphetamine-like products, it appears to be a safe alternative to stimulants in the treatment of ADHD. In adolescents who have comorbid substance abuse problems, bupropion might be the first-line treatment (Riggs et al. 1998).

Two important uses of bupropion are as an adjunct to SSRI treatment to augment the antidepressant effect and as an adjunct to counteract the sexual side effects of SSRIs. Bupropion does appear to augment SSRI antidepressant effects and is generally less complicated to use than is either lithium or thyroid supplements. The STAR*D study found that bupropion added to an SSRI was helpful but that it was no more helpful than a parallel nonrandomized track in which buspirone was added (Trivedi et al. 2006). (Bupropion augmentation is discussed in greater detail in Chapter 9: "Augmentation Strategies for Treatment-Resistant Disorders.")

Bupropion is unique among the antidepressants in that it is probably not effective in the treatment of anxiety disorders. One pilot study of bupropion in the treatment of panic disorder yielded negative findings (Sheehan et al. 1983). To our knowledge, no recent studies have examined the efficacy of bupropion in the treatment of panic disorder. Many anxious patients find bupropion too activating and prefer other agents.

Bupropion's metabolism is probably dependent on a number of hepatic enzymes; therefore, interactions with the SSRIs may be less problematic than once thought. Still, there has been at least one case report of a seizure being associated with the combination of fluoxetine and bupropion.

Side Effects

Bupropion has a favorable side-effect profile, in part because of its low affinity for muscarinic, α-adrenergic, and histaminic receptors. The only side effects of the sustained-release bupropion that occurred reliably more commonly than with placebo in clinical trials of 100–300 mg/day were insomnia, dry mouth, and tremor. The insomnia is best managed by moving the evening dose to earlier in the afternoon. A separation of at least 8 hours between the morning and evening dose is advised.

Bupropion does not induce orthostatic hypotension or stimulate appetite. Some investigators have argued that bupropion could be particularly useful in patients who gain weight while taking other agents. There are reports that patients with sexual dysfunction who are taking other antidepressants do better with bupropion, and, again, the drug has been reported to counteract SSRI-induced sexual dysfunction.

Seizures for the immediate-release formulation of the drug have been reported at the rate of 4 per 1,000 at dosages less than 450 mg/day; this risk increased to 4 per 100 when the dosage was increased above 450 mg/day. The sustained-release formulation, which has largely supplanted the immediate-release formulation, appears to carry a seizure risk of about 1 per 1,000 patients at dosages less than 400 mg/day. This risk is similar to the seizure risk associated with most antidepressants. The risk of seizures appears to be enhanced in patients with a prior history of seizure disorders, head injury, bulimia, and anorexia. Concurrent use of alcohol, stimulants, or cocaine also enhances the risk of seizures in these patients. The manufacturer also cautions that single doses of the drug should never exceed 150 mg for the immediate-release formulation and 200 mg for the sustained-release preparation. The XL formulation may be taken as a single dose of up to 450 mg.

Overdose

Bupropion has proved relatively safe in overdose. However, there have been cases of completed suicide with bupropion alone (Rohrig and Ray 1992). In some cases, patients who overdosed on bupropion had significant neurological complications, including seizures and status epilepticus (Spiller et al. 1994; Storrow 1994). Thus, some caution should be exercised in prescribing large supplies of bupropion for suicidal patients.

Drug Interactions

Serious drug interactions are uncommon with bupropion. Bupropion is metabolized by the cytochrome P450 2B6 enzyme, which is responsible for metabolizing very few drugs (orphenadrine and cyclophosphamide). Thus, potential pharmacokinetic interactions with other antidepressants or general medicines are unlikely.

Any drug that lowers the seizure threshold should be used cautiously with bupropion. Thus, drugs such as clozapine, theophylline, and clomipramine should be used cautiously or avoided with bupropion. Likewise, it may be prudent to avoid the use of bupropion in patients who are dependent on alcohol or benzodiazepines, since sudden discontinuation of these drugs in the context of concurrent bupropion use can increase seizure risk.

The use of an MAOI and bupropion is contraindicated. There appears to be an enhanced risk of general toxicity with phenelzine and bupropion and a greater risk of hypertensive crises.

Dosage and Administration

Bupropion has a relatively wide usual dosage range (i.e., 200–450 mg/day). The modal optimum dosage range in our experience has been 300 to 400 mg/day. Bupropion is available in an immediate-release formulation (75-mg and 100-mg tablets); in a sustained-release preparation (Wellbutrin SR) (100-mg, 150-mg, and 200-mg tablets) given twice daily; and in an extended-release once-daily formulation (150-mg and 300-mg tablets).

Mirtazapine

Mirtazapine (Remeron), which was released in the United States in 1996, is chemically related to mianserin, a drug that has been used for a number of years in Europe. Mirtazapine is FDA approved for the treatment of depression but appears to be useful for a variety of other disorders. Although it did not emerge as among the more popular antidepressants during the late 1990s, mirtazapine has established an important niche in clinical practice. Mirtazapine has been available generically since 2004.

Pharmacological Effects

Mirtazapine has a tetracyclic chemical structure (Figure 3–5) but is unrelated to the TCAs. Its mechanism of action is fairly unusual among the available antidepressants. It appears to be an antagonist of central presynaptic α_2-adrenergic receptors. As an α_2-adrenergic receptor blocker, mirtazapine acts to increase norepinephrine release. The increased noradrenergic tone results in a rapid increase in synaptic 5-HT levels by mobilizing 5-HT release secondary to stimulation of α_1-adrenergic receptors on 5-HT cell bodies. Mirtazapine also blocks 5-HT$_2$ and 5-HT$_3$ receptors. Mirtazapine is not a specific reuptake blocker of any monoamine neurotransmitter. However, it does appear to be a potent antagonist of H$_1$ receptors—a feature that confers some of the drug's more problematic side effects. Mirtazapine does not have particularly strong anticholinergic effects and does not significantly block postsynaptic α-adrenergic receptors. As a result, postural hypotension is generally not associated with mirtazapine use.

Mirtazapine is available in 7.5-mg, 15-mg, 30-mg, and 45-mg tablets. A quick-dissolving wafer formulation (Remeron SolTabs) has been released.

Mirtazapine

Figure 3–5.   Chemical structure of mirtazapine.

Mirtazapine is well absorbed from the GI tract and extensively metabolized to at least four active products. Each of these metabolites, including the most common, desmethylmirtazapine, is less active than the parent drug. Mirtazapine is metabolized by cytochrome P450 2D6, 3A3/4, and 1A2 enzymes but is neither an inducer nor an inhibitor of these hepatic enzymes (Fawcett and Barkin 1998). Thus, it can be taken safely with other psychotropic agents.

Indications

In premarketing trials of mirtazapine, which involved several thousand patients, the drug appeared to be as effective as the TCAs amitriptyline and clomipramine. Both outpatients with milder depression and more severely depressed inpatients respond to mirtazapine. Compared with trazodone, mirtazapine appears to be superior in the treatment of depressed inpatients (van Moffaert et al. 1995). Mirtazapine has also been studied in treating brief recurrent depression, which meets all of the DSM-IV (American Psychiatric Association 1994) criteria for major depression except for the time criterion. Brief depression lasts less than 2 weeks but tends to recur many times in the course of a year. Mirtazapine at low doses appears, on the basis of case reports, to effectively treat these depressive episodes (Stamenkovic et al. 1998). Other subtypes of depression, including atypical depression and seasonal depression, may also be responsive to mirtazapine (Falkai 1999).

More recent studies have directly compared mirtazapine with SSRIs in the treatment of depression (Fava et al. 2001; Leiononen et al. 1999; Quitkin et al. 2001; Wheatley et al. 1998). Mirtazapine was reported to be comparable in efficacy to fluoxetine, paroxetine, and citalopram and in each study was slightly, though not significantly, more effective. Compared with the SSRIs, mirtazapine may have more rapid anxiolytic and antidepressant effects (Thompson 1999). With mirtazapine, in contrast to citalopram and paroxetine, the antidepressant and antianxiety effects are sometimes seen by the second week. A meta-analysis by Thase (2003) found that mirtazapine was significantly more effective than SSRIs. However, another, more recent meta-analysis failed to show an efficacy advantage of mirtazapine over the SSRIs (Papakostas et al. 2008). Thus, the advantages of mirtazapine over SSRIs may be more in side-effect profile (fewer sexual side effects, more sedating at night) than in efficacy.

Since mirtazapine, with its greater propensity for sedation and weight gain, is often used after SSRIs, the STAR*D study evaluated the utility of mirtazapine for achieving remission after the failure of two trials (Fava et al. 2006b). Mirtazapine was as effective (or ineffective) as nortriptyline in achieving remission after two failed antidepressant trials. The remission rate for mirtazapine on the HRSD at this late stage of the study was only 8%.

Additionally, the dropout rate from adverse effects with mirtazapine appears to be usually similar to that with the SSRIs.

We reported on a comparison of paroxetine and mirtazapine in elderly depressive patients (Schatzberg et al. 2002). Mirtazapine was associated with significantly earlier response and fewer dropouts due to adverse events than was paroxetine.

Preliminary data from open-label trials suggest that mirtazapine is useful for most of the anxiety disorders that are responsive to SSRIs or venlafaxine. For example, mirtazapine may be useful in the treatment of panic disorder, with or without concurrent depression (Carpenter et al. 1999b). Patients with depression and comorbid GAD appear to do well when taking mirtazapine at dosages of 15–45 mg/day (Goodnick et al. 1999). Pilot studies of mirtazapine for PTSD also appeared promising (Connor et al. 1999).

Another potential use for mirtazapine is in augmenting antidepressant effects. Because of its low risk of pharmacokinetic interaction, mirtazapine should be relatively easy to combine with many antidepressants. The drug, with its complex pharmacology, may complement antidepressants that act more specifically. Preliminary data have shown that mirtazapine effectively augments SSRIs (Carpenter et al. 1999a). In the STAR*D trial, the combination of mirtazapine (average dosage=36 mg/day) with venlafaxine (average dosage=210 mg/day) resulted in remission-level responses in just 13% of patients who had failed three consecutive antidepressant trials (McGrath et al. 2006). This result was similar to the remission rate found for tranylcypromine in patients who had failed three trials. However, the venlafaxine-mirtazapine combination was better tolerated than the tranylcypromine.

Mirtazapine had been reported to help reverse SSRI-induced sexual side effects (Farah 1999), but a double-blind trial failed to show benefits of mirtazapine in treating sexual side effects (Michelson et al. 2000). In addition, the drug has been reported to help improve negative symptoms in schizophrenia (Berk et al. 2001) and to ameliorate antipsychotic-induced extrapyramidal symptoms.

As reported earlier, mirtazapine has been used as an effective anti-nausea medication in chemotherapy patients (Kim et al. 2008) and postoperative anesthesia medication (Chen et al. 2008). Compared with the more commonly used $5-HT_3$ antagonists such as ondansetron (Zofran), generic mirtazapine is a fraction of the cost and may provide additional benefits, such as sedation and anti-anxiety effects. While anecdotal experience suggests mirtazapine might be as useful an anti-nausea medication as other $5-HT_3$ antagonists, no comparison study has ever been done.

Side Effects

Mirtazapine has generally been well tolerated in clinical studies. The most common side effects are dry mouth, sedation, somnolence, and weight gain. More than half of all patients treated with mirtazapine, compared with less than 20% of patients treated with placebo, experienced somnolence. Somnolence is more evident at lower doses than at higher doses because antihistaminic effects predominate relative to noradrenergic or serotonergic effects at dosages below 15 mg/day. Thus, vis-à-vis sedation, a starting dosage of 30 mg/day is often better and usually not more poorly tolerated than a dosage of 7.5 mg/day. A trial in Europe did compare mirtazapine at dosages of 15 mg/day and 30 mg/day and found no differences in sedation between the two groups.

Weight gain and increased appetite are clear problems for some patients taking mirtazapine. In short-term trials of 6–12 weeks, about 20% of patients treated with mirtazapine reported increased appetite, and 7.5% of patients had an increase in weight of at least 7%. In our clinical experience, at least 20% of patients gain weight with long-term use of mirtazapine. The most reliable strategy for controlling weight when taking mirtazapine is controlling appetite and exercise. The notion that higher doses of mirtazapine may be less problematic for weight gain is less clear than the effects on somnolence. Some clinicians anecdotally report that the use of H_2 antagonists, such as ranitidine 150 mg bid, mitigates the weight gain associated with mirtazapine, but this approach is untested. Likewise, some clinicians use stimulants or sibutramine (Orlistat) to help control weight. However, sibutramine is a serotonergic drug and may increase the risk of serotonergic side effects, while stimulants generally require triplicate form prescriptions and have an established abuse potential. Weight gain in the elderly appears to be less common.

The effects of mirtazapine on cholesterol and triglycerides have become better recognized in recent years. About 15% of patients demonstrate a significant (>20%) increase in cholesterol, and 6% of patients experience a significant increase in triglycerides. It is thus worthwhile to obtain fasting triglyceride and cholesterol levels at baseline and periodically with treatment, especially for patients with known hypercholesterolemia or who have a history of high triglyceride levels. Concurrent use of an HMG-CoA (3-hydroxy-3-methylglutaryl-coenzyme A) reductase inhibitor such as atorvastatin (Lipitor) has been anecdotally reported to reduce the cholesterol and lipid effects of mirtazapine at dosages of 10–80 mg/day. Unless the benefits of mirtazapine are substantial, however, it may be easier to switch to another agent if there are clinically significant increases in cholesterol or triglyceride levels.

Along with bupropion and nefazodone, mirtazapine is one of the few antidepressants that have limited sexual side effects. Switching from an SSRI to mirtazapine appears to resolve sexual dysfunction associated with the use of an SSRI (Koutouvidis et al. 1999). There are case reports that indicate that adding mirtazapine at dosages of 15–30 mg/day to an SSRI can mitigate SSRI-induced sexual side effects (Koutouvidis et al. 1999). However, a more recent double-blind trial of mirtazapine in treating SSRI-induced sexual side effects showed no benefit over placebo (Michelson et al. 2002).

Orthostatic hypotension, or conversely hypertension, is occasionally seen in patients treated with mirtazapine. About 7% of patients experience significant dizziness, and some of this may be from postural changes. It is worthwhile to occasionally monitor blood pressure in patients treated with mirtazapine, particularly elderly patients. Other rare but significant side effects associated with mirtazapine include elevations in hepatic transaminases in about 2% of patients—a rate similar to that seen with SSRIs. Worries about agranulocytosis at the time of release of the drug to the market have not been borne out.

Overdose

Mirtazapine appears to be fairly safe in overdose. We are unaware of fatal overdoses with mirtazapine in doses of up to 2 g. The most common effect of overdose with mirtazapine is sedation. Gastric lavage and supportive management have thus far been adequate in dealing with overdoses.

Drug Interactions

As indicated earlier, mirtazapine has a low risk of pharmacokinetic interactions. The most common interaction is synergism with other CNS depressants. Concurrent benzodiazepines, barbiturates, or alcohol increases the risk of significant somnolence and sedation. The combination of mirtazapine and a CNS depressant also has an additive effect on motor impairment.

The proserotonergic effects of mirtazapine impart a potential risk of serotonin syndrome, although this risk is largely obviated via its blocking 5-HT_2 and 5-HT_3 postsynaptic receptors. The α_2-noradrenergic effects pose a risk of hypertensive crises when the drug is used in combination with an MAOI. As a result, mirtazapine should be discontinued for at least 2 weeks before an MAOI is started and vice versa.

Dosage and Administration

Although the recommended starting dosage is 15 mg/day, we now advise starting most patients at 30 mg/day. Geriatric patients and those with severe insomnia should be started at 15 mg/day. Mirtazapine is administered once a day, about 1 hour before bedtime. The dose may then be increased by 15 mg every 2 weeks to the maximum recommended dosage of 45 mg/day. In Europe, the maximum dosage of the same drug is 60 mg/day, and we will sometimes push the dose to this level in patients with treatment-resistant conditions.

Tricyclic and Tetracyclic Antidepressants

Structures

The chemical structures of TCAs and related compounds are remarkably similar (Figure 3–6). Desipramine and nortriptyline are demethylated metabolites of imipramine and amitriptyline, respectively. Amoxapine is a derivative of the antipsychotic loxapine and has an additional fourth ring off a side chain. Maprotiline is a four-ring compound, with the fourth ring arising perpendicular to the traditional three rings. Its side chain is identical to that of desipramine.

Pharmacological Effects

The pharmacological effects of the tricyclic and tetracyclic antidepressants are highly similar. Initially, particular emphasis was placed on their relative effects in blocking the reuptake of norepinephrine or 5-HT. These differences came to underlie various theories on the biology of depression, particularly the low-norepinephrine hypothesis versus the low-5-HT hypothesis. In recent years, theories have become more complex as the pharmacological effects of these drugs have been shown to go beyond their mere immediate reuptake-blocking effects to include later secondary effects on pre- and postsynaptic receptors, on second-messenger systems, and on other neurotransmitter systems. Such effects may account for differences among the various drugs in both their range of efficacy and their side effects. At one time, the relative effects of norepinephrine reuptake–blocking versus 5-HT reuptake–blocking were used to explain the relative sedative properties (5-HT) versus activating properties (norepinephrine) of these drugs. Sedation, which early on was ascribed to serotonergic and anticholinergic effects, has in part been ascribed to the antihistamine (H_1 receptor) actions of TCAs. Some investigators have argued that weight gain could also be due to H_1 receptor–blocking effects. Anticholinergic effects include dry mouth, constipation, urinary hesitancy, blurred vision, and confusion. The H_2 receptor–blocking effects may play a role in these drugs promoting healing of peptic ulcers.

The relative norepinephrine reuptake–blocking effects, compared with 5-HT reuptake–blocking effects, of the non-MAOI antidepressants are summarized in Table 3–7. The relative effects of these agents on acetylcholine, α_1, H_1, 5-HT$_1$, and 5-HT$_2$ receptors are summarized in Table 3–8. These poten-

Tricyclic antidepressants (TCAs): overview	
Efficacy	Second- or third-line agents for MDD (FDA approved for all) Panic disorder OCD (FDA approved for clomipramine) Pain syndromes Migraine prophylaxis Enuresis (FDA approved for imipramine)
Side effects	Dry mouth, constipation, urinary retention, blurred vision, confusion Weight gain Sedation Sexual dysfunction Orthostasis Tachycardia Cardiac conduction abnormalities
Dosage and administration	Individualize with low hs dosing (25–50 mg) for imipramine and amitriptyline. Increase by 25–50 mg every 3–7 days to target dosage of 150–300 mg/day. (Nortriptyline should be started at 10–25 mg and increased, as needed, to a maximum dosage of 150 mg/day.) Monitor levels and ECGs after dose stabilized.
Safety in overdose	Lethal in overdose (induces arrhythmias). Lavage and monitor on a cardiac bed for QRS widening.
Discontinuation	Flulike and GI symptoms from cholinergic rebound. Reduce by 25–50 mg every 3 days.
Drug interactions	CNS depressants: ↑ sedation, ataxia Anticoagulants: ↑ warfarin levels Antipsychotics: ↑ TCA and antipsychotic levels Cimetidine: ↑ TCA levels Clonidine: hypertensive crisis (**avoid**) L-Dopa: TCAs ↓ absorption MAOIs: serotonin syndrome (avoid clomipramine; imipramine and amitriptyline may be used with close monitoring) Stimulants: ↑ TCA levels Oral contraceptives: ↑ TCA levels Quinidine: ↑ arrhythmias (**avoid**) SSRIs: ↑ TCA levels Sympathomimetics: ↑ arrhythmias, hypertension, tachycardia

Note.   CNS = central nervous system; ECG = electrocardiogram; FDA = U.S. Food and Drug Administration; GI = gastrointestinal; MAOI = monoamine oxidase inhibitor; MDD = major depressive disorder; OCD = obsessive-compulsive disorder; SSRI = selective serotonin reuptake inhibitor.

Imipramine

Trimipramine

Amitriptyline

Desipramine

Doxepin

Nortriptyline

Protriptyline

Maprotiline

Amoxapine

Clomipramine hydrochloride

Figure 3–6. Chemical structures of tricyclic and tetracyclic antidepressants.

Table 3–7.   Norepinephrine (NE) and serotonin (5-HT) reuptake–blocking effects of the non-MAOI antidepressants

Antidepressant	NE	5-HT
amitriptyline	+	++
amoxapine	++	+
bupropion	+/−	0
citalopram/escitalopram	0	+++
clomipramine	++	+++
desipramine	+++	+
doxepin	+	+
fluoxetine	0	+++
fluvoxamine	0	+++
imipramine	+	++
maprotiline	++	0
mirtazapine	+	−
nefazodone	0/+	+
nortriptyline	++	+
paroxetine	+[a]	+++
protriptyline	+++	+
sertraline	0	+++
trazodone	0	+
trimipramine	0	0
venlafaxine	+	++

Note.   Data are approximations of relative activity from in vivo, in vitro, and clinical studies. Data on clomipramine include results on desmethylclomipramine on both active metabolites with pronounced effects on noradrenergic systems. In certain in vivo models, the tricyclic antidepressants (other than clomipramine) and trazodone have been reported not to block 5-HT uptake. MAOI = monoamine oxidase inhibitor. Strength of effect represented on a scale from 0 (no effect) to +++ (marked effect). +/− indicates marginal effect.
[a]Effect at high doses.

cies represent best estimates based on receptor-binding and clinical studies. Note that the TCAs currently available in the United States are relatively weak 5-HT reuptake blockers. Clomipramine is the one exception to this rule. Indeed, in some in vivo models, TCAs—other than clomipramine—are devoid of 5-HT-blocking effects, as is trazodone. Moreover, recent research points to some of the antidepressants as having 5-HT receptor–blocking effects, suggesting that some are 5-HT antagonists. Taken together, laboratory data suggest that the tricyclics—other than clomipramine (see Chapter 6: "Antianxiety Agents")—are weak serotonergic agents. In contrast, the SSRIs are relatively pure 5-HT re-

Table 3–8. Relative receptor-blocking effects of antidepressants

Antidepressant	ACh	α_1	H_1	5-HT$_1$	5-HT$_2$
amitriptyline	+++	+++	++	+/−	+/−
amoxapine	+	++	+	+/−	+++
bupropion	0	0	0	0	0
citalopram/escitalopram	0	0	0	0	
clomipramine	+	++	+	0	+
desipramine	+	+	+	0	+/−
doxepin	++	+++	+++	+/−	+/−
fluoxetine	0	0	0	0	+/−
fluvoxamine	0	0	0	0	0
imipramine	++	+	+	0	+/−
maprotiline	+	+	++	0	+/−
mirtazapine	0	0	+++	+	+
nefazodone	0	+	0	+	++
nortriptyline	+	+	+	+/−	+
paroxetine	+	0	0	0	0
protriptyline	+++	+	+	0	+
sertraline	0	0	0	0	0
trazodone	0	++	+/−	+	++
trimipramine	++	++	+++	0	+/−
venlafaxine	0	0	0	0	0

Note. Data are approximations of relative activity from in vivo, in vitro, and clinical studies. ACh = muscarinic acetylcholine receptor; α_1 = α_1-adrenergic receptor; H_1 = histamine$_1$ receptor; 5-HT$_1$ = serotonin$_1$ receptor; 5-HT$_2$ = serotonin$_2$ receptor. Strength of effect represented on scale from 0 (no effect) to +++ (marked effect). +/− indicates marginal effect.

uptake blockers, with little in the way of antagonist effects. Thus, these drugs offer an alternative for the clinician. The tricyclic and tetracyclic antidepressants are virtually devoid of dopamine reuptake–blocking effects. Of the available antidepressants, only sertraline and bupropion have such effects, and the effects are somewhat weak. Variations in biological effects help in drug selection, in terms of both clinical efficacy and side effects. The types of side effects that are seen with tricyclic and tetracyclic compounds are summarized in Table 3–9.

Table 3–9.   Common or troublesome side effects of tricyclic and tetracyclic drugs

Anticholinergic	Central nervous system
Dry mouth	Tremor
Constipation	Sedation
Blurred vision	Stimulation
Urinary hesitancy	Myoclonic twitches
Esophageal reflux	Seizure (maprotiline)
Cardiovascular	Extrapyramidal symptoms (amoxapine)
Orthostatic hypotension	Other
Palpitations	Perspiration
Conduction slowing	Weight gain
Hypertension	Sexual dysfunction
	Impotence

Indications

The principal indication for TCAs and related compounds approved by the FDA for marketing is major depression. Other FDA-approved indications include anxiety (for doxepin) and childhood enuresis (for imipramine as an adjunctive treatment). Nonapproved but common uses include insomnia (particularly for amitriptyline and doxepin), headache (most commonly for amitriptyline, imipramine, and doxepin), agoraphobia with panic attacks (for imipramine and clomipramine particularly), chronic pain syndromes (most frequently for doxepin and maprotiline), and bulimia (for imipramine and desipramine). Imipramine has also been reported to be effective in treating GAD, and trimipramine and doxepin were once thought to be effective in treating peptic ulcers. The most recently released TCA, clomipramine, has potent anti–obsessive-compulsive effects, as do the SSRIs, and is FDA approved for that use. Obviously, these drugs exert rather wide pharmacological effects, which account for their potentially broad range of actions. (For further discussion of the use of TCAs in the treatment of anxiety disorders, see the section on antidepressants in Chapter 6: "Antianxiety Agents.")

Currently, eight tricyclic and two tetracyclic antidepressants are available in the United States. One tricyclic, clomipramine, is approved for the treatment of OCD but not for depression. It is used worldwide, however, as a major antidepressant, particularly in cases of refractory depression. Generic and brand names, formulations and strengths, and therapeutic dosage ranges of the tricyclic and tetracyclic antidepressants are listed in Table 3–10.

The original patents have expired on all of these drugs, and generic preparations are now available. In the United States, use of generic compounds has not been without controversy. Although generic drugs offered a savings for the consumer, some clinicians questioned their pharmacological equivalence. One difficulty stemmed from the FDA definition of bioequivalence, which relies heavily on the demonstration that an identical dosage of a generic preparation produces blood levels within a specified range (20%–30%) above and below those produced by the original compound. Even with approved generic preparations, some studies had suggested that they were not truly equivalent to standard brands. Moreover, pharmaceutical companies were not required to prove that their generic preparations had equivalence in clinical or biological potency. This area appears to be less of a problem at present, since generic drug manufacturers have improved their production methods.

Blood Levels

In past decades, considerable attention has been paid to the use of drug blood levels to monitor treatment with various psychotropic agents. Currently, blood levels are most commonly used in patients treated with TCAs, neuroleptics, clozapine, lithium carbonate, and anticonvulsants. Blood levels have not proved to be useful with the SSRIs and most newer antidepressants. Likewise, blood levels for benzodiazepines are neither widely available nor commonly used. Drug concentrations are determined primarily in serum (e.g., for lithium carbonate and anticonvulsants) or plasma (e.g., for TCAs). In addition to measuring the concentration of neuroleptics in blood, some laboratories measure the relative binding to dopamine receptors (so-called radioreceptor assays). However, this practice has not been widely adopted.

Generally, TCA serum levels are determined in blood drawn 8–12 hours after the patient's last dose, in an effort to avoid false peaks in blood levels that would occur if blood were drawn immediately after a patient had taken the medication. Also, plasma levels are most accurate when the blood is drawn after the patient has achieved steady state—the point at which a specific dose of drug given over a several-day period produces a consistent blood level. For most TCAs, this period is approximately 5–7 days.

Table 3–10.   Tricyclic and tetracyclic antidepressants: names, formulations and strengths, and dosages

Generic name	Brand name[a]	Formulations and strengths	Therapeutic dosage range (mg/day)[b]
Tricyclics			
amitriptyline	Elavil	Tablets: 10, 25, 50, 75, 100, 150 mg	150–300
clomipramine	Anafranil	Capsules: 25, 50, 75 mg	100–250
desipramine	Norpramin	Tablets: 10, 25, 50, 75, 100, 150 mg	150–300
doxepin	Sinequan	Capsules: 10, 25, 50, 75, 100, 150 mg	150–300
		Oral solution: 10 mg/mL (120-mL bottle)	
imipramine	Tofranil	Tablets: 10, 25, 50 mg	150–300
imipramine pamoate	Tofranil-PM[c]	Capsules: 75, 100, 125, 150 mg	150–300
nortriptyline	Aventyl, Pamelor	Capsules: 10, 25, 50, 75 mg	50–150
		Oral solution: 10 mg/5 mL (480-mL bottle)	
protriptyline	Vivactil	Tablets: 5, 10 mg	15–60
trimipramine maleate	Surmontil	Capsules: 25, 50, 100 mg	150–300
Tetracyclics			
amoxapine	Asendin	Tablets: 25, 50, 100, 150 mg	150–400
maprotiline	Ludiomil	Tablets: 25, 50, 75 mg	150–225

[a]All the tricyclic and tetracyclic antidepressants shown are available generically.
[b]Dosage ranges are approximate. Many patients respond at relatively low dosages (even dosages below those in the ranges given in table); others may require higher dosages.
[c]Sustained release.

Plasma levels can be particularly useful barometers of drug metabolism. There is approximately a 30-fold difference among human subjects in plasma levels of TCAs produced by a single, fixed milligram-per-kilogram dose of a drug, reflecting the degree to which the slowest and fastest metabolizers differ in drug absorption and metabolism. The TCAs are metabolized in part via the cytochrome P450 2D6 enzyme. Approximately 5%–7% of the Caucasian population is deficient in this enzyme. In addition, metabolism of the TCAs is affected by age and by inhibition or activation by other drugs. Obviously, slow metabolizers (such as elderly persons) are at a higher risk for attaining toxic levels of drugs; fast metabolizers may have difficulty building drug levels. Most patients, however, fall in the middle range of the normal bell-shaped curve distribution.

The clearest use of TCAs is for patients with more severe major depression. There is little or no relationship between TCA level and clinical response in patients with nonendogenous depression or in those with dysthymia. Two types of "positive" relationships between TCA level and clinical response in endogenously depressed patients have been described in the literature. Glassman et al. (1977) reported a sigmoidal relationship between response and imipramine plus desipramine levels; clinical response increases with plasma level up to approximately 250 ng/mL and then levels off thereafter (Figure 3–7). Glassman et al. reported rates of response of 30%, 67%, and 93% for patients with plasma levels in the ranges of less than 150, 150–225, and greater than 225 ng/mL, respectively. For nortriptyline, a curvilinear relationship has been described, as indicated in Figure 3–8. Response increases with plasma level and then plateaus in the range of approximately 50–150 ng/mL, with a decrease in response at plasma levels greater than 150 ng/mL. The critical range of 50–150 ng/mL has been called the "therapeutic window." Nonresponding patients with plasma levels of approximately 150 ng/mL may respond to a lowering of dosage and plasma level into the window. The decreased responsivity at levels above the window is not due to side effects. Therapeutic windows have at times been described for other drugs, but these windows are not as clear as that seen with nortriptyline. Approximate therapeutic plasma levels for tricyclic and tetracyclic drugs are summarized in Table 3–11.

A number of medications may increase or decrease plasma levels—generally by interfering with or augmenting liver microsomal enzyme activity. For example, nicotine, barbiturates (including butalbital [Fiorinal]), chloral hydrate, phenytoin, and carbamazepine induce breakdown of TCAs, and clinicians should keep this in mind when prescribing TCAs for patients who are

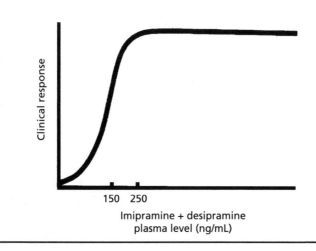

Figure 3–7.   Sigmoidal relationship between clinical response and imipramine plus desipramine plasma levels.

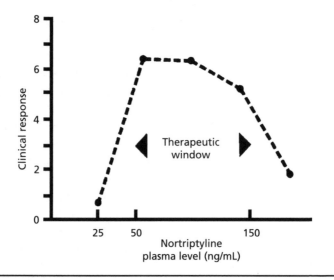

Figure 3–8.   Curvilinear relationship between clinical response and nortriptyline plasma levels.

Table 3–11. Approximate therapeutic serum level ranges for tricyclic and tetracyclic drugs

Drug	Serum level (ng/mL)
amitriptyline	100–250[a]
amoxapine	Unknown
desipramine	150–300
doxepin	120–250[a]
imipramine	150–300[a]
maprotiline	150–250
nortriptyline[b]	50–150
protriptyline	75–250
trimipramine	Unknown

[a]Total concentration of drug and demethylated metabolite.
[b]Has a clear therapeutic window.

taking these compounds. In contrast, antipsychotics (particularly phenothiazines), the SSRIs, methylphenidate, disulfiram, and fenfluramine increase plasma levels by slowing drug metabolism in the liver. (Fenfluramine [Pondimin] was withdrawn from the market in 1997, when "fen-phen" was found to be associated with heart valve disease.) The SSRIs have become the agents one worries most about, because they are potent competitive inhibitors of the cytochrome P450 2D6 enzyme and thus may substantially increase TCA plasma levels. Conversely, TCAs increase phenothiazine plasma levels. Benzodiazepines and antiparkinsonian medications have little or no effect on TCA levels.

A number of issues arise when one considers plasma level data. For one, studies generally use fixed milligram-per-kilogram dosing, and consequently it is possible that a patient with a given TCA plasma level (e.g., 250 ng/mL) taking the drug at a given dosage (e.g., 300 mg/day of imipramine) might well have responded to a lower dosage and at a lower plasma level. In a sense, then, plasma levels can be viewed as barometers of the adequacy of treatment. Patients who are not responding to a 4- to 6-week trial of imipramine but who have attained a plasma level of 150 ng/mL or less may respond to an increase in dosage and plasma level to greater than 200 ng/mL. On the other hand, other patients who are responding at exactly the same dosage and plasma level do not need to have the dosage or plasma level increased, even if the plasma level is below the therapeutic range. Some investigators have advocated determining the plasma level for any patient who is responding to a TCA in order to record that patient's therapeutic plasma level while taking that drug. This could prove important if the patient has a recurrence and requires retreatment. Sometimes a routine check of a TCA blood level in a patient who is clinically much improved and has only minor side effects reveals a plasma level of greater than 400 ng/mL, and the patient relapses when the dose is decreased to bring down the plasma level. This result suggests that for that particular patient, a very high plasma level is necessary for improvement. Indeed, there was a prospective report that some patients require very high dosages and blood levels for an adequate response, although there is an inherent risk with this approach.

So far, only amitriptyline shows clear toxicity related to plasma levels around 500 ng/mL. Obviously, clinical judgment is necessary. An ECG is useful with patients who do well only at very high plasma levels of the drug, to ensure that cardiac conduction is not seriously affected—that is, to ensure that no intracardiac conduction slowing takes place.

Formerly, the variation in TCA assays among laboratories was of major importance, because clinicians were unable to interpret a given value in their laboratories. Major national efforts to cross-validate results from laboratories have helped, and this problem appears to have resolved.

In summary, plasma levels can provide useful clinical information if the clinician keeps these issues in mind.

Side Effects

A review in the *Physicians' Desk Reference* (PDR) of the package-insert information on each of the TCAs and related agents indicates their myriad side effects. The side effects can be grouped broadly by categories: anticholinergic, cardiovascular, and so forth (Table 3–9). This organization is somewhat artificial, because a single side effect (e.g., sedation) may actually be due to any number of distinct neurochemical effects (e.g., histamine blockade, increased 5-HT availability, 5-HT$_2$ antagonism) or combinations of effects. In addition, some side effects may reflect drug action either in the brain or at the periphery or both (e.g., orthostatic hypotension).

How can clinicians help in the management of side effects? In some patients, particularly those with complicating medical illness, side reactions may not be entirely controllable or manageable. There are, however, some things that can be done, particularly for less severe reactions in medically healthy patients.

One very important issue is *attitude*. Early on, some psychiatrists commonly had rather negative views about medication, which were communicated indirectly or overtly to the patient, particularly if the impetus to try medications had arisen from the patient and not the physician. In our experience, such attitudes can be troubling to the patient, who must rely on the physician's belief in the importance of medication trials and in being able to deal with the side effects. The imperative for clinicians to develop well-reasoned and balanced views about prescribing drugs has obviated this problem somewhat in recent years.

A general principle of drug prescribing is that some side effects can be managed by reducing the dosage or can be avoided by increasing the dosage slowly. In our experience, this is particularly true for the early emergence of "spaciness," depersonalization, confusion, orthostatic hypotension, or marked sedation. If these reactions persist in the presence of more moderate dose escalation, a switch to another TCA or another class of drug may be necessary. In dealing with anticholinergic side effects or sedation, switching to desipramine seems reasonable. For patients who develop orthostatic hypotension, nortriptyline is often a useful alternative, because it tends to produce orthostatic changes at plasma levels above the so-called therapeutic window. Thus, nortriptyline is more easily tolerated than imipramine, whose orthostatic effects are often produced at low plasma levels (see subsection on TCA blood levels earlier in this section). Nortriptyline has been used successfully in several studies on poststroke and geriatric depression.

Peripheral anticholinergic side effects have also been reported as being ameliorated by administering bethanechol, a procholinergic drug, at dosages of 25–50 mg tid or qid, and generally continuing for as long as the patient continues to take TCAs. This drug can be particularly helpful to patients with urinary hesitancy. In cases of anticholinergic deliria, physostigmine (a centrally acting procholinergic agent) may be administered either intravenously or intramuscularly to clarify the diagnosis.

Blurred vision as a result of TCAs can be treated with 4% pilocarpine drops or with oral bethanechol. Patients otherwise doing well with maintenance TCA treatment, and therefore likely to be taking the drug for some time, may require a change in their eyeglass prescription to correct the blurring of vision.

For severe dry mouth, a 1% pilocarpine solution can be created by mixing the 4% solution available as eyedrops with three parts water. This solution can be swished around the mouth for a few minutes, 30–60 minutes before an increase in salivation is needed. For example, patients may use this mouthwash before having to give a lecture. Bethanechol in 5-mg or 10-mg tablets may be administered sublingually for a similar effect. Although we know of no studies, anticholinergic effects may be ameliorated with cholinesterase inhibitors.

An important, possibly antihistaminic, side effect of TCAs is weight gain—particularly seen with amitriptyline and doxepin—which can be difficult to control pharmacologically. Often, patients who demonstrate this side effect while taking one TCA will continue to gain weight when switched to another, related drug. In some patients, switching to one of the newer antidepressants may be the only way to maintain an antidepressant effect and promote weight reduction, because MAOIs also cause weight gain. Unfortunately, some patients still continue to gain weight while receiving the drug to which they are showing an antidepressant response. In such cases, support and advice regarding dieting may be the only recourse. Addition of topiramate may facilitate weight loss.

The two tetracyclic agents, maprotiline and amoxapine, have been reported to produce troublesome side effects—seizures and extrapyramidal symptoms—that have been less frequently reported with the standard TCAs. Induced seizures have been reported in a number of single case reports of patients taking maprotiline. Our group reported on a series of 11 patients with maprotiline-related seizures at one hospital and a study of all U.S. maprotiline-related seizures (Dessain et al. 1986). In our series, prolonged treatment (longer than 6 weeks) at high dosages (225–400 mg/day) appeared to be a major factor. This was confirmed in the U.S. survey. In addition, rapid dose escalation—with the dosage reaching 150 mg/day within 7 days—was a major factor in the general survey. When these two factors were eliminated, the risk of seizures appeared to approximate that associated with classic antidepressants (approximately 0.2%). The manufacturer of maprotiline altered its dosage guidelines, recommending beginning treatment at 75 mg/day for 2 weeks, a maximum dosage of 225 mg/day for up to 6 weeks, and maintenance at 175 mg/day or less. The previous dosage schedule was similar to that of imipramine.

Amoxapine has been reported to produce a number of side effects associated with dopamine receptor blockade. These side effects are similar to those more commonly found with the neuroleptic loxapine—for example, galactorrhea, akathisia, and other extrapyramidal symptoms and even a few cases of dyskinesia. Amoxapine is metabolized to a 7-OH metabolite. In some individuals, alternate hydroxylation at the 8 position results in the accumulation of a neuroleptic metabolite. Generally speaking, we recommend tapering or stopping medications if these symptoms occur (see subsection on blood levels earlier in this section).

Overdose

Overdoses can result in death. Tricyclics have narrow safety margins, and intracardiac slowing and arrhythmias may result in death when overdoses are taken. In addition, patients taking overdoses can demonstrate confusion, deliria, and loss of consciousness.

Dosage and Administration

Having evaluated a depressed patient, the clinician must determine whether TCAs are an appropriate treatment. In the first edition of this manual, we subscribed to the approach of using a TCA first in the treatment of endogenous or major depression. As a consequence of the superior safety and tolerability of the newer agents, particularly the SSRIs, the TCAs were relegated to second-line status in the second edition. However, some investigators continue to suspect that the TCAs are superior to the newer agents in the treatment of more serious, melancholic depressive episodes. Although it has been difficult to demonstrate greater efficacy for TCAs (see "Indications" subsection in section on SSRIs earlier in this chapter), the jury is still out. Because the vast majority of studies on inpatients and those with melancholic depression have employed TCAs, these agents still need to be considered early in the treatment of more serious depression.

The choice of which TCA to use is somewhat a matter of personal preference. There is really considerable overlap among these various drugs, although some are a bit more stimulating (desipramine and protriptyline) and others are more sedating (amitriptyline and doxepin). Among the secondary amines, desipramine and nortriptyline have become two of the most popular TCAs with which to begin treatment. These two drugs have the most favorable side-effect profiles in the TCA group. In addition, these two drugs have reliable plasma level data regarding clinical response. On the other hand, amitriptyline has a very poor side-effect profile secondary to its anticholinergic and antihistaminic side effects and may not be the best first choice for many patients, especially elderly ones. With any of these drugs, the clinician is best advised to start with a relatively low dose, which can then be increased slowly.

For imipramine, the starting doses and regimens vary. One common imipramine regimen is to prescribe 75 mg/day during week 1 and to increase the dosage weekly, as needed, to 150 mg/day during week 2, 225 mg/day during week 3, and 300 mg/day during week 4. Another approach is to start at 50 mg/day, increasing the dosage by 25 mg every few days, as tolerated, to 150 mg/day; and then, after about 2 weeks, to increase the dosage from 150 mg/day, at a rate of 50 mg every 3 days, to 300 mg/day. (Similar dosage regimens are recommended for other uses of the drug, such as for panic and pain.)

In prescribing imipramine for some patients, particularly elderly patients (who may be especially intolerant or taking other medications), it seems reasonable to begin at 25 mg on day 1 and to increase to 50 mg on day 2, allowing the patient to become acclimated to a single small dose. We also advise a more conservative schedule of increases for elderly patients, keeping the dosage at 50 mg/day for 1 week and thereafter increasing it at a rate of 25 mg every 2 days to 150 mg/day. After 7 days at 150 mg/day, the dosage can be increased further as tolerated. Elderly patients present a somewhat distinctive problem regarding drug-drug interactions (see Chapter 12, "Pharmacotherapy in Special Situations"). The not uncommon medical problems of elderly persons and their relatively slow drug metabolism usually dictate conservative management. However, clinicians must be careful: some elderly patients are not slow metabolizers, but instead require reasonably high dosages and therefore are at risk of being undertreated. The degree of side effects can be a useful barometer of the ability to tolerate a given dosage, and plasma levels may aid in prescribing optimal doses (see subsections on TCA blood levels and side effects earlier in this section).

For doxepin, amitriptyline, and trimipramine, dosage ranges similar to those for imipramine are recommended in both younger and older patients. Trimipramine has a relatively low side-effect profile in elderly patients and has a rapid effect on promoting sleep.

Protriptyline and nortriptyline are prescribed in rather different ways. For younger patients, protriptyline is generally started at 15 mg/day (5 mg tid) in week 1, with an increase each week of 5–10 mg in the daily dose, to a maximum dosage of 60 mg/day. For elderly patients, protriptyline is generally begun at 10 mg/day, aiming for a maximum dosage of 30–40 mg/day. Nortriptyline, which is the only TCA that clearly has a so-called therapeutic window, can be ineffective if plasma levels are either too low or too high. The therapeutic dosage range for nortriptyline in adults is 50–150 mg/day. We recommend starting at 50 mg/day and weekly increasing the daily dosage by 50 mg to 100 mg/day. (In elderly patients, begin at 25 mg/day and increase the dosage to 50 mg/day after 3–4 days.) After 3 weeks, a decrease in dosage may actually be helpful—a situation rather different from that of the other TCAs (see subsection on TCA blood levels earlier in this section).

Amoxapine's starting dosage in healthy adults is 150 mg/day, with a maximum dosage of 400 mg/day. A few patients have been treated with up to 600 mg/day. However, this dosage increases the risk of seizures. This drug may be particularly effective in treating psychotic depression (Anton and Sexauer 1983).

Maprotiline's starting and maximum dosages are 75 and 225 mg/day, respectively. To avoid seizures, the starting dose of maprotiline should be maintained for 2 weeks, and after 6 weeks of treatment, the dosage should be reduced to a maximum of 175 mg/day (Dessain et al. 1986).

Discontinuation

In discontinuing or tapering TCAs, it is most prudent to do so at a maximum rate of 25–50 mg every 2–3 days. Many patients will demonstrate symptoms of cholinergic rebound if the TCA is discontinued too abruptly. These symptoms include nausea, queasy stomach, cramping, sweating, headache, neck pain, and vomiting. We have observed several patients who experienced intense GI symptoms during and after TCA withdrawal. For these patients, propantheline bromide (15 mg tid prn) was extremely helpful. Moreover, Nelson et al. (1983) reported that some patients demonstrate "rebound" hypomania or mania with sudden cessation of TCAs, an observation confirmed by others.

When the issue of rebound symptoms versus a medical illness or recurrence of psychiatric symptoms is in doubt, a single dose of the discontinued drug will often relieve the symptoms rapidly, confirming the diagnosis of a withdrawal syndrome. There is one report in which withdrawal mania responded to reinstitution of desipramine therapy (Nelson et al. 1983).

Monoamine oxidase inhibitors (MAOIs): overview	
Efficacy	Third-line agents for MDD (FDA approved for resistant depression) Social anxiety Panic disorder Second-line agents for Parkinson's disease (selegiline has FDA approval)
Side effects	Weight gain Orthostasis Sexual dysfunction Dry mouth Insomnia/somnolence Headache
Safety in overdose	Can be lethal in overdose. Hypertensive crisis, stroke, and myocardial infarction have been reported. Manage with lavage, emesis induction, and close management of blood pressure and airway.
Dosage and administration	Phenelzine: start at 15 mg bid or tid and increase by 15 mg per week to target dosage of 60–90 mg/day.
	Tranylcypromine: start at 10 mg bid or tid and increase by 10 mg per week to target dosage of 40–60 mg/day.
	Isocarboxazid: start at 10 mg bid and increase dosage, if the drug is tolerated, by 10 mg every 2–4 days to 40 mg/day by end of first week. Maximum recommended dosage is 60 mg/day, administered in divided doses.
	Selegiline transdermal system (Emsam): start with 6-mg patch daily for 4 weeks and then increase to 9-mg patch for 2 weeks, and then 12-mg patch as needed. No dietary restrictions at 6 mg/day.
Discontinuation	Flulike symptoms, hallucinations, hypomania, and dysphoria reported with sudden dis- continuation. Taper dose by 25% per week.

(continued)

Monoamine oxidase inhibitors (MAOIs): overview *(continued)*	
Drug interactions	Foods containing high levels of tyramine **(contraindicated)** (see Table 3–14): hypertensive crisis β-Blockers: ↑ hypotension, bradycardia Oral hypoglycemics: ↑ hypoglycemic effects Bupropion **(contraindicated):** hypertensive crisis, seizure Carbamazepine **(contraindicated):** hypertensive crisis Meperidine **(contraindicated):** serotonin syndrome Nefazodone: possible serotonin syndrome Sympathomimetics: hypertensive crisis SSRIs **(contraindicated):** serotonin syndrome TCAs: clomipramine **contraindicated** Mirtazapine **(contraindicated):** hypertensive crisis SNRIs **(contraindicated):** serotonin syndrome

Note. FDA = U.S. Food and Drug Administration; MDD = major depressive disorder; SNRI = serotonin-norepinephrine reuptake inhibitor; SSRI = selective serotonin reuptake inhibitor; TCA = tricyclic antidepressant.

Monoamine Oxidase Inhibitors

Pharmacological Effects

The first-generation MAOIs—isocarboxazid, phenelzine, and tranylcypromine—have few direct effects on reuptake or receptor blockade. Instead, they inhibit MAO in various organs, exerting greater effects on monoamine oxidase A (MAO-A)—for which norepinephrine and 5-HT are primary substrates—than on MAO-B, which acts primarily on other amines (e.g., phenylethylamine) and dopamine. Also, MAO-A is found in the gut mucosa and is responsible for degrading various amines that can act as false neurotransmitters and produce hypertensive crises (see later in this section). Isocarboxazid, phenelzine, and tranylcypromine are so-called irreversible inhibitors. When the enzyme is inhibited by these agents, protein regeneration is required before MAO enzymatic activity is restored. Selegiline (Eldepryl), a selective ir-

Figure 3–9. Chemical structures of monoamine oxidase inhibitors (MAOIs).

reversible MAO inhibitor used in the treatment of Parkinson's disease, exerts its effects on MAO-B and is generally thought to have a very low risk of producing hypertensive crises. However, at the low dosages used in treating parkinsonian patients (5–10 mg/day), this drug is a weak antidepressant, and data from Sunderland et al. (1989) suggested that at higher antidepressant dosages, the drug affects both MAO-A and MAO-B and thus does not protect against hypertensive crises. More information on selegiline is provided in the section "Selective and Reversible Monoamine Oxidase Inhibitors" later in this chapter.

There are two structural classes of MAOIs: the hydrazines (i.e., phenelzine) and the nonhydrazines (tranylcypromine and selegiline) (Figure 3–9; Table 3–12).

Table 3–12. Monoamine oxidase inhibitors (MAOIs): names, formulations and strengths, and dosages

Generic name	Brand name	Tablets and capsules	Oral concentrate	Usual therapeutic dosage (mg/day)[a]
phenelzine	Nardil	Tablet: 15 mg	None	45–90
selegiline	Eldepryl	Capsule: 5 mg	None	20–50
	Carbex	Tablet: 5 mg		
	Emsam	Patch: 6 mg/24 hr, 9 mg/24 hr, 12 mg/24 hr		
tranylcypromine	Parnate	Tablet: 10 mg	None	30–60
isocarboxazid	Marplan	Tablet: 10 mg	None	30–60

[a]Dosage ranges are approximate. Many patients respond at relatively low dosages (even dosages below those in the ranges given in table).

Indications

The primary PDR clinical indication for MAOIs is for treatment of depression refractory to TCA therapy. With so many other safer antidepressants currently available, MAOIs are now typically indicated when several trials have failed. Still, some patients respond better to MAOIs than to any other class of agents. Phenelzine has an FDA-approved indication for anxious depression. Although the British had emphasized frequently that the MAOIs were not particularly helpful in treating the severe forms of major depression referred to in the past as endogenous, the American experience, including our own, had been entirely different. These drugs were lifesavers for many severely depressed patients, particularly those whose depression did not respond to TCAs.

Why the discrepancy? For one, there was little doubt that MAOIs were effective in patients with panic attacks or with anxious or atypical depression. However, their effectiveness in patients with melancholic or endogenous depression may require the prescription of considerably higher dosages than those used in the early British trials, in which relatively low dosages were used. Another difficulty with determining ranges of efficacy revolves around the occurrence of pronounced obsessionality, agitation, and anxiety in many endogenously depressed patients, who may have, in the early studies, been misdiagnosed as only anxiously depressed.

Investigators at Columbia University have attempted to define an atypical depressive syndrome that preferentially responds to phenelzine and other MAOIs such as moclobemide. Their data suggest that patients with atypical depression respond better to MAOIs than to TCAs. The SSRIs are also effective in treating atypical depression. Because the SSRIs are considerably safer than the MAOIs, the use of MAOIs in the treatment of atypical depression has dropped off considerably since the introduction of fluoxetine. MAOIs are also effective in the treatment of social phobia.

Side Effects

Common side effects of MAOIs are listed in Table 3–13. Because MAOIs do not block acetylcholine receptors, they produce less dry mouth, blurred vision, constipation, and urinary hesitancy than do TCAs. However, we have seen patients who have developed urinary hesitancy, presumably as a result of an increase in noradrenergic activity. When the problem occurs, a reduction in

Table 3–13. Common or troublesome side effects of monoamine oxidase inhibitors (MAOIs)

Orthostatic hypotension
Hypertensive crises (interactions with foodstuffs[a] or medications)
Hyperpyrexic reactions
Anorgasmia or sexual impotence
Insomnia during night
Sedation (particularly in daytime; due to insomnia during night)
Stimulation during day
Muscle cramps and myositis-like reactions
Urinary hesitancy[b]
Constipation[b]
Dry mouth[b]
Weight gain
Myoclonic twitches
Skin irritation at patch site (Emsam)

[a]See Table 3–14.
[b]Less than with tricyclic antidepressants.

dosage may help. We have been less impressed with the adjunctive use of bethanechol with MAOIs than with its use with TCAs.

The most common side effect of MAOIs is dizziness, particularly of the
orthostatic type. This side effect appears to be somewhat more common with
MAOIs than with TCAs. Dose reduction may help; but, again, we have often
found reduction in the dose to be problematic, because too great a reduction
may lead to reemergence of depressive symptoms. Alternative approaches include 1) maintenance of adequate hydration—about eight glasses of fluid a day—
and increased salt intake; 2) use of support stockings, "bellybinders," or corsets;
and 3) addition of a mineralocorticoid (fludrocortisone [Florinef]). Although
this mineralocorticoid has been used in patients with orthostatic hypotension
not induced by medication, we have rarely found it to be helpful in the usual
daily dose of 0.3 mg. We have been told by colleagues that fludrocortisone can
be effective at a total daily dose of 0.6–0.8 mg. An intriguing report appeared
before our second edition, pointing to the use of small amounts of cheese to help
maintain blood pressure—a counterintuitive but imaginative solution. However, most clinicians were wary of the understandable risk of hypertensive crises
with cheese, particularly when one did not really know the tyramine content of

the foodstuff. We are not aware of any recent reports on this. Similarly, one would intuit that adding a stimulant (D-amphetamine or methylphenidate) to an MAOI would result in marked surges of blood pressure. In fact, however, Feighner et al. (1985) reported that the addition of stimulants for patients receiving MAOIs or MAOI-TCA combinations normalized blood pressure in depressed patients with serious orthostatic hypotension or brought out a clinical response in patients who had previously not had any response. There were no incidents of hypertensive crises; in fact, several of the patients developed orthostatic hypotension. Daily dosages used were 5–20 mg of D-amphetamine and 10–15 mg of methylphenidate. These authors recommended beginning at a dosage of 2.5 mg/day of either drug. We have heard of several clinicians in the community who have used these approaches successfully, but we have also heard of occasional hypertensive crises when stimulants were used in combination with MAOIs.

Sedation and activation are also potential problems, the latter being more common. Activation takes two forms: stimulation during the day (particularly with tranylcypromine) and insomnia at night. Tranylcypromine's stimulatory effects have been related to its having a structure similar to that of amphetamines, although this pharmacological link has not been clearly established. Overstimulation can be ameliorated somewhat by dose reduction, although the side effect is not easily eliminated. If a dose reduction does not result in a decrease in stimulation, patients may need to be switched to another medication.

Phenelzine is, overall, far less stimulating and more sedating than tranylcypromine. As such it offers a major alternative for daytime overstimulation. However, phenelzine may produce both insomnia and secondary daytime sedation. Oddly, one often encounters insomnia in patients who are nevertheless showing a good clinical response to the drug, making it a particularly difficult side effect to manage. Changing the dosage regimen may be helpful. Patients who are not taking phenelzine in the evening may benefit from switching drug taking to the evening hours. Conversely, patients who are taking much of the drug in the evening may respond by taking it earlier in the day. These manipulations can be helpful, although in our experience they are highly variable in their efficacy. Some patients may ultimately require hypnotic agents to overcome persistent insomnia. By the second edition of this manual, we had become very impressed with the addition of low doses of amitriptyline, trimipramine, or trazodone (50–100 mg at bedtime) to counteract MAOI-induced sleep disturbances. Caution should still be exercised in using trazodone or the TCAs with MAOIs because of the slight risk of developing a serotonin syndrome. With trazodone, we recommend trying doses of 50–100 mg per night. An increase to 150 mg hs can be tried if there has been no response at a lower dose and the medication has been well tolerated.

As the dose of an MAOI is increased to high levels in an attempt to achieve a therapeutic effect, patients occasionally become "intoxicated"—drunk, ataxic, confused, and sometimes euphoric. This is a sign of overdose, and the dose should be reduced. Some patients develop muscle pains or paresthesias—probably the result of the MAOIs interfering with pyridoxine (vitamin B_6) metabolism. Pyridoxine administered at dosages of approximately 100 mg/day can be helpful.

A particularly bothersome side effect is anorgasmia, which in some patients lessens over time. We have not been impressed with any pharmacological attempts to counteract this side effect, although cyproheptadine has been said to be helpful. Agents such as buspirone and bupropion are best avoided in combination with MAOIs.

Overdose

Overdoses are not necessarily lethal. Patients will show sedation and orthostasis. However, overdoses commonly involve other medications, resulting in serotonin syndromes or hypertensive reactions.

Drug Interactions

The greatest side-effect problems with MAOIs involve untoward interactions with certain foodstuffs or cold remedies, which may produce hypertensive crises with violent cerebrovascular accidents, or serotonin syndromes—consisting of hyperpyrexia, mental status changes, myoclonus, and delirium—that can lead to coma and death. MAO in the intestinal tract degrades tyramine. When MAO is inhibited by MAOIs, the individual is at risk for absorbing large amounts of tyramine and probably other substances (e.g., phenylethylamine), which can act as false neurotransmitters or indirect agonists and elevate blood pressure. Fortunately, dietary restrictions can markedly reduce the risk (Table 3–14). Various prohibited foods are included in lists in the PDR. These lists have been reviewed by several investigators, and relative risks have been attributed to many of the foods. As a general rule, we have begun to specifically advise patients to avoid eating Chinese food because of the ingredients used (e.g., soy sauce, sherry).

Table 3–14.   Foods to be avoided with monoamine oxidase inhibitors (MAOIs)

Foods definitely to be avoided:
  Beer, red wine
  Aged cheeses (cottage and cream cheese are allowed)
  Dry sausage
  Fava or Italian green beans
  Brewer's yeast
  Smoked fish
  Liver (beef or chicken)

Foods that may cause problems in large amounts but are otherwise less problematic:
  Alcohol
  Ripe avocado
  Yogurt
  Bananas (ripe)
  Soy sauce

Foods that were thought to be problems but are probably not problematic in usual
      quantities:
  Chocolate
  Figs
  Meat tenderizers
  Caffeine-containing beverages
  Raisins

Source.   Based on McCabe and Tsuang 1982.

The serotonin syndrome is generally not due to interaction with foodstuffs. It represents increased central 5-HT activity and may be particularly provoked by the addition of certain medications.

In some cases of either hypertensive or hyperpyrexic reactions, the exact cause is not clear. Of particular importance regarding medication interactions is warning patients to check with their physician before taking other medications along with the MAOIs. Meperidine (Demerol), epinephrine, local anesthetics (containing sympathomimetic agents), and decongestants can be particularly dangerous.

Frequently, we are asked which decongestant or antihistamine can be used with the MAOIs. Unfortunately, there is little in the way of prospective data. Diphenhydramine is used by many practitioners, with apparent success. One problem, however, with this approach is that some over-the-counter diphenhydramine elixirs contain pseudoephedrine, and at least one untoward interaction with the latter agent has been seen by our group. Another option is nasal sprays, but with this form, too, some patients may show increases in blood pressure.

Another issue has to do with general anesthesia—during ECT or surgery—in patients treated with MAOIs. Although at first glance this seems a frightening prospect, there have been many patients who have successfully undergone procedures requiring general anesthesia without consequence. Indeed, Dr. George Murray informed us, for the second edition of this manual, that Massachusetts General Hospital had collected reports on some 2,000 such cases. Obviously, anesthesiologists need to be apprised of a patient's medications in order to determine the safest approach. To this end, it is probably wise to have patients taking MAOIs carry a MedAlert Card. Still, in many settings, surgeons and anesthesiologists advise patients to stop taking MAOIs before undergoing surgery. Further study is needed to determine the most prudent approach to this knotty problem.

If a patient develops a surge in blood pressure with violent headaches, he or she should be instructed to go to a local emergency room. Phentolamine (Regitine), a central α-blocker, can be administered intravenously to reverse the acute rise in blood pressure. Years ago, some psychopharmacologists recommended that patients take oral chlorpromazine when headache occurred. We have stopped this practice unless patients have not had a documented increase in blood pressure, because some patients will display marked headaches secondary to a lowering of blood pressure. Instead, we provide our patients with nifedipine, a calcium channel blocker, in case they experience marked increases in blood pressure; 10 mg per hour until relief occurs (generally one or two doses) appears to be very helpful. To enhance absorption, patients should be instructed to bite into the capsule before swallowing. This approach may prove problematic in elderly patients, because acute lowering of blood pressure and myocardial infarction have been reported with this approach for these patients.

We advise patients with headaches to have their blood pressure checked. In addition, routine monitoring of blood pressure with an MAOI, particularly during the first 6 weeks of treatment, seems prudent (for both the hypotensive and the hypertensive effects of the drug).

Dosage and Administration

The traditional therapeutic dosage ranges of these three MAOIs are as follows: phenelzine, 45–90 mg/day; tranylcypromine, 30–60 mg/day; oral selegiline,

20–50 mg/day. Some patients require treatment at the higher end of the dosage range. For example, 90 mg/day of phenelzine is commonly required in a patient with severe depressive illness.

A patient treated with phenelzine should start taking the medication at 30 mg/day, and the dosage should be increased to 45 mg/day after 3 days. Thereafter, the dosage can be increased at a rate of 15 mg per week to 90 mg/day. We have seen patients who require as much as 120 mg/day; however, many patients cannot tolerate the orthostatic side effects of these drugs. Some investigators have recommended a dosage of 1 mg/kg per day of the drug as a guideline for adequacy of treatment.

For tranylcypromine, a starting dosage of 20 mg/day for 3 days seems reasonable. The dosage can then be increased to 30 mg/day for 1 week, with increases of 10 mg per week to 50–60 mg/day. The manufacturer's current recommended maximum dosage of the drug is 40 mg/day. One investigator, Dr. Jay Amsterdam, reported that extremely high dosages of the drug (110–130 mg/day) may help patients with even the most refractory depression. There is some thought that at such high dosages the drug is exerting alternative, additional effects—possibly acting as a reuptake blocker (Amsterdam and Berwish 1989). Once a patient has responded, the medication should be maintained for a length of time similar to that recommended for the TCAs.

Discontinuation

The currently available MAOIs irreversibly bind MAO to such a degree that it takes approximately 2 weeks after the MAOI is stopped for the enzyme to regenerate. During this time, tyramine and drug interactions may occur. Thus, it is important to inform patients that they should maintain their dietary and drug restrictions for 2 weeks after the MAOI is discontinued. In addition, these drugs should be tapered to avoid rebound hypomania. Rarely, the withdrawal of an MAOI elicits a psychiatric excitement or psychosis resembling a delirium more than mania. If the clinician wants to switch a patient from one MAOI to another, care must be taken to avoid drug-drug interactions. The clinician should taper the first MAOI and allow for a 10- to 14-day drug-free period before beginning another MAOI. Some patients have experienced severe untoward reactions in switching from one MAOI to another, particularly from phenelzine to tranylcypromine—perhaps reflecting the latter's amphetamine-like properties. In general, a good reason to switch from one MAOI to another is intolerance to side effects. If an adequate trial of an MAOI fails, there is little evidence that switching to another MAOI helps.

When a transition between a TCA and an MAOI is being made, the PDR recommends that patients stop taking all medications between trials for 10–14 days. Many clinicians, however, have reported that a briefer drug-free period (i.e., 1–5 days) is sufficient for the transition from a TCA to an MAOI. For the transition from an MAOI to a TCA, the 10- to 14-day period is generally recommended. The difference in these strategies is probably due to the 10- to 14-day period needed to regenerate MAO.

However, patients taking MAOIs should wait 2 weeks before starting fluoxetine. For the transition from fluoxetine to an MAOI, a 5-week period is recommended by the manufacturer because of the long half-life of the demethylated metabolite norfluoxetine. For the other SSRIs, a 2-week washout is adequate before starting an MAOI. Likewise, a 1- to 2-week washout should ensue before switching to an MAOI from venlafaxine and bupropion. The 5-HT$_2$ antagonists nefazodone and trazodone appear to require very short washouts; 1 week is quite enough.

Selective and Reversible Monoamine Oxidase Inhibitors

As described earlier, all of the currently available MAOIs at antidepressant doses are nonselective and irreversible inhibitors of MAO; that is, they irreversibly inhibit both MAO-A and MAO-B, and for enzyme activity to commence, new MAO must be generated. Drugs that selectively block MAO-B, such as selegiline, may substantially decrease the risk of hypertensive crises, because they do not substantially affect MAO in the gut. Similarly, a reversible inhibitor of MAO-A would have a low affinity for MAO and would be readily displaced by pressor amines, thus reducing the risk of a hypertensive crisis. Two RIMAs, moclobemide and brofaromine, were under investigation, but interest in marketing these drugs in the United States has waned considerably.

The FDA approved selegiline in 1991 for use in Parkinson's disease under the trade name Eldepryl. Much of the earlier clinical and scientific literature refers to selegiline by its earlier name, L-deprenyl. Selegiline has proved a useful drug in Parkinson's disease and may be the only antiparkinsonian drug that has neuroprotective qualities and modestly affects the progression of the illness. At the dosages used in Parkinson's disease, 5–10 mg/day, the drug is a selective but irreversible inhibitor of MAO-B. Unfortunately, currently available studies of the use of selegiline in depression suggest that dosages of 20–60 mg/day are required to relieve depression. At these higher dosages, both MAO-A and MAO-B are inhibited and hypertensive crises following ingestion of tyramine in foods are possible. One such case, albeit mild, has been reported in a patient treated with 20 mg/day of selegiline.

Over the past several years, a transdermal form of selegiline has also been studied for the treatment of depression. A selegiline transdermal system, marketed under the brand name Emsam, was approved by the FDA in February 2006.

There are numerous published clinical studies of the use of selegiline in depression (Agosti et al. 1991; Mann et al. 1989; Sunderland et al. 1994). These studies can be interpreted as confirming the clear therapeutic effect of selegiline in patients with atypical and chronic depression and more serious depression. Furthermore, the Sunderland et al. study suggests that at a dosage of 60 mg/day, selegiline is useful for and well tolerated by geriatric patients with treatment-resistant depression. The drug is of substantial clinical interest because its pattern of side effects at dosages up to 40 mg/day appears quite favorable compared with that of the older MAOIs. Selegiline does not seem to cause clinically significant orthostatic hypotension or sexual dysfunction, and it may cause less insomnia than the older drugs. Several patients who were unable to tolerate the side effects of older MAOIs have tolerated selegiline quite well. It should be noted, however, that most published selegiline trials have lasted only 4–6 weeks, and some patients treated with the older MAOIs develop clinically intolerable side effects only after taking the drug for 2–3 months. Psychiatrists already experienced in the MAOI management of patients may find selegiline worth trying in cases of treatment-resistant conditions. Patients who have a good antidepressant response to MAOIs but who are experiencing intolerable side effects may be the best candidates for selegiline.

Oral selegiline is currently not approved for use in depression. But transdermal selegiline is approved for the treatment of depression. Because selegiline is metabolized to R isomers of amphetamine and methamphetamine in the body and is a dopamine reuptake inhibitor, we strongly urge a 2-week interval between stopping an older MAOI and starting selegiline. Patients treated with transdermal selegiline at dosages higher than 6 mg/day should adhere to the usual restrictions of a low-tyramine diet. That being said, we have done studies of transdermal selegiline at dosages higher than 6 mg/day and have not observed any dietary effects. Three other comments are worth making. First, measuring platelet MAOI in patients who are taking selegiline is probably not useful, because almost complete inhibition occurs after 1 week at a dosage of 10 mg/day. Second, the drug is very expensive: a local drugstore charges around $5 per 5-mg pill. Finally, selegiline should not be stopped abruptly, because it is associated with a discontinuation syndrome consisting of nausea, dizziness, and hallucinations.

At least two studies have demonstrated efficacy of transdermal selegiline against placebo in major depression (Amsterdam 2003; Bodkin and Amsterdam 2002). Of interest is that in patch delivery, selegiline in brain may be a far more potent MAO-A inhibitor, and this may confer greater efficacy. The drug (in a patch) may earn FDA approval for acute and chronic major depression either with or without atypical features. The transdermal formulation bypasses gut and liver and allows for higher plasma levels with a low risk of foodstuff interactions. The drug is available in patches of 20, 30, and 40 mg/cm^2 (6, 9, and 12 mg/24 hours, respectively) applied daily. In clinical trials, the starting daily dose was typically 20 mg (6 mg/24 hours), and the daily dose was then increased by 10 mg (3 mg/24 hours) every 1–2 weeks to a maximum of 40 mg (12 mg/24 hours). The package insert indicates that dietary modifications are required for patients using EmSam 9 and 12 mg/24 hours, which pose greater risk of tyramine interaction than with the 6 mg/24 hours patch. This observation is based on a study in healthy control subjects in which a high-tyramine diet was associated with mild increases in blood pressure with the 9- and 12-mg patches. The risk of untoward interactions is largely theoretical. We have done studies that used the 9- and 12-mg doses without a restricted diet and have observed no increases in blood pressure.

Rash has been the primary side effect that was observed to be greater with transdermal selegiline than with placebo. While most patients do not have substantial reactions to the patch, some skin reactions can be quite intense. We have seen a few patients with erythema that extends far beyond the patch site, and pruritis is not uncommon. Oral diphenhydramine seems to help with the itching. After site reactions, insomnia is the next most common side effect and is consistent with the amphetamine-like effects of the drug. Standard sleep medications such as zolpidem or temazepam appear to be helpful and are well tolerated. While sleep does seem to normalize after the patient has taken the drug for a few weeks, just taking the patch off at night also seems to help. Unfortunately, taking half the dose might also decrease the efficacy of the transdermal selegiline. The patch, designed for 24-hour delivery, needs to be changed daily. Some patients have taken to cutting the 6 mg/24 hour patch in half if they cannot tolerate a full dose. Although cutting the patch should reduce the daily dose in proportion to the amount cut (since surface area of the patch is directly related to total drug dose), the manufacturer recommends against cutting the patch because compromising the integrity of the patch could affect reliability of transdermal drug delivery. The risk of a serotonin syndrome when transdermal selegiline is used in combination with a serotonergic drug appears reduced but not eliminated. Thus, the drug should not be combined with SSRIs, SNRIs, or most TCAs. However, orthostasis, weight gain, and sexual dysfunction appear to be much less of a problem with transdermal selegiline than with oral MAOIs.

Given the ease of use and better tolerability of transdermal selegiline versus oral MAOIs, we are typically using it before considering other MAOIs. The patient profile that may best fit with transdermal selegiline includes patients who have experienced failed trials with one or more classes of antidepressants, depressed patients with prominent fatigue or cognitive deficits, and patients with atypical depression.

Moclobemide is the best-studied RIMA. Its actions on MAO are easily reversed (i.e., do not require regeneration of the enzyme). Moclobemide has a half-life of only 1–3 hours. It is available in Europe, Canada, and other parts of the world, but not in the United States. Several thousand depressed patients have been enrolled in moclobemide studies over the past 10 years, and it has been found to be effective in a wide spectrum of depressive illnesses, including melancholic, endogenous, atypical, psychotic (in combination with a neuroleptic), and bipolar subtypes (Fitton et al. 1992).

Moclobemide appears to be effective in elderly as well as younger patients and may be effective in the treatment of social phobia. In unpublished South American trials, moclobemide appeared to be as effective as—if not more effective than—imipramine and superior to placebo. However, one meta-analysis in Europe (Lotufo-Neto et al. 1999) suggested that moclobemide was not a particularly effective antidepressant in comparison with imipramine and placebo. In another South American study, moclobemide was significantly more effective than placebo in the treatment of social phobia.

The primary advantages of moclobemide over standard MAOIs are its tolerability and its safety. Nausea is the only side effect reported more commonly for moclobemide than for placebo. Significant orthostasis and other cardiovascular side effects are usually not seen. Furthermore, moclobemide has proved safe in overdoses to 20 g.

Because moclobemide does not increase tyramine sensitivity (Cusson et al. 1991), the risk of dietary interactions appears low. In Europe, the only significant dietary restriction is avoiding large amounts of aged cheeses after taking a dose of the drug. Moclobemide is usually given after meals or at bedtime to minimize dietary interactions.

The risk of serious drug interactions also appears to be lower with moclobemide. However, serious interactions have been reported with meperidine, clomipramine, and possibly the SSRIs. There is one report that moclobemide has been administered safely with fluvoxamine and fluoxetine (Dingemanse 1993). It is unlikely that moclobemide will be introduced soon in the United States because of a number of failed trials, but it is available through pharmacies in Europe and Canada. Development of another RIMA, brofaromine, was also canceled because of an apparent lack of sufficient efficacy.

Norepinephrine Reuptake Inhibitors: Reboxetine and Atomoxetine

Reboxetine, a selective NRI antidepressant, has been in use for many years in Europe and South America. Similarly, atomoxetine (Strattera) is an NRI approved for the treatment of ADHD. Neither of these agents is approved for the treatment of depression in the United States, but both have been studied as potential antidepressants here. The American experience with both atomoxetine and reboxetine as antidepressants or adjunctive treatments to serotonergic antidepressants has been uneven. Monotherapy trials based in the United States have not been consistent in showing a benefit for either NRI in the treatment of depression. For reboxetine, a U.S. trial with statistically significant results was reported, but the effect size was small. Atomoxetine monotherapy trials have generally failed. Likewise, although some small open-label studies have found benefit of atomoxetine or reboxetine added to an SSRI in the treatment of resistant depression (Carpenter et al. 2005; Lucca et al. 2000; Papakostas et al. 2006), a study by Michelson et al. (2006) failed to demonstrate efficacy for atomoxetine augmentation in patients who did not respond to sertraline.

Although neurotransmitter systems are clearly interconnected, it is equally evident that not everyone who responds to one antidepressant will respond to another. The role of NRIs in the treatment of depression remains unclear.

Pharmacological Effects

Reboxetine and atomoxetine enhance central norepinephrine neurotransmission by selectively blocking the reuptake of norepinephrine. They are therefore *selective* NRIs. There is evidence that reboxetine directly modulates the activity of the norepinephrine-rich locus coeruleus in the brain.

Alterations in the noradrenergic system have long been noted in depressed patients. For example, levels of MHPG, the main metabolite of norepinephrine, are often increased in the urine, plasma, and cerebrospinal fluid of depressed patients relative to control subjects. Abnormalities have been noted in depressed patients in various norepinephrine receptors, including presynaptic α_2 receptors and postsynaptic α_1 and β receptors. Most antidepressants, even the SSRIs, are known to have specific effects on norepinephrine receptors. For example, most antidepressants are known to downregulate postsynaptic β receptors with chronic administration. In fact, this reduction in β receptors takes several weeks and is correlated with the typical lag time of 3–6 weeks needed for antidepressants to be effective.

Many symptoms of depression may be more closely related to norepinephrine function than to serotonin function. For example, symptoms such as fatigue, hypersomnia, motoric retardation, and anhedonia have been hypothesized to be more related to alterations in norepinephrine than to 5-HT, although both are clearly important (Montgomery 1998). There is a strong interrelationship between the noradrenergic and serotonergic systems.

Whether a selective NRI is more useful in treating some types of depression than other classes of agents remains to be seen. However, the selectivity of reboxetine in norepinephrine reuptake makes it unique among the antidepressants in the United States and Europe.

Indications

The only well-studied indication for reboxetine is for the treatment of major depression. European studies have compared reboxetine with various antidepressants and placebo. For the treatment of general depression, reboxetine appeared to be at least as effective as desipramine and fluoxetine (Massana 1998; Massana et al. 1999). Reboxetine, however, appeared to be superior to fluoxetine in improving social functioning. In addition, reboxetine was significantly better than fluoxetine in reducing symptoms of severe depression and melancholic depression. As expected, 1-year data showed that reboxetine is significantly more effective than placebo in preventing relapse and recurrence. The anecdotal experience of some psychiatrists overseas is that reboxetine is not a particularly robust antidepressant. In fact, Cipriani and colleagues (2009) found that of 12 newer-generation antidepressants available in Europe, reboxetine was consistently the least efficacious agent. Still, there may be some patients who respond better to noradrenergic agents than do others.

Although a noradrenergic agent would not necessarily be expected to be an effective treatment for panic disorder, it is clear that noradrenergic agents such as nortriptyline and desipramine are effective antipanic drugs. In double-blind studies comparing reboxetine with placebo in the treatment of panic disorder, reboxetine appeared to be effective. However, the effects were not seen until after 5 weeks of continuous treatment, and relatively higher doses of the drug may be required.

Two large-scale U.S. studies produced mixed results. In one, reboxetine had minimal, although statistically significant, benefit over placebo. Paroxetine appeared to produce greater benefit. In the other, no difference was seen between reboxetine and placebo. These studies held up any expected FDA approval for reboxetine.

Atomoxetine is approved only for the treatment of ADHD in both children and adults. The manufacturer, Eli Lilly, studied atomoxetine as a potential antidepressant without demonstrating consistent benefit. Atomoxetine has also been investigated in the treatment of pediatric enuresis (Shatkin 2004), Tourette's syndrome (Niederhofer 2006), and obesity (Gadde et al. 2006).

Side Effects

A specific norepinephrine reuptake blocker would be expected to have a side-effect profile that is different from those of other classes of antidepressants. Compared with the SSRIs, reboxetine and atomoxetine are less likely to produce nausea, diarrhea, somnolence, and sexual side effects (Mucci 1997). Unlike the TCAs, reboxetine does not have particularly strong anticholinergic effects. Thus, relative to the TCAs, reboxetine and atomoxetine are less associated with some antimuscarinic effects. However, common anticholinergic-like side effects, such as dry mouth, are also mediated by the noradrenergic system or by a change in noradrenergic/anticholinergic balance. Among the side effects that have been reported more commonly with reboxetine than with the SSRIs are dry mouth, constipation, urinary hesitancy, and hypotension. Urinary hesitancy is much more common in males treated with the NRIs than in those treated with fluoxetine, and caution should be taken in older men. Anecdotally, α_1 antagonists such as prazosin and tamsulosin may reverse the urinary hesitancy associated with the NRIs (Kasper and Wolf 2002). In rare cases, reboxetine was associated with scrotal shrinkage, reflecting muscle contraction, though this was not a serious issue with the drug.

The cardiovascular effects of the NRIs appear to be limited, with only 3% of patients reporting hypertension versus 1% of subjects receiving placebo. Increased heart rate was no more common than with placebo, but hypotension, although mild, was more common in patients treated with reboxetine than in those treated with fluoxetine or placebo.

Overdose

Like many of the newer antidepressants, reboxetine and atomoxetine appear to be relatively safe in overdose. There have been no fatal overdoses attributed to NRI overdose alone at the time of this writing. However, NRI overdoses are associated with emesis, confusion, and tachycardia.

Dosage and Administration

The starting adult dosage for reboxetine is typically 4 mg bid. For most patients, the starting dose will be the therapeutic dose. If no response is seen by 3–4 weeks, the dosage may be increased to the maximum dosage of 10 mg/day. The half-life of the drug suggests bid dosing, although qd dosing can be tried. In elderly patients, the typical starting dosage is 2 mg bid, with the maximum dosage of 6 mg/day.

Atomoxetine in the treatment of adult attention-deficit disorder is typically started at 40 mg/day, and the dosage is then increased to 80 mg/day after at least 3 days at the lower dosage. The usual maximum dosage is 100 mg/day.

Drug Interactions

Because of the lack of significant cytochrome P450 enzyme effects, reboxetine has very little in the way of pharmacokinetic interactions with other drugs. There may be a synergistic effect in combining NRIs with other stimulating agents such as amphetamine or bupropion. In addition, there can be synergistic effects of NRIs with a pressor agent or albuterol. The combination of NRIs and other antidepressants is largely untested but makes intuitive sense in the treatment of resistant depression. At least one study of the combination of sertraline and reboxetine in rats indicated that the combined drugs produced more rapid changes in serotonin and norepinephrine receptors than could be produced by either drug alone (Harkin et al. 1999).

The use of an NRI with an MAOI is generally contraindicated. Although a serotonin syndrome is unlikely, it is still possible that an NRI will interact with an MAOI in ways that might be problematic. There is some speculation that reboxetine might mitigate the hypertensive effects of dietary tyramine in patients taking MAOIs (Dostert et al. 1997).

Discontinuation

Because of its short half-life, reboxetine may pose a greater risk of causing discontinuation symptoms. At this time, specific syndromes have not been associated with the abrupt discontinuation of an NRI. However, given the pharmacokinetic profile of this drug, it would be prudent to discontinue it gradually. A suggested taper schedule is to decrease the total daily dose by no more than 2–4 mg each week.

Melatonin Agonist–5-HT$_{2C}$ Antagonist

Agomelatine represents one of the more novel approaches to the pharmacotherapy of depression. The drug's 5-HT$_{2C}$ antagonist pharmacology provides both antidepressant and anxiolytic properties, while the melatonin MT$_1$ and MT$_2$ agonist properties provide for sleep induction without much sedation. A disturbance of circadian rhythms has long been recognized in mood disorders, most notably in sleep and the diurnal variation common to melancholic depression. It remains to be seen whether a potent melatonin agonist has other benefits in the treatment of depression.

Agomelatine has demonstrated anxiolytic and antidepressant properties in animal models (Papp et al. 2006). Preliminary clinical trials have demonstrated that dosages above 25 mg/day appear effective in the treatment of depression (Loo et al. 2002a, 2002b). The first phase III trial to be completed was very encouraging. Agomelatine 25–50 mg/day was superior to placebo in the treatment of depression and was well tolerated (Kennedy and Emsley 2006). An analysis of more severely depressed patients within the sample of 212 patients studied indicated that this subset also appeared to respond to agomelatine. Thus, there is some hope that agomelatine may prove to be useful in severely depressed patients and perhaps patients with treatment-resistant depression. To date, five double-blind trials have indicated that agomelatine looks about as effective as comparators (venlafaxaine, paroxetine) and more effective than placebo (Dolder et al. 2008). There are also preliminary reports of agomelatine being useful in bipolar depression and seasonal affective disorder.

Even if agomelatine proves no more efficacious than currently available treatments, its favorable side-effect profile may be a distinct advantage over the side-effect profiles of many available antidepressants. Agomelatine's specific receptor effects are associated with fewer sexual side effects and less daytime sedation than those of most serotonergic antidepressants (Dubocovich 2006). In addition, there is no evidence of weight gain or of a discontinuation syndrome when the drug is stopped abruptly. The most common side effects of agomelatine reported thus far are headache, GI upset, and nasopharyngitis.

It is anticipated that the target dosage of agomelatine will be 25 mg/day, with some patients benefiting from a dosage of up to 50 mg/day. We can imagine the combination of agomelatine with either SSRIs, bupropion, or SNRIs in the treatment of resistant depression, but no studies have yet evaluated the augmenting benefit of agomelatine. The drug has been approved in Europe but, as of this writing, not in the United States.

Gepirone

Gepirone is an older agent that has been studied in the treatment of anxiety disorders and, more recently, in depression. Gepirone is in the same chemical class as buspirone but is a more potent 5-HT_{1A} agonist. An extended-release formulation of gepirone received a nonapprovable letter in 2004 but could be approved in the future with additional studies. Buspirone, now available generically, was never fully embraced by psychiatrists as an effective anxiolytic. Nonetheless, the drug was effective for some patients and was particularly popular in primary care settings. The exact place for gepirone in psychiatric practice remains to be seen. In the more than 20 years that gepirone has been studied, its efficacy has been established in generalized anxiety. Studies have also suggested that gepirone, compared with placebo, is effective in the treatment of major depression (Wilcox et al. 1996). It may be as effective as imipramine in depressed patients (Feiger 1996). Some of the comparisons with placebo have been significant but not robust. However, gepirone appears to have more robust separations from placebo in the treatment of atypical depression. In one earlier trial, there was a 62% response rate in patients with atypical depression treated for 8 weeks with up to 120 mg/day of gepirone versus only a 20% response rate in placebo-treated patients (McGrath et al. 1994). Subsequent work also supported the idea that gepirone may be selectively more effective in patients with atypical depression (Quitkin and Gibertine 2001).

Gepirone has generally been well tolerated in clinical trials. The most common side effect was dizziness, with some nausea, headache, and lightheadedness reported. Gepirone is probably weight neutral. The most effective dosage range with the extended-release form for the treatment of depression has been 40–80 mg/day.

We would consider gepirone as an alternative to bupropion or mirtazapine, in patients concerned about sexual side effects. In addition, it might be a first-line alternative to the SSRIs in patients with atypical depression. The role of gepirone as an augmenting agent to the SSRIs has not been assessed but intuitively makes some sense. It has never received FDA approval in the United States, and it is unclear whether it ever will.

Novel Antidepressants

A number of antidepressants that have had truly novel mechanisms of actions have been investigated in the past 10 years. Most have failed. Other novel agents will emerge, but the antidepressants with some type of monoamine action have been, by far, the most consistently effective.

Among the monoamine agents a class of great interest are the *triple reuptake inhibitors*. These drugs block the reuptake of dopamine in addition to 5-HT and norepinephrine. It is speculated that the dopamine-enhancing effects of these drugs might lead to earlier response and greater efficacy in some patients. Two triple reuptake drugs that are in early development are DOV 216303 and tesofensine. Tesofensine has shown consistent benefits as an anorexiant in early trials. Patients have lost an average of 14 kg at 24 weeks while taking 0.5 mg of tesofensine. This drug may also help with glucose control in type 2 diabetes and help the motor symptoms of Parkinson's disease. However, few data exist on its utility as an antidepressant other than from animal studies, in which the results are promising. Like tesofensine, DOV 216303 has shown antidepressant effects in animal models and appears well tolerated in Phase I trials. A concern about the dopamine reuptake inhibitors is abuse potential. Studies with tesofensine thus far have not indicated tolerance or withdrawal.

Another novel approach to the treatment of depression has been the use of cortisol-specific agents. Depression—particularly more serious forms of depression such as psychotic depression—is known to be associated with abnormalities in the hypothalamic-pituitary-adrenal axis, including changes in cortisol levels and secretion and increases in levels of corticotropin-releasing factor (CRF). Cortisol and its analogs, the glucocorticoids, are known to produce mood, cognitive, and psychotic symptoms that mimic, to some degree, what is observed in serious forms of depression. Cortisol synthesis inhibitors such as ketoconazole have shown some benefits in a subset of patients with hypercortisolemia. However, ketoconazole can be quite toxic at the doses required to inhibit cortisol synthesis. CRF1 antagonists have shown efficacy in early trials, but no large controlled trial has yet to show benefit of these agents. In fact, a recent report on a Pfizer CRF1 antagonist in major depression was negative. We have studied the glucocorticoid receptor antagonist mifepristone and have shown benefits in the treatment of psychotic symptoms of psychotic depression in early pilot trials and a multicenter Phase II trial. (Two of us [A.F.S. and C.D.] have a conflict of interest in owning equity in the company pursuing this indication.) However, three subsequent trials have failed to replicate the earlier findings. Additional controlled trials with mifepristone guided by blood levels and CRF antagonists are currently under way. Thus, the clinical efficacy of cortisol-specific treatments of depression awaits further study.

Another line of antidepressant research has involved the use of peptide hormone antagonists, including substance P antagonists, as antidepressants. In preliminary studies, two substance P antagonists developed by Merck were found to be superior to placebo in the treatment of major depression (Kramer et al. 1998, 2004). The drug also was well tolerated and had few side effects. However, subsequent trials of MK-0869, unfortunately, failed in all five Phase III trials (Keller et al. 2006), and the drug is no longer in development. Nonetheless, other pharmaceutical companies have developed substance P antagonists that are currently being studied in major depression and social phobia. Our hunch is that these drugs may prove to be more effective in treating anxiety disorders than treating depression. Other peptide hormone neurotransmitters that are being investigated for developing agents with antidepressant effects include somatostatin and cholecystokinin.

Yet another group of investigational drugs targets the glutamatergic system. Glutamate receptors have long been thought to play a part in the pathophysiology of depression. N-methyl-D-aspartate (NMDA) antagonists, and AMPA and kainate receptor agonists have antidepressant effects in animal models. Ketamine, which is thought to act on NMDA receptors, has been shown in small studies to have antidepressant effects in patients with resistant depression when given as a single intravenous dose. Unfortunately, ketamine can have untoward effects on perception, cognition, and blood pressure. These effects, along with the route of administration (intravenous), limit the utility of ketamine. Also, it is possible that chronic administration of ketamine may be toxic. Another glutamate-specific drug, riluzole, is a functional antagonist of glutamate receptors that is approved for use in the treatment of amyotrophic lateral sclerosis. Riluzole has shown benefit in the treatment of resistant depression in four small open-label studies. Although riluzole is effective orally, it is probably also not a practical drug, given its great expense. Controlled studies are anticipated with riluzole, but the only data available are from these open studies, which have involved about 50 patients total to date.

Inflammatory cytokines are thought to play a role in the pathophysiology of depression. Cytokines such as interleukin-6 and tumor necrosis factor–α are known to be increased in depression. These elevations appear to play a role in increasing CRF and cortisol levels in depression. In animal models, acute administration of these cytokines induces anhedonia, decreased libido, and decreased social interaction. It makes sense, therefore, that an anti-inflammatory drug might have antidepressant properties. In a study of etanercept, a tumor necrosis factor (TNF)–specific agent being investigated for the treatment of psoriasis, patients treated with the drug had significantly greater improvement in mood on the Beck Depression Inventory than did the patients receiving placebo. This benefit was independent of the magnitude of response obtained for the psoriasis. A variety of other drugs, including the TNF antibody infliximab, may be candidates for investigation in the treatment of depression.

Thus, there are many new targets for the treatment of depression. So far, however, monoamine drugs have been the only consistent class of drugs to show benefits in the treatment of major depression. Since many patients do not respond adequately to monoamine drugs, it is the hope of clinicians and patients everywhere that new advantageous agents will become available in the coming years.

Bibliography

Agosti V, Stewart JW, Quitkin FM: Life satisfaction and psychosocial functioning in chronic depression: effect of acute treatment with antidepressants. J Affect Disord 23:35–41, 1991

Aguglia E, Casacchia M, Cassano GB, et al: Double-blind study of the efficacy and safety of sertraline versus fluoxetine in major depression. Int Clin Psychopharmacol 8:197–202, 1993

Aizenberg D, Zemishlany Z, Weizman A: Cyproheptadine treatment of sexual dysfunction induced by serotonin reuptake inhibitors. Clin Neuropharmacol 18:320–324, 1995

Altamura AC, Pioli R, Vitto M, et al: Venlafaxine in social phobia: a study in selective serotonin reuptake inhibitor non-responders. Int Clin Psychopharmacol 14:239–245, 1999

American Psychiatric Association: Diagnostic and Statistical Manual of Mental Disorders, 4th Edition. Washington, DC, American Psychiatric Association, 1994

Amsterdam JD: A double-blind, placebo-controlled trial of the safety and efficacy of selegiline transdermal system without dietary restrictions in patients with major depressive disorder. J Clin Psychiatry 64:208–214, 2003

Amsterdam JD, Berwish NJ: High dose tranylcypromine therapy for refractory depression. Pharmacopsychiatry 22:21–25, 1989

Amsterdam JD, Hornig-Rohan M, Maislin G: Efficacy of alprazolam in reducing fluoxetine-induced jitteriness in patients with major depression. J Clin Psychiatry 55:394–400, 1994a

Amsterdam JD, Maislin G, Potter L: Fluoxetine efficacy in treatment resistant depression. Prog Neuropsychopharmacol Biol Psychiatry 18:243–261, 1994b

Ansseau M, Darimont P, Lecoq A, et al: Controlled comparison of nefazodone and amitriptyline in major depressive inpatients. Psychopharmacology (Berl) 115:254–260, 1994

Anton RF, Sexauer JD: Efficacy of amoxapine in psychotic depression. Am J Psychiatry 140:1344–1347, 1983

Aranda-Michel J, Koehler A, Bejarano PA, et al: Nefazodone-induced liver failure: report of three cases. Ann Intern Med 130 (4, part 1):285–288, 1999

Aranow RB, Hudson JL, Pope HG, et al: Elevated antidepressant plasma levels after addition of fluoxetine. Am J Psychiatry 146:911–913, 1989

Archer DF, Dupont CM, Constantine GD, et al: Desvenlafaxine for the treatment of vasomotor symptoms associated with menopause: a double-blind, randomized, placebo-controlled trial of efficacy and safety. Am J Obstet Gynecol 200(3):238.e1–238.e10, 2009

Arminen SL, Ikonen U, Pulkkinen P, et al: A 12-week double-blind multi-centre study of paroxetine and imipramine in hospitalized depressed patients. Acta Psychiatr Scand 89:382–389, 1994

Armitage R, Rush AJ, Trivedi M, et al: The effects of nefazodone on sleep architecture in depression. Neuropsychopharmacology 10:123–127, 1994

Asakura S, Tajima O, Koyama T: Fluvoxamine treatment of generalized social anxiety disorder in Japan: a randomized double-blind, placebo-controlled study. Int J Neuropsychopharmacol 10:263–274, 2007

Åsberg M, Cronholm B, Sjoqvist F, et al: Relationship between plasma level and therapeutic effect of nortriptyline. Br Med J 3:331–334, 1971

Ashton AK, Bennett RG: Sildenafil treatment of serotonin reuptake inhibitor–induced sexual dysfunction (letter). J Clinical Psychiatry 60:194–195, 1999

Ashton AK, Rosen RC: Bupropion as an antidote for serotonin reuptake inhibitor–induced sexual dysfunction. J Clin Psychiatry 59:112–115, 1998

Balon R: Intermittent amantadine for fluoxetine-induced anorgasmia. J Sex Marital Ther 22:290–292, 1996

Banasr M, Soumier A, Hery M, et al: Agomelatine, a new antidepressant, induces regional changes in hippocampal neurogenesis. Biol Psychiatry 59:1087–1096, 2006

Banham ND: Fatal venlafaxine overdose (letter; comment). Med J Aust 169:445, 448, 1998

Barbey JT, Roose SP: SSRI safety in overdose. J Clin Psychiatry 59 (suppl 15):42–48, 1998

Beasley C Jr, Dornseif BE, Bosomworth JC, et al: Fluoxetine and suicide: a meta-analysis of controlled trials of treatment for depression. BMJ 23:685–692, 1991 [also see comments] [erratum: BMJ 23:968, 1991]

Beasley C Jr, Potvin JH, Masica DN, et al: Fluoxetine: no association with suicidality in obsessive-compulsive disorder. J Affect Disord 24:1–10, 1992

Belanoff J, Flores B, Kalezhan M, et al: Rapid reversal of psychotic major depression using mifepristone. J Clin Psychopharmacol 21:516–521, 2001

Belanoff JK, Rothschild AJ, Cassidy F, et al: An open label trial of C-1073 (mifepristone) for psychotic major depression. Biol Psychiatry 52:386–392, 2002 [also see comment]

Bell IR, Cole JO: Fluoxetine induces elevation of desipramine levels and exacerbation of geriatric nonpsychotic depression (letter). J Clin Psychopharmacol 8:447–448, 1988

Bellino S, Paradiso E, Bogetto F: Efficacy and tolerability of pharmacotherapies for borderline personality disorder. CNS Drugs 22:671–692, 2008

Benazzi FL: Nefazodone withdrawal symptoms. Can J Psychiatry 43:194–195, 1998 [also see comment: Can J Psychiatry 44:286–287, 1999]

Berk M, Ichim C, Brook S: Efficacy of mirtazapine add-on therapy to haloperidol in the treatment of negative symptoms of schizophrenia: a double-blind, randomized, placebo-controlled study. Int Clin Psychopharmacol 16:87–92, 2001

Bertschy G, Vandel S, Vandel B, et al: Fluvoxamine-tricyclic antidepressant interaction: an accidental finding. Eur J Clin Pharmacol 40:119–120, 1991

Bhagwagar Z, Cowen PJ: "It's not over when it's over": persistent neurobiological abnormalities in recovered depressed patients. Psychol Med 38:307–313, 2008

Bhatara VS, Bandettini FC: Possible interaction between sertraline and tranylcypromine. Clin Pharm 12:222–225, 1993

Bhattacharjee C, Smith M, Todd F, et al: Bupropion overdose: a potential problem with the new "miracle" anti-smoking drug. Int J Clin Pract 55:221–222, 2001

Bielski RJ, Cunningham L, Horrigan JP, et al: Gepirone extended-release in the treatment of adult outpatients with major depressive disorder: a double-blind, randomized, placebo-controlled, parallel-group study. J Clin Psychiatry 69:571–577, 2008

Bielski RJ, Ventura D, Chang CC: A double-blind comparison of escitalopram and venlafaxine extended release in the treatment of major depressive disorder. J Clin Psychiatry 65:1190–1196, 2004

Black DW, Wesner R, Gabel J: The abrupt discontinuation of fluvoxamine in patients with panic disorder. J Clin Psychiatry 54:146–149, 1993

Bodkin JA, Amsterdam JD: Transdermal selegiline in major depression: a double-blind, placebo-controlled, parallel-group study in outpatients. Am J Psychiatry 159:1869–1875, 2002

Borys DJ, Setzer SC, Ling LJ, et al: Acute fluoxetine overdose: a report of 234 cases. Am J Emerg Med 10:115–120, 1992

Boyd IW: Venlafaxine withdrawal reactions. Med J Aust 169:91–92, 1998

Brown WA, Harrison W: Are patients who are intolerant to one SSRI intolerant to another? J Clin Psychiatry 56:30–34, 1995

Buckley NA, McManus PR: Fatal toxicity of serotoninergic and other antidepressant drugs: analysis of United Kingdom mortality data. BMJ 325(7376):1332–1333, 2002 [also see comment]

Cankurtaran ES, Ozalp E, Soygur H, et al: Mirtazapine improves sleep and lowers anxiety and depression in cancer patients: superiority over imipramine. Support Care Cancer 16:1291–1298, 2008

Cantwell DP: ADHD through the life span: the role of bupropion in treatment. J Clin Psychiatry 59 (4, suppl):92–94, 1998

Carpenter LL, Jocic Z, Hall JM, et al: Mirtazapine augmentation in the treatment of refractory depression. J Clin Psychiatry 60:45–49, 1999a

Carpenter LL, Leon Z, Yasmin S, et al: Clinical experience with mirtazapine in the treatment of panic disorder. Ann Clin Psychiatry 11:81–86, 1999b

Carpenter LL, Milosavljevic N, Schecter JM, et al: Augmentation with open-label atomoxetine for partial or nonresponse to antidepressants. J Clin Psychiatry 66:1234–1238, 2005

Chen CC, Lin CS, Ko YP, et al: Premedication with mirtazapine reduces preoperative anxiety and postoperative nausea and vomiting. Anesth Analg 106:109–113, 2008

Chouinard G, Goodman W, Greist J, et al: Results of a double-blind placebo-controlled trial of a new serotonin uptake inhibitor, sertraline, in the treatment of obsessive-compulsive disorder. Psychopharmacol Bull 26:279–284, 1990

Cipriani A, Furukawa TA, Salanti G, et al: Comparative efficacy and acceptability of 12 new-generation antidepressants: a multiple-treatments meta-analysis. Lancet 373:746–758, 2009

Claghorn J: A double-blind comparison of paroxetine and placebo in the treatment of depressed outpatients. Int Clin Psychopharmacol 6 (suppl 4):25–30, 1992

Claghorn JL, Feighner JP: A double-blind comparison of paroxetine with imipramine in the long-term treatment of depression. J Clin Psychopharmacol 13 (6, suppl 2):23S–27S, 1993

Clayton AH, Warnock JK, Kornstein SG, et al: A placebo-controlled trial of bupropion SR as an antidote for selective serotonin reuptake inhibitor–induced sexual dysfunction. J Clin Psychiatry 65:62–67, 2004

Clerc GE, Ruimy P, Verdeau-Palles J: A double-blind comparison of venlafaxine and fluoxetine in patients hospitalized for major depression and melancholia. The Venlafaxine French Inpatient Study Group. Int Clin Psychopharmacol 9:139–143, 1994

Cohn CK, Shrivastava R, Mendels J, et al: Double-blind, multicenter comparison of sertraline and amitriptyline in elderly depressed patients. J Clin Psychiatry 51 (12, suppl):28–33, 1990

Cole JO, Bodkin JA: Antidepressant drug side effects. J Clin Psychiatry 51 (1, suppl):21–26, 1990

Connor KM, Davidson JR, Weisler RH, et al: A pilot study of mirtazapine in posttraumatic stress disorder. Int Clin Psychopharmacol 14:29–31, 1999

Cooper GL: The safety of fluoxetine—an update. Br J Psychiatry 153 (suppl 3):77–86, 1988

Cougnard A, Verdoux H, Grolleau A, et al: Impact of antidepressants on the risk of suicide in patients with depression in real-life conditions: a decision analysis model. Psychol Med 9:1–9, 2008

Cusson JR, Goldenberg E, Larochelle P: Effect of a novel monoamine-oxidase inhibitor, moclobemide, on the sensitivity to intravenous tyramine and norepinephrine in humans. J Clin Pharmacol 31:462–467, 1991

Dalfen AK, Stewart DE: Who develops severe or fatal adverse drug reactions to selective serotonin reuptake inhibitors? Can J Psychiatry 46:258–263, 2001

Dallal A, Chouinard G: Withdrawal and rebound symptoms associated with abrupt discontinuation of venlafaxine (letter). J Clin Psychopharmacol 18:343–344, 1998

Daniels RJ: Serotonin syndrome due to venlafaxine overdose. J Accid Emerg Med 15:333–334, 1998

Danish University Antidepressant Group: Paroxetine: a selective serotonin reuptake inhibitor showing better tolerance but weaker antidepressant effect than clomipramine in a controlled multicenter study. J Affect Disord 18:289–299, 1990

Davidson JR, DuPont RL, Hedges D, et al: Efficacy, safety, and tolerability of venlafaxine extended release and buspirone in outpatients with generalized anxiety disorder. J Clin Psychiatry 60:528–535, 1999

Davidson JR, Weisler RH, Butterfield MI, et al: Mirtazapine vs placebo in posttraumatic stress disorder: a pilot trial. Biol Psychiatry 53(2):188–191, 2003

Davis JL, Smith RL: Painful peripheral diabetic neuropathy treated with venlafaxine HCl extended release capsules (letter; see comments). Diabetes Care 22:1909–1910, 1999

DeBattista C, Doghramji K, Menza MA, et al: Adjunct modafinil for the short-term treatment of fatigue and sleepiness in patients with major depressive disorder: a preliminary double-blind, placebo-controlled study. J Clin Psychiatry 64:1057–1064, 2003

DeBattista C, Lembke A, Solvason HB, et al: A prospective trial of modafinil as an adjunctive treatment of major depression. J Clin Psychopharmacol 24:87–90, 2004

DeBattista C, Solvason B, Poirier J, et al: A placebo-controlled, randomized, double-blind study of adjunctive bupropion sustained release in the treatment of SSRI-induced sexual dysfunction. J Clin Psychiatry 66:844–848, 2005

DeBattista C, Belanoff J, Glass S, et al: Mifepristone versus placebo in the treatment of psychosis in patients with psychotic major depression. Biol Psychiatry 60:1343–1349, 2006

den Boer JA, Bosker FJ, Meesters Y: Clinical efficacy of agomelatine in depression: the evidence. Int Clin Psychopharmacol 21 (suppl 1):S21–S24, 2006

Dessain EC, Schatzberg AF, Woods BT, et al: Maprotiline treatment in depression: a perspective on seizures. Arch Gen Psychiatry 43:86–90, 1986

Detke MJ, Lu Y, Goldstein DJ, et al: Duloxetine, 60 mg once daily, for major depressive disorder: a randomized double-blind, placebo-controlled trial. J Clin Psychiatry 63:308–315, 2002

Diaz-Martinez A, Benassinni O, Ontiveros A, et al: A randomized, open-label comparison of venlafaxine and fluoxetine in depressed outpatients. Clin Ther 20:467–476, 1998

Dingemanse J: An update of recent moclobemide interaction data. Int Clin Psychopharmacol 7:167–180, 1993

Dolder CR, Nelson M, Snider M: Agomelatine treatment of major depressive disorder. Ann Pharmacother 42:1822–1831, 2008

Doogan DP, Langdon CJ: A double-blind, placebo-controlled comparison of sertraline and dothiepin in the treatment of major depression in general practice. Int Clin Psychopharmacol 9:95–100, 1994

Dostert P, Benedetti MS, Poggesi I: Review of the pharmacokinetics and metabolism of reboxetine, a selective noradrenaline reuptake inhibitor. Eur Neuropsychopharmacol 7 (suppl 1):S23–S35 [discussion S71–S73], 1997

Dubocovich ML: Agomelatine targets a range of major depressive disorder symptoms. Curr Opin Investig Drugs 7(7):670–80, 2006

Dunner DL: An overview of paroxetine in the elderly. Gerontology 1:21–27, 1994

Einarson TR, Arikian SR, Casciano J, et al: Comparison of extended-release venlafaxine, selective serotonin reuptake inhibitors, and tricyclic antidepressants in the treatment of depression: a meta-analysis of randomized controlled trials. Clin Ther 21:296–308, 1999

Ellingrod VL, Perry PJ: Venlafaxine: a heterocyclic antidepressant. Am J Hosp Pharm 51:3033–3046, 1994

Falkai P: Mirtazapine: other indications. J Clin Psychiatry 60 (suppl 17):36–40 [discussion 46–48], 1999

Farah A: Relief of SSRI-induced sexual dysfunction with mirtazapine treatment (letter). J Clin Psychiatry 60:260–261, 1999

Fava M, Rosenbaum JF, McGrath PJ, et al: Lithium and tricyclic augmentation of fluoxetine treatment for resistant major depression: a double-blind, controlled study. Am J Psychiatry 151:1372–1374, 1994

Fava M, Dunner DL, Greist JH, et al: Efficacy and safety of mirtazapine in major depressive disorder patients after SSRI treatment failure: an open-label trial. J Clin Psychiatry 62:413–420, 2001

Fava M, Nurnberg HG, Seidman SN, et al: Efficacy and safety of sildenafil in men with serotonergic antidepressant-associated erectile dysfunction: results from a randomized, double-blind, placebo-controlled trial. J Clin Psychiatry 67:240–246, 2006a

Fava M, Rush AJ, Wisniewski SR, et al: A comparison of mirtazapine and nortriptyline following two consecutive failed medication treatments for depressed outpatients: a STAR*D report. Am J Psychiatry 163:1161–1172, 2006b

Fawcett J, Barkin RL: Review of the results from clinical studies on the efficacy, safety and tolerability of mirtazapine for the treatment of patients with major depression. J Affect Disord 51:267–285, 1998

Feiger AD: A double-blind comparison of gepirone extended release, imipramine, and placebo in the treatment of outpatient major depression. Psychopharmacol Bull 32:659–665, 1996

Feiger A, Kiev A, Shrivastava RK, et al: Nefazodone versus sertraline in outpatients with major depression: focus on efficacy, tolerability, and effects on sexual function and satisfaction. J Clin Psychiatry 57 (2, suppl):53–62, 1996

Feiger AD, Tourian KA, Rosas GR, et al: A placebo-controlled study evaluating the efficacy and safety of flexible-dose desvenlafaxine treatment in outpatients with major depressive disorder. CNS Spectr 14:41–50, 2009

Feighner JP, Aden GC, Fabre LF, et al: Comparison of alprazolam, imipramine and placebo in the treatment of depression. JAMA 249:3056–3064, 1983

Feighner JP, Herbstein J, Damlouji N: Combined MAOI, TCA, and direct stimulant therapy of treatment-resistant depression. J Clin Psychiatry 46:206–209, 1985

Fisher S, Bryant SG, Kent TA: Postmarketing surveillance by patient self monitoring: trazodone vs fluoxetine. J Clin Psychopharmacol 13:235–242, 1992

Fitton A, Faulds D, Goa KL: Moclobemide: a review of its pharmacology and therapeutic use in depressive illness. Drugs 43:561–596, 1992

Fluoxetine Bulimia Nervosa Collaborative Study Group: Fluoxetine in the treatment of bulimia nervosa: a multicenter, placebo-controlled, double-blind trial. Arch Gen Psychiatry 49:139–147, 1992

Fontaine R, Ontiveros A, Elie R, et al: A double-blind comparison of nefazodone, imipramine, and placebo in major depression. J Clin Psychiatry 55:234–241, 1994

Frank E, Kupfer DJ, Perl JM, et al: Three-year outcomes for maintenance therapy of recurrent depression. Arch Gen Psychiatry 47:1093–1104, 1990

Friel PN, Logan BK, Fligner CL: Three fatal drug overdoses involving bupropion. J Anal Toxicol 17(7):436–438, 1993

Gadde KM, Yonish GM, Wagner HR 2nd, et al: Atomoxetine for weight reduction in obese women: a preliminary randomised controlled trial. Int J Obes (Lond) 30:1138–1142, 2006

Gambi F, De Berardis D, Campanella D, et al: Mirtazapine treatment of generalized anxiety disorder: a fixed-dose, open-label study. J Psychopharmacol 19:483–487, 2005

Gelenberg AJ, Lydiard RB, Rudolph RL, et al: Efficacy of venlafaxine extended-release capsules in nondepressed outpatients with generalized anxiety disorder: a 6-month randomized controlled trial. JAMA 283:3082–3088, 2000

Gittelman DK, Kirby MG: A seizure following bupropion overdose (letter). J Clin Psychiatry 54:162, 1993

Glassman A, Perel J, Shostak M, et al: Clinical implication of imipramine plasma levels for depressive illness. Arch Gen Psychiatry 34:197–204, 1977

Golden RN, Rudorfer MV, Sherer M, et al: Bupropion in depression I: biochemical effects and clinical response. Arch Gen Psychiatry 45:139–143, 1988

Goldstein D, Bitter I, Lu Y, et al: Duloxetine in the treatment of depression: a double-blind, placebo-controlled comparison with paroxetine. Eur Psychiatry 17 (suppl 1): 98, 2002

Goldstein MG: Bupropion sustained release and smoking cessation. J Clin Psychiatry 59 (4, suppl):66–72, 1998

Goodnick PJ: Pharmacokinetics of second generation antidepressants: bupropion. Psychopharmacol Bull 27:513–519, 1991

Goodnick PJ, Puig A, DeVane CL, et al: Mirtazapine in major depression with comorbid generalized anxiety disorder. J Clin Psychiatry 60:446–448, 1999

Gorwood P, Corruble E, Falissard B, et al: Toxic effects of depression on brain function: impairment of delayed recall and the cumulative length of depressive disorder in a large sample of depressed outpatients. Am J Psychiatry 165:731–739, 2008

Grimsley SR, Jann MW: Paroxetine, sertraline, and fluvoxamine: new selective serotonin reuptake inhibitors. Clin Pharm 11:930–957, 1992

Gupta S, Ghaly N, Dewan M: Augmenting fluoxetine with dextroamphetamine to treat refractory depression. Hosp Community Psychiatry 43:281–283, 1992

Gupta S, Droney T, Masand P, et al: SSRI-induced sexual dysfunction treated with sildenafil. Depress Anxiety 9:180–182, 1999

Hamilton MS, Opler LA: Akathisia, suicidality, and fluoxetine. J Clin Psychiatry 53:401–406, 1992 [also see comments]

Hammad TA, Laughren T, Racoosin J: Suicidality in pediatric patients treated with antidepressant drugs. Arch Gen Psychiatry 63:332–339, 2006a

Hammad TA, Laughren TP, Racoosin JA: Suicide rates in short-term randomized controlled trials of newer antidepressants. J Clin Psychopharmacol 26:203–207, 2006b

Hamner MB, Frueh BC: Response to venlafaxine in a previously antidepressant treatment-resistant combat veteran with post-traumatic stress disorder. Int Clin Psychopharmacol 13:233–234, 1998

Haria M, Fitton A, McTavish D: Trazodone: a review of its pharmacology, therapeutic use in depression and therapeutic potential in other disorders. Drugs Aging 4:331–355, 1994

Harkin A, Kelly JP, McNamara M, et al: Activity and onset of action of reboxetine and effect of combination with sertraline in an animal model of depression. Eur J Pharmacol 364:123–132, 1999

Harris MG, Benfield P: Fluoxetine: a review of its pharmacodynamic and pharmacokinetic properties, and therapeutic use in older patients with depressive illness. Drugs Aging 6:64–84, 1995

Henry JA: Overdose and safety with fluvoxamine. Int Clin Psychopharmacol 6 (suppl 3):41–45 [discussion 45–47], 1991

Hidalgo R, Hertzberg MA, Mellman T, et al: Nefazodone in post-traumatic stress disorder: results from six open-label trials. Int Clin Psychopharmacol 14(2):61–68, 1999

Hirschfeld RM: Efficacy of SSRIs and newer antidepressants in severe depression: comparison with TCAs. J Clin Psychiatry 60:326–335, 1999

Holliday SM, Benfield P: Venlafaxine: a review of its pharmacology and therapeutic potential in depression. Drugs 49:280–294, 1995

Holliday SM, Plosker GL: Paroxetine: a review of its pharmacology, therapeutic use in depression and therapeutic potential in diabetic neuropathy. Drugs Aging 3: 278–299, 1993

Howland RH: Pharmacotherapy of dysthymia: a review. J Clin Psychopharmacol 11:83–92, 1991

Jacobsen FM: Fluoxetine-induced sexual dysfunction and an open trial of yohimbine. J Clin Psychiatry 53:119–122, 1992 [also see comments]

Jaffe PD, Batziris HP, van der Hoeven P, et al: A study involving venlafaxine overdoses: comparison of fatal and therapeutic concentrations in postmortem specimens. J Forensic Sci 44:193–196, 1999

Jermain DM, Preece CK, Sykes RL, et al: Luteal phase sertraline treatment for premenstrual dysphoric disorder: results of a double-blind, placebo-controlled, crossover study. Arch Fam Med 8:328–332, 1999

Johnson H, Bouman WP, Lawton J: Withdrawal reaction associated with venlafaxine. BMJ 317(7161):787, 1998

Kaizar EE, Greenhouse JB, Seltman H, et al: Do antidepressants cause suicidality in children? A Bayesian meta-analysis. Clin Trials 3(2):73–90 [discussion 91–98], 2006

Kamath J, Handratta V: Desvenlafaxine succinate for major depressive disorder: a critical review of the evidence. Expert Rev Neurother 8:1787–1797, 2008

Kasper S, Wolf R: Successful treatment of reboxetine-induced urinary hesitancy with tamsulosin. Eur Neuropsychopharmacol 12:119–122, 2002

Kast RE, Foley KF: Cancer chemotherapy and cachexia: mirtazapine and olanzapine are 5-HT3 antagonists with good antinausea effects. Eur J Cancer Care (Engl) 16:351–354, 2007

Katona CL, Abou-Saleh MT, Harrison DA, et al: Placebo-controlled trial of lithium augmentation of fluoxetine and lofepramine. Br J Psychiatry 166:80–86, 1995

Kavoussi RJ, Liu J, Coccaro EF: An open trial of sertraline in personality disordered patients with impulsive aggression. J Clin Psychiatry 55:137-141, 1994

Kaye WH, Weltzin TE, Hsu LK, et al: An open trial of fluoxetine in patients with anorexia nervosa. J Clin Psychiatry 52:464–471, 1991

Keller M, Montgomery S, Ball W, et al: Lack of efficacy of the substance P (neurokinin 1) receptor antagonist aprepitant in the treatment of major depressive disorder. Biol Psychiatry 59:216–223, 2006

Keller MB, Trivedi MH, Thase ME, et al: The Prevention of Recurrent Episodes of Depression with Venlafaxine for Two Years (PREVENT) Study: outcomes from the 2-year and combined maintenance phases. J Clin Psychiatry 68:1246–1256, 2007

Keller Ashton A, Hamer R, Rosen RC: Serotonin reuptake inhibitor–induced sexual dysfunction and its treatment: a large-scale retrospective study of 596 psychiatric outpatients. J Sex Marital Ther 23:165–175, 1997

Kennedy SH, Emsley R: Placebo-controlled trial of agomelatine in the treatment of major depressive disorder. Eur Neuropsychopharmacol 16(2):93–100, 2006

Keppel Hesselink JM, de Jongh PM: Sertraline in the prevention of depression (comment). Br J Psychiatry 161:270–271, 1992

Khan A, Khan S: Placebo response in depression: a perspective for clinical practice. Psychopharmacol Bull 41:91–98, 2008

Kiayias JA, Vlachou ED, Lakka-Papadodima E: Venlafaxine HCl in the treatment of painful peripheral diabetic neuropathy (letter; see comment). Diabetes Care 23: 699, 2000

Killen JD, Robinson TN, Ammerman S, et al: Randomized clinical trial of the efficacy of bupropion combined with nicotine patch in the treatment of adolescent smokers. J Consult Clin Psychol 72:729–735, 2004

Kim SW, Shin IS, Kim JM, et al: Effectiveness of mirtazapine for nausea and insomnia in cancer patients with depression. Psychiatry Clin Neurosci 62:75–83, 2008

Kline NS: Clinical experience with iproniazid (Marsilid). J Clin Exp Psychopathol 19 (2, suppl 1): 72–78 [discussion 78–79], 1958

Kornstein SG: Maintenance therapy to prevent recurrence of depression: summary and implications of the PREVENT Study. Expert Rev Neurother 8:737–742, 2008

Kotlyar M, Golding M, Brewer ER, et al: Possible nefazodone withdrawal syndrome (letter). Am J Psychiatry 156:1117, 1999

Koutouvidis N, Pratikakis M, Fotiadou A: The use of mirtazapine in a group of 11 patients following poor compliance to selective serotonin reuptake inhibitor treatment due to sexual dysfunction. Int Clin Psychopharmacol 14:253–255, 1999

Kramer MS, Cutler N, Feighner J, et al: Distinct mechanism for antidepressant activity by blockade of central substance P receptors. Science 281:1640–1645, 1998 [also see comments]

Kramer MS, Winokur A, Kelsey J, et al: Demonstration of the efficacy and safety of a novel substance P (NK1) receptor antagonist in major depression. Neuropsychopharmacology 29:385–392, 2004

Kuhn R: Uber die behandlung depressiver zustande mit einem iminodibenzylderivat (G22355). Schweiz Med Wochenschr 87:1135–1140, 1957

Kuhn R: The treatment of depressive states with G22 355 (imipramine hydrochloride). Am J Psychiatry 115:459–464, 1958

Kupfer DJ, Frank E, Perel JM, et al: Five-year outcome for maintenance therapies in recurrent depression. Arch Gen Psychiatry 49:769–773, 1992

Labbate LA, Pollack MH: Treatment of fluoxetine-induced sexual dysfunction with bupropion: a case report. Ann Clin Psychiatry 6:13–15, 1994

Landen M, Eriksson E, Agren H, et al: Effect of buspirone on sexual dysfunction in depressed patients treated with selective serotonin reuptake inhibitors. J Clin Psychopharmacol 19:268–271, 1999

Lauber C: Nefazodone withdrawal syndrome (letter). Can J Psychiatry 44:285–286, 1999

Leaf EV: Comment: venlafaxine overdose and seizure. Ann Pharmacother 32:135–136, 1998

Leiononen E, Skarstein J, Behnke K, et al: Efficacy and tolerability of mirtazapine versus citalopram: a double-blind, randomized study in patients with major depressive disorder. Int Clin Psychopharmacol 14:329–337, 1999

Lenderking WR, Tennen H, Nackley JF, et al: The effects of venlafaxine on social activity level in depressed outpatients. J Clin Psychiatry 60:157–163, 1999

Liappas J, Paparrigopoulos T, Tzavellas E, et al: Mirtazapine and venlafaxine in the management of collateral psychopathology during alcohol detoxification. Prog Neuropsychopharmacol Biol Psychiatry 29(1):55–60, 2005

Liebowitz MR, Quitkin FM, Stewart JW: Antidepressant specificity in atypical depression. Arch Gen Psychiatry 45:129–137, 1988

Lohoff FW, Rickels K: Desvenlafaxine succinate for the treatment of major depressive disorder. Expert Opin Pharmacother 9:2129–2136, 2008

Lonnqvist J, Sihvo S, Syvalahti E, et al: Moclobemide and fluoxetine in atypical depression: a double-blind trial. J Affect Disord 32:169–177, 1994

Loo H, Dalery J, Macher JP, et al: Pilot study comparing in blind the therapeutic effect of two doses of agomelatine, melatoninergic agonist and selective 5HT2C receptors antagonist, in the treatment of major depressive disorders [in French]. Encephale 28:356–362, 2002a

Loo H, Hale A, D'haenen H: Determination of the dose of agomelatine, a melatoninergic agonist and selective 5-HT(2C) antagonist, in the treatment of major depressive disorder: a placebo-controlled dose range study. Int Clin Psychopharmacol 17:239–247, 2002b

Lotufo-Neto F, Trivedi M, Thase ME: Meta-analysis of the reversible inhibitors of monoamine oxidase type A moclobemide and brofaromine for the treatment of depression. Neuropsychopharmacology 20:226–247, 1999

Louie AK, Lewis TB, Lannon RA: Use of low-dose fluoxetine in major depression and panic disorder. J Clin Psychiatry 54:435–438, 1993

Lucca A, Serretti A, Smeraldi E: Effect of reboxetine augmentation in SSRI resistant patients. Hum Psychopharmacol 15:143–145, 2000

Luckhaus C, Jacob C: Venlafaxine withdrawal syndrome not prevented by maprotiline, but resolved by sertraline (letter). Int J Neuropsychopharmacol 4(1):43–44, 2001

Mainie I, McGurk C, McClintock G, et al: Seizures after bupropion overdose (letter). Lancet 357(9268):1624, 2001

Maletic V, Robinson M, Oakes T, et al: Neurobiology of depression: an integrated view of key findings. Int J Clin Pract 61:2030–2040, 2007

Mann JJ, Aarons SF, Wilner PJ, et al: A controlled study of the antidepressant efficacy and side effects of (–)-deprenyl: a selective monoamine oxidase inhibitor. Arch Gen Psychiatry 46:45–50, 1989

Massana J: Reboxetine versus fluoxetine: an overview of efficacy and tolerability. J Clin Psychiatry 59 (suppl 14):8–10, 1998

Massana J, Moller HJ, Burrows GD, et al: Reboxetine: a double-blind comparison with fluoxetine in major depressive disorder. Int Clin Psychopharmacol 14:73–80, 1999

McCabe BT, Tsuang MT: Dietary consideration in MAO inhibitor regimens. J Clin Psychiatry 43:178–181, 1982

McGrath PJ, Quitkin FM, Harrison W, et al: Treatment of melancholia with tranylcypromine. Am J Psychiatry 141:288–289, 1984

McGrath PJ, Stewart JW, Quitkin FM, et al: Gepirone treatment of atypical depression: preliminary evidence of serotonergic involvement. J Clin Psychopharmacol 14:347–352, 1994

McGrath PJ, Stewart JW, Fava M, et al: Tranylcypromine versus venlafaxine plus mirtazapine following three failed antidepressant medication trials for depression: a STAR*D report. Am J Psychiatry 163:1531–1541, 2006

McKenzie MS, McFarland BH: Trends in antidepressant overdoses. Pharmacoepidemiol Drug Saf 16:513–523, 2007

Mendlewicz J: Efficacy of fluvoxamine in severe depression. Drugs 2:32–37 [discussion 37–39], 1992

Michelson D, Bancroft J, Targum S, et al: Female sexual dysfunction associated with antidepressant administration: a randomized, placebo-controlled study of pharmacologic intervention. Am J Psychiatry 157:239–243, 2000

Michelson D, Kociban K, Tamura R, et al: Mirtazapine, yohimbine or olanzapine augmentation therapy for serotonin reuptake–associated female sexual dysfunction: a randomized, placebo-controlled trial. J Psychiatr Res 36:147–152, 2002

Michelson D, Adler LA, Amsterdam JD, et al: Addition of atomoxetine for depression incompletely responsive to sertraline: a randomized, double-blind, placebo-controlled study, in 2006 Syllabus and Proceedings Summary, American Psychiatric Association 159th Annual Meeting, New York, May 20–25, 2006. Arlington, VA, American Psychiatric Association, 2006, p 74

Mitchell AJ: The role of corticotropin releasing factor in depressive illness: a critical review. Neurosci Biobehav Rev 22:635–651, 1998

Modell JG, Rosenthal NE, Harriett AE, et al: Seasonal affective disorder and its prevention by anticipatory treatment with bupropion XL. Biol Psychiatry 58:658–667, 2005

Monoamine oxidase inhibitors and anesthesia: update. Int Drug Ther Newsl 24:13–14, 1989

Monteleone P, Gnocchi G: Evidence for a linear relationship between plasma trazodone levels and clinical response in depression in the elderly. Clin Neuropharmacol 13 (suppl 1):84–89, 1990

Montgomery SA: Chairman's overview: the place of reboxetine in antidepressant therapy. J Clin Psychiatry 59 (suppl 14):26–29, 1998

Montgomery SA, Baldwin DS, Blier P, et al: Which antidepressants have demonstrated superior efficacy? A review of the evidence. Int Clin Psychopharmacol 22:323–329, 2007 (Erratum in Int Clin Psychopharmacol 23:61, 2008)

Mooney JJ, Schatzberg AF, Cole JO, et al: Enhanced signal transduction by adenylate cyclase in platelet membranes of patients showing antidepressant responses to alprazolam: preliminary data. J Psychiatr Res 19:65–75, 1985

Mucci M: Reboxetine: a review of antidepressant tolerability. J Psychopharmacol 11 (suppl 4):S33–S37, 1997

Muehlbacher M, Nickel MK, Nickel C, et al: Mirtazapine treatment of social phobia in women: a randomized, double-blind, placebo-controlled study. J Clin Psychopharmacol 25:580–583, 2005

Murdoch D, McTavish D: Sertraline: a review of its pharmacodynamic and pharmacokinetic properties, and therapeutic potential in depression and obsessive-compulsive disorder. Drugs 44:604–624, 1992

Murphy GM Jr, Kremer C, Rodrigues HE, et al: Pharmacogenetics of antidepressant medication intolerance. Am J Psychiatry 160:1830–1835, 2003 [also see comment]

National Center for Health Statistics: Health, United States, 2007, With Chartbook on Trends in the Health of Americans. Hyattsville, MD, Centers for Disease Control and Prevention, U.S. Department of Health and Human Services, 2007. Available at: http://www.cdc.gov/nchs/data/hus/hus07.pdf. Accessed August 5, 2009.

Nefazodone for depression. Med Lett Drugs Ther 37:33–35, 1995

Nelson JC, Shottenfeld RS, Conrad CD: Hypomania after desipramine withdrawal. Am J Psychiatry 140:624–625, 1983

Nemeroff CB: The clinical pharmacology and use of paroxetine, a new selective serotonin reuptake inhibitor. Pharmacotherapy 14:127–138, 1994

Nemeroff CB, Entsuah RA, Willard B, et al: Venlafaxine and SSRIs pooled remission analysis (NR263), in 2003 New Research Program and Abstracts, American Psychiatric Association 156th Annual Meeting, San Francisco, CA, May 17–22, 2003. Washington, DC, American Psychiatric Association, 2003

Niederhofer H: Is atomoxetine also effective in patients suffering from Tourette syndrome? J Child Neurol 21(9):823, 2006

Nierenberg AA: The treatment of severe depression: is there an efficacy gap between the SSRIs and TCA antidepressant generations? J Clin Psychiatry 55 (9, suppl): 55–61 [discussion 60–61, 98–100], 1994

Nierenberg AA, Keck PE: Management of monoamine oxidase inhibition–associated insomnia with trazodone. J Clin Psychopharmacol 9:42–45, 1989

Nierenberg AA, Cole JO, Glass L: Possible trazodone potentiation of fluoxetine: a case series. J Clin Psychiatry 53:83–85, 1992

Nierenberg AA, Feighner JP, Rudolph R, et al: Venlafaxine for treatment-resistant unipolar depression. J Clin Psychopharmacol 14:419–423, 1994

Nierenberg AA, McLean NE, Alpert JE, et al: Early nonresponse to fluoxetine as a predictor of poor 8-week outcome. Am J Psychiatry 152:1500–1503, 1995

Nierenberg AA, Farabaugh AH, Alpert JE, et al: Timing of onset of antidepressant response with fluoxetine treatment. Am J Psychiatry 157:1423–1428, 2000

Norden MJ: Fluoxetine in borderline personality disorder. Prog Neuropsychopharmacol Biol Psychiatry 13:885–893, 1989

Norden MJ: Buspirone treatment of sexual dysfunction associated with selective serotonin reuptake inhibitors. Depression 2:109–112, 1994

Norton PA, Zinner NR, Yalcin I, et al: Duloxetine versus placebo in the treatment of stress urinary incontinence. Am J Obstet Gynecol 187:40–48, 2002

Nurnberg HG, Hensley PL, Lauriello J, et al: Sildenafil for women patients with antidepressant-induced sexual dysfunction. Psychiatr Serv 50:1076–1078, 1999a

Nurnberg HG, Lauriello J, Hensley PL, et al: Sildenafil for iatrogenic serotonergic antidepressant medication–induced sexual dysfunction in 4 patients. J Clin Psychiatry 60:33–35, 1999b

Nurnberg HG, Thompson PM, Hensley PL: Antidepressant medication change in a clinical treatment setting: a comparison of the effectiveness of selective serotonin reuptake inhibitors. J Clin Psychiatry 60:574–579, 1999c

Nurnberg HG, Gelenberg A, Hargreave TB, et al: Efficacy of sildenafil citrate for the treatment of erectile dysfunction in men taking serotonin reuptake inhibitors. Am J Psychiatry 158:1926–1928, 2001

Nurnberg HG, Hensley PL, Heiman JR, et al: Sildenafil treatment of women with antidepressant-associated sexual dysfunction: a randomized controlled trial. JAMA 300:395–404, 2008

Olfson M, Marcus SC, Shaffer D: Antidepressant drug therapy and suicide in severely depressed children and adults: a case-control study. Arch Gen Psychiatry 63:865–872, 2006

Oslin DW, Ten Have TR, Streim JE, et al: Probing the safety of medications in the frail elderly: evidence from a randomized clinical trial of sertraline and venlafaxine in depressed nursing home residents. J Clin Psychiatry 64:875–882, 2003

Otani K, Tanaka O, Kaneko S, et al: Mechanisms of the development of trazodone withdrawal symptoms. Int Clin Psychopharmacol 9:131–133, 1994

Pande AC, Sayler ME: Severity of depression and response to fluoxetine. Int Clin Psychopharmacol 8:243–245, 1993

Papakostas GI, Petersen TJ, Burns AM, et al: Adjunctive atomoxetine for residual fatigue in major depressive disorder. J Psychiatr Res 40(4):370–373, 2006

Papakostas GI, Thase ME, Fava M, et al: Are antidepressant drugs that combine serotonergic and noradrenergic mechanisms of action more effective than the selective serotonin reuptake inhibitors in treating major depressive disorder? A meta-analysis of studies of newer agents. Biol Psychiatry 62:1217–1227, 2007

Papakostas GI, Homberger CH, Fava M: A meta-analysis of clinical trials comparing mirtazapine with selective serotonin reuptake inhibitors for the treatment of major depressive disorder. J Psychopharmacol 22:843–848, 2008

Papp M, Litwa E, Gruca P, Mocaer E: Anxiolytic-like activity of agomelatine and melatonin in three animal models of anxiety. Behav Pharmacol 17(1):9–18, 2006

Paris PA, Saucier JR: ECG conduction delays associated with massive bupropion overdose. J Toxicol Clin Toxicol 36:595–598, 1998

Patten SB: The comparative efficacy of trazodone and imipramine in the treatment of depression. Can Med Assoc J 146:1177–1182, 1992

Pearlstein TB, Stone AB: Long-term fluoxetine treatment of late luteal phase dysphoric disorder. J Clin Psychiatry 55:332–335, 1994

Pernia A, Mico JA, Calderon E, et al: Venlafaxine for the treatment of neuropathic pain. J Pain Symptom Manage 19:408–410, 2000

Pescatori ES, Engelman JC, Davis G, et al: Priapism of the clitoris: a case report following trazodone use. J Urol 149:1557–1559, 1993

Phanjoo A: The elderly depressed and treatment with fluvoxamine. Int Clin Psychopharmacol 6 (suppl 3):33–37 [discussion 37–39], 1991

Pinzani V, Ginies E, Robert L, et al: Venlafaxine withdrawal syndrome: report of six cases and review of the literature [in French]. Rev Medecine Interne 21:282–284, 2000

Pope HG, Hudson JI, Jonas JM, et al: Bulimia treated with imipramine: a placebo-controlled, double-blind study. Am J Psychiatry 140:554–558, 1983

Price J, Grunhaus LJ: Treatment of clomipramine-induced anorgasmia with yohimbine: a case report. J Clin Psychiatry 51:32–33, 1990

Prien RF, Kupfer DJ, Mansky PA, et al: Drug therapy in the prevention of recurrences in unipolar and bipolar affective disorders. Arch Gen Psychiatry 41:1096–1104, 1984

Quitkin F, Gibertine M: Patients with probable atypical depression are responsive to the 5-HT$_{1a}$ partial agonist, gepirone-ER. Presentation at the annual meeting of the American College of Neuropsychopharmacology, San Juan, Puerto Rico, 2001

Quitkin F, Rabkin A, Klein DF: Monoamine oxidase inhibitors. Arch Gen Psychiatry 36:749–760, 1979

Quitkin FM, Rabkin JG, Ross D, et al: Duration of antidepressant drug treatment: what is an adequate trial? Arch Gen Psychiatry 41:238–245, 1984

Quitkin FM, McGrath PJ, Stewart JW, et al: Chronological milestones to guide drug change: when should clinicians switch antidepressants? Arch Gen Psychiatry 53:785–792, 1996

Quitkin FM, Taylor BP, Kremer C: Does mirtazapine have a more rapid onset than SSRIs? J Clin Psychiatry 62:358–361, 2001

Raby WN: Treatment of venlafaxine discontinuation symptoms with ondansetron (letter). J Clin Psychiatry 59:621–622, 1998

Raskin J, Wiltse CG, Siegal A, et al: Efficacy of duloxetine on cognition, depression, and pain in elderly patients with major depressive disorder: an 8-week, double-blind, placebo-controlled trial. Am J Psychiatry 164:900–909, 2007

Reimherr FW, Chouinard G, Cohn CK, et al: Antidepressant efficacy of sertraline: a double-blind, placebo- and amitriptyline-controlled, multicenter comparison study in outpatients with major depression. J Clin Psychiatry 51 (12, suppl):18–27, 1990 [also see comments]

Richelson E: Synaptic pharmacology of antidepressants: an update. McLean Hospital Journal 13:67–88, 1988

Richelson E, Nelson A: Antagonism by antidepressants of neurotransmitter receptors of normal human brain in vitro. J Pharmacol Exp Ther 230:94–102, 1984

Rickels K, Schweizer E: Clinical overview of the selective serotonin reuptake inhibitors. J Clin Psychiatry 51 (12, suppl):9–12, 1990

Rickels K, Chung HR, Csanolsi IB, et al: Alprazolam, diazepam, imipramine, and placebo in outpatients with major depression. Arch Gen Psychiatry 44: 862–866, 1987

Rickels K, Downing R, Schweizer E, et al: Antidepressants for the treatment of generalized anxiety disorder: a placebo-controlled comparison of imipramine, trazodone, and diazepam. Arch Gen Psychiatry 50:884–895, 1993

Rickels K, Schweizer E, Clary C, et al: Nefazodone and imipramine in major depression: a placebo-controlled trial. Br J Psychiatry 164:802–805, 1994

Riggs PD, Leon SL, Mikulich SK, et al: An open trial of bupropion for ADHD in adolescents with substance use disorders and conduct disorder. J Am Acad Child Adolesc Psychiatry 37:1271–1278, 1998

Rinne T, van den Brink W, Wouters L, et al: SSRI treatment of borderline personality disorder: a randomized, placebo-controlled clinical trial for female patients with borderline personality disorder. Am J Psychiatry 159:2048–2054, 2002

Rohrig TP, Ray NG: Tissue distribution of bupropion in a fatal overdose. J Anal Toxicol 16:343–345, 1992

Roose SP, Glassman AH: Cardiovascular effects of tricyclic antidepressants in depressed patients with and without heart disease. J Clin Psychiatry 50 (July suppl):1–18, 1989

Roose SP, Glassman AH, Attia E, et al: Selective serotonin reuptake inhibitor efficacy in melancholia and atypical depression. Paper presented at the 147th annual meeting of the American Psychiatric Association, Philadelphia, PA, May 21–26, 1994

Rosen R, Shabsigh R, Berber M, et al, Vardenafil Study Site Investigators: Efficacy and tolerability of vardenafil in men with mild depression and erectile dysfunction: the Depression-Related Improvement With Vardenafil for Erectile Response Study. Am J Psychiatry 163:79–87, 2006

Rothschild AJ: Fluoxetine-nortriptyline therapy of treatment-resistant major depression in a geriatric patient. J Geriatr Psychiatry Neurol 7:137–138, 1994

Rothschild AJ, Locke CA: Reexposure to fluoxetine after serious suicide attempts in three patients. J Clin Psychiatry 52:491–493, 1991

Rothschild AJ, Samson JA, Bessette MP, et al: Efficacy of the combination of fluoxetine and perphenazine in the treatment of psychotic depression. J Clin Psychiatry 54:338–342, 1993

Rush AJ, Trivedi MH, Wisniewski SR, et al., STAR*D Study Team: Bupropion-SR, sertraline, or venlafaxine-XR after failure of SSRIs for depression. N Engl J Med 354:1231–1242, 2006

Russell IJ, Mease PJ, Smith TR, et al: Efficacy and safety of duloxetine for treatment of fibromyalgia in patients with or without major depressive disorder: results from a 6-month, randomized, double-blind, placebo-controlled, fixed-dose trial. Pain 136:432–444, 2008

Rynn M, Russell J, Erickson J, et al: Efficacy and safety of duloxetine in the treatment of generalized anxiety disorder: a flexible-dose, progessive-titration, placebo-controlled trial. Depress Anxiety 25:182–189, 2008

Sacchetti E, Conte G, Guarneri L: Are SSRI antidepressants a clinically homogeneous class of compounds? Lancet 344:126–127, 1994

Sackeim HA, Roose SP, Burt T: Optimal length of antidepressant trials in late-life depression. J Clin Psychopharmacol 25 (4, suppl 1):S34–S37, 2005

Sarchiapone M, Amore M, De Risio S, et al: Mirtazapine in the treatment of panic disorder: an open-label trial. Int Clin Psychopharmacol 18(1):35–38, 2003

Sargant W: The treatment of anxiety states and atypical depressions by the monoamine oxidase inhibitor drugs. J Neuropsychiatry 3 (suppl 1):96–103, 1962

Schatzberg AF: Trazodone: a 5-year review of antidepressant efficacy. Psychopathology 20 (suppl 1):48–56, 1987

Schatzberg AF, Cole JO: Benzodiazepines in depressive disorders. Arch Gen Psychiatry 35:1359–1365, 1978

Schatzberg AF, Rosenbaum AH, Orsulak PJ, et al: Toward a biochemical classification of depressive disorders, III: pretreatment urinary MHPG levels as predictors of response to maprotiline. Psychopharmacology (Berl) 75:34–38, 1981

Schatzberg AF, Kremer C, Rodrigues HE, et al: Double-blind, randomized comparison of mirtazapine and paroxetine in elderly depressed patients. Am J Geriatr Psychiatry 10:541–550, 2002

Schneier FR, Liebowitz MR, Davies SO, et al: Fluoxetine in panic disorder. J Clin Psychopharmacol 10:119–121, 1990

Schwartz D, Blendl M: Sedation and anxiety reducing properties of trazodone, in Trazodone: Modern Problems in Pharmacopsychiatry, Vol 9. Edited by Ban TA, Silvestrini B. Basel, Switzerland, S Karger, 1974, pp 29–46

Seagraves RT, Lee J, Stevenson K, et al: Tadalafil for treatment of erectile dysfunction in men on antidepressants. J Clin Psychopharmacol 27:62–66, 2007

Shatkin JP: Atomoxetine for the treatment of pediatric nocturnal enuresis. J Child Adolesc Psychopharmacol 14:443–447, 2004

Sheehan DV, Davidson J, Manshreck TC, et al: Lack of efficacy of a new antidepressant (bupropion) in the treatment of panic disorder with phobias. J Clin Psychopharmacol 3:28–31, 1983

Shrivastava RK, Cohn C, Crowder J, et al: Long-term safety and clinical acceptability of venlafaxine and imipramine in outpatients with major depression. J Clin Psychopharmacol 14:322–329, 1994

Shrivastava RK, Shrivastava S, Overweg N, et al: Amantadine in the treatment of sexual dysfunction associated with selective serotonin reuptake inhibitors (letter). J Clin Psychopharmacol 15:83–84, 1995

Simon GE, VonKorff M, Heiligenstein JH, et al: Initial antidepressant choice in primary care: effectiveness and cost of fluoxetine vs. tricyclic antidepressants. JAMA 275:1897–1902, 1996

Simon GE, Savarino J, Operskalski B, et al: Suicide risk during antidepressant treatment. Am J Psychiatry 163(1):41–47, 2006

Sondergard L, Kvist K, Andersen PK, et al: Do antidepressants precipitate youth suicide? A nationwide pharmacoepidemiological study. Eur Child Adolesc Psychiatry 15:232–240, 2006a

Sondergard L, Kvist K, Andersen PK, et al: Do antidepressants prevent suicide? Int Clin Psychopharmacol 21:211–218, 2006b

Spar E: Plasma trazodone concentrations in elderly depressed inpatients: cardiac and short-term efficacy. J Clin Psychopharmacol 7:406–409, 1987

Spiegel K, Kalb R, Pasternak GW: Analgesic activity of tricyclic antidepressants. Ann Neurol 13:462–465, 1983

Spiller HA, Ramoska EA, Krenzelok EP, et al: Bupropion overdose: a 3-year multicenter retrospective analysis. Am J Emerg Med 12:43–45, 1994

Stamenkovic M, Pezawas L, de Zwaan M, et al: Mirtazapine in recurrent brief depression. Int Clin Psychopharmacol 13:39–40, 1998

Stark P, Fuller RW, Wong DT: The pharmacologic profile of fluoxetine. J Clin Psychiatry 46:7–13, 1985

Stein MB, Liebowitz MR, Lydiard R, et al: Paroxetine treatment of generalized social phobia (social anxiety disorder): a randomized controlled trial. JAMA 280:708–713, 1998

Steiner M, Steinberg S, Stewart D, et al: Fluoxetine in the treatment of premenstrual dysphoria. Canadian Fluoxetine/Premenstrual Dysphoria Collaborative Study Group. N Engl J Med 332:1529–1534, 1995 [also see comments]

Stokes PE: Fluoxetine: a five-year review. Clin Ther 15:216–243 [discussion 215], 1993

Storrow A: Bupropion overdose and seizure. Am J Emerg Med 12:183–184, 1994

Stuppaeck CH, Geretsegger C, Whitworth AB, et al: A multicenter double-blind trial of paroxetine versus amitriptyline in depressed inpatients. J Clin Psychopharmacol 14:241–246, 1994

Sunderland T, Cohen RM, Thompson KE, et al: L-Deprenyl treatment of older depressives (NR159), in 1989 New Research Program and Abstracts, American Psychiatric Association 142nd Annual Meeting, San Francisco, May 6–11, 1989. Washington, DC, American Psychiatric Association, 1989, p 101

Sunderland T, Cohen RM, Molchan S, et al: High-dose selegiline in treatment-resistant older depressive patients. Arch Gen Psychiatry 51:607–615, 1994

Taylor MJ, Rudkin L, Hawton K: Strategies for managing antidepressant-induced sexual dysfunction: systematic review of randomised controlled trials. J Affect Disord 88:241–254, 2005

Teicher MH, Cohen BM, Baldessarini RJ, et al: Severe daytime somnolence in patients treated with an MAOI. Am J Psychiatry 145:1552–1556, 1988

Teicher MH, Glod C, Cole JO: Emergence of intense suicidal preoccupation during fluoxetine treatment. Am J Psychiatry 147:207–210, 1990

Teicher MH, Glod CA, Cole JO: Antidepressant drugs and the emergence of suicidal tendencies. Drug Saf 8:186–212, 1993

Thase ME: Effectiveness of antidepressants: comparative remission rates. J Clin Psychiatry 64 (suppl 2):3–7, 2003

Thase ME: Are SNRIs more effective than SSRIs? A review of the current state of the controversy. Psychopharmacol Bull 41:58–85, 2008

Thase ME, Blomgren SL, Birkett MA, et al: Fluoxetine treatment of patients with major depressive disorder who failed initial treatment with sertraline. J Clin Psychiatry 58:16–21, 1997

Thase ME, Entsuah AR, Rudolph RL: Remission rates during treatment with venlafaxine or selective serotonin reuptake inhibitors. Br J Psychiatry 178:234–241, 2001

Thompson C: Mirtazapine versus selective serotonin reuptake inhibitors. J Clin Psychiatry 60 (suppl 17):18–22 [discussion 46–48], 1999

Tignol J, Stoker MJ, Dunbar GC: Paroxetine in the treatment of melancholia and severe depression. Int Clin Psychopharmacol 7:91–94, 1992

Tollefson GD, Rampey A Jr, Potvin JH, et al: A multicenter investigation of fixed-dose fluoxetine in the treatment of obsessive-compulsive disorder. Arch Gen Psychiatry 51:559–567, 1994

Trivedi MH, Fava M, Wisniewski SR, et al, STAR*D Study Team: Medication augmentation after the failure of SSRIs for depression. N Engl J Med 354(12):1243–1252, 2006

van Bemmel AL, Havermans RG, van Diest R: Effects of trazodone on EEG sleep and clinical state in major depression. Psychopharmacology (Berl) 107:569–574, 1992 van Laar MW, van Willigenburg AP, Volkers ER: Acute and subchronic effects of nefazodone and imipramine on highway driving, cognitive functions, and daytime sleepiness in healthy adult and elderly subjects. J Clin Psychopharmacol 15:30–40, 1995

van Moffaert M, de Wilde J, Vereecken A, et al: Mirtazapine is more effective than trazodone: a double-blind controlled study in hospitalized patients with major depression. Int Clin Psychopharmacol 10:3–9, 1995

Vartiainen H, Leinonen E: Double-blind study of mirtazapine and placebo in hospitalized patients with major depression. Eur Neuropsychopharmacol 4:145–150, 1994

Volicer L, Rheaume Y, Cyr D: Treatment of depression in advanced Alzheimer's disease using sertraline. J Geriatr Psychiatry Neurol 7:227–229, 1994

Walker PW, Cole JO, Gardner EA, et al: Improvement in fluoxetine-associated sexual dysfunction in patients switched to bupropion. J Clin Psychiatry 54:459–465, 1993

Walsh BT, Kaplan AS, Attia E, et al: Fluoxetine after weight restoration in anorexia nervosa: a randomized controlled trial. JAMA 295(22):2605–2612, 2006 [erratum: JAMA 296(8):934, 2006]

Weilburg JB, Rosenbaum JF, Biederman J, et al: Fluoxetine added to non-MAOI antidepressants converts nonresponders to responders: a preliminary report. J Clin Psychiatry 50:447–449, 1989

Weinmann S, Becker T, Koesters M: Re-evaluation of the efficacy and tolerability of venlafaxine vs SSRI: meta-analysis. Psychopharmacology (Berl) 196:511–520, 521–522 (discussion), 2008

Weisler RH, Johnston JA, Lineberry CG, et al: Comparison of bupropion and trazodone for the treatment of major depression. J Clin Psychopharmacol 14:170–179, 1994

Wheadon DE, Rampey A Jr, Thompson VL, et al: Lack of association between fluoxetine and suicidality in bulimia nervosa. J Clin Psychiatry 53:235–241, 1992

Wheatley D: Triple-blind, placebo-controlled trial of Ginkgo biloba in sexual dysfunction due to antidepressant drugs. Hum Psychopharmacol 19(8):545–548, 2004

Wheatley DP, van Moffaert M, Timmerman L, et al: Mirtazapine: efficacy and tolerability in comparison with fluoxetine in patients with moderate to severe major depressive disorder. J Clin Psychiatry 59:306–312, 1998

Wilcox CS, Ferguson JM, Dale JL, et al: A double-blind trial of low- and high-dose ranges of gepirone-ER compared with placebo in the treatment of depressed outpatients. Psychopharmacol Bull 32:335–342, 1996

Wolfe F, Cathey MA, Hawley DJ: A double-blind placebo-controlled trial of fluoxetine in fibromyalgia. Scand J Rheumatol 23:255–259, 1994

Wolfersdorf M, Barg T, Konig F, et al: Paroxetine in the treatment of inpatients with non-delusional endogenous or neurotic depression. Schweiz Arch Neurol Psychiatr 145:15–18, 1994

Yoon SJ, Pae CU, Kim DJ, et al: Mirtazapine for patients with alcohol dependence and comorbid depressive disorders: a multicentre, open label study. Prog Neuropsychopharmacol Biol Psychiatry 30:1196–1201, 2006

Young AH, Gallagher P, Watson S, et al: Improvements in neurocognitive function and mood following adjunctive treatment with mifepristone (RU-486) in bipolar disorder. Neuropsychopharmacology 29:1538–1545, 2004

Zisook S, Rush AJ, Haight BR, et al: Use of bupropion in combination with serotonin reuptake inhibitors. Biol Psychiatry 59:203–210, 2006

Zobel AW, Nickel T, Kunzel HE, et al: Effects of the high-affinity corticotropin-releasing hormone receptor 1 antagonist R121919 in major depression: the first 20 patients. J Psychiatr Res 34:171–181, 2000

4

Antipsychotic Drugs

Observations in the late nineteenth century that aniline dyes had calming and sedating effects ultimately led to the development of the first phenothiazine, promethazine. In 1952, a related phenothiazine, chlorpromazine, was investigated as an antiautonomic drug to protect the body against its own excessive compensatory reactions during major surgery. It spread into psychiatry from the field of anesthesia after an initial clinical report by Delay et al. (1952) demonstrated the drug's favorable side-effect profile and its efficacy in treating acute psychosis. Endless subsequent double-blind studies have served chiefly to confirm the effects already obvious to the original French clinicians.

We now know substantially more about the side effects and limitations of the currently available antipsychotic drugs and more about their mechanisms of action. We are beginning to understand dose-response relationships and have second-generation antipsychotics (SGAs) that now represent the most commonly prescribed antipsychotics. There is considerable, growing debate as to whether the benefits of the second-generation agents over their first-generation counterparts are outweighed by their cost and side effects.

The second-generation, or atypical, antipsychotics, which include cloza-pine, olanzapine, risperidone, quetiapine, ziprasidone, aripiprazole—and, more recently, paliperidone, iloperidone, and asenapine—have now largely sup-planted the first-generation, "typical" antipsychotics such as perphenazine and haloperidol. The concept of atypicality arose from the finding that the SGAs had a greater serotonin (5-HT)/dopamine (DA) ratio than did earlier drugs and might be associated with improved efficacy (particularly for so-called negative symptoms) and reduced extrapyramidal side effects. For example, greater serotonergic effects of SGAs were thought to be associated with fewer extrapyramidal symptoms (EPS) and greater efficacy in reducing cognitive and negative symptoms. However, recent data have not always found that the second-generation, atypical agents are that different from the first-generation, typical agents. Thus, the atypicals may not be that "atypical" after all (Gründer at al. 2009).

The SGAs, like the first-generation antipsychotics, are a heterogeneous group of agents, each with potential advantages and disadvantages over indi-vidual, first-generation drugs. For example, the rate of EPS does appear to be lower in most SGAs compared with the first-generation drugs. However, the Clinical Antipsychotic Trials of Intervention Effectiveness (CATIE; Lieber-man et al. 2005) did not show clear advantages of the SGAs over perphena-zine, including in rates of EPS. However, the relatively short duration of the CATIE trial might prevent a clear determination of EPS, such as parkinsonism and tardive dyskinesia, that may take years to develop. Also, in the CATIE, patients with a history of EPS while taking neuroleptics were not randomly assigned to the typical agent, potentially affecting incidence of EPS in the per-phenazine cell.

On the other hand, the rates of tardive dyskinesia associated with typical antipsychotics might have been inflated historically by the high doses of these agents that were used. For example, haloperidol in early trials and in clinical use was commonly given at a dosage of 20 mg/day or higher. We now know that 2–5 mg/day of haloperidol results in the 80% binding to D_2 receptors needed for efficacy. Since doses resulting in >80% binding increase EPS with-out necessarily increasing efficacy, the real rates of tardive dyskinesia in the first-generation drugs are probably less than the 4% per year rate that is frequently quoted. Some clinicians, particularly in primary care settings, have mistakenly assumed that there is no risk for akathisia, dystonias, and tardive dyskinesia with the SGAs. Although the risk of EPS with SGAs is somewhat smaller than the risk with typical antipsychotics, the risk is not negligible, particularly with risperidone at higher doses.

The SGAs are thought to have a number of other advantages over the typical antipsychotic agents. As indicated above, the SGAs may be somewhat more helpful than typical agents in treating the negative symptoms of schizophrenia. The negative symptoms result in considerably more disability for patients with schizophrenia than do positive symptoms such as hallucinations and delusions. Results from CATIE and the European Cost Utility of the Latest Antipsychotic Drugs in Schizophrenia Study (CUtLASS) trial do not necessarily support the benefit of SGAs over first-generation agents in treating negative symptoms. Likewise, a meta-analysis of randomized controlled trials to date did not find that the SGAs had any greater efficacy than the first-generation agents in reducing negative symptoms (Leucht et al. 2009c). In addition, the SGAs may have benefit in treating the cognitive disturbance and executive dysfunction that can be so disabling in schizophrenia patients. Some but not all studies suggest a modest advantage of the SGAs versus the first-generation antipsychotics. However, these apparent benefits have not translated into evidence that the SGAs are superior to the typical agents on measures of quality of life (Jones et al. 2006). Clozapine has shown clear utility in the treatment of schizophrenia that has not responded to typical agents. Both CATIE and CUtLASS appear to confirm this finding. It was this utility in patients with treatment-refractory schizophrenia that ultimately led to the approval of clozapine in the United States. Finally, the SGAs appear to have more mood-stabilizing and perhaps mood-elevating properties than do typical antipsychotics. While the typical agents such as chlorpromazine are clearly effective antimanic agents, evidence that the typical agents are effective in the maintenance treatment of bipolar disorder or are effective in treating bipolar depression is lacking. Depressive symptoms in schizophrenia are often improved by SGAs more than by the older drugs. In fact, clozapine became the first drug with a specific indication for reducing suicidality in patients with schizophrenia.

While there may be some benefits of the SGAs in schizophrenia, the effect size of the SGAs in treating this disorder is probably no greater than that seen with the first-generation agents. In a meta-analysis of 127 comparison trials,

Davis and colleagues (2003) found that only clozapine had a robustly larger effect size than haloperidol in the treatment of schizophrenia. More recent studies have confirmed these earlier findings (Leucht et al. 2009a, 2009b). The rest of the SGAs, while impacting somewhat different aspects of the illness, had an overall effect that was about equal to that of haloperidol. However, the utility of second-generation (atypical) versus first-generation (typical) agents in the treatment of mood disorders may be a different matter.

It is now clear that virtually all of the SGAs are effective antimanic drugs and probably work faster than and at least as well as mood-stabilizing agents such as lithium in this regard (see Chapter 5, "Mood Stabilizers"). The use of second-generation agents in mood disorders appears to have eclipsed their use in schizophrenia some time ago. Olanzapine, already approved by the U.S. Food and Drug Administration (FDA) for the treatment of acute mania, has also received FDA approval for the maintenance monotherapy of bipolar disorder. In addition, olanzapine was approved in a combination formulation with fluoxetine (Symbyax) first for the treatment of bipolar depression and recently for refractory depression. Olanzapine and other SGAs such as quetiapine are also increasingly being used as adjunctive and augmentation agents in the treatment of unipolar depression. Quetiapine has recently been approved as a monotherapy for bipolar depression. The role of the SGAs in the treatment of mood disorders continues to be defined (see Chapter 5).

While the $D_2/5\text{-}HT_2$ antagonists offer many advantages over the typical antipsychotics, they have some distinct disadvantages as well. Among them is cost. The SGAs cost many times what older drugs do, and some county mental health programs, such as in San Francisco County, California, have restricted drugs such as olanzapine from their formularies because they can no longer afford them. As reported earlier, it is difficult to demonstrate a clear advantage of the SGAs in efficacy (for the treatment of schizophrenia, at least) to justify the enormously greater costs. Another important disadvantage of the $D_2/5\text{-}HT_2$ antagonists is their metabolic effect. In 2003, the FDA advised all manufacturers of SGAs that their labels should be changed to reflect that these drugs are associated with an enhanced risk of hyperglycemia and diabetes. While the extent of the metabolic risks associated with the SGAs continues to be debated, there is little doubt that some enhanced risk of weight gain and metabolic effects occurs with most, though probably not all, of the second-generation agents.

General Principles of Antipsychotic Use

The Drugs

There are, at the time of this writing, 21 antipsychotic drugs available for prescription use in the United States: 12 first-generation antipsychotic agents and 9 second-generation antipsychotic agents (Table 4–1; Figure 4–1). One of the first-generation agents, pimozide, is FDA approved for use only in Tourette's disorder and is now rarely used because of the known risk of QTc prolongation. Likewise, droperidol, another agent with a black box warning of QTc prolongation, is approved only for parenteral use in anesthesia. Studies done on the rate of arrhythmias in droperidol-treated patients since the black box warning in 2001 have not necessarily supported an enhanced risk (Nuttal et al. 2007).

All the antipsychotic agents, except clozapine, are reasonably potent postsynaptic dopamine receptor blockers (dopamine antagonists). Although it is conceivable that the antipsychotic effects of these drugs might be attributable to some other mechanism, it seems unlikely. While some of the efficacy of the SGAs may be due to 5-HT_2 antagonism or the blockade of other dopamine receptors, agents that purely block 5-HT_2 or dopamine receptors other than D_2 have often failed as effective antipsychotics.

All the effective antipsychotic drugs, except clozapine, act on the nigrostriatal system in the predicted manner and can potentially produce EPS. For an antipsychotic to be effective, it generally requires a dopamine antagonism of 60%–80% of dopamine D_2 receptors. Lower levels of dopamine antagonism tend not to be associated with antipsychotic properties, whereas higher levels tend to produce more extensive EPS. Positron emission tomography (PET) studies indicate that a dosage of about 2.5–6.0 mg/day of haloperidol results in occupation of about 60%–80% of D_2 receptors (Remington and Kapur 1999). These studies also indicate that the standard therapeutic dosages of olanzapine (10–20 mg/day) and risperidone (2–6 mg/day) also result in a 60%–80% binding of D_2 receptors. Only clozapine fails to show a D_2 binding affinity of less than 60% at therapeutic dosages. In typical antipsychotics, dosages higher than these are not clearly associated with improvement in psychosis but do increase the risk of EPS (Kapur et al. 1999). The lack of parkinsonian side effects may also reflect the limited time these agents occupy dopamine receptors. More recently, SGAs have been thought to bind less tightly—

Table 4–1.   Antipsychotic drugs: names, formulations, and strengths

Generic name	Brand name	Formulations and strengths
aripiprazole	Abilify	Tablets: 2, 5, 10, 15, 20, 30 mg
	Abilify Disc Melt	Orally disintegrating tablets: 10, 15 mg
		Oral solution: 1 mg/mL (150 mL)
		Injection: 9.75 mg/1.3 mL
asenapine	Saphris	Tablets (sublingual): 5, 10 mg
chlorpromazine	Thorazine[a]	Tablets: 10, 25, 50, 100, 200 mg
		Injection: 25 mg/mL (1-mL and 2-mL ampules)
clozapine	Clozaril[a,b]	Tablets: 12.5, 25, 50, 100, 200 mg
	FazaClo	Orally disintegrating tablets: 12.5, 25, 50, 100 mg
droperidol	Inapsine[a]	Injection: 2.5 mg/mL (1- and 2-mL ampules and vials)
fluphenazine	Prolixin[a]	Tablets: 1, 2.5, 5, 10 mg
		Concentrate: 5 mg/mL (120-mL bottle)
		Elixir: 2.5 mg/5 mL (60-mL and 473-mL bottles)
		Injection: 2.5 mg/mL (10-mL multidose vial)
fluphenazine decanoate	Prolixin Decanoate[a]	Injection: 25 mg/mL (5-mL multidose vial)
haloperidol	Haldol[a]	Tablets: 0.5, 1, 2, 5, 10, 20 mg
		Concentrate: 2 mg/mL
		Injection: 5 mg/mL (1-mL ampule and single-dose vial; 10-mL multidose vial)
haloperidol decanoate	Haldol Decanoate[a]	Injection: 50 mg/mL (1-mL ampule and 5-mL multidose vial), 100 mg/mL (5-mL multidose vial)
iloperidone	Fanapt	Tablets: 1, 2, 4, 6, 8, 10, 12 mg
loxapine	Loxitane[a]	Capsules: 5, 10, 25, 50 mg
molindone	Moban[a]	Tablets: 5, 10, 25, 50 mg

Table 4–1. Antipsychotic drugs: names, formulations, and strengths *(continued)*

Generic name	Brand name	Formulations and strengths
olanzapine	Zyprexa	Tablets: 2.5, 5, 7.5, 10, 15, 20 mg
	Zydis	Orally disintegrating tablets: 5, 10, 15, 20 mg
	Zyprexa Intramuscular	Injection: 10-mg vial (before reconstitution)
paliperidone	Invega	Tablets (extended release): 1.5, 3, 6, 9 mg
paliperidone palmitate	Invega Sustenna	Injection: 39, 78, 117, 156, 234 mg
perphenazine	Trilafon[a]	Tablets: 2, 4, 8, 16 mg
		Concentrate: 16 mg/5 mL (120-mL bottle)
pimozide	Orap	Tablets: 1, 2 mg
quetiapine	Seroquel	Tablets: 25, 50, 100, 200, 300, 400 mg
	Seroquel XR	Tablets (extended release): 50, 150, 200, 300, 400 mg
risperidone	Risperdal	Tablets: 0.25, 0.5, 1, 2, 3, 4 mg
		Oral solution: 1 mg/mL (30-mL bottle)
	Risperdal M-TAB	Orally disintegrating tablets: 0.5, 1, 2, 3, 4 mg
	Risperdal Consta	Long-acting injectable: 12.5, 25, 37.5, 50 mg
thioridazine	Mellaril[a]	Tablets: 10, 25, 50, 100 mg
		Concentrate: 30 mg/mL (120-mL bottle)
thiothixene	Navane[a]	Capsules: 1, 2, 5, 10 mg
trifluoperazine	Stelazine[a]	Tablets: 1, 2, 5, 10 mg
ziprasidone	Geodon	Tablets: 20, 40, 60, 80 mg
		Injection: 20-mg vial (before reconstitution)

[a]Available in generic form.
[b]Use of clozapine must be registered with the manufacturer's monitoring national registry (see subsection "Clozapine" in this chapter).

A. Phenothiazines

1. Aliphatic

Promazine*

Chlorpromazine

Triflupromazine

2. Piperidine

Thioridazine

Mesoridazine*

Figure 4–1.   Chemical structures of antipsychotic drugs.
*No longer available in the United States.

3. Piperazine

Fluphenazine

Prochlorperazine

Trifluoperazine

Perphenazine

B. Butyrophenone-like

Haloperidol

Droperidol

Pimozide

Figure 4–1. Chemical structures of antipsychotic drugs *(continued)*.

C. Thioxanthenes

Chlorprothixene*

Thiothixene

D. Indole

Molindone

E. Dibenzazepines

Clozapine

Loxapine

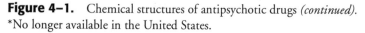

Figure 4–1.   Chemical structures of antipsychotic drugs *(continued).*
*No longer available in the United States.

F. Benzisoxazole

Risperidone

G. Thienobenzodiazepine

Olanzapine

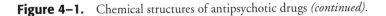

Figure 4–1. Chemical structures of antipsychotic drugs *(continued).*

or for briefer periods—to D_2 receptors than do typical agents, resulting in fewer EPS.

Clozapine, with its risk of agranulocytosis, has been known to be unique in its action on psychosis for over 30 years and to be relatively free of EPS other than akathisia. Until recently, however, no really comparable drug had been discovered to replace it, despite the efforts of many major pharmaceutical firms. Olanzapine appears quite similar to clozapine in its pharmacological effects but superior in side-effect profile. In the CATIE and CUtLASS trials, olanza-

H. Other

Ziprasidone

Aripiprazole

Asenapine

Figure 4–1.   Chemical structures of antipsychotic drugs *(continued)*.

H. Other, continued

Iloperidone

Paliperidone

Figure 4–1. Chemical structures of antipsychotic drugs *(continued)*.

pine did seem to do better on measures of efficacy in schizophrenia relative to other SGAs and some first-generation agents. However, clozapine tends to be even more consistently effective in patients who have failed to respond to other antipsychotic agents.

Efficacy

All the available antipsychotic drugs have been clearly shown to be more effective than placebo in treating schizophrenia, both acutely and chronically.

Most major studies on typical antipsychotics were done many years ago and used some variant of DSM-II criteria (American Psychiatric Association 1968). They involved an unknown but possibly large proportion of acute patients who might be judged, by DSM-IV (American Psychiatric Association 1994) standards, to have schizophreniform, bipolar, or schizoaffective disorder. It is therefore clinically sensible to assume that all the drugs are effective in all these DSM-IV conditions and to include mania as a proven indication as well. The SGAs have all been studied with DSM-III-R and DSM-IV criteria for schizophrenia and bipolar disorder.

In many respects, the nature and timing of clinical response to antipsychotics are unsatisfactory. In large-scale 6-week placebo-controlled trials involving hospitalized patients, 75% of drug-treated patients showed at least moderate improvement, whereas only 25% of placebo-treated patients did as well, and some got worse. However, most patients never achieve complete remission, and few are able to function at a fully effective level on return to the community. Some SGAs may be better than first-generation agents in improving social functioning. Studies of quality of life of patients who are administered clozapine for treatment-refractory schizophrenia have sometimes shown a dramatic improvement in work-related activity and a substantial decrease in the rate of rehospitalization. About 30% of patients who do not respond to first-generation antipsychotics will respond to clozapine in a 12-week trial. In addition, another 15%–30% of patients who do not respond in the first few months will respond in 6–12 months (Meltzer 1997; Meltzer et al. 1989).

Antipsychotics tend to act in a slow, approximate manner. A few patients show rapid, excellent response, but most get better more slowly, and some do not respond at all or do so only very slowly. Sometimes the response is so slow and variable that clinicians, in an understandable but probably misguided effort to speed clinical response, may prescribe very high drug dosages early in treatment. In recent studies, as well as in studies done over four decades ago, improvement increased relatively rapidly between the first and sixth week of taking the drug. Thereafter, modest further improvement occurred between the sixth and thirteenth week, with little additional improvement by the twenty-sixth week. These changes are, of course, *average* improvement—individual patients may improve more or less, earlier or later. Similarly, once a patient's condition has improved, it is difficult to find the minimal effective maintenance dose in any reliable way. One might imagine that the physician could gradually reduce the dosage from that at which the patient had recovered. Unfortunately, when patients whose condition is stable are shifted from an antipsychotic drug to placebo abruptly, some experience relapse relatively soon, but others experience relapse at a leisurely and completely unpredictable rate over months and even years. In only a few cases is the relapse so rapid that a minimum maintenance dosage can be easily determined.

Reviews of the antipsychotic discontinuation literature by Baldessarini and Viguera (1995) and Gilbert et al. (1995) show that relapse rates are higher in the first 3 months after abrupt discontinuation of neuroleptics. Nonadherence with prescribed SGAs, quite common in schizophrenia, also consistently results in higher relapse rates and greater likelihood of hospitalization (Sun et al. 2007). The reviews also show that slowly tapering antipsychotics (or stopping depot antipsychotics, with their long half-lives) not only substantially decreases the early relapse rate but also leaves more patients with stable functioning in the community 2 years later than does rapid termination of neuroleptic therapy. It appears that abrupt discontinuation of antipsychotic medication by treaters or, unilaterally, by patients is almost as bad for patients with chronic schizophrenia as abrupt discontinuation of lithium carbonate is for patients with bipolar disorder (Suppes et al. 1993).

This newer look at old data, supported by a study by Green et al. (1990), throws into question many old reports about the differences between drug and placebo observed in follow-up studies designed to assess the relative values of active and inert therapies for chronic psychosis. If abrupt termination of drug therapy artificially increases relapse rates, much work needs to be reassessed or redone.

The value of depot drugs in the long-term management of chronic psychosis also needs more positive consideration (Glazer and Kane 1992). In past years, clinicians working with intermittent antipsychotic medication strategies for patients with chronic schizophrenia claimed that identifying the individual patient's unique signs of impending relapse (e.g., poor sleep, pacing, special fears or worries) could enable the treating psychiatrist to reinstitute antipsychotic medication rapidly and thus avert a full psychotic episode (Carpenter and Heinrichs 1983; Herz et al. 1982). Enlisting both patient and family to identify such early warning signs and symptoms and to watch for their reemergence may be beneficial. This technique could be applied as well to gradual dose-tapering strategies. For this strategy to work well, careful patient monitoring by both family or caretakers and mental health professionals would be necessary. Unfortunately, studies attempting to demonstrate the efficacy of this approach have not been successful. Intermittent medication strategies have been repeatedly shown to be less effective than low, fixed, steady dosage regimens (Carpenter et al. 1990; Herz et al. 1991). Moreover, one trial indicated that higher doses of maintenance depot haloperidol were more effective in preventing relapse than were lower doses (Kane et al. 2002). Still, lower doses are clearly better tolerated than higher doses and are more effective than placebo in preventing relapse. The availability of a long-acting form of risperidone (Risperdal Consta) now provides clinicians with an SGA that can be given twice a month. An FDA panel suggested that a depot form of olanzapine receive a qualified approval. However, concerns about excessive sedation have prevented approval of depot olanzapine as of this writing.

Acute Antipsychotic Treatment

The decision of which antipsychotic agent to administer for a first break of psychosis or in the emergency room (ER) setting has become more complex with the availability of the SGAs. In general, second-generation agents are now the first-line antipsychotics in the treatment of most psychotic episodes. While studies such as CATIE and CUtLASS 1 have failed to show any efficacy benefit of the SGAs over first-generation antipsychotics in the treatment of schizophrenia, clinicians have not generally embraced the first-generation agents again. There are a number of factors that might explain why clinicians have been hesitant to return to the older agents despite enormous savings in the cost of medications. One is concern about the risk of EPS, particularly tardive dyskinesia. While CATIE did not show great differences between perphenazine and second-generation drugs, perphenazine and risperidone were somewhat more likely to be associated with akathisia (Miller et al. 2005). The rates of tardive dyskinesia and dystonia in the CATIE trial were equivalent in the SGAs and perphenazine. However, as alluded to earlier, the CATIE trial may not have been long enough to show differences in rates of tardive dyskinesia. The known rates of tardive dyskinesia in the SGAs in long-term schizophrenia trials do appear to be lower than those reported in trials of first-generation agents in schizophrenia, even after the more aggressive dosing is taken into account. The overall rate of tardive dyskinesia in the SGAs seems to be around 1% per year or less, while the reported rates of tardive dyskinesia for even midpotency first-generation drugs appear to be at least twice as high or greater. Even if the overall rate of tardive dyskinesia turns out to be only 2% per year in first-generation drugs instead of the 4% per year that is often quoted, a twofold increase in the tardive dyskinesia rates would be enough to scare many clinicians from using the first-generation agents. Since the standard of care is currently to use SGAs, the application of first-generation drugs for cost savings presents a legal dilemma should a patient develop an irreversible tardive dyskinesia while taking a first-generation drug.

That being said, the available evidence suggests that the first-generation drugs are underutilized in favor of much more expensive, but no more efficacious, second-generation drugs. We are more inclined to use first-generation agents than SGAs as the first intervention in some situations. The first is in the management of acutely agitated psychotic patients. The combination of a high-potency agent such as intramuscular haloperidol and a benzodiazepine is an inexpensive and long-proven strategy for treating severe agitation in emergency settings. While often inadequate for long-term use, the brief use of a typical antipsychotic in the ER or intensive care unit (ICU) is often warranted. The availability of intramuscular preparations of aripiprazole, ziprasidone, and olanzapine for the treatment of acute agitation is an important development in emergency psychiatry. The intramuscular second-generation agents produce less EPS and may work more rapidly than does haloperidol alone. However, these intramuscular forms of the SGAs have been somewhat slow to catch on in ER settings, perhaps due to the cost, the relative inconvenience, and the availability of effective older options such as the combination of benzodiazepines and high-potency typical antipsychotic drugs. Intramuscular aripiprazole, olanzapine, and ziprasidone clearly cause less dystonia and parkinsonism than does intramuscular haloperidol. However, the intramuscular SGAs are not devoid of EPS and are associated with akathisia. Patients clearly at risk for dystonia (e.g., agitated young males) or parkinsonism (e.g., geriatric patients) might be better treated with intramuscular SGAs as the initial intervention. We sometimes employ intramuscular haloperidol in the emergency setting while simultaneously initiating orally administered second-generation agents for long-term management.

Choosing among the SGAs is a matter of best matching patient characteristics to the side-effect profiles of the various agents. For rapid oral titration in the treatment of an acutely psychotic patient, the best choices currently are risperidone, aripiprazole, and olanzapine (in orally disintegrating tablets; Risperdal M-TAB, Abilify Disc Melt, and Zydis).

Quetiapine and clozapine require more time to achieve a therapeutic dose than other SGAs and so may be less advantageous in the acute setting. As in the emergency setting, we sometimes employ a high-potency antipsychotic such as orally administered haloperidol concurrently with upward titration of quetiapine. Then, at about 2–4 weeks, we taper the haloperidol and continue the titration of the SGA.

Choosing among the first-generation antipsychotics follows the same principle of matching patient characteristics to the side-effect profiles of agents. We tend to favor midpotency first-generation drugs such as perphenazine and molindone as the best balance of side effects, including EPS, and weight gain. The clinician might guess that a sedating drug like chlorpromazine may elicit a better response in an anxious, excited, acutely psychotic patient, or the clinician might judge that a less sedating drug like haloperidol is a better choice because relatively larger doses are likely to be better tolerated. Either choice is acceptable. A small series of studies by Van Putten (1978) showed that if the first dose of an antipsychotic was judged even slightly helpful by a patient, that patient had a good response to the drug over a 4-week trial. On the other hand, if the first dose was unpleasant because of oversedation or early signs of akathisia, the patient did badly during a 4-week trial, even if antiparkinsonian drugs and dosage adjustment were used to their best advantage. It may be— although no one has tried such an irregular approach—that one should give acutely ill patients a different drug every day until one is found that the patient does not dislike. The inverse of this approach is to take good drug histories, whenever possible, and to avoid using drugs that the patient remembers to have been unpleasant.

Antipsychotic drugs differ in the dosages and formulations in which they are available. Thioridazine and pimozide, and some SGAs, are not available in parenteral forms. Generic, and therefore less expensive, forms are available for chlorpromazine, trifluoperazine, haloperidol, thioridazine, and most first-generation antipsychotics. Among the second-generation agents, only clozapine and risperidone are available generically. Olanzapine's patent expires in 2011. So far there is no evidence that generic forms of antipsychotic drugs are significantly different from the original product, but some patients strongly prefer the old standby. Haloperidol may have a special tactical advantage in being

Table 4–2.   Antipsychotic drug potency

Generic name	Brand name	Chlorpromazine equivalence
aripiprazole	Abilify	10 mg
chlorpromazine	Thorazine	100 mg
clozapine	Clozaril	50 mg
fluphenazine hydrochloride	Prolixin	2 mg
fluphenazine decanoate	Prolixin Decanoate	0.25 cc/month
haloperidol	Haldol	2 mg
loxapine	Loxitane	10 mg
molindone	Moban	10 mg
olanzapine	Zyprexa	~5 mg
perphenazine	Trilafon	10 mg
prochlorperazine	Compazine	15 mg
quetiapine	Seroquel	63 mg
risperidone	Risperdal	0.5 mg
thioridazine	Mellaril	100 mg
thiothixene	Navane	4 mg
trifluoperazine	Stelazine	5 mg

available as a tasteless, colorless elixir, whereas the chlorpromazine and thioridazine elixirs taste very medicinal. A list of available formulations and strengths of antipsychotic agents is presented in Table 4–1. The cost of each agent per 100 tablets is given in Appendix A.

Several experts have tried to compare the potencies of the various available antipsychotic agents. Our version of the comparative potencies of the various available antipsychotics, based on D_2 binding data, is presented in Table 4–2.

Early Intervention in First-Episode Psychosis

There is some evidence that the earlier the treatment of a first-episode psychosis, the more favorable the long-term outcome. As with depression, some loss of gray matter has been noted in schizophrenia to commence with the beginning of psychosis (Pantellis et al. 2003). Gray matter loss has been noted in early schizophrenia in the cingulate gyrus, orbital frontal cortex, and cerebellar cortex, among other areas, that progresses over time. In addition, there is often a loss of function in patients with schizophrenia that precedes the emergence of psychotic symptoms. Thus, there is hope that early intervention might improve long-term outcome or even prevent the full-blown development of schizophrenia in patients with prodromal symptoms.

In general, there appears to be a negative relationship between time to treatment of a first-episode psychosis and outcome across a number of measures. For example, the shorter the duration of untreated psychotic symptoms, the greater the response to antipsychotics (Perkins et al. 2005). The longer the patient stays psychotic, the less likely medications will be successful in alleviating symptoms. This appears to be true for response to both positive and negative symptoms, but the effects are most notable in the treatment of positive symptoms. Shorter duration of illness to first treatment may also be associated with improvement in functional outcome and cognition and a reduced risk of relapse.

Does early treatment in first-episode psychotic patients impact the progressive morphological changes that have been observed in schizophrenia? There is some suggestion that early treatment might have a neuroprotective effect that presumably could be associated with improved prognosis. Lieberman and colleagues (2003) randomly assigned a group of 300 patients with first-episode psychosis to treatment with either haloperidol or olanzapine. The patients treated with olanzapine did not appear to show morphological changes, whereas the patients treated with haloperidol did. Over the course of 2 years, the olanzapine-treated patients did not have loss in frontal gray matter as did the haloperidol-treated patients. In addition, there was a modest increase in volume in the temporal areas in the patients treated with olanzapine but not in the patients treated with haloperidol. The implications of this study are unclear, but the findings suggest that early intervention may impact cortical areas in important ways and that different antipsychotics might act differently. More generally, intervening early and attempting to prevent relapse in schizophrenia may substantially improve long-term outcome. The possibility that we might prevent the syndrome of schizophrenia altogether through early identification of at-risk children and adolescents is intriguing. However, the tools for identifying at-risk patients and the interventions that might prevent schizophrenia from emerging are not yet developed.

Inpatient Treatment

In the age of managed care, with dwindling length of hospital stays, there is considerable pressure to move acutely psychotic patients out of the hospital rapidly. Unfortunately, as previously described, all antipsychotics work in a slow, approximate manner. There is no evidence that pushing doses higher than that which is known to produce a 60%–80% D_2 receptor blockade speeds response. Controlled acute-treatment drug studies generally fail to find an antipsychotic dosage so low that improvement does not occur, whereas such studies find that very high dosages are often less effective than lower dosages. So far, we know of no study of acutely psychotic inpatients that has found a dosage too low to be effective. The psychiatrist faced with a disturbed patient and a concerned or even frightened ward staff who ordinarily use high antipsychotic dosages and frequent prn medication may be hard put to keep to a low-, steady-dosage regimen, however sensible, but we strongly believe that the latter alternative is best. Again, using oral and parenteral benzodiazepines such as lorazepam may be more useful than administering higher dosages of an antipsychotic, and the former may provide more benefit to both patient and staff.

Choosing the "right" drug for the patient may not be possible, and the actual drug used may often be irrelevant, since all available first- and second-generation antipsychotics are essentially equivalent in average efficacy. Nevertheless, for patients who previously received antipsychotic therapy, it is well worth getting a detailed drug history from them and from their family and past physicians. The point is to know the drugs that the patient has received and responded to—or those that the patient has had bad reactions to or disliked actively—and to try to choose a drug that the patient will both accept and respond to.

If a patient's condition does not improve with an adequate dosage of an antipsychotic, several approaches are available, although the reasons for selecting a specific one remain obscure. A different antipsychotic drug can be tried, of course. However, in the absence of undesirable side effects, it is always difficult to be sure whether a shift to a different drug at a more or less equivalent dosage will be better than continuing the original drug for a longer period. Pragmatically, 2 weeks without response in markedly psychotic patients and 5–6 weeks in patients with milder symptoms or with detectable but quite inadequate improvement generally forces the clinician to make a change. Again, the choice of the second drug is determined more clearly by the patient's past untoward reactions to specific antipsychotics than by any rational strategy based on the patient's specific pattern of psychopathology. Some clinicians end up selecting the last drug that worked for them for a patient with a similar treatment-resistant condition. Because, for patients who are not experiencing a response, higher dosages of the original antipsychotic have usually already been tried without benefit, it is better to use the time of change to see whether a substantially lower equivalent dosage of the new drug is any better. Again, if the second drug is well tolerated, it should be continued for several weeks. The only situation in which changing drugs can be dramatic is a shift to parenteral or depot medication in a patient who has not actually been taking his or her oral medication. As Donald Klein once said, "The first thing to do when a drug isn't working is to make sure the patient is actually taking it!" When the patient is taking a substantial dose of an antipsychotic and his or her condition is not improving, it is possible that akinesia, akathisia, or confusion due to the anticholinergic effects of antiparkinsonian drugs may be responsible. One can decrease the dosage rapidly and expect some rebound agitation, followed, sometimes, by significant improvement.

It is still unclear whether antipsychotic plasma levels are of major value in titrating dose, but there are enough suggestions of the existence of a therapeutic window with some antipsychotics that the clinician can try, with caution, using plasma levels as a gauge of clinical response in patients who are not experiencing improvement. Therapeutic ranges of antipsychotics, except for haloperidol and perhaps clozapine, really do not exist, but laboratories can provide commonly observed blood level ranges. If a patient's blood level (12 hours after an oral dose or 1 week after a depot injection) is either very high or almost undetectable, appropriate changes can be tried. If the patient is already on a very high dosage of a neuroleptic and the laboratory finds almost none of the agent in the blood, one should change drugs (or laboratories) or double-check that compliance is not a factor. We worry about escalating antipsychotics to huge dosages on the basis of laboratory data alone unless one has access to an outstandingly competent laboratory.

At this time, the best evidence for rational relationships between plasma levels and clinical response exists for haloperidol. There may even be a curvilinear relationship between blood levels of haloperidol and clinical response such that levels below 4 ng/mL or above 26 ng/mL are associated with poorer clinical response compared with levels within the "therapeutic window" of 4–26 ng/mL. However, not all studies agree, and clinicians wanting to use this guideline must determine for themselves whether the levels are useful. The other drug for which there may be a clinically useful therapeutic window is clozapine. A number of studies suggest that therapeutic response is correlated with clozapine serum levels above 350 ng/mL (Liu et al. 1996; Van der Zwaag et al. 1996). The clinically convincing event occurs when a patient who has not experienced a response improves when a level of antipsychotic that is outside the therapeutic window is adjusted to fall within it. However, in therapeutic drug monitoring of clozapine, serum levels generally do not add much to clinical care. The problem is that there is such great inter-individual variability in clozapine serum levels that they do not adequately predict either response or toxicity.

For a patient whose condition does not appear to be responding to treatment, careful reevaluation for overt and covert side effects is necessary. Adding (or removing) antiparkinsonian drugs or other medications designed to alleviate specific side effects or shifting to another antipsychotic may be helpful. Even having the patient take the whole dose at bedtime may help by decreasing daytime sedation or inertia. Reconsidering diagnosis is also helpful. For some patients who were initially assumed to have schizophrenia, a diagnosis of psychotic depression or bipolar disorder may turn out to be more accurate, and the addition of an antidepressant or lithium may be indicated. Some patients with treatment-resistant DSM-IV schizophrenia who have few or no affective symptoms can experience improvement when lithium or valproate is added to an antipsychotic, although this approach rarely results in a full remission. Other augmentation strategies, including the combination of two antipsychotics, may be helpful (see Chapter 9: "Augmentation Strategies for Treatment-Resistant Disorders").

If a patient's psychosis is unremitting and serious and is quite probably either worse or no better while the patient is taking antipsychotic drugs, the clinician should have the patient stop taking all antipsychotics to make sure that his or her condition is not made worse by them. Moreover, the use of antipsychotics in the face of little apparent response needs to be justified because of the risk of EPS and metabolic side effects. Unfortunately, some patients are simply not responsive to available treatments for psychosis. The failure to respond to multiple antipsychotics should prompt a reevaluation of the diagnosis and consideration of comorbidities that might affect response such as active substance abuse.

Maintenance Drug Therapy

For a patient who has recovered from a first psychotic episode, there is no evidence regarding how long to continue antipsychotic therapy. Probably stopping the drug 2 days after the patient appears much better will lead to a return of psychosis, whereas tapering off medication after 3 months might be tolerated by many patients—perhaps 85%—without relapse rapidly ensuing. Nonetheless, schizophrenia is a chronic illness characterized by exacerbations and relative remissions, so maintenance pharmacotherapy is almost always required. At some point, the drug action shifts from being directly antipsychotic to preventing relapse. In principle, and generally in practice, patients with schizophrenia reach a stable level of remission—often with residual psychotic symptoms that do not improve with increased medication and that may not worsen when the drug is stopped. In fact, in the short run, some patients feel "better"—more alert and energetic—without medication. However, the risk of relapse is a good deal greater when patients are not taking medication.

Antipsychotic drugs are clearly effective in the prevention of relapse of schizophrenia. Unfortunately, as many as 25%–50% of patients will experience a relapse within 2 years despite good compliance with their antipsychotic medication. In one major study, one-half of the antipsychotic-treated schizophrenic patients experienced a relapse by the end of the 2-year study period. About 85% of the placebo-treated patients relapsed over the same period. Recent studies of olanzapine in maintenance treatment suggest that approximately 20% of patients experience a relapse within 1 year while taking the drug, whereas about 70% experience a relapse with placebo treatment (Tran et al. 1998). The rate of relapse with olanzapine in these studies (20%) was better than the rate of relapse with haloperidol (30%) during the same time period. It is clear that antipsychotics are more effective than placebo, but many patients experience a relapse despite adequate drug therapy.

At this time, SGAs are generally the treatment of choice for maintenance therapy of schizophrenia. Reduced risk of tardive dyskinesia, improved cognitive function, and perhaps greater efficacy in treating negative symptoms have resulted in the SGAs being the maintenance treatment of choice for schizophrenia. However, the biggest single drawback to use of second-generation agents in maintenance therapy is their greater proclivity for producing significant weight gain compared with first-generation antipsychotic agents (Allison et al. 1999). Weight gain is terribly problematic in patients treated with clozapine or olanzapine. At this time, among the SGAs, risperidone, ziprasidone, and aripiprazole appear to have the lowest propensity to cause weight gain, although risperidone does produce some weight gain. In addition, a few patients will respond better to first-generation dopamine receptor antagonists than to second-generation agents. For these patients, maintenance with the lowest effective dosage of a first-generation agent is warranted.

Perhaps one-fifth of all patients whose condition is stabilized while taking an antipsychotic medication show signs of increasing psychosis as the drug is tapered—strong evidence that the medication is necessary. For the first-episode patient in full remission, prolonged antipsychotic treatment is not indicated, but generally it has seemed sensible for the patient to continue taking a very gradually decreasing dosage of the drug with which he or she improved. The tapering should last at least 3 months after discharge or from the point of marked improvement. If the patient is expected to be under stress in the next 6–9 months (e.g., completing school, starting a new job, getting divorced), we favor continuing the neuroleptic until the stress point is well past and the patient is generally coping adequately. Recent data suggest that in patients with schizophrenia, maintenance therapy, even after the first episode, could alter the course of the illness in a positive manner. Thus, maintenance therapy is beginning to be used earlier in the course of the illness, even after a single episode.

For patients with a history of two or more psychotic episodes that appear to have occurred after withdrawal of antipsychotics (either by the clinician or by the patient), prolonged maintenance antipsychotic therapy is indicated. Systematic large-scale studies are under way that may modulate our old beliefs. Kane's work suggests that as little as about 2.5 mg (0.1 mL) of fluphenazine decanoate every 2 weeks (10% of the fluphenazine decanoate dosage at which the patient's condition was clinically stable) is more effective than placebo, though less effective than the full (100%) dose, in preventing relapse (Kane et al. 1983). The 10% dose illustrates current problems in weighing the risks and benefits of a low-dose approach: the patients taking this dose appear to feel better and function a bit better than patients on the 100% dose, and their condition is judged to be better by their families. They also develop fewer dyskinetic movements. However, they more often experience relapse into psychosis. Is this outcome "better" or "worse" overall? Several studies suggested that a 20% dose (e.g., about 5 mg every 2 weeks) was as effective as the full dose at preventing relapse for the first year. In the second year, the group on the 20% dose had more relapses than the group on the full dose. At this time, for patients with schizophrenia, we favor long-term maintenance at their full antipsychotic dose if possible. Patients who do not tolerate standard doses of classic antipsychotics should be switched to standard doses of SGAs. For patients who are unable to tolerate standard doses, we suggest a gradual taper of the antipsychotic dose over 6–9 months to the lowest dose that controls symptoms.

Among the typical antipsychotics, only fluphenazine and haloperidol are available in long-acting or depot preparations in the United States. Risperidone was the first SGA to also be available in a long-acting form (Risperdal Consta). This form of risperidone requires injections every 2 weeks but appears to be effective. Some patients in the risperidone long-acting trials at Stanford experienced minor irritation around the injection site, but the drug was remarkably well tolerated by most patients over several years. A number of other depot drugs (fluspirilene, flupentixol, perphenazine), as well as an oral tablet (penfluridol) that lasts a week, are available in Europe and, in some cases, Canada. Depot fluphenazine and haloperidol are available in the decanoate form.

Because one of the main reasons antipsychotics do not work is that patients dislike them and refuse to take them, depot antipsychotics have the great advantage that a known amount of drug is administered reliably and that the staff is immediately aware when an injection is missed. Several controlled studies have failed to show, however, that depot fluphenazine is any more effective than oral fluphenazine in averting psychotic relapse in aftercare patients. Our interpretation of these counterintuitive data is that research studies with dedicated nurses, excellent outreach, weekly medication monitoring, and all patients getting both pills and injections provide an excellent but unrealistic level of aftercare that ensures both pill taking and injection taking. In more typical, understaffed aftercare programs, depot fluphenazine injections are likely to be much easier to monitor and to be better monitored than pill taking. More "naturalistic" studies would probably have shown depot drugs to be more effective at averting relapse, especially in patients with a history of noncompliance. It is not uncommon to find that patients who have repeatedly stopped taking oral antipsychotic medication after hospital discharge and have vociferously objected to taking medication will cooperate faithfully with a depot antipsychotic regimen, presenting themselves for the injection on time, month after month. The reasons for this improved compliance are unclear. One possibility is that patients who stop oral antipsychotic medications feel "better" in a few days as the side effects wear off. Some patients even become transiently euphoric before going on to become grossly psychotic. Stopping oral medication may therefore be reinforcing to the patient, whereas delaying depot injections is not. Intermittent treatment with antipsychotics should be avoided in most patients with schizophrenia. A depot formulation of risperidone is now available.

Other problems in maintenance antipsychotic therapy are evident. First, maintenance therapy averts relapse in about 50%–75% of the patients on that regimen. Second, it is often very hard to determine whether the patient experienced a relapse because the antipsychotic medication was stopped or whether the patient stopped the medication because he or she began to experience a relapse. Third, many patients with chronic schizophrenia who are well stabilized in the community become very rigid about their treatment; they become upset (and experience a relapse) if their medication is changed. We have had several long-term aftercare patients who had been taking antipsychotics for more than 5 years who relapsed with as little as a 40% decrease in their antipsychotic dose. In another study, investigators withdrew active medication in patients with schizophrenia who had been stable in the community for 5 years and found an 80% relapse rate over the following year; this finding suggests that low-dose maintenance drug therapy may be necessary for prolonged periods (Hogarty et al. 1995). Again, the newer agents may provide better efficacy and lower risk of tardive dyskinesia. Given the evidence that abrupt stopping of oral antipsychotics may precipitate relapse, more extensive use of depot antipsychotics is indicated for patients with schizophrenia or schizoaffective disorder.

Trials of withdrawing medication to demonstrate continued need for it are not indicated in cases of recurring schizophrenia. However, these trials may be required in order to defend the use of maintenance antipsychotic therapy in patients with mental retardation, psychotic depression or other depressive conditions, dementia (in elderly patients), and borderline personality disorder (BPD) or other personality disorders. There is a growing body of evidence that a variety of psychosocial therapies can reduce relapse rates (or, better, postpone relapse) in patients with chronic schizophrenia who also are receiving drug therapy. However, none of these therapies substantially modify the deficits in interpersonal functioning present in patients with chronic schizophrenia, regardless of whether they are taking medication. Further, these therapies work best in the first year of a long-term study and less well as time progresses. At least part of this problem is that patients seem "better" and push themselves or are pushed into rehabilitation, social programs, or work programs that make demands that are beyond their coping abilities and that lead to relapse (Hogarty et al. 1995).

Use in Other Psychiatric Disorders

Bipolar Disorder

Until the year 2000, virtually all the literature on large-scale studies of prophylactic treatment for patients with bipolar disorder concerned lithium or valproic acid. However, increasing evidence from clinics serving such patients suggests that many of them end up receiving, and probably require, long-term antipsychotic therapy to remain stable in the community (Sernyak and Woods 1993; White et al. 1993). Two pivotal trials of olanzapine in delaying the onset of mood episodes in patients with bipolar I disorder have demonstrated the clear utility of the drug in the maintenance treatment of bipolar disorder (Citrome et al. 2006; Tohen et al. 2006). Aripiprazole has also demonstrated its utility in maintenance treatment. A study on olanzapine in combination with a mood stabilizer indicated that the combination significantly protected against symptoms but not syndrome relapse when compared with mood stabilizers alone (Tohen et al. 2004).

Clozapine has proved effective in both open and controlled trials of the treatment of schizoaffective disorder and treatment-resistant bipolar disorder (Frye et al. 1998; Green et al. 2000; Mahmood et al. 1997; Suppes et al. 1999). In a large chart review at McLean Hospital of patients receiving clozapine, patients presenting with manic symptoms did better than those presenting with depression.

At this time, all of the SGAs except clozapine have at least two trials supporting their efficacy in treating acute mania. Olanzapine, quetiapine, ziprasidone, aripiprazole, and risperidone have FDA approval for this indication.

Another application of the antipsychotics is in the treatment of bipolar depression. Olanzapine in combination with fluoxetine became the first drug (in a combination capsule, Symbyax) approved for the treatment of bipolar depression. However, even olanzapine alone has notable effects in bipolar depression. Symbyax is available in olanzapine-fluoxetine combinations of 6 mg/25 mg, 6 mg/50 mg, 12 mg/25 mg, and 12 mg/50 mg. The recommended starting dose is 6 mg/25 mg, with adjustment as needed. Quetiapine now has demonstrated utility as a monontherapy in the treatment of bipolar depression and has been approved by the FDA for this indication. The approved dosage range is 300–600 mg/day, although there were no differences between the two dosages in efficacy (Endicott et al. 2008; Thase et al. 2006).

SGAs already are far more commonly used in the treatment of mood disorders than they are in the treatment of schizophrenia. It is likely that the application of these drugs in the treatment of different phases of bipolar disorder will continue to expand (see Chapter 5, "Mood Stabilizers").

Unipolar Depression

In psychotic depression, there is good evidence that the combination of perphenazine and amitriptyline is superior to either drug alone. There is no reason to believe that there is anything magical about this pair of drugs; probably any antidepressant plus any antipsychotic would work about as well. Very few studies of psychotic depression have involved SGAs. The initial trials with the combination of fluoxetine and olanzapine compared with olanzapine monotherapy and placebo showed good efficacy for the combination in one trial but a lack of efficacy in a second one (Rothschild et al. 2004). Olanzapine alone failed to separate from placebo. In a recent National Institute of Mental Health (NIMH)–sponsored trial, the combination did separate from placebo, but it took 6 weeks to see significance (Andreescu et al. 2007). There is limited evidence that amoxapine alone can be useful in the treatment of psychotic depression. ECT is undeniably effective in treating psychotic depression— perhaps more effective than tricyclic antidepressant (TCA)–antipsychotic combinations. The dosages of antipsychotics used in psychotic depression are often quite high (e.g., 48–72 mg of perphenazine); it is unclear whether such high dosages are necessary. In one double-blind study (Shelton et al. 2001), olanzapine in combination with fluoxetine was reported to be significantly more effective than placebo. Some analyses have not concluded that the combination of an antipsychotic to an antidepressant is any better than an antidepressant alone (Wijkstra et al. 2005). However, there is little evidence that antipsychotics, including the SGAs, are useful in the monotherapy of psychotic depression.

When first-generation antipsychotics are used in treating depression, the medical record should reflect the reasons clearly. With continued use for several months, the risks of dyskinesia must be noted and the need for maintenance neuroleptic use must be specifically justified. Many early malpractice suits for tardive dyskinesia involved depressed patients who developed dyskinesia while taking typical antipsychotics. Data from McLean Hospital suggested that patients with unipolar or bipolar depression, whether psychotic or nonpsychotic, develop dyskinesia twice as early as, and with half the drug exposure of, patients with schizophrenia. There are limited data on rates of tardive dyskinesia in long-term use of SGAs in the adjunctive treatment of major depression. However, the rates of tardive dyskinesia in 1-year open-label treatment of adjunctive aripiprazole for depression were less than 1%. Of the available first-generation antipsychotics, only thioridazine is approved by the FDA for use in depression—specifically, moderate to marked depression with anxiety or agitation. There are occasional depressed patients who appear to be uniquely responsive to antipsychotics and fail to improve while taking more conventional antidepressants.

The use of SGAs in the adjunctive treatment of depression has been increasing steadily since 2000. A number of studies now suggest benefit of adding olanzapine, quetiapine, and aripiprazole to antidepressants in the treament of depression (Berman et al. 2009; Garakani et al. 2008; Marcus et al. 2008; Thase et al. 2006). Aripiprazole was approved for the adjunctive treatment of depression in 2007, and olanzapine in combination with fluoxetine was approved for the treatment of resistant depression in 2009. As of this writing, an FDA advisory panel recommended against the approval of quetiapine as a monotherapy for depression out of safety concerns, but the panel was more favorably inclined to recommend approval of quetiapine as an adjunctive agent for resistant depression. The data indicating efficacy of the SGAs in the treatment of major depression are now more extensive than those for any augmenting agents used in the treatment of depression. For example, there are more studies of lithium in the augmentation of antidepressant response, but all of the lithium studies combined have a subject enrollment that is a fraction of the number of patients studied with the newer antipsychotics. The advantage of the SGAs over some traditional augmenting agents such as lithium is greater safety (especially in overdose) and more limited blood monitoring.

Since there are no randomized studies to date comparing the SGAs with other common augmenting strategies such as lithium, thyroid hormone, bupropion, and stimulants, it is difficult to compare efficacy among the adjunctive treatments. However, the antipsychotics studies have been fairly consistent in showing adjunctive benefit. There are many unanswered question with adjunctive SGAs in the treatment of major depression. For example, it is not clear what the optimal duration of treatment with antipsychotics is or what the long-term safety of these drugs is in a depressed population.

There may be some advantages, at least from a metabolic perspective, of aripiprazole over other SGAs in the long-term management of depressed patients. At this time there are not any substantial data supporting the use of SGAs other than aripiprazole, quetiapine, and olanzapine in the adjunctive treatment of depression. To date, only quetiapine XR has demonstrated benefit in the monotherapy of major depression. Results from four randomized controlled trials enrolling about 2,000 patients have suggested that quetiapine at dosages averaging 150–300 mg/day is effective in the monotherapy of depression. Quetiapine is unlikely to ever be a first-line agent in the treatment of depression because of the weight gain and metabolic concerns, but it could be a second-line agent and is likely to see some utility as an adjunctive treatment. (see Chapter 9, "Augmentation Strategies for Treatment-Resistant Disorders").

Anxiety Disorders

Another potential indication for the SGAs is in the treatment of generalized anxiety disorder (GAD). Quetiapine has been studied in controlled trials in the treatment of GAD, and the data were reviewed by an FDA advisory panel in 2009. Four trials have, to date, shown benefit of quetiapine over placebo and benefit comparable to that of approved GAD drugs, including paroxetine and escitalopram. The trials have typically involved dosages of 50, 150, and 300 mg/day over 8 weeks of treatment. While the FDA advisory panel agreed the data supported the efficacy of quetiapine in the treatment of GAD, they did recommend against the approval of quetiapine because of safety concerns in this population. While metabolic issues might be an acceptable trade-off in a more serious illness such as bipolar disorder or schizophrenia, the panel was not convinced this was a reasonable trade-off in GAD. One advantage over traditional agents for the treatment of GAD, such as the antidepressants, is a more rapid onset of action. Quetiapine is also a non–habit-forming alternative to the benzodiazepines, On the other hand, quetiapine may carry greater risks of weight gain, EPS, and metabolic issues than the alternatives. As noted in Chapter 3 ("Antidepressants"), TCAs, selective serotonin reuptake inhibitors (SSRIs), and venlafaxine carry less risk and are probably at least as effective as antipsychotic drugs. Recent reviews suggest that both first- and second-generation antipsychotics may be effective for a wide range of anxiety problems (see Gao et al. 2006). However, the risks and benefits of all available treatments for GAD should be assessed in a given patient before deciding on a treatment.

One situation in which an antipsychotic might be particularly useful in treating an anxiety disorder is when patients present with obsessive-compulsive disorder (OCD) plus schizotypal personality or schizophrenia. In such cases, the OCD is reported to show little or no response to standard drug or behavior therapies. There are suggestions that occasional patients do respond when risperidone or a first-generation antipsychotic is added, but the situation is far from clear. Some patients with schizophrenia can develop OCD symptoms while taking an SGA, perhaps because of its 5-HT$_2$ antagonism. Adjunctive use of pimozide and other antipsychotics clearly helps with tics associated with OCD and Tourette's disorder. There is evidence that the addition of olanzapine or risperidone to an SSRI helps some OCD patients. Risperidone has the best track record as an augmenting agent for OCD, but olanzapine is at least as effective as risperidone (Hollander et al. 2003; Koran et al. 2000; Mottard and de la Sablonniere 1999). The most recent work on quetiapine as an augmentor of SSRIs in OCD is mixed (Kordon et al. 2008; Vulink et al. 2009).

We have occasionally used SGAs in the treatment of panic disorder. There are case reports of the utility of olanzapine in the treatment of panic disorder, and we have seen patients who could not tolerate or respond to SSRIs or venlafaxine who have done well with olanzapine monotherapy for their panic symptoms (Mandalos and Szarek 1999). Likewise, aripiprazole has been used to augment antidepressants in patients with panic disorder who have failed to respond to antidepressant monotherapy (Hoge et al. 2008). Still, olanzapine or other SGAs should be considered only if other strategies fail.

Antipsychotics have long been used in the treatment of posttraumatic stress disorder (PTSD). There is no evidence that antipsychotics help much for some of the core symptoms of PTSD, including intrusive ideation and hypervigilance. However, antipsychotics can be useful adjunctive agents for the management of agitation, irritable aggression, anxiety, and sleep difficulties in some patients. In addition, PTSD patients seem to benefit from second-generation agents in a reduction of reexperiencing symptoms. Because of the sleep and anti-agitation benefits of olanzapine, we often add 5–10 mg of the drug at night to an SSRI or mood stabilizer. Risperidone 1–3 mg in divided doses also seems very helpful for some combat veterans with irritable aggression (Monnelly and Ciraulo 1999; Pivac et al. 2004; States and Dennis 2003).

Anxiety frequently accompanies bipolar disorder. The SGAs clearly help mitigate associated symptoms in bipolar patients. For example, Hirschfeld and colleagues (2006) found that quetiapine at 300 and 600 mg/day was significantly better than placebo in improving anxiety symptoms in patients with bipolar I depression. However, the efficacy of quetiapine for anxiety in bipolar II patients was less convincing.

Personality Disorders

Antipsychotics have been employed in the treatment of patients with borderline and schizotypal personality disorders for many years. However, relatively few studies have been done to support this practice. The paucity of studies is due in part to the difficulties of doing pharmacological trials in patients with personality disorders. Comorbidity with Axis I disorders is common and complicates the selection of patients for studies and the interpretation of study results.

Schizotypal patients may represent one end of the schizophrenia spectrum and often benefit from antipsychotics. Schizotypal personality in younger patients is often perceived as a prodrome of schizophrenia. The only controlled trial of treating schizotypal personality patients with a second-generation agent, risperidone, reported that a daily dose of 0.5–2 mg was beneficial (Koenigsberg et al. 2003). Earlier uncontrolled studies with typical antipsychotics also showed benefits.

Until the past 10 years, much of the work with BPD involved typical antipsychotics. A number of open-label and controlled trials suggested that haloperidol can target the impulsive aggression that BPD patients may exhibit. However, the typical antipsychotics did little to help with the dysphoria and affective instability common to BPD patients. Long-term treatment with haloperidol has generally been poorly tolerated, often discontinued, and only modestly helpful (Cornelius et al. 1993).

The SGAs have started to be more comprehensively studied in recent years in the treatment of persons with BPD, and growing evidence suggests these agents have an important role to play in the treatment of some patients. For example, olanzapine may produce greater global benefits in BPD patients than does fluoxetine (Zanarini et al. 2004). Furthermore, the addition of olanzapine to dialectical behavior therapy (DBT) in patients with BPD seems to facilitate the rapid reduction of irritability and aggression (Linehan et al. 2008). However, not all placebo-controlled studies of olanzapine in BPD have demonstrated benefits. In the largest controlled trial in patients with BPD to date, Schulz and colleagues (2008) did not find olanzapine more effective than placebo in a 12-week study of more than 300 borderline patients. Smaller trials involving risperidone, aripiprazole, and quetiapine have suggested benefits in treating BPD but tend to favor improvement in aggression and impulsivity over improvement of other symptoms. We tend to find that the combination of an SSRI and an SGA is often the optimal pharmacological approach in treating BPD patients. The SSRI-SGA combination seems to treat the dysphoria, mood instability, and impulsivity with good tolerability. Combinations such as paroxetine with risperidone or fluoxetine with olanzapine anecdotally seem well tolerated and effective. The self-identity issues in borderline patients can make weight gain a sensitive issue in prescribing olanzapine, quetiapine, or clozapine. Some data show that risperidone and clozapine are useful in treating self-mutilative behavior and aggression in patients with BPD (Benedetti et al. 1998; Chengappa et al. 1999; Frankenburg and Zanarini 1993). Studies with SGAs have shown more consistent, albeit often modest, effects on treating the core symptoms of BPD. Double-blind studies, while few, have generally suggested benefits of SGAs. For example, in a double-blind trial, aripiprazole was more effective than placebo in treating anxiety, depressive symptoms, and anger in borderline patients (Nickel et al. 2006). Likewise, the addition of olanzapine to DBT was more effective than a placebo added to DBT in addressing core borderline symptoms (Soler et al. 2005).

A reasonable interpretation of these results is that antipsychotics have a stabilizing effect on irritability, mood lability, and impulsivity and that they decrease anxiety. They may have a use in the early stages of a more comprehensive treatment program for patients with BPD such as with DBT. As of this writing, the second-generation agents have shown more consistent benefit in the treatment of borderline symptoms than have the first-generation agents. Thus, given what appears to be a lower long-term risk of some EPS and a broader spectrum of activity for borderline symptoms, the SGAs should generally be used over the first-generation antipsychotics for the treatment of borderline symptoms.

Other States

Antipsychotics are widely used for agitated organic states such as delirium, Alzheimer's dementia, and mental retardation, with varying degrees of benefit. Sometimes the antipsychotics cause more harm (through side effects) than good, and their use is strictly empirical—valuable only if they help (see Chapter 12, "Pharmacotherapy in Special Situations"). In conditions such as depression, anxiety, personality disorder, and organic brain syndromes, for which efficacy of these agents is not firmly established, other drug therapies or no drug therapy may be preferable. The use of antipsychotics should never be routine, and their effects and their effectiveness for each particular patient should always be carefully monitored and documented.

Since the SGAs were introduced, there has been a marked increase in their use for dementia. It has been difficult to demonstrate clear benefit of the second-generation drugs in the treatment of psychosis associated with dementia. Thus, despite many controlled trials, no antipsychotic is approved in the management of elderly dementia patients, and it is unlikely that any will be. The FDA has placed a class warning around increased mortality in geriatric patients with dementia treated with antipsychotics. When the data are pooled together, there is about a 1.7-fold increase in mortality in antipsychotic versus placebo-treated patients. This mortality appears to be associated with several causes, including cardiovascular events, cerebrovascular accidents (CVAs), and infection-related deaths. That being said, there are few good options or reasonable alternatives to the antipsychotics in the treatment of psychosis or agitation associated with dementia. Benzodiazepines, anticonvulsants, and other drugs all have significant limitations in the population of elderly dementia patiants. In comparative studies among the SGAs in dementia patients (CATIE AD; Sultzer et al. 2008), the antipsychotics do seem to have better effects than placebo on some symptoms, including anger, aggression, and paranoid ideas. Overall, the antipsychotics studied—risperidone, olanzapine, and quetiapine—did not make much of a difference relative to placebo in improving functioning or quality of life. There was some greater efficacy of risperidone and olanzapine than for quetiapine in this study. We have found that 2.5–7.5 mg of olanzapine given at bedtime is often helpful for treating agitation and insomnia in patients with dementia. We have been less impressed with the prn use of olanzapine for achieving rapid improvement in agitation. However, carefully done studies have called into question the efficacy of the SGAs in the treatment of agitation and behavioral dyscontrol associated with dementia (Schneider et al. 2006). Given the black box warning of increased mortality associated with the SGAs in geriatric patients, it is unclear whether the benefits outweigh the risks. The use of antipsychotics in patients with dementia should be assessed on a case-by-case basis.

Some studies have found a slightly higher rate of CVAs in dementia patients treated with olanzapine or risperidone. This finding led to an FDA warning, and the risk of CVA is now listed as a potential adverse event in the package inserts of both olanzapine and risperidone. SGAs could conceivably increase the risk of stroke by increasing other risk factors for CVAs, such as obesity and diabetes. However, large-scale analyses of geriatric patients in the community have not found an increased rate of CVAs in patients treated with risperidone or olanzapine (Herrmann et al. 2004). Although the increased risk of CVA associated with SGAs is, at best, small, nonetheless, as with younger patients, monitoring geriatric patients treated with SGAs for changes in weight, glucose levels, and triglyceride levels is worthwhile.

In addition to the treatment of dementia patients, the SGAs are being applied with some success in patients with other conditions. In 2006, for example, risperidone became the first medication approved for use in treating the self-aggression and anger associated with pediatric autism (McDougle et al. 2005). Previous work with haloperidol in the treatment of autism showed modest benefits but significant EPS. Risperidone appears to be better tolerated. Another potential application of SGAs is in the treatment of anorexia nervosa. No pharmacotherapy has been demonstrated to help anorexia on a consistent basis at this time. However, early open-label trials, case reports, and at least one controlled trial suggest that olanzapine and quetiapine may help reduce the anxiety and obsessiveness around food and body image while contributing to weight gain (Dennis et al. 2006; Mondraty et al. 2005; Powers et al. 2007).

Second-Generation (Atypical) Antipsychotics

Clozapine

Clozapine (Clozaril) has been available in the United States for about 20 years for use with patients who have treatment-resistant schizophrenia or patients who are unable to tolerate the side effects of first-generation antipsychotics. Clozapine was in many ways the best new development in the treatment of schizophrenia since chlorpromazine was discovered. The drug does have problems and dangers, it does not work for everyone, and patients who are helped substantially may still be far from well. However, it is thus far the only antipsychotic drug that has been shown in controlled studies to be clearly more effective than older antipsychotics in resistant schizophrenia. It is also thus far the only antipsychotic drug that causes essentially no pseudoparkinsonism or dystonia and that is, apparently, unlikely to cause tardive dyskinesia.

Clozapine has been in clinical use in Europe for more than 30 years. It was withdrawn from general use after deaths from agranulocytosis were reported in Finland in the mid-1970s. Over the intervening years, no other antipsychotic with similar properties was found, perhaps because clozapine has an odd mix of pharmacological effects: more dopamine$_1$ (D$_1$) than D$_2$ effects, more effect on cortical and limbic dopaminergic systems than on the basal ganglia, and greater serotonergic (5-HT$_2$), histaminic, and α-adrenergic blocking activity than other available neuroleptics. Evidence from early (pre-1978) multicenter trials showed clozapine to be more effective than haloperidol or chlorpromazine, leading Sandoz Pharmaceuticals to remarket the drug under controlled conditions in some European countries. In the United States, the FDA insisted that clozapine's efficacy in treating patients with demonstrably treatment-resistant schizophrenia be proved. Such proof was obtained, and the resulting study was published (Kane et al. 1988). Patients with chronic schizophrenia who had failed on at least three adequate neuroleptic trials and had not had a remission in 5 years participated in the study. About one-third of

Second-generation (dopamine-serotonin antagonist) antipsychotics: overview	
Efficacy	Schizophrenia (FDA approved for all) Treatment-resistant schizophrenia (clozapine) Mania (FDA approved for olanzapine, quetiapine, and ziprasidone) Bipolar depression (FDA approved for quetiapine) Depression/anxiety/agitation (efficacy established but not FDA approved for these purposes)
Side effects	Weight gain Gastrointestinal effects Insulin resistance Sedation Akathisia Orthostatic hypotension Bradykinesia Tachycardia Dizziness ↑ Triglycerides (except ziprasidone) EPS, NMS (rare) Agranulocytosis (clozapine) (rare) Seizures (clozapine)
Safety in overdose	Seizures with clozapine in overdose. Respiratory depression in combination with other CNS depressants. QT interval changes. Lavage and vital sign support.
Dosage and administration	Clozapine: 12.5–25 mg; then increase dosage 25–50 mg per week, as needed and tolerated, to 300–600 mg/day Risperidone: 0.5–1 mg bid to 3 mg bid by end of first week, as tolerated Olanzapine: 2.5–5 mg hs; increase by 5 mg every week to 20 mg hs Quetiapine: 25 mg bid; increase total daily dose by 50 mg, as needed and tolerated, to 300–600 mg/day Ziprasidone: 20 mg qd or bid; increase by 20–40 mg per week, to a maximum dosage of 80 mg bid Aripiprazole: 15 mg qd; increase up to 30 mg/day after 1 week
	Full benefits in 4 weeks to 6 months

Second-generation (dopamine-serotonin antagonist) antipsychotics: overview *(continued)*	
Discontinuation	Mild cholinergic rebound, faster relapse. Taper as slowly as titrated up.
Drug interactions	Fluvoxamine (1A2 inhibitor): ↑ second-generation antipsychotic levels EtOH: ↑ sedation and orthostasis Antihypertensives: may ↑ orthostasis Carbamazepine: ↓ serum levels of olanzapine; ↓ clozapine levels; ↑ hematological adverse events with clozapine CNS depressants: ↑ sedation Ciprofloxacin (Cipro) (potent 1A2 inhibitor): ↑ second-generation antipsychotic levels

Note. CNS = central nervous system; EPS = extrapyramidal symptoms; EtOH = ethanol; FDA = U.S. Food and Drug Administration; NMS = neuroleptic malignant syndrome.

the patients improved after taking clozapine for 4 weeks, compared with 2% of patients who improved after taking chlorpromazine (Kane et al. 1988).

Clozapine may differ from first-generation antipsychotics by modestly reducing negative symptoms (e.g., withdrawal, lack of motivation). However, recent studies such as CATIE and CUtLASS have cast doubt on the real-world effectiveness of second-generation drugs in the treatment of negative symptoms. The debate continues regarding whether typical antipsychotics actually cause negative symptoms or whether such symptoms are an integral part of schizophrenia. In addition, clozapine may also affect other dimensions of schizophrenia, such as suicidality. One large study indicated that patients with schizophrenia or schizoaffective disorder who were treated with clozapine (average dosage=274 mg/day) were less likely than were olanzapine-treated patients to attempt suicide or require emergency intervention for a perceived risk of attempting suicide (Meltzer et al. 2003). The risk of completing suicide was low and not statistically different between drugs. The finding of reduced suicidal behavior led to a unique FDA approval for clozapine for decreasing recurrent suicidal behavior in patients with schizophrenia or schizoaffective disorder. Although other SGAs, such as olanzapine, also appear to reduce suicidal behavior in some patients relative to first-generation agents such as haloperidol, clozapine may have unique properties in reducing suicidal behavior. Clozapine may be better than any of the other SGAs in reducing impulsive aggression, and it this property that may account for its reported ability to reduce self-aggression, self-mutilation, and suicide attempts. Although the side-effect profile of clozapine will typically prevent its use as a first- or second-line agent, we have seen a number of cases in which clozapine was used effectively to reduce self-destructive behavior in schizophrenia, bipolar disorder, and even BPD patients.

Because of its tendency to cause serious agranulocytosis—affecting as many as 1.2% of all treated patients in the United States—clozapine is marketed under a unique system: all patients who are to begin taking clozapine must be cleared through a national registry (one of five currently in existence), and the physician and the pharmacy are responsible for obtaining weekly white blood cell counts (WBCs) for all these patients for the first 6 months of treatment, twice monthly for the next 6 months, and then monthly after the first year. Limited amounts of clozapine are dispensed at the time the blood is drawn.

Currently, there are five pharmaceutical companies that market clozapine: Novartis Pharmaceuticals, Mylan Laboratories, IVAX Pharmaceuticals, Caraco Pharmaceutical Laboratories, and AzurPharma. Each company employs its own registry for monitoring, tracking, and reporting patients' WBCs and absolute neutrophil counts (ANCs). All registries must conduct a rechallenge status check from the National Non-Rechallenge Masterfile, which is maintained by Novartis, on all patients who are beginning clozapine or restarting clozapine. The National Non-Rechallenge Masterfile is a national database that identifies patients whose reported WBCs and ANCs are below critical levels, who require termination of clozapine therapy, and who should not be reexposed to clozapine. The five clozapine registries are as follows: Clozaril National Registry (Novartis Pharmaceutical Corporation; 1-800-448-5938: www.clozarilregistry.com); Clozapine Patient Registry (IVAX) (1-800-507-8334; www.clozapineregistry.com); Clozapine Prescription Access System (CPAS) (Mylan; 1-800-843-9915; www.mylan-clozapine.com); Caraco Clozapine Distribution System (CCDS) (Caraco; 1-888-835-2237; www. caracoclozapine.com); and FazaClo Patient Registry (AzurPharma; 1-877-329-2256; www.fazaclo.com/registry_contents.asp).

This system of laboratory monitoring contributes to the expense of prescribing clozapine, but a generic form of clozapine has reduced the pill costs considerably. However, because the onset of agranulocytosis is unpredictable—some patients show slow, steady decreases in WBC, whereas others experience an abrupt plunge in WBC, resulting in agranulocytosis—the purpose is to catch all new cases rapidly and to institute medical treatment early to avoid the deaths that were observed in Europe before this adverse effect was recognized. A few deaths have occurred in the United States under weekly monitoring. The agranulocytosis associated with clozapine use is believed to be an autoimmune reaction, not a direct toxic effect on the bone marrow. It is not dose related. Most cases occur in the second through fourth months of treatment, but some reactions have occurred as late as 18 months after the drug was begun. Patients developing agranulocytosis once will rapidly develop it again if the drug is restarted.

Clozapine is available generically in 12.5-mg, 25-mg, 50-mg, 100-mg, and 200-mg tablets, and in 12.5-mg, 25-mg, and 100-mg scored disintegrating tablets. The starting dosage is 25 mg at bedtime, and the manufacturer recommends dosing bid, but many patients end up taking the whole dose at bedtime. The dosage should be increased slowly and cautiously from 25 mg/day to 200 mg/day over the first 2–3 weeks, then stabilized at that dosage for a few weeks, with further increases as tolerated. Most patients respond well to dosages between 300 and 500 mg/day. If clear improvement has not occurred, the dosage can be gradually increased to 900 mg/day. However, because drug-related grand mal seizures occur quite frequently (in about 15% of patients) at dosages over 550 mg/day, anticonvulsants should probably be added. Phenytoin or valproate, in standard anticonvulsant doses, has been used for this purpose at McLean Hospital.

Sedation is one major side effect limiting dosage increases. Many patients develop tolerance to this effect, but some do not. Cardiovascular side effects, both severe orthostatic hypotension and marked tachycardia (up to 130–140 bpm), can occur early in clozapine treatment. These side effects require very slow dose increases and, sometimes, the use of counteractive medications such as modafinil. A few patients develop unpleasant gastrointestinal distress and flulike symptoms early in treatment and refuse to take the drug again. Drug-induced fevers of around 100°F can occur early in treatment but pass and are not serious. Blood counts should be obtained, but in local experience with more than 300 patients, they have always been normal or elevated. Hypersalivation at night, causing wet pillowcases, is common; clonidine can be helpful in counteracting this side effect. Enuresis occasionally occurs.

Although the manufacturer has strongly urged that other antipsychotics be withdrawn from patients before clozapine is begun, this advice is hard to follow with many psychotic patients. We have almost always added low doses of clozapine to ongoing antipsychotic therapy, then tapered the prior antipsychotic once the clozapine dosage reached 200 mg/day. We have combined clozapine, generally without incident, with benzodiazepines, lamotrigine, lithium, valproic acid, TCAs, trazodone, other SGAs (such as aripiprazole), high-potency first-generation (typical) agents, fluoxetine, and even ECT. Since approximately 40%–70% of patients with resistant schizophrenia will also be resistant to clozapine as well, augmenting strategies are often attempted. The evidence to date suggests that augmentation of clozapine with agents such as lamotrigine, amisulpride, and ethyl-eicosapentaenoic acid might benefit some patients with resistant schizophrenia (Kontaxakis et al. 2005; Mouaffak et al. 2006). Some patients taking SSRIs and clozapine may develop high clozapine levels and sedation. We recommend periodically checking clozapine levels when the two are combined. Fluvoxamine may be particularly problematic, since it is a more potent cytochrome P450 1A2 inhibitor. We have seen several cases of neuroleptic malignant syndrome (NMS) associated with clozapine use, particularly in patients on concurrent lithium. As indicated earlier, lithium is sometimes thought to predispose patients to NMS. The NMS associated with clozapine may be milder than with first-generation agents and tends not to be characterized by rigidity, fevers, and as high of elevations in creatine phosphokinase. Rather, the presentation of NMS in clozapine-treated patients may include delirium, autonomic instability, and milder EPS (Hasan and Buckley 1998; Karagianis et al. 1999). Drugs that are known to induce agranulocytosis, such as carbamazepine, should be avoided.

The course of improvement with clozapine treatment is somewhat unpredictable. Patients who clearly show a substantial decrease in psychotic symptoms may do so in the first few weeks of treatment or as late as 3–6 months or more later. Some patients—a third or more in our experience—show marked improvement, although most are not totally free of psychotic residua. Schizoaffective patients may experience more complete improvement than schizophrenic patients, although schizoaffective patients often have better remissions before clozapine treatment. Psychotic and nonpsychotic patients with treatment-resistant mania also usually respond. Patients who take clozapine for 1 or more years may show gradual, continuing improvement. Even minimally improved psychotic patients may be less impulsively angry, violent, or argumentative and may show a gratifying absence of distressing akathisia, parkinsonism, and akinesia. At McLean Hospital, many such patients have continued to be administered clozapine because they are less distressed by their symptoms and are less of a management problem, even though they are still grossly impaired by psychotic symptoms.

Tardive dyskinesia may be unchanged initially by clozapine treatment, but it often fades over time to near the vanishing point. In some patients the dyskinesia improves early, whereas in others it improves only very slowly. It is unclear whether clozapine suppresses dyskinesia or allows it to fade as it might in patients who are no longer taking antipsychotics.

Long-term side effects of maintenance clozapine therapy are not known, although in the United States, a handful of patients have been taking the drug continuously for over 20 years without known adverse effects (including tardive dyskinesia). With long-term treatment with clozapine, the majority of patients gain weight, whereas a few lose a little weight. There is a controversy about whether clozapine is likely to cause diabetes and ketoacidosis. A consensus development conference on antipsychotic drugs and obesity and diabetes concluded that clozapine appeared to be associated with an increased risk for diabetes (American Diabetes Association et al. 2004). However, this conclusion has not been uniformly adopted.

All the SGAs, especially clozapine, olanzapine, and quetiapine, have been thought to be associated with an increased risk of of hyperglycemia and diabetes, and this is now reflected as a warning in the package inserts of all SGAs. Aripiprazole and ziprasidone may carry lesser risks. Risperidone appears to be intermediate in risk between olanzapine and ziprasidone. There have been a number of cases of diabetic ketoacidosis reported with the use of clozapine and other SGAs. However, the extent of the enhanced risk of diabetes with the SGAs is much debated. Schizophrenia, itself, enhances the risk of diabetes, and typical antipsychotics also increase the risk of diabetes. Whatever the extent of the risk, there is little doubt that several of the second-generation agents are associated with considerable weight gain and a risk of obesity. Obesity in turn is thought to be a clear risk factor for insulin resistance, hyperglycemia, and type 2 diabetes. However, there are cases of diabetes in antipsychotic-treated patients that have occurred independently of weight gain, and we have reported that the insulin resistance that occurs with SGAs is not correlated with acute changes in weight. Thus, the disorder and the drug appear to be associated with insulin resistance independently of weight (Meltzer et al. 2005; Reaven et al. 2009), as evidenced by obesity, high blood pressure, and high triglyceride levels. The syndrome generally does not result in diabetes but appears to place subjects at risk for cardiovascular disease. The acute diabetic ketoacidosis appears to be unrelated to the longer-term weight gain and insulin subsensitivity and may be an idiosyncratic reaction.

In the same way as we taught our residents to routinely monitor patients who were taking typical antipsychotics for signs of EPS and tardive dyskinesia, we now teach our residents to monitor patients who are taking SGAs for signs of a metabolic syndrome. We agree with the American Psychiatric Association/ American Diabetes Association recommendations (Table 4–3) on screening patients. A scale and blood pressure cuff are useful pieces of monitoring equipment to keep in the office. The patients most likely to run into trouble with a metabolic syndrome or diabetes are those with the greatest risk factors for these conditions before pharmacotherapy. Thus, it is important to pay special attention to patients with baseline obesity, dyslipidemias, and a family or personal history of diabetes. If the patient has gained more than 5% of body weight or has a BMI over 30, we may check glucose and lipid levels as frequently as every month until we are convinced that the patient is medically stable. A finger stick is probably more useful than a hemoglobin A_{1c} (HbA_{1c}), unless the patient is already diabetic. The HbA_{1c} is somewhat too global and blunt an assessment to tell us what is happening on a day-to-day basis. A fasting glucose or a finger stick is probably the most useful assessment to obtain in monitoring glucose levels. However, the clinician must keep in mind that patients often maintain fasting glucose levels constant while they become insulin resistant. The resistance may be better monitored by increasing triglyceride or decreasing high-density lipid levels. In addition to screening glucose and lipid levels, we monitor weight and blood pressure and elicit symptoms of diabetes (polydipsia, polyuria, hyperphagia) every few months, and we repeat screening labs 3 months after the initation of therapy. Thereafter, we repeat screening labs once a year or as indicated.

The major problem in monitoring clozapine therapy over time, in addition to monitoring metabolic effects, is the necessity of keeping alert to decreases in the leukocyte count. Our experience suggests that a fair number of patients will worry the clinician by regularly—or occasionally for a few weeks—running WBCs between 3,000 and 4,200 cells/mm^3. Others will show dramatic

Table 4–3. APA/ADA recommendations for screening patients who are taking second-generation antipsychotics

Screen prior to initiating the antipsychotic

Personal or family history of obesity, diabetes, high cholesterol levels, high blood pressure, or heart disease

Weight and height (BMI > 25)

Waist circumference (>40 inches in males; >35 inches in females)

Blood pressure (>130/85)

Fasting blood glucose levels (>110)

Fasting cholesterol levels (HDL < 40; total >200)

Fasting triglyceride levels (>175)

Note. Abnormal levels indicated in parentheses. ADA = American Diabetes Association; APA = American Psychiatric Association.

decreases, say from 8,000 to 5,000 cells/mm^3, from one week to the next. In patients who appear to be benefiting from treatment or who have not been taking clozapine long enough for the outcome to be at all clear, we have gone to twice-weekly complete blood counts (CBCs) until the count has risen again. Getting several weekly CBCs before starting clozapine treatment helps the physician identify patients who are likely to run low leukocyte counts even in the absence of clozapine. One worries less about such patients if the low count is a known characteristic. Should agranulocytosis clearly occur or should the count drop below 3,000 cells/mm^3 or an ANC drop below 2,000/mm^2, the drug should be stopped. Guidelines for monitoring of clozapine use are given in Table 4–4.

In assessing patients with treatment-resistant conditions reported to have stopped taking clozapine because of leukopenia, it is worth determining exactly what happened. Physicians sometimes stop clozapine because patients have a transiently low WBC (3,000–3,999 cells/mm^3); such patients never actually had agranulocytosis. These patients often respond to a second trial of clozapine without ever developing true agranulocytosis. In complex cases, consultation may be helpful before clozapine is restarted. In our opinion, clozapine is useful in treating all patients requiring antipsychotics who have failed to respond to several other antipsychotics; in those with tardive dyskinesia; and in those who have severe, uncontrollable EPS, especially akathisia.

Table 4–4.   Guidelines for clozapine monitoring

Event	Required action	Results	Further action
WBC is 3,500[a] or has dropped significantly,[b] or immature cell forms are present	Repeat WBC and differential count; advise patient to immediately report appearance of fever, sore throat, or other signs of infection.	If repeat WBC is 3,000–3,500 and absolute neutrophil count[c] (ANC) > 2,000 and no immature cell forms, continue clozapine therapy.	Twice-weekly WBC and differential until WBC > 3,500 and cell differential normal.
WBC < 3,500 or ANC < 2,000 and no signs of agranulocytosis	Interrupt clozapine therapy and notify registry. WBC with differential weekly until WBC count ≥ 3,000 and ANC ≥ 2,000.	WBC ≥ 3,000 and ANC ≥ 2,000, and no symptoms of infection are present.	May restart clozapine with twice-weekly WBC until WBC ≥ 3,500, then WBC weekly for 6 months.
WBC < 2,000 or ANC < 1,500 (agranulocytosis) with signs of infection (fever, malaise, weakness, lethargy); this constitutes a medical emergency	Immediately and permanently discontinue clozapine. Monitor patient closely for fever and other signs of infection. Order daily tests until WBC and differential return to normal (WBC ≥ 3,000 and ANC ≥ 2,000).	If WBC > 3,000, repeat posttreatment WBC and differential weekly for 52 weeks.	Consult hematologist for treatment options. Pharmacist notifies registry of discontinuation and provides serial WBC results.

Table 4–4.   Guidelines for clozapine monitoring *(continued)*

Frequency of monitoring	
Initiation of therapy	Weekly for 6 months
6–12 months of therapy with WBC $\geq$ 3,500/mm^2 and ANC $\geq$ 2,000/mm^2	Every 2 weeks for 6 months
12 months of continuous therapy with normal WBC and ANC	Every 4 weeks thereafter
Discontinuation of therapy	Weekly for at least 4 weeks from day of discontinuation or until WBC and ANC are 3,500 and 2,000/mm^2, respectively, or higher

Note.   ANC=absolute neutrophil count; WBC=white blood cell count.
[a]WBC and ANC per mm^3.
[b]"Dropped significantly" is defined as a single drop or a cumulative drop of 3,000 mm^3 or more, or ANC of 1,500 or more within 3 weeks.
[c]ANC/mm^3 = WBC (mm^3) × neutrophil (%). Example: If WBC=7,500/mm^3 and neutrophils=35%, ANC=7,500 × 0.35 = 2,625 mm^3.
Source.   Adapted from Wyatt RD, Chew RH: *Wyatt's Practical Psychiatric Practice: Forms and Protocols for Clinicians*, 3rd Edition. Washington, DC, American Psychiatric Publishing, 2005, p. 40. Copyright 2005, American Psychiatric Publishing, Inc. Used with permission.

The combined cost of the required weekly WBCs and the drug is relatively high. However, most insurance carriers may cover all or a portion of the costs; the fiscal cost-benefit ratio for patients in public or private institutions has been determined, and the results favor the use of clozapine. For example, under Medicare Part D, clozapine is covered by most Prescription Drug Plans (PDPs) under a tiered system, depending on the plan. Now that clozapine is available generically, virtually all county mental health programs are purchasing the generic formulation at great savings over the name brand.

Risperidone

Risperidone (Risperdal) was the next SGA introduced in the United States after clozapine. The drug exerts relatively more D_2 than D_1 antagonism. It also has antagonist effects at $5\text{-}HT_2$ and possibly $5\text{-}HT_1$ receptors. Several multisite collaborative double-blind studies have documented risperidone's apparent effectiveness in treating patients with schizophrenia and its unusual dose-response relationship: 6 mg/day is more effective and associated with fewer side effects than larger dosages, whereas 2 mg/day has been shown to be ineffective. The 6-mg (3 mg bid) dosage is at least as effective as 20 mg of haloperidol. However, the double-blind data regarding side effects are misleading. Although risperidone did not appear to produce much in the way of EPS in comparison to placebo, both "treatments" were associated with more EPS than one might anticipate. Also, a fairer trial would compare 3–6 mg of risperidone with 3.5–7.0 mg of haloperidol, since these are the levels at which both drugs block D_2 receptors at 60%–80% efficiency. At these lower doses, it is unclear whether risperidone maintains a significant edge over haloperidol regarding the rates of EPS.

Risperidone is indicated in the treatment of schizophrenia, schizoaffective disorder, acute mania, and mixed states (Hirschfeld et al. 2004). Risperidone was also approved both as a monotherapy and as an adjunctive agent in the treatment of acute mania and is approved in the treatment of irritability and mixed states in patients with autism. The utility of risperidone as a maintenance treatment or a treatment for bipolar depression is as yet unclear. As reported earlier in this chapter, risperidone also has shown benefits in the augmentation treatment of unipolar depression.

In relatively short double-blind studies with healthy patients receiving only risperidone, the dosage could be raised from 1 mg bid to 2 mg bid to 3 mg bid over a few days without adverse effects. In clinical practice, one may need to raise the dosage more slowly. At McLean Hospital, risperidone seemed the ideal drug as a first-line treatment for psychotic patients until worrisome adverse effects began to be noticed: EPS, orthostatic hypotension, agitation, oversedation, and so forth. Orthostasis has been particularly problematic in some patients and occasionally results in syncope and falls. Our experience is that dystonias are somewhat less common with risperidone relative to first-generation antipsychotics. However, bradykinesia and akathisia are often seen with risperidone treatment. Some of these adverse events might have been avoided if the dose had been raised more slowly or more attention had been paid to pharmacokinetic interactions with other drugs, especially SSRIs. We have seen that the combination of an SSRI and risperidone may enhance the orthostatic side effects of the drug. Risperidone appears more likely to raise prolactin levels than does olanzapine. All in all, local enthusiasm over risperidone has abated somewhat, although the drug is widely used nationally.

In addition, the proportion of patients who clearly do much better while taking risperidone than while taking other, typical antipsychotics seems a good deal less impressive than was the case with clozapine. We suspect that we have not yet learned how best to use risperidone. Staying low in dose and going slow with everybody, but even lower and slower with older patients or patients taking multiple medications, seems wise. In elderly patients, starting risperidone at a dosage of 0.5 mg qd or bid and slowly titrating the drug upward appears prudent, and we tend to keep the dosage below 1–2 mg/day for the first 2 weeks in an attempt to limit side effects.

Clozapine has always seemed more effective than older antipsychotics. Risperidone seems more like a somewhat improved haloperidol: it is as effective as haloperidol but has fewer of the side effects typically associated with the latter drug if the dose is kept low. Our impression has been that clinicians who try to switch patients from clozapine to risperidone are often disappointed in the outcome. Still, at least one study has suggested that over a 1-year period, risperidone was equal in efficacy to clozapine and much better tolerated (Azorin et al. 2001).

Recent studies have not found risperidone or other SGAs to have that many advantages over first-generation agents. For example, in the CATIE trial (Lieberman et al. 2005; Stroup et al. 2006), risperidone was about as well tolerated and effective as perphenazine. However, the trial has been criticized for employing doses of risperidone and other agents that may have been too low. For example, in the CATIE trial, many patients were treated with risperidone at dosages (< 3 mg/day) that are often considered to be too low. Dosage ranges were selected in part by the manufacturers.

The virtues of risperidone seem to disappear when the dosage is increased because the patient is not improving fast enough to suit managed care or hospital administration. In affective psychotic patients, risperidone may be more effective for depression and may be more likely to cause mania, whereas clozapine is more effective for mania-like states and may be effective for depression.

Risperidone may turn out, in the long run—if used wisely and well—to be the ideal first-line antipsychotic, to lead to better control of both negative and positive symptoms, and to cause less tardive dyskinesia and NMS. However, compared with other SGAs, risperidone causes more EPS particularly when the dosage is pushed much beyond 6 mg/day. The cumulative risk of tardive dyskinesia with risperidone treatment for 1 year is around 0.5%–1% in younger patients and perhaps as high 2.6 % in older patients. A long-acting depot formulation, Risperdal Consta, is available for maintenance therapy. Typical dosages range from 25 to 50 mg every 2 weeks.

Weight gain while taking risperidone is generally much less of a problem than it is with clozapine, olanzapine, or quetiapine. Our sense is that weight gain with risperidone is probably more comparable to that seen with aripiprazole and ziprasidone. That said, there have been cases of diabetic ketoacidosis associated with risperidone use, and we employ the same screening methods for all patients taking SGAs at this point.

Some final thoughts about risperidone use:

1. In changing patients from a typical antipsychotic (or clozapine), it is unwise to discontinue the older antipsychotic, wait 2 weeks, and then start risperidone. Phasing the new drug in slowly while phasing the older drug out should lessen the chance of relapse.

2. Adding risperidone to clozapine has already been tried with some benefit, particularly in patients with an incomplete response and/or oversedation while taking clozapine.

3. Dosages of 6 mg/day or less tend to avoid EPS better than do higher dosages.

Paliperidone

In 2006, 9-hydroxyrisperidone (paliperidone; Invega), the active metabolite of risperidone, was approved in the United States for the acute and maintenance treatment of schizophrenia. Like risperidone, paliperidone is a $D_2/5\text{-HT}_2$ antagonist with some α_1- and α_2-adrenergic and H_1 antagonism as well. An initial application of the use of paliperidone for use in acute mania was withdrawn because of insufficient data. In 2009, a submission was filed with the FDA for paliperidone in the monotherapy and adjunctive treatment of schizoaffective disorder. If approved for this indication, paliperidone would represent the first drug indicated for the treatment of schizoaffective disorder. In a 6-week randomized controlled trial involving more than 300 patients (Kane et al. 2007), patients treated with 12 mg/day of adjunctive paliperidone ER showed significantly greater benefit on the primary outcome measure (Positive and Negative Syndrome Scale; PANSS) than did patients receiving placebo. Both the 6 and 12 mg/day groups, however, experienced greater benefits than the placebo-treated groups on secondary measures, including the Young Mania Rating Scale and the Hamilton Depression Rating Scale. A second 6-week, international study of paliperidone ER (Marder et al. 2007) also demonstrated the efficacy of paliperidone ER in the monotherapy of schizoaffective disorder.

Schizoaffective disorder is in some ways the poor stepchild of schizophrenia, with relatively few carefully controlled studies completed to date. Historically, schizoaffective disorder has been treated with the combination of antipsychotics and mood stabilizers or antidepressants. The paliperidone studies provide additional evidence that a combination strategy is useful but that monotherapy with an antipsychotic may be as useful in many schizoaffective patients. The manufacturer of paliperidone received FDA approval, in July 2009, for a long-acting, injectable formulation of the drug in the maintenance treatment of schizophrenia. Paliperidone palmitate (Invega Sustenna) is a once-a-month injectable that was studied in trials of 9- and 24-week duration. The dosages in these studies were 25 mg, 50 mg, and 150 mg per injection. Patients treated with the paliperidone injection received greater benefit on the PANNS than did subjects receiving placebo. In addition, paliperidone palmitate was more effective than placebo in preventing relapse in the 24-week trial.

The primary advantage of both paliperidone ER and the injectable formulation over risperidone and its formulations is convenience for some patients. Oral risperidone may require twice-daily dosing in some patients versus once-daily for paliperidone. Likewise, paliperidone palmitate is injected once a month versus twice a month for risperidone. The primary disadvantage of paliperidone relative to rispiridone is cost. A generic formulation of risperidone was approved by the FDA in 2008, and the cost will come down further as other generic formulations become available. At this time, there are few data to suggest either efficacy or side-effect advantages of the metabolite over its parent drug. Since the long-acting injectable form of risperidone will not be generic, the even longer-acting paliperidone palmitate might be the better choice for many patients.

Iloperidone

Iloperidone (Fanapt) was approved unexpectedly by the FDA in 2009 for the treatment of schizophrenia. Iloperidone was originally developed many years years ago by Roussel. Early trials suggested that it was not as effective as haloperidol or risperidone in the treatment of schizophrenia, and the drug was shelved in 1996. The rights to iloperidone were sold to Novartis, then Titan Pharmaceuticals, and finally to Vanda. In 2007, Vanda received a nonapprovable letter from the FDA with both safety and efficacy issues raised about iloperidone. Nonetheless, additional data resulted in Vanda's getting approval for the drug in 2009.

Iloperidone, like other SGAs, is primarily thought to act as a $D_2/5\text{-}HT_2$ antagonist. The drug also has some activity at the α_2, $5\text{-}HT_1$, D_1, D_2, D_3, D_4, and D_6 receptors. Iloperidone is well absorbed orally and has a peak serum plasma level in 2–4 hours. It has a half-life of around 24–36 hours in most subjects. Iloperidone is a substrate for both CYP 2D6 and 3A4. Thus, drugs such as fluoxetine can more than double serum levels of iloperidone, and carbamazepine can substantially reduce serum levels. Thus adjustments in dosing may be necessary for patients who are concurrently taking drugs that are 2D6 or 3A4 inhibitors or inducers.

The efficacy of iloperidone was established in two Phase III trials in the United States. In a 6-week trial ($N=706$), two doses of iloperidone (12–16 and 20–24 mg/day) were superior to placebo and equal to an active comparator at the endpoint in the treatment of schizophrenia (Potkin et al. 2008). Likewise, in a second 4-week trial (N=604), 12 mg bid was superior to placebo in treating both positive and negative symptoms of schizophrenia (Kane et al. 2008).

The most common side effects in the clinical trials were dizziness, dry mouth, fatigue, somnolence, tachycardia, orthostatic hypotension, and weight gain. Tachycardia, dizziness, and weight gain appear to be dose-related, with higher doses (24 mg/day) causing more problems than lower doses (12 mg/day). The weight gain and metabolic effects seem more in line with what has been observed with risperidone than with what has been reported with either olanzapine or clozapine. Across short- and long-term trials, the average weight gain was about 2 kg.

There are at least two disadvantages of iloperidone over other SGAs at this time. One is the slow dosing titration that is required to limit the hypotension seen in clinical trials. About 5% of patients taking iloperidone at a dosage of 24 mg/day experienced hypotension, and more aggressive titration was associated with greater risk of hypotension and syncope. The recommended starting dosage is 1 mg bid, with doubling of the dose daily to a target dosage of 6–12 mg bid (12–24 mg/day). In the clinical trials, the comparison antipsychotic often seemed to work more rapidly because little titration was required for haloperidol or risperidone. A second disadvantage is that iloperidone can prolong QT intervals. At the higher dosage, there was an increase in QTc intervals by 9 msec. Drugs that inhibited 2D6 and 3A4 further prolonged QTc interval. Thus, caution must be exercised in combining iloperidone with CYP450 inhibitors, as well as drugs that are known to prolong QTc intervals, including quinidine, chlorpromazine, and thioridazine.

It is unclear to us exactly where iloperidone is going to fit in the treatment of schizophrenia. It is not going to be a first-line agent because of the dosing and QTc issues. Iloperidone is going to be more expensive than either first-generation drugs or generic SGAs. Patients who cannot tolerate or respond to other SGAs might be a candidate for iloperidone.

Olanzapine

Olanzapine (Zyprexa) was introduced to the U.S. market in 1996. Like other SGAs, it has a high binding ratio of 5-HT$_2$ to D$_2$ receptors. The receptor-binding affinities of olanzapine appear to lie somewhere between the very broad receptor effects of clozapine and the more narrow receptor binding of risperidone. Like clozapine, olanzapine is an antagonist of dopamine receptors (D_1–D_4) and the 5-HT_2 receptor. In addition, it is antihistaminic, is anticholinergic, and blocks α_1-adrenergic receptors. Olanzapine is metabolized primarily via the cytochrome P450 enzymes 1A2 and, to a lesser extent, 2D6. Olanzapine appears to be at least as effective as haloperidol in the short-term treatment of schizophrenia. It may be better than haloperidol in improving negative symptoms, concurrent depression and suicidality, and cognition. In addition, in pre-marketing studies, olanzapine 10–20 mg/day was associated with significant improvement in positive symptoms, including delusions, hallucinations, and thought disorder.

Olanzapine is still among the most commonly used second-generation agents even though it is also among the most expensive. The CATIE trial suggested that olanzapine might be somewhat more efficacious overall than other second-generation agents in that it was less likely to be discontinued (Stroup et al. 2006). A full 64% of patients discontinued olanzapine before the 18-month trial was completed, versus 74%–82% of patients discontinuing the comparator antipsychotics. Olanzapine was also more likely than the comparison agents (perphenazine, risperidone, quetiapine, and ziprasidone) to be associated with metabolic side effects.

Olanzapine is now approved for the treatment of a variety of disorders other than schizophrenia. Olanzapine was the first SGA approved for the treatment of acute mania. It probably works faster and at least as effectively as does lithium or valproate. In addition, olanzapine became the third drug, after lithium and lamotrigine, to show benefit in the prevention of mania and depression in bipolar I patients. Olanzapine, when combined with fluoxetine, became the first drug approved for the treatment of bipolar depression. Olanzapine by intramuscular injection has been approved for the acute treatment of agitation in patients with schizophrenia and bipolar disorder. As previously reported, olanzapine also appears to have·a role in treating psychotic depression, and as an augmenting agent in treating unipolar depression (see subsection "Unipolar Depression" earlier in this chapter).

It remains unclear whether olanzapine is as useful as clozapine in the treatment of refractory schizophrenia, even though comparison studies have generally found the drugs to be equally effective in this context (Bitter et al. 2004; Tollefson et al. 2001). However, the CATIE trial suggested the superiority of clozapine to olanzapine in treating resistant schizophrenia (McEvoy et al. 2006). Olanzapine is a fairly "dirty" drug, in that it affects multiple neurotransmitter systems, but it is not quite as "dirty" as clozapine. It is this "dirtiness" that contributes to clozapine's toxicity but that may also be important in the efficacy of the drug in more refractory cases.

Head-to-head trials of olanzapine and risperidone in refractory depression also suggest that the drugs are probably equally effective but differ in side-effect profiles. Olanzapine is associated with more weight gain and sedation, whereas risperidone is more likely to increase prolactin levels and produce EPS.

Olanzapine appears to have a clear advantage over high-potency typical agents such as haloperidol in that it is associated with less EPS. In the CATIE trial (Lieberman et al. 2005), however, the rate of EPS with perphenazine was about the same as it was with the SGAs, including olanzapine. Olanzapine has been shown in multiple studies to produce less EPS than does haloperidol. In acute trials, the only extrapyramidal symptom reliably noted at a greater rate than with placebo was akathisia, and the incidence of this effect increases with dose. At least 10% of patients will develop akathisia in an acute 6-week trial at dosages of 10 to 15 mg/day. We have found that propranolol 10 mg bid or tid can help with this problem. However, some patients have a significant worsening of postural hypotension with even small additions of β-blockers, so caution is advised. Dystonic reactions and dyskinesias appear to be quite uncommon with olanzapine at usual dosages. However, patients do tend to report more severe parkinsonian symptoms with increasing dosages of the drug, including feeling stiffer and more slowed down. About 20% of patients will report Parkinson's-type symptoms at dosages above 10 mg/day. Anticholinergic agents clearly help if parkinsonism develops.

The rate of tardive dyskinesia with olanzapine appears markedly less than that of first-generation agents but is not zero as it appears to be with clozapine. Tardive dyskinesia occurs at a rate of around 0.5%–1% per year of treatment, which is 10–15 times less frequent than with haloperidol at comparison doses. Even with less aggressive dosing of haloperidol, say 2–5 mg/day, the rates of tardive dyskinesia in olanzapine-treated patients appear to be a fraction of those reported with haloperidol. We recommend periodically assessing patients who are taking any antipsychotic for signs of tardive dyskinesia and doing this at regular intervals.

NMS appears to be uncommon but not unheard of with olanzapine use. There are several reports in the literature of olanzapine inducing NMS, including in patients who had previously developed NMS while taking first-generation agents. Our limited experience with NMS in olanzapine-treated patients is that, as with clozapine, the presentation may be atypical, with fewer and less severe EPS than are seen with first-generation antipsychotics.

Anticholinergic side effects such as constipation and dry mouth occur in 5%–10% of patients taking olanzapine at therapeutic dosages. Like risperidone and clozapine, olanzapine produces α-adrenergic blockade, resulting in a dose-related increase in orthostasis and dizziness. We suggest monitoring orthostatic blood pressures, particularly with older patients and those with a history of postural hypotension. Support stockings help orthostasis in older patients. These orthostatic effects are not nearly as dramatic as the effects that can occur with clozapine.

The most problematic side effects with long-term, maintenance use of olanzapine are weight gain and sedation. At least 29% of patients will gain more than 7% of their body weight in a 6-week trial, and 5.4 kg, or about 12 lb, is the average weight gain with long-term use (Allison et al. 1999). However, we have seen some patients gain 50 lb or more in a year. This weight gain is terribly distressing for many patients. Large weight gains have been thought to be associated with insulin resistance and dyslipidemias, although the former has not been clearly demonstrated. As with other SGAs, patients taking olanzapine should be screened and monitored for metabolic symptoms (see overview of SGAs and Table 4–3 earlier in this chapter).

The weight gain associated with olanzapine appears to be, at least in part, from an increased appetite, and we warn patients that olanzapine can result in their desire to eat more. Most of the weight gain that occurs with olanzapine appears to occur in the first 6 months, with gain then appearing to plateau for up to 3 years. Patients with body mass indexes (BMIs) < 23 (i.e., thinner patients) have been thought to be most at risk for gaining substantial weight, but this may be an artifact of starting at a lower weight. Obese patients tend to gain much less weight and eventually may actually lose weight. Counting calories or participating in a food monitoring system such as that offered by Weight Watchers can be very helpful, as can be more rigorous and regular exercise. Pharmacologically, three strategies are worth considering: Topiramate appears to be useful at dosages of 50–100 mg/day as an appetite suppressant. Eli Lilly has found that the H_2 antagonist famotidine at a dosage of 600 mg/day appears to prevent the weight gain to some extent. Animal data suggest that amantadine may also help patients lose weight gained while taking olanzapine. One earlier report indicates that metformin can help mitigate weight gain associated with antipsychotic use (Morrison et al. 2002). More recent blinded studies with metformin have shown conflicting results. Wu and colleagues (2008) found that the addition of metformin 750 mg/day to olanzapine and other SGAs resulted in a significantly decreased probability that the patient would gain more than 7% of body weight over 12 weeks. On the other hand, Baptista and colleagues (2008) found that the addition of metformin 850–1,700 mg/day plus sibutramine 10–20 mg/day did not result in less weight gain in olanzapine-treated patients, nor did the combination affect other metabolic parameters. The use of metformin is an interesting approach, since it may help address the insulin resistance associated with antipsychotic use. We have used metformin at dosages of 500 mg bid or tid with mixed success in inducing weight loss or preventing weight gain. The clinical data for this approach remain limited.

Olanzapine is very sedating for many patients and should be taken at bedtime if possible. About 40% of patients will report daytime somnolence at a dosage of 15 mg/day. Taking the olanzapine on an empty stomach about an hour before bedtime may increase the nighttime sedation and reduce the daytime somnolence. The use of modafinil in doses of 100–200 mg in the morning may help mitigate the somnolence.

There are no reported cases of agranulocytosis, and no blood count monitoring is recommended. Still, some reversible neutropenias and hemolytic anemias have been seen in olanzapine-treated animals. Significant elevations in hepatic transaminases (to greater than three times the upper limit of normal) occur in about 2% of patients, but 5% or more of patients have minor elevations. We are unaware of any serious hepatic problems associated with olanzapine, and monitoring of hepatic enzymes is not indicated.

Olanzapine appears to be fairly safe in overdose. Up to 1 month's supply (300 mg) has been taken with no ill effects other than drowsiness and slurred speech. Because overdoses often involve multiple drugs, including alcohol, there may be the risk of synergistic central nervous system depression effects, resulting in more serious outcomes, but none have been reported.

Olanzapine is usually started at 2.5–5 mg/day, and the dosage is usually increased to 10 mg/day in the first week. Some patients will complain of somnolence and constipation even at 5 mg/day. Patients have not found it easy to break the tablets, and the manufacturer suggests that doing so breaks the film that protects the active drug from the oxidative effects of exposure to the environment. The result can be that the drug loses its potency if broken and not taken within a few hours. The drug is now available in 2.5-mg, 5-mg, 7.5-mg, 10-mg, 15-mg, and 20-mg tablets. Some patients require the usual maximum dosage of 20 mg/day, although we know of some cases in which dosages of 30–40 mg/day have been used successfully. Lieberman has collected a series of patients with refractory conditions in whom responses occurred only when dosages of approximately 60–80 mg/day were used. Unfortunately, the pricing structure is such that at dosages greater than 20 mg/day, the drug becomes very expensive. An intramuscular formulation of olanzapine is available for acute management at doses of 2.5–10 mg per day. In addition, a depot form of olanzapine is under development.

Quetiapine

Quetiapine (Seroquel) was released in the United States in 1998 and is now the most commonly prescribed SGA in the United States. Like clozapine, the drug appears to have low affinity for D_1 and D_2 receptors but relatively high affinity for D_4 receptors (Seeman and Tallerico 1999). Clozapine, olanzapine, and quetiapine all seem to have more pronounced effects on mesolimbic dopamine activity than on nigrostriatal pathways, a phenomenon that accounts for their low tendency to produce EPS. Like other SGAs, quetiapine appears to have high affinity for $5-HT_2$ receptors. Quetiapine does not appear to have very significant anticholinergic or antihistaminic effects, but it does block α_1-adrenergic receptors to some extent. One potential drawback of the current preparation of quetiapine is its very short half-life—the average half-life is about 2–3 hours—and quetiapine therefore needs to be given at least two times a day. For chronically psychotic patients, this multiple dosing is less than ideal and might result in compliance problems. Fortunately, a sustained-release preparation—quetiapine extended-release tablets—is now available.

Quetiapine has been studied in large groups of schizophrenic patients and has been compared with placebo, chlorpromazine, and haloperidol. In general, quetiapine has been consistently more effective than placebo and at least as effective as comparison drugs in controlling positive symptoms (Gray 1998). After several weeks of treatment, quetiapine appears also to improve negative symptoms. Although quetiapine appears to be a generally effective and well-tolerated antipsychotic, it has not been studied or marketed with the same vigor as have risperidone and olanzapine. Thus, it currently is used much less frequently than either of these drugs; however, its use recently has been increasing sharply.

As with other SGAs, quetiapine is effective in the acute treatment of mania and was approved in 2004 for this indication (Ghaemi and Katzow 1999). Adding quetiapine to a mood stabilizer such as lithium is more effective in treating bipolar disorder than using lithium alone (Sachs et al. 2004). There are data suggesting quetiapine at dosages of 300–600 mg/day is an effective treatment for the anxiety component of bipolar depression (Gao et al. 2006). However, quetiapine seems to have good antidepressant properties in bipolar depression as well. FDA approval has been granted to quetiapine as the first monotherapy for the treatment of depression. It joins Symbyax as the only approved treatments for bipolar depression. Additionally, early work suggests that quetiapine may be a useful maintenance treatment in bipolar disorder. The use of quetiapine as adjunctive treatment and as a monotherapy in the treatment of unipolar depression appears to be effective but is most likely to be approved only as an adjunctive agent in resistant depression (for discussion, see subsection "Unipolar Depression" earlier in this chapter). Finally, quetiapine has shown efficacy in the treatment of GAD but has not yet been approved secondary to safety concerns raised by the FDA.

Quetiapine has been examined in the treatment of childhood autism but appears to be poorly tolerated and not very effective in this population. Risperidone, which is the only drug approved in the treatment of autism-related behavioral symptoms, appears to be a better choice. Studies are under way to examine the utility of quetiapine in treating psychotic depression and impulsive aggression. At least one study reported success with quetiapine in the treatment of some dimensions of borderline personality (Hilger et al. 2003).

The most common side effects of quetiapine, compared with placebo, are somnolence and dizziness. Quetiapine can produce orthostatic hypotension in about 7% of patients, and 1% may experience frank syncope with rapid titration of the dose. Thus, for outpatients, we tend to use a starting dosage of 50–100 mg/day and increase the dosage in increments of about 100 mg/day, with the goal of achieving a therapeutic dosage of 400–800 mg/day by the end of the second week of treatment. For inpatients, we start at 100 mg and then increase the dosage more aggressively, in increments of 100–200 mg, with a target dosage of 400–800 mg/day by day 6 for patients with schizophrenia or bipolar disorder. It is a good idea to check orthostatic blood pressures daily with a more aggressive titration.

Somnolence is experienced by at least 18% of patients taking quetiapine in 6-week clinical trials, but our experience is that as many as 50% of patients complain of somnolence when the dosage is increased above 400 mg/day. Since we have found that most patients with schizophrenia require total daily doses above 300 mg, somnolence is a problem for many patients. We try to shift most of the dose to the evening, so a 400-mg total daily dose is divided into 100 mg in the morning and 300 mg in the evening. This seems to work out for most patients and does not appear to detract from the efficacy of the drug. (Again, modafinil at dosages of 100–200 mg/day can help with the daytime somnolence.) For bipolar depression, the target dosage for quetiapine will be 300 mg/day. While 600 mg/day was also found to be effective, it was no more effective than 300 mg/day and was less well tolerated (Thase et al. 2006).

The weight gain associated with quetiapine seems to be less than that seen with olanzapine and clozapine but more than that seen with ziprasidone and risperidone. About one-fourth of patients experience an increase in body weight of greater than 7% in 3- to 6-week trials, but this may be an underestimate of what can be expected at higher daily doses. As with other SGAs, monitoring and controlling food intake are the keys to weight management with this drug.

The concern about cataracts in patients treated with quetiapine was probably overstated. While dogs did develop cataracts with chronic quetiapine therapy, postmarketing surveillance has not revealed an increased rate of cataract formation in human patients. Infrequent cataract formation has been associated with a number of first-generation antipsychotics and SGAs. The manufacturer recommends ocular examinations every 6 months, but few practitioners follow this recommendation, and we have seen little evidence thus far that it is warranted.

A small percentage of quetiapine-treated patients also exhibit transient and asymptomatic increases in liver enzymes. There have been no reports thus far of hematological abnormalities, but a reversible sinus tachycardia has often been seen.

EPS are not common with quetiapine. As with olanzapine, there have been rare reports of tardive dyskinesia, and these reports are expected to increase as more patients use quetiapine for longer periods of time. Although no clear estimates of the frequency of tardive dyskinesia with quetiapine are available, the frequency is unlikely to be any higher than the low frequency of tardive dyskinesia seen with olanzapine (0.5%–1% per year). The risk of serious complications from an overdose of quetiapine is small. We are unaware of any fatalities with overdoses up to 10 g. A sustained-release formula of quetiapine is currently under development.

Ziprasidone

In the year 2000, ziprasidone (Geodon), another SGA, was released to the U.S. market. Ziprasidone is already fairly popular in Sweden, where it was released in 1998, and has an efficacy and side-effect profile that will all but ensure a niche for it in the increasingly crowded U.S. market for SGAs.

Ziprasidone, like other SGAs, has a complex pharmacology. It appears to be an agonist at the 5-HT_{1A} receptor and an antagonist of 5-HT_{1D} and 5-HT_{2C} receptors. Ziprasidone has been shown to enhance the release of dopamine in the dorsolateral prefrontal cortex and block the reuptake of both norepinephrine and serotonin (Markowitz et al. 1999). These attributes should make ziprasidone a good antidepressant and anxiolytic as well as an effective antipsychotic. The drug appears to show relatively weak affinity for muscarinic and α-adrenergic receptors.

In studies of schizophrenia and schizoaffective disorder, ziprasidone appeared to be as effective as 15 mg of haloperidol in improving positive psychotic symptoms, as measured by the Brief Psychiatric Rating Scale or the Positive and Negative Syndrome Scale for schizophrenia (Goff et al. 1998). However, ziprasidone was superior to haloperidol in its effects on negative symptoms and depression. The CATIE trial, on the other hand, did not find advantages in the efficacy of ziprasidone compared with the the midpotency agent perphenazine (Lieberman et al. 2005; Stroup et al. 2006). As expected, ziprasidone has been shown to substantially reduce depressive symptoms, as measured by the Montgomery-Åsberg Depression Rating Scale, in patients with schizophrenia or schizoaffective disorder. The pharmacology of ziprasidone suggests that it should have antidepressant and anxiolytic effects in nonpsychotic patients as well.

Ziprasidone is an effective antimanic drug and is now FDA approved for this indication. Two double-blind trials have demonstrated that ziprasidone at dosages of 80–160 mg/day is effective in the treatment of mania (Keck et al. 2003b). Ziprasidone appears to separate from placebo in mania very early (i.e., within 3 days) Also, preliminary studies indicate that ziprasidone may help in bipolar depression. The intramuscular form of ziprasidone is rapidly effective for treating agitation in psychotic patients, including bipolar manic patients. Preliminary studies of ziprasidone augmentation of antidepressants have not necessarily shown benefits for the treatment of unipolar depression.

Ziprasidone appears to be well tolerated. Most notable is that ziprasidone is unique among the second-generation agents in not being associated with significant weight gain (Allison et al. 1999). This feature alone should make ziprasidone extremely popular, since clozapine and olanzapine have been so problematic in this regard. As with other SGAs, ziprasidone is associated with a low incidence of EPS, much like with olanzapine and probably better than with risperidone, although head-to-head trials have not been completed.

The most common side effects observed in clinical trials with ziprasidone are drowsiness, dyspepsia, dizziness, constipation, and nausea. Ziprasidone causes weight loss and a decrease in triglycerides (Simpson et al. 2004). There appears to be a dose-related increase in α-adrenergic blockade that can result in dizziness and orthostatic hypotension. Still, these α-adrenergic receptor–blocking effects are much less common than with clozapine and probably similar to what is seen with risperidone and olanzapine. Ziprasidone is associated with mild to moderate QTc interval prolongation in about 4%–5% of patients taking the drug. The clinical significance of this finding is still unclear, as is the issue of whether it is prudent to follow the electrocardiogram (ECG) in some patients. Postmarketing surveillance has not found a a clinically significant effect of QTc prolongation in ziprasidone-treated patients. Concerns regarding conduction effects of the drug have limited its adoption as a first-line therapy in the United States. In general, we tend not to follow ECGs routinely in ziprasidone-treated patients. However, patients with a known history of arrhythmia should have a baseline and repeat ECG.

Ziprasidone has a short half-life (5 hours) that necessitates twice-a-day dosing. The dosage range that appears most effective in clinical studies is 60–80 mg bid or 120–160 mg/day (Keck et al. 1998). The drug should be started at a dosage of 40 mg bid and the dosage increased to 80 mg bid after 1 week. This strategy was used in the mania studies and can now be applied in treating patients with schizophrenia. Earlier experience suggested that initiation of ziprasidone at a dosage of 40 mg/day was not particularly effective. Another major advantage that ziprasidone has over other SGAs is that it is now available in an intramuscular formulation. The usual dose of the intramuscular form is 10 mg every 2 hours as needed, to a maximum dosage of 40 mg/day. In acute emergency situations, SGAs have generally not been preferred because oral dosing requires more time to achieve maximum benefits. Through the intramuscular route, ziprasidone can be administered quickly and reliably. Preliminary reports suggest that intramuscular ziprasidone is as effective as intramuscular haloperidol in treating acute psychosis and agitation but less likely to cause EPS.

Aripiprazole

Aripiprazole (Abilify) is a second-generation antipsychotic with a somewhat unique pharmacological profile. It is a partial agonist at the D_2 and $5\text{-}HT_{1A}$ receptors and also has $5\text{-}HT_2$ properties found with other SGAs. Among the other pharmacological properties of aripiprazole is its affinity as a presynaptic D_2 autoreceptor agonist. Thus, it can enhance as well as inhibit dopamine release in specific regions of the brain. Aripiprazole's pharmacological profile should indicate that it has antipsychotic, antimanic, and antidepressant properties. It was the first adjunctive treatment approved, in 2007, for unipolar major depression.

Aripiprazole is approved for the treatment of schizophrenia and was the latest second-generation agent to be approved in the United States. At least four controlled trials have confirmed the role of aripiprazole in the treatment of schizophrenia. In a meta-analysis of 1,545 patients in placebo-controlled trials, aripiprazole was more effective than placebo and at least as effective as risperidone and haloperidol (Carson et al. 2002). Aripiprizole was the only SGA that was not evaluated in the CATIE trial. Thus, we do not know how it fares in a more real-world setting compared with other SGAs and with perphenazine. In industry-sponsored trials, aripiprazole was superior to haloperidol in the treatment of negative symptoms. Also, aripiprazole was as effective as haloperidol in preventing relapse in 1-year studies of schizophrenia but resulted in a lower dropout rate secondary to a better side-effect profile. Aripiprazole is one of the only antipsychotics to be approved in the acute and maintenance treatment of adolescents with schizophrenia. There are relatively few controlled trials of antipsychotics in adolescents with schizophrenia. Studies with 13- to 17-year-olds with schizophrenia indicate that aripiprazole is effective at fixed dosages of 10 or 30 mg/day. The higher dosage is not significantly more effective than the lower dosage. The starting dosage in treating adults with schizophrenia is 5–10 mg/day, with a maximum recommended dosage of 30 mg/day. If the patient is activated at a dosage of 10 mg/day, a lower dosage should be tried (e.g., 5 mg/day). In adolescents, the starting dose is 2 mg, with most patients showing benefits at 10 mg/day. The maximum recommended dosage in adolescents with schizophrenia is 30 mg/day.

As of this writing, multiple placebo-controlled trials have shown benefit for aripiprazole in treating acute mania. The antimanic effects of aripiprazole were superior to those of placebo, and the effects were seen within 4 days (Keck et al. 2003a). Aripiprazole appeared to significantly reduce the irritability, lability, and aggressiveness associated with acute mania. Studies have also been completed that indicate that aripiprazole is an effective maintenance treatment in bipolar I disorder. It appears to delay the onset of mania in bipolar I patients. Aripiprazole is thus one of only a handful of agents to have received FDA approval for use in the maintenance treatment of bipolar disorder. In the maintenance trials, aripiprazole clearly delayed time to the next manic episode. The effects of aripiprazole on preventing depression could not be adequately evaluated in these pivotal trials. Aripiprazole is also one of two SGAs, along with risperidone, to be approved in children. Studies in acute bipolar 1 disorder in patients ages 10 to 17 years, indicate that aripiprazole is effective at dosages of 10 and 30 mg/day. The efficacy of aripiprazole as a maintenance treatment in children with bipolar disorder is not yet established.

Aripiprazole has been evaluated in the treatment of bipolar depression in adults but has not shown reliable benefit in randomized controlled trials, at least as a monotherapy. It is anticipated, but not definitively proven, that aripiprazole should be useful as an adjunctive treatment for bipolar depression just as it is for unipolar depression.

Aripiprazole has a long half-life—about 50–80 hours—and steady state is therefore not achieved for about 2 weeks. The long half-life allows once-a-day dosing. Long-acting depot forms of aripiprazole for maintenance therapy in schizophrenia and short-acting intramuscular forms for acute agitation are under development.

The side-effect profile of aripiprazole may be significantly better than that of most other SGAs. The data over 1 year suggest that aripiprazole should be fairly weight neutral, as is ziprasidone, and aripiprazole lacks any significant effect on QTc intervals. Aripiprazole is one of the few antipsychotics, first- or second-generation, that does not increase prolactin levels and that may even lower these levels. In terms of EPS, there is some question as to whether aripiprazole may have a greater tendency to cause akathisia, but the answer to this question awaits head-to-head comparison trials. Agitation and akathisia certainly seem to occur in some of our aripiprazole-treated patients. The most common side effects seen with aripiprazole in Phase III trials were nausea, tremor, insomnia, headache, and agitation.

The side-effect profile of aripiprazole varies by the age of the patient and the indication for which it is applied. For example, sedation and EPS are much bigger problems in children and adolescents treated with aripiprazole than they are with adults. On the other hand, akathisia is three times more common in depressed adult patients treated with aripiprazole, even at lower doses, than it is in patients with schizophrenia.

In adults with depression, the typical starting adjunctive dosage is 2–5 mg/day. We have seen patients for whom 2 mg is an adequate dose. On the other hand, we have also seen depressed patients who tolerate and respond to the medication at dosages much higher than the maximum recommended dosage of 15 mg/day. For adults with bipolar disorder, we still tend to start at doses lower than the manufacturer recommends: 5 or 10 mg, with titration to 30 mg as tolerated and needed. The same holds true for adults with schizophrenia.

First-Generation (Typical) Antipsychotics

Approximately 15 first-generation antipsychotics are still on the U.S. market, with haloperidol being the most commonly prescribed. These drugs differ from the increasingly dominant SGAs in their considerably higher ratio of D_2-to-$5-HT_2$ antagonism. They may also occupy dopamine receptors for longer periods.

The first-generation antipsychotics continue to have a number of advantages over SGAs. A significant advantage is cost. Most of the first-generation antipsychotics are available generically at a fraction of the cost of newer drugs. Studies such as CATIE and CUtLASS 1 have challenged the idea that the typical agents are less effective or even more poorly tolerated in the treatment of

Typical (D$_2$ antagonist) antipsychotics: overview

Efficacy	Schizophrenia (positive symptoms) (FDA-approved indication) Tourette's disorder (pimozide; FDA-approved indication) Mania (FDA-approved indication for chlorpromazine only) Psychotic depression (with antidepressant) Drug-induced psychosis Agitation,[a] nausea, hiccups (not FDA approved for these purposes; off-label)
Side effects	EPS (more common in high-potency drugs) NMS (rare) Dry mouth, constipation, urinary retention, sedation, weight gain (more common in low-potency drugs) Skin and eye complications QT interval prolongation (thioridazine)
Dosage and administration	Individualize dosing. 50–150 mg chlorpromazine equivalents (see Table 4–2) to start, with maximum total daily dose of 300–600 mg chlorpromazine equivalents (e.g., 6–12 mg haloperidol).
Safety in overdose	CNS depression, hypotension, ECG changes, EPS. Manage with vital sign support, gastric lavage. Do not induce emesis secondary to aspiration risk.
Drug interactions	CNS depressants: ↑ sedation Antacids: ↓ antipsychotic absorption Carbamazepine: ↓ antipsychotic levels SSRIs: ↑ antipsychotic levels Nicotine: ↓ antipsychotic levels Meperidine: ↑ sedation, hypotension β-Blockers: ↑ hypotension; may ↑ antipsychotic and β-blocker levels TCAs: may ↑ antipsychotic and TCA levels Valproic acid: chlorpromazine may ↑ valproic acid levels

Note. CNS = central nervous system; ECG = electrocardiogram; EPS = extrapyramidal symptoms; FDA = U.S. Food and Drug Administration; NMS = neuroleptic malignant syndrome; SSRI = selective serotonin reuptake inhibitor; TCA = tricyclic antidepressant.
[a]Agitation associated with psychosis: FDA-approved indication for intramuscular olanzapine only.

schizophrenia. Finally, the high-potency agents are considerably less likely to cause weight gain than most SGAs. In fact, molindone tends to be associated with less weight gain than other first-generation antipsychotics or SGAs. In some patients, weight gain and its complications may pose a greater long-term risk to the patient than do EPS.

Still, the relative lower rates of EPS, particularly tardive dyskinesia, and perhaps somewhat better efficacy in treating negative and cognitive symptoms with second-generation agents have made them preferred agents for the long-term management of psychosis. Despite these advantages of SGAs, many patients with schizophrenia remain on first-generation antipsychotics, and this will continue to be the case until we have agents that are clearly superior.

Although there is no evidence that one first-generation antipsychotic works any better than another, some patients clearly do take to one agent more than another. As is true for other classes of psychotropic agents, choosing a first-generation antipsychotic has more to do with the side-effect profile of the drug than with other factors. Low-potency agents such as chlorpromazine have the advantage of causing less severe EPS but more sedation, weight gain, and postural hypotension than higher-potency agents. On the other hand, high-potency antipsychotics such as haloperidol and fluphenazine tend to be preferred over low-potency agents despite their greater proclivity for EPS. The antihistaminic and anticholinergic effects of low-potency agents may be more problematic for the day-to-day functioning of many patients. The art of using these drugs involves choosing the right agent and then managing the inevitable side effects of the drug.

Side Effects

Sedation

Sedation, often accompanied by fatigue, can be useful early in treatment but a liability after the patient has improved. All antipsychotics can be sedating in some patients at some dosage, but chlorpromazine is generally the most sedating. Its sedative effects are often judged to be very unpleasant by non–psychiatrically ill volunteers receiving even 25 mg or 50 mg of the drug in a single dose, but these effects are sometimes accepted or even welcomed by some patients with psychosis or personality disorders. Thioridazine, chlorprothixene, and loxapine are also often relatively sedating, whereas the other high-potency antipsychotics are often less or not at all sedating. In one acute-dosing strategy, the antipsychotic dosage is gradually raised until the psychosis is controlled; at that point the patient develops increased sedation, which then requires dosage reduction. In chronic administration, sedation and fatigue overlap with akinesia, a side effect characterized by inertia, inactivity, and lack of spontaneous movement. Akinesia will often abate when an antiparkinsonian drug is added; it will often abate more slowly when the dosage is lowered.

When antipsychotics are used as prn medication (orally or parenterally), it is likely that sedation is the main effect produced, even though a decrease in psychosis may be desired. As has been discussed, a benzodiazepine (e.g., lorazepam 1–2 mg) may be more appropriate for this purpose. Unfortunately, the short-term (or long-term) utility of prn medication of any sort has never been seriously studied.

Autonomic Effects

All antipsychotics can cause postural hypotension, but this problem is presumed to be more common and severe with the low-potency drugs, at least with chlorpromazine and thioridazine, and more dangerous in elderly or medically ill patients. All first-generation antipsychotics also have anticholinergic effects, which are most striking with thioridazine but are also clearly present with chlorpromazine, mesoridazine, and trifluoperazine; they are also present, but to a lesser degree, with the other drugs. Dry mouth, constipation, and urinary hesitancy can occur, as can visual blurring. When antipsychotics are combined with other anticholinergic drugs (antiparkinsonian or TCA drugs), delirium or bowel stasis can occur. Constipation is a milder form of this effect. Retrograde ejaculation is fairly common with thioridazine and can occur with other drugs in this class. This effect can progress to impotence. It is worth inquiring about sexual effects, since patients may be upset by such effects but hesitant to mention them spontaneously.

Endocrine Effects

The direct effect of first-generation antipsychotic drugs is an increase in blood prolactin level. There is a large and complex literature on this effect, because prolactin level has been proposed as an alternative to measuring antipsychotic blood level directly. Attempts to use prolactin level as a guide to adequate dosage in newly hospitalized patients have not been validated to date, but one study suggested that aftercare patients with a low prolactin level were more likely to relapse than those with a higher level. Hyperprolactinemia can cause breast enlargement and galactorrhea in both female and male patients and may play a role in the impotence in male patients and the amenorrhea in female patients that are occasionally seen with these drugs. To reduce prolactin levels, dopaminergic drugs such as amantadine (200–300 mg/day) or bromocriptine (7.5–15 mg/day) can be tried.

Weight gain, often quite excessive, can occur with all antipsychotic drugs. It is unclear whether it is a result of increased appetite or decreased activity. Molindone is believed to be less likely to cause weight gain and may even cause modest weight loss, again for unknown reasons. Although all antipsychotics except thioridazine are good antiemetics, nausea and vomiting are sometimes seen as side effects, for reasons not yet determined.

Skin and Eye Complications

A variety of allergic skin rashes can occur with antipsychotics (as with all other drugs) but are more common with chlorpromazine. Chlorpromazine with prolonged high-dose administration can cause pigmentation of areas exposed to light and pigment deposits in the eye, chiefly in the back of the cornea and the front of the lens. These deposits almost never affect vision and do not require regular slit lamp examinations. However, patients showing an opaque pupil when a light is shone into the eye should have an ophthalmological evaluation. These deposits probably occur only with chlorpromazine but could conceivably occur with other drugs. Retinal pigmentation occurs only with thioridazine (but has never been reported, so far, with thioridazine's metabolite mesoridazine), and its serious and irreversible effect on vision requires that thioridazine dosage be kept at or below 800 mg/day. Chlorpromazine often causes skin photosensitivity, manifested as severe sunburn in exposed skin areas after relatively brief (30–60 minutes) exposure to direct sunlight. A sunscreen containing para-aminobenzoic acid (PABA), which screens out ultraviolet rays, will help avoid this effect. Other antipsychotics may cause photosensitivity, and patients taking them are generally advised to wear sunscreen. Sun sensitivity can best be determined by cautious exposure to the sun in gradually increased durations. Many patients will prove to tolerate the sun normally. Chlorpromazine should be avoided in patients who are likely to spend long periods outdoors at work or for pleasure. Patients taking chlorpromazine for prolonged periods of time can develop a slate-gray to purplish pigmentation of skin areas exposed to sunlight that probably fades slowly once the drug is stopped.

Other or Rare Complications

Agranulocytosis has been associated with chlorpromazine and thioridazine and could presumably occur with other first-generation antipsychotics. Its incidence is low—perhaps 1 case in 5,000 patients treated. Agranulocytosis usually appears in the first 3 months of treatment. Monitoring for agranulocytosis does not require frequent or regular blood counts. However, patients developing a sore throat and fever in the first few months of therapy require an emergency WBC to rule out this rare but serious complication. Leukopenias in the range of 3,000–4,000/mm^3 also occur and are not generally serious, whereas agranulocytosis, often defined as a WBC of less than 2,000/mm^3 with less than 500/mm^3 of polymorphonuclear leukocytes, is very serious and requires immediate medical attention by a hematologist. Needless to say, clinicians should seriously consider stopping a drug if the WBC is less than 3,000/mm^3. See the section on clozapine earlier in this chapter for discussion of the particular problem of clozapine-associated agranulocytosis.

A form of allergic obstructive hepatitis was reported relatively frequently in the early days of chlorpromazine use, with an incidence of 2%–3%, but this disease has been much more rarely encountered in recent years. Even when this allergic obstructive hepatitis occurred more frequently, it was a relatively mild, transient disorder that did not lead to hepatic necrosis or permanent liver damage. Liver problems occur so rarely with other antipsychotics as to make one believe that the occasionally abnormal liver function tests seen in patients taking these drugs are due to some intercurrent, unrelated event or drug. Such abnormalities, unless progressive and severe, are not a reason for discontinuing an effective antipsychotic in a patient who needs the drug, although internists tend to blame the antipsychotic, without an adequate basis, when abnormal liver function tests are observed.

Seizures can also occur in patients treated with antipsychotics. Only promazine (no longer used) caused them with any frequency. We know of no good data available on the comparative effects of all antipsychotic drugs on seizure threshold, but we tend to suspect loxapine and chlorpromazine of being involved in the rare antipsychotic-related seizures seen at McLean Hospital, and we presume that the high-potency drugs are less likely to cause seizures. Certainly, patients with known epilepsy who are receiving anticonvulsants often receive antipsychotics without any obvious effect on seizure frequency. Seizures associated with clozapine use are discussed earlier in this chapter.

Sudden death has been associated with antipsychotic use in healthy young adults. The mechanisms suggested include QTc prolongation, torsades de pointes, ventricular fibrillation, and aspiration of food or of vomitus during a grand mal seizure, but no clear etiology has been proved. Several first-generation antipsychotics, including thioridazine, mesoridazine, and droperidol, now contain black box warnings in the package inserts. The use of these drugs has dropped dramatically since these warnings were established. Occasional sudden deaths have been reported among patients in seclusion rooms during summer months. This may be due to the effect of the antipsychotic on heat regulation. Since sudden, unpredictable deaths occurred in young psychiatric patients before antipsychotic drugs were discovered, their connection with medication remains tenuous. Over the last 30 years we have heard of more sudden deaths associated with thioridazine (four) than with any other antipsychotic, but even with this drug such occurrences are very rare. As a result of a study focusing primarily on QTc prolongation in SGAs, thioridazine and its metabolite mesoridazine (Serentil) received, in 2000, a black box warning from the FDA about QTc prolongation. As a result, thioridazine and mesoridazine are unlikely to be used much.

Neurological Effects

Although dopamine receptor blockade in the striatum is the most popular mechanism invoked for all neurological side effects of antipsychotic drugs, and anticholinergic antiparkinsonian drugs are the conventional remedy, the presumed cholinergic-dopaminergic imbalance is probably only a partial explanation.

Dystonia.   One of the earliest forms of EPS, dystonia, often manifested by tonic muscle spasm in the tongue, jaw, and neck, usually occurs in the first few hours or days after taking an antipsychotic. It can present as a very frightening opisthotonos of the whole body with extensor rigidity or as only mild tongue stiffness. In one small study, dystonia appeared as antipsychotic blood levels were dropping, not rising, making one wonder whether in this case the dystonia might have been a rebound effect as dopamine blockade was waning.

In any event, dystonia can be fairly effectively averted by prophylactic anti-parkinsonian use and rarely occurs with thioridazine. It is more common in younger males but can occur in either sex at any age.

Once present, the dystonia can be rapidly relieved by intravenous antiparkinsonian drugs (only diphenhydramine and benztropine are readily available for parenteral use) or, less rapidly, by intramuscular medication. However, such diverse drugs as diazepam, amobarbital, and caffeine sodium benzoate, and even hypnosis, have been said to relieve it as well. Once the dystonia has resolved and the patient is protected by oral antiparkinsonian medication, the offending antipsychotic can be continued without recurrence of the dystonia. However, patients often feel less apprehensive if a different antipsychotic drug is substituted. Some patients on depot fluphenazine develop recurrences of dystonia with succeeding injections.

Oculogyric crises, manifested by forced eye rotation, usually upward, are conventionally classified with the dystonias, but they fairly frequently occur—even recur—later in treatment, when more conventional dystonia is rare.

Pseudoparkinsonism.   Some time in the early stages of treatment, usually between 5 days and 4 weeks, the patient can develop signs of parkinsonism. In contrast to idiopathic Parkinson's disease, pill-rolling tremor is very rare, but muscle stiffness, cogwheel rigidity, stooped posture, masklike facies, and even drooling are quite common. Micrographia occurs and can help differentiate antipsychotic-induced tremor from lithium-induced tremor. Patients rarely develop such severe parkinsonian rigidity that they become incapacitated or even immobilized. When they do, such patients are sometimes misdiagnosed as having catatonia. Patients with such severe rigidity do not respond readily to even massive doses of antiparkinsonian drugs; the condition may require as long as 2 weeks to clear after the antipsychotic drug is stopped. Often, milder degrees of pseudoparkinsonism are seen for prolonged periods in patients taking long-term maintenance medication and can contribute to passive inactivity in such patients.

Akinesia.   Akinesia, a reduction in spontaneous or voluntary movement, can be seen in patients taking maintenance antipsychotic medication in the absence of signs of parkinsonism. Regular coarse tremor can also be seen in the absence of any other parkinsonian signs. Both conditions respond to either administration of antiparkinsonian drugs or reduction in antipsychotic dose.

Akinesia, as well as pseudoparkinsonism and depression, can be confused with the negative symptoms of schizophrenia. One approach to differentiating apathy and alogia due to psychosis from neurological side effects is to institute a therapeutic trial of a drug such as biperiden for 2 weeks. If the negative symptoms disappear, they were presumably a side effect of a antipsychotic, not a result of the psychotic disorder. A trial of an antidepressant can serve the same purpose if depressive symptoms are suspected.

Work at McLean Hospital has suggested that selegiline (Eldepryl), the monoamine oxidase B (MAO-B) inhibitor used to treat conventional parkinsonism, is also beneficial at a dosage of 5 mg bid in schizophrenic patients with negative symptoms who are taking antipsychotics. If the selegiline dosage does not exceed 10 mg/day (or 6 mg/day for the transdermal patch), the special diet required with monoamine oxidase inhibitor (MAOI) use is not necessary. A placebo-controlled trial of this use has been completed, and the drug seems to work. If selegiline does "work," it may be hard to tell whether it is effective because it reduces parkinsonian symptoms, reduces depression, or improves negative symptoms directly.

Akathisia. Akathisia, the inner-driven restlessness caused by antipsychotics, is the least understood and most troublesome of the neurological side effects of these agents. It ranges from an unpleasant subjective feeling of muscular discomfort to an agitated, desperate, markedly dysphoric pacing with hand wringing and weeping. Between these extremes, patients find themselves unable to sit still for long, having to stand up and move around or continually shift their position. Akathisia is sometimes mistaken for psychotic agitation and treated inappropriately by an increase in antipsychotic dose. It can be experienced even after the first dose of an antipsychotic but can become a clinical problem at any time in the first few weeks of medication use.

Akathisia occurs with thioridazine and olanzapine, as well as with the other older drugs, and may even occur with clozapine and risperidone. It is less responsive to antiparkinsonian drugs than are other neurological side effects and is the bane of maintenance medication, being a common basis for patients' refusing to stay on such a regimen. Studies suggest that propranolol at dosages of 30–120 mg/day sometimes suppresses akathisia when neither antiparkinsonian drugs nor benzodiazepines, such as lorazepam, work. Its efficacy casts some doubt on the theory that dopamine receptor blockade is the mechanism underlying akathisia.

Regular, rhythmic leg jiggling—up and down or, less commonly, to and fro—is often seen in patients treated with antipsychotics and is probably, but not certainly, a variant of akathisia, although some consider it a form of tremor. Patients with this phenomenon are often unaware of it or not bothered by it. The best basis for differential diagnosis of akathisia is to ask the patient whether the restlessness is a muscle feeling or a head feeling—the first being akathisia and the second anxiety. If there is any doubt, it is safer to assume that akathisia exists, because overdosing with antipsychotics is vastly more common than underdosing.

The drug therapy of akathisia often requires polypharmacy. Antiparkinsonian drugs, β-blockers, and benzodiazepines can all be helpful in some patients, but more than one of these agents may be required. Lowering the antipsychotic dosage should also be considered.

Use of Antiparkinsonian Drugs

For decades there have been impassioned arguments pro and con about the prophylactic use of antiparkinsonian drugs (Stanilla and Simpson 1995). Many senior clinicians claim that patients' acceptance of a drug is enhanced and unpleasant side effects are averted by routine administration of antiparkinsonian agents to all patients starting (or restarting) to take an antipsychotic drug. Others, however, assert that two drugs together (an antipsychotic drug and an antiparkinsonian drug) can be more toxic than an antipsychotic alone and that an antiparkinsonian should only be added when neurological side effects appear.

We believe there is enough evidence that antiparkinsonian drugs avert neurological side effects to use them routinely in treating most acutely psychotic patients under age 45 who are starting to take a first-generation antipsychotic, unless the anticholinergic side effects are contraindicated. In the less common situation, in which cautious trials of antipsychotics at very low dosages (e.g., haloperidol 1–3 mg/day) are undertaken, prophylactic antiparkinsonian drugs are unnecessary. If routine antiparkinsonian medication is not used prophylactically in the acute treatment of patients, prn orders for such patients should be written. After 4 weeks to 6 months of long-term maintenance antipsychotic therapy, the antiparkinsonian drugs can be shifted to a prn basis or withdrawn.

A few patients (approximately 15%) will redevelop clear neurological side effects—and even more (approximately 30%) will feel "better" (less anxious or depressed or inert)—while continuing to take antiparkinsonian drugs. Some patients with chronic schizophrenia are delighted to stop their antipsychotic but demand to continue their antiparkinsonian drug (Wojcik 1979). Very rarely, patients use trihexyphenidyl or other antiparkinsonian agents to get high, but far more patients taking antipsychotics do better taking antiparkinsonians than not taking them. Rarely, patients develop an anticholinergic delirium or intestinal stasis while taking antiparkinsonian drugs; dry mouth and blurred vision are more common side effects.

Dosage ranges of available antiparkinsonian drugs are given in Table 4–5. Probably, if blood level determinations either of the drug itself or of anticholinergic levels by radioreceptor assay were generally available, dosage might be adjusted more rationally. Currently, if a patient has neither relief of neurological side effects nor dry mouth, a cautious increase in dose—even over the maximum recommended in the *Physicians' Desk Reference* (PDR)—can be considered, although decreasing the antipsychotic dose may be even more rational.

Most of the antiparkinsonian drugs are assumed to work by their anticholinergic effects and are probably equivalent to one another, although we have seen, in rare cases, syndromes that respond uniquely to the anticholinergic antihistamine diphenhydramine or to ethopropazine. No controlled comparative studies of these drugs exist to guide the clinician. Probably diphenhydramine is more sedating, trihexyphenidyl slightly more stimulating, and biperiden more neutral in this dimension (Table 4–5). Amantadine, which is presumed to work as a dopamine receptor agonist, can be used at dosages of 200–300 mg/day. It is probably as effective as the anticholinergic antiparkinsonian drugs, but it has no proven advantages. Tolerance to its antiparkinsonian effects may also be more of a problem than with anticholinergic antiparkinsonian agents. However, it may be useful when galactorrhea develops because it reduces blood prolactin levels. Although one might expect a dopamine receptor agonist to be a stimulant, patients sometimes find amantadine to be sedating. Bromocriptine, another dopamine receptor agonist, is available for prescription use and has been studied extensively in idiopathic Parkinson's disease. It may well prove useful in treating drug-induced pseudoparkinsonism and probably does not aggravate psychosis in patients whose dosage of antipsychotic has been stabilized. L-Dopa has not been systematically studied in pseudoparkinsonism. It probably works too slowly and can sometimes aggravate psychosis. The standard antiparkinsonian drugs generally have no obvious effect on the psychosis; findings from the few controlled studies comparing antipsychotic drugs with and without added antiparkinsonian agents are equivocal.

Anticholinergic effects of the antiparkinsonian drugs can cause cognitive impairment in non–psychiatrically ill subjects and in patients with schizophrenia. The magnitude and clinical importance of this effect are unclear, but it is possible that mild memory problems caused by anticholinergic drug effects might well be overlooked in patients who were already cognitively impaired or sedated. It is well to remember that patients with idiopathic parkinsonism can become delirious at higher dosages of all antiparkinsonian drugs, including amantadine, and these patients should be watched for signs of organicity if these drugs are pushed to higher dosages.

Two newer antiparkinsonian drugs are worth mentioning. Pramipexole (Mirapex) and ropinirole (ReQuip) represent a new class of dopamine receptor agonists. Pramipexole was studied in the treatment of depression and psychosis, but its only FDA-approved indication is for the treatment of Parkinson's disease. Although our experience with these drugs is limited, we have seen patients with schizophrenia who respond to the antiparkinsonian effects of these drugs and do not appear to develop psychotic symptoms at lower doses (<1 mg/day of pramipexole). There is some evidence that these dopamine receptor agonists may also help with the negative symptoms of schizophrenia. One problem with pramipexole and ropinirole is that they are quite expensive, and third-party payers such as Medicare will typically not cover them for treatment of antipsychotic-induced parkinsonism. Another problem is that dopamine receptor agonists have been associated with visual hallucinations in some patients; about 3% of Parkinson's patients develop visual hallucinations while taking dopamine receptor agonists.

Tardive Dyskinesia

Some patients exposed to antipsychotic drugs develop abnormal, involuntary, irregular choreiform or athetoid movements. These movements most commonly include tongue overactivity (darting, writhing, twisting, or repeated protrusion) and finger movements (choreiform or hand clenching). Chewing or lateral jaw movements, lip puckering, facial grimacing, torticollis or retrocollis, trunk twisting, pelvic thrusting, respiratory grunting, athetoid arm and shoulder move-

Table 4–5. Antiparkinsonian drugs: names, formulations and strengths, and dosage ranges

Generic name	Brand name	Formulations and strengths	Usual dosage range (mg/day)
Primarily anticholinergic			
benztropine	Cogentin[a]	Tablets: 0.5, 1, 2 mg Injection: 1 mg/mL (2-mL ampule)	2–6
biperiden	Akineton	Tablet (HCl): 2 mg	2–8
diphenhydramine	Benadryl[b]	Tablet: 25 mg Capsules: 25, 50 mg Elixir and syrup: 12.5 mg/5 mL (120-mL and 480-mL bottles) Injection: 50 mg/mL (1-mL single-dose vial; 10-mL multidose vial; 1-mL prefilled syringe)	50–300
procyclidine	Kemadrin	Tablet: 5 mg	10–20
trihexyphenidyl	Artane[b]	Tablets: 2, 5 mg Elixir: 2 mg/5 mL (480-mL bottle)	4–15
Dopaminergic			
amantadine	Symmetrel[b]	Tablet and capsule: 100 mg Syrup: 50 mg/5 mL (480-mL bottle)	100–300

[a]Tablets only available in generic form.
[b]Available in generic form.

ments, and a variety of toe, ankle, and leg movements all occur in a variety of combinations. These are hard to distinguish, at times, from mannerisms associated with schizophrenia and are essentially impossible to distinguish on the basis of phenomenology alone from other, rarer causes of dyskinesia.

Patients with typical movements of the sort described above are still referred to as having *tardive dyskinesia.* Those with major athetoid dystonic movements and sustained postures of the face, neck, arms, or trunk are referred to as having *tardive dystonia,* often a more severe and more incapacitating condition. Athetoid dystonic movements often coexist with the more typical tongue and lip movements of tardive dyskinesia. Tardive dystonia is more likely to be ameliorated by antiparkinsonian drugs than is conventional tardive dyskinesia. *Tardive akathisia,* a syndrome of forced motor restlessness persisting long after antipsychotic drugs have been stopped, can also occur. It is even less common than tardive dystonia. So-called *tardive Tourette's disorder* has also been described.

The severity of tardive dyskinesia ranges from minimal tongue restlessness and finger movements to gross, incapacitating, disfiguring movements. Most identifiable cases are mild and not noticed by either the patient or the family or are passed off as minor tics or restlessness by both. Even clearly visible dyskinesias are often of little real consequence, but in about 3% of cases the dyskinesia is sufficiently severe to cause social or functional problems. Most patients and families seen in the Tardive Dyskinesia Clinic at McLean Hospital are much more concerned about the possible ultimate consequences of currently very mild dyskinesia than about the minor movements with which the patient presents at the time of consultation.

It is currently impossible to predict which patients will develop dyskinesia, early or late, mild or severe. However, the best available data suggest that there is a rate of development of dyskinesia of about 4%–7% per year over the first 5 years of exposure with first-generation agents and that patients over age 55 and patients with affective disorders may be at greater risk (Cole et al. 1992; Jeste et al. 1995). In chronically institutionalized psychotic patients, dyskinesia prevalence rates are often on the order of 20%–40%. At the extremes, a few patients develop persistent dyskinesia after only a few weeks of exposure to antipsychotics, but antipsychotic use up to 6 months is generally considered safe. In our experience, about one-half the patients who develop overt dyskinesia do so while taking the antipsychotic at stable maintenance dosages, whereas about one-quarter first manifest dyskinesia when the antipsychotic is tapered or stopped (covert dyskinesia). Dyskinesia fades away in some patients when their antipsychotics are stopped or weeks, months, or years later. Some patients lose their dyskinesia even while continuing to take medication at a stable maintenance dosage. There is a significant rate of occurrence of dyskinesia in individuals never exposed to antipsychotics—from 1% to 5%, increasing with advancing age; therefore, not all dyskinesias in patients taking antipsychotics are due to the drug. Unfortunately, no one can tell which cases are idiopathic. Neither are there any strong, consistent treatment factors related to dyskinesia. Duration of antipsychotic treatment correlates more commonly with dyskinesia than does total dose.

There is no clear evidence that any one first-generation or typical antipsychotic is less commonly related to tardive dyskinesia development than another. Clozapine appears far less likely to cause tardive dyskinesia; for risperidone, the jury is still out. Basic research data on dopamine receptor overproliferation caused by antipsychotics in laboratory animals have been used to claim that drugs such as thioridazine or molindone should be less likely to cause tardive dyskinesia than other antipsychotics. However, we have seen a number of cases of tardive dyskinesia in patients exposed only, or almost only, to thioridazine and two cases in patients mainly taking molindone. We also saw one patient who had been taking various antipsychotics for years but who developed tardive dyskinesia after a year of taking risperidone alone. In our experience, periods of withdrawal from antipsychotics are not related to tardive dyskinesia development, and lithium exposure does not seem to slow the emergence of dyskinesia.

Antiparkinsonian drug exposure is a more complicated issue. In two cohorts of 100 patients each studied at McLean Hospital because of recent onset of tardive dyskinesia, more months taking antiparkinsonian drugs was significantly correlated with slower onset of the disorder; this finding was replicated in both cohorts. In contrast, Jeste et al. (1995), in an older population in whom antipsychotic drugs were generally avoided, found that the use of antiparkinsonian drugs increased the risk of developing tardive dyskinesia. Kane (1995) found that patients who had severe neurological side effects from antipsychotics tended to be at high risk for development of tardive dyskinesia. Antiparkinsonian drugs are clearly able to exacerbate preexisting dyskinesia. Our interpretation of this mixture of messages is that prophylactic antiparkinsonian drug use in younger patients is safe and may even be prophylactic against tardive dyskinesia, whereas severe neurological side effects and older age coupled with antiparkinsonian use may make tardive dyskinesia onset more likely. Therefore, the clinician must seriously consider the risks and benefits of extended treatment with antipsychotics in all patients likely to continue taking medication for longer than a few months. This issue must be discussed with the patient and his or her family unless there are defensible clinical reasons for not doing so. Either way, everything should be documented in the patient's chart, and the process should be redone if signs of dyskinesia are noted. (See Chapter 1: "General Principles of Psychopharmacological Treatment" for further discussion of this issue.)

To date, the available long-term (2- to 10-year) follow-up studies suggest that tardive dyskinesia is not generally a progressive disorder and can improve or vanish over time, even in those taking antipsychotics. With chronically psychotic patients, the best clinical decision is often to continue the antipsychotic, but this decision must be based on the available facts in each case.

There is no effective or standard treatment for tardive dyskinesia. Trying to slowly taper the antipsychotic dose is often recommended. Lithium is often added, and the use of reserpine has its advocates. A shift to a different antipsychotic is also sometimes suggested. Findings from a series of positive small studies suggest that vitamin E (400 IU tid) may gradually decrease dyskinesia, particularly if the dyskinesia has been present less than 5 years (Adler et al. 1993; Gardos and Cole 1995). Higher doses of vitamin E tend to cause diarrhea.

A variety of unusual drugs have been tried in the treatment of tardive dyskinesia, most in single small studies. One of the more interesting is buspirone used in large doses (Moss et al. 1992). The only drug with substantial evidence (two controlled studies and a large-scale open study) of efficacy in tardive dyskinesia is clozapine (Gardos and Cole 1995). Despite this amount of work, one cannot predict which patients will benefit and whether their dyskinesia will improve slowly or rapidly. It also is not clear whether the improvement in tardive dyskinesia with clozapine treatment is due to the clozapine itself or to the discontinuation of the first-generation agent. An interesting option for the treatment of tardive dyskinesia may be gabapentin. One study suggested that 900–1,800 mg of gabapentin seemed to attenuate tardive dyskinesia in a group of patients with affective disorders who had been treated with first-generation antipsychotics (Hardoy et al. 1999).

Tardive dyskinesia is remarkably heterogeneous in its response to drug therapies. Although the condition is often assumed to be due to dopaminergic overactivity and should therefore be suppressed by dopamine-blocking agents and aggravated by anticholinergic antiparkinsonian drugs, some patients show exactly the opposite responses, and pseudoparkinsonism paradoxically often coexists with dyskinesia. Benzodiazepines often mildly alleviate dyskinetic movements. A vast range of other centrally active drugs have been tried and have sometimes helped. Luckily, most cases of dyskinesia are not serious enough to warrant special treatment. If special treatment is needed, clozapine seems to be the most effective therapy, but a potentially dangerous one; vitamin E seems helpful and benign. Olanzapine requires further study. Beyond these, the clinician and the patient can often work out a medication regimen unique to each patient, which, over time, seems to help.

Neuroleptic Malignant Syndrome

Neuroleptic malignant syndrome is a potentially life-threatening complication of antipsychotic drug use. Estimates of its incidence vary from study to study, but a rate of 1% of all psychiatric admissions in which the patients are treated with neuroleptics seems reasonable, although rates as low as 0.07% and as high as 2.4% have been reported. Although criteria for the diagnosis of NMS have fluctuated from article to article, there is general agreement that all patients with NMS have hyperthermia, severe EPS, and autonomic dysfunction. The operational criteria for diagnosis of NMS currently in use at McLean Hospital are presented in Table 4–6, which provides a good description of the range of signs and symptoms that may be present (see also Chapter 10, "Emergency Department Treatment").

Misdiagnosis can obviously occur when patients have both fever caused by infection and pseudoparkinsonism, but the severe muscle rigidity often seen in NMS is rare as an accompanying feature of incidental infection. Serum creatine kinase levels can be increased by intramuscular injections or by violent physical struggling, but rarely to a level as high as 1,000 IU/mL. Neuroleptics can affect temperature-regulating brain centers and can therefore be associated with heatstroke, particularly in hot weather or in hot seclusion rooms, in the absence of other manifestations of NMS. A neuroleptic-induced catatonia, really a severe parkinsonian rigidity, can occur in the absence of fever.

Table 4–6. Operational criteria for diagnosis of neuroleptic malignant syndrome

The following three items are all required for a definite diagnosis:

1. Hyperthermia: oral temperature of at least 38.0°C in the absence of another known etiology
2. Severe extrapyramidal effects characterized by two or more of the following: lead-pipe muscle rigidity, pronounced cogwheeling, sialorrhea, oculogyric crisis, retrocollis, opisthotonos, trismus, dysphagia, choreiform movements, festinating gait, and flexor-extensor posturing
3. Autonomic dysfunction characterized by two or more of the following: hypertension (at least 20-mm rise in diastolic pressure above baseline), tachycardia (at least 30 bpm), prominent diaphoresis, and incontinence

In retrospective diagnosis, if one of the three items listed above has not been specifically documented, a probable diagnosis is still permitted if the remaining two criteria are clearly met and the patient displays one of the following characteristic signs: 1) clouded consciousness as evidenced by delirium, mutism, stupor, or coma; 2) leukocytosis (>15,000 white blood cells/mm^3); 3) serum creatine kinase level greater than 1,000 IU/mL.

NMS itself usually develops over 1–3 days in patients taking antipsychotics. Many cases develop in the first week, and most within the first month, of treatment with antipsychotics. There is weak evidence that concomitant treatment with lithium may predispose patients to develop NMS. NMS has been observed with essentially all widely used neuroleptics, although thioridazine is perhaps underrepresented. The dose does not seem to be a major factor, although lower doses seem likely to be safer. Depot neuroleptics do not seem to be more likely to cause NMS, but their prolonged duration of action will make the syndrome last about twice as long (Glazer and Kane 1992).

The best treatment is early identification, stopping neuroleptics, and, in moderate to severe cases, rapid transfer to a medical center. The dopamine agonist bromocriptine, at a dosage of 5 mg every 4 hours, can often relieve muscle rigidity and reduce fever. Dantrolene is used in ICUs to reduce muscle spasm. Anticholinergic antiparkinsonian drugs are probably not helpful. Symptomatic treatment (e.g., cooling the body) is helpful.

The syndrome can recur after it appears to have been brought under control, so patients should be observed carefully for 1 month after the condition is first noted. Neuroleptics should be avoided during that period. We have successfully used ECT in treating persistently manic patients who have recently experienced an episode of NMS. In many, but not all, patients, neuroleptics can be restarted cautiously at much lower dosages without the recurrence of NMS. It is not clear whether thioridazine is safer than one-quarter the dosage of the original offending medication. It seems sensible to avoid depot antipsychotics in patients with a history of NMS.

Long-Acting Injectable Antipsychotics

Adherence to a regimen of oral medications is difficult for many patients with schizophrenia and bipolar disorder. In the comparative efficacy trial, CATIE and Step BD, over 75% of patients eventually discontinued their oral medications. Long-acting injectables may be an alternative to daily oral medications for some patients. The primary advantage of injectables is their once- or twice-a-month dosing. On the other hand, disadvantages may include cost, the pain and inconvenience of having to come in regularly for an injection, and the persistence of side effects.

Depot haloperidol is still a commonly used long-acting injectable. It has been available as an alternative to depot fluphenazine. It is claimed that depot haloperidol's half-life is long enough that an injection every 4 weeks is adequate. If one assumes that 60–70 mg of orally ingested haloperidol actually survives passage through the gut and the liver to become bioavailable, a monthly injection of 20 times the daily oral dose is indicated. If a patient is treated with 10 mg/day of haloperidol, 200 mg/month of haloperidol decanoate could be given. The comparable conversion figure for fluphenazine is much lower—12.5 mg (0.5 mL) of the decanoate form every 3 weeks for patients taking 10 mg/day of oral fluphenazine. Our guess is that a lower haloperidol decanoate conversion figure will eventually prove adequate.

Dose-ranging studies of haloperidol decanoate suggest that the relapse rates for patients with schizophrenia taking 50 or 100 mg every 4 weeks are only a little higher than the relapse rates for patients taking 200 mg every 4 weeks.

The 25-mg dose was clearly inadequate for controlling psychotic symptoms. In the few controlled studies comparing the two depot drugs, haloperidol has tended to be slightly more effective with slightly fewer EPS. Studies comparing oral with depot haloperidol show fewer side effects for the depot preparation; the opposite is true for the fluphenazine formulations. The clinician working in a setting where depot antipsychotics are commonly used should probably try depot haloperidol in a few patients and make up his or her own mind about its utility and consumer acceptance.

Two SGAs are available for use as a long-acting injectable, and one other is in development. A long-acting injectable form of risperidone (Risperdal Consta) was approved in 2003 for the maintenance treatment of schizophrenia. The pivotal trials of the long-acting injectable form at 25 mg every 2 weeks for 12 weeks showed that the active drug was almost three times more likely than a placebo injection to lead to improvement on a standard psychosis scale (the PANSS). Since then, a number of controlled trials at doses of 25–75 mg every 2 weeks have shown that the long-acting injectable form of risperidone is effective and may have some tolerability advantages over the oral form. For example, the rate of EPS, including tardive dyskinesia, may be lower for the injectable form than for the oral form (Rainer 2008). In 1-year trials, the risperidone injection was associated with a tardive dyskinesia rate of about 1%, which is certainly no higher than, and probably lower than, the rate with the oral medicine. In addition, the rate of tardive dyskinesia with the long-acting injectable form of risperidone appears to be considerably lower than the rate reported with haloperidol decanoate or with fluphenazine decanoate. On the other hand, the long-acting injectable form of risperidone is much more expensive than the oral generic risperidone and has shown mixed results, compared with oral medications, in some outcome measures, such as decreased time in the hospital and decreasing overall healthcare costs (Taylor et al. 2009a, 2009b).

A long-acting injectable form of paliperidone (Invega Sustenna) was approved by the FDA, in July 2009, in the maintenance treatment of schizophrenia. Paliperidone palmitate is a once-a-month injection whose efficacy appears to be similar to that of Risperdal Consta. Administration starts with two subsequent injections 1 week apart in the deltoid. The starting dose is typically 234 mg at day 1 and 156 mg at day 8 (Hu 2009).

The long-acting injectable form of an SGA in development is olanzapine pamoate. Olanzapine pamoate has shown efficacy as a once-a-month or twice-a-month injection in the maintenance treatment of schizophrenia. In one 24-week trial, 150 or 300 mg of olanzapine pamoate every 2 weeks or 405 mg every 4 weeks was comparable in efficacy to daily oral olanzapine 10–20 mg/day. Likewise, a 160-week open-label follow-up reported that the long-acting injectable form of olanzapine was significantly different than oral olanzapine in being less likely to be discontinued, less likely to be associated with weight gain >7%, and possibly lower rates of EPS. The major problem noted in clinical trials with the long-acting injectable form of olanzapine has been post-injection delirium and sedation syndrome (PDSS). Accidental injection of olanzapine into the intravascular space may lead to a prolonged oversedation and delirium. In all the olanzapine trials, about 1.4% of patients to date have experienced this syndrome, which can range from mild confusion and gait disturbance to coma. All patients have recovered, but it may take days to weeks before full recovery is seen. It is the potential for PDSS that has kept olanzapine pamoate from the market thus far. Special precautions in the injection of olanzapine pamoate may mitigate the risk of PDSS further, but it remains to be seen whether the risk can be mitigated enough to allow approval of the drug.

Adjunctive Treatment of Negative and Cognitive Symptoms

Negative or deficit symptoms contribute significantly to the morbidity associated with schizophrenia. Symptoms such as affective flattening, social withdrawal, executive dysfunction, anhedonia, and poverty of speech and thought content appear to be much more disabling to patients with schizophrenia than are positive symptoms. Although some authors suggest that the negative symptoms are largely related to the negative effects of first-generation antipsychotics, such symptoms were reported in the literature more than 100 years ago, before the availability of neuroleptics.

The pathophysiology of negative symptoms is still unknown. One theory that has gained popularity in recent years is that negative symptoms are related to a relative deficiency of dopamine in the prefrontal cortex. There are reports of levodopa, amphetamine, amantadine, and bromocriptine all being helpful in the negative symptoms of schizophrenia. On the other hand, some investigators have not found these dopamine agonists helpful (Silver and Geraisy 1995). A potential problem with these approaches is the possibility of worsening the psychosis in some patients. However, low doses of stimulants have been used over the years to counteract the sedation and malaise associated with first-generation antipsychotics and clozapine, and these stimulants do not appear to exacerbate psychosis as often as might be expected. Another approach is to use a drug such as selegiline to increase the availability of dopamine generally while also using a first-generation antipsychotic. Bodkin et al. (1996) found that selegiline 5 mg bid over 6 weeks significantly improved negative symptoms and EPS in a group of 21 schizophrenia and schizoaffective disorder patients while having no effect on positive symptoms. At these low doses, one would not anticipate significant interactions with second-generation, serotonergic antipsychotics, but caution should be exercised. Finally, low doses of first-generation antipsychotics may actually increase the availability of dopamine synaptically by stimulating presynaptic dopamine autoreceptors to release more dopamine. There have been some anecdotal reports of both worsening of positive symptoms and improvement of negative symptoms with low-dose antipsychotics. Amisulpride, a dopamine-blocking benzamide antipsychotic not yet available in the United States, was found in a placebo-controlled study to significantly improve negative symptoms of schizophrenia at low doses (Boyer et al. 1995). At high doses, amisulpride and first-generation antipsychotics may worsen negative symptoms by dampening dopaminergic tone throughout the prefrontal cortex.

The FDA and NIMH have sought to improve treatments for the cognitive deficits because these deficits are directly related to the disability seen in schizophrenia. The Measurement and Treatment Research to Improve Cognition in Schizophrenia initiative (MATRICS) seeks to identify the cognitive deficits, develop better measurement tools for assessing cognition in schizophrenia, and encourage clinical trial design for assessing new agents to target these cognitive deficits. A number of potential drug targets are currently being evaluated in the treatment of cognitive deficits in schizophrenia. Among the more promising targets are acetylcholine receptor subtypes. Agonists of the α_7 nicotinic receptor have shown initial promise in the improving cognitive deficits. An experimental α_7 agonist DMXB-A showed significant cognitive benefit in a proof of concept study with 12 patients with schizophrenia (Green 2007). Likewise, one acetylcholine esterase inhibitor, galantamine, has shown benefit in some, but not all, studies of treating cognitive deficits in schizophrenia (Gray and Roth 2007). On the other hand, rivastigmine and donepezil have not shown much benefit as adjunctive agents in treating cognitive deficits.

Noradrenergic neurotransmission also appears to be important in cognition. α_2-adrenergic receptor agonists such as guanfacine and clonidine have shown some benefit in enhancing cognition in small trials (Friedman et al. 2001). Guanfacine continues to be investigated in improving cognition in schizophrenia, as it is less likely to induce hypotension than is clonidine.

The role of serotonin in the pathophysiology of positive and negative symptoms has gained significant attention with the success of clozapine. As described earlier, all the SGAs have in common a high ratio of 5-HT$_2$-to-D$_2$ affinities relative to first-generation antipsychotics. Certain 5-HT$_2$ agonists such as lysergic acid diethylamide (LSD) can produce hallucinations and other psychotic symptoms, whereas 5-HT$_2$ antagonists seem to improve psychosis. Even though serotonin has a putative effect on dopamine, which can contribute to its favorable effect on positive symptoms and the occasional worsening of EPS, serotonergic agents also appear to help with negative symptoms. All the SGAs share the ability to improve negative symptoms, and this is believed to be due in part to their 5-HT$_2$ antagonism. Of interest is a report that mirtazapine reduced negative symptoms in schizophrenia patients who were taking haloperidol (Berk et al. 2001). In addition, several studies suggest that the SSRIs may improve negative symptoms in schizophrenic patients. For example, Spina et al. (1994), in a placebo-controlled study of 34 patients with schizophrenia, found that adding 20 mg/day of fluoxetine to first-generation antipsychotics substantially improved negative symptoms. Likewise, paroxetine 30 mg/day appears effective in improving negative symptoms (Jockers-Scherubl et al. 2005). However, SSRIs may also increase the toxicity of first-generation antipsychotics and SGAs through competitive inhibition of the cytochrome P450 enzyme 2D6. We have occasionally used sertraline 50–100 mg/day as an adjunctive agent in treating negative symptoms and have found it modestly helpful. A number of other antidepressant treatments, including transdermal selegiline (Bodkin et al. 2005), mirtazapine (Zoccali et al. 2004), and transcranial magnetic stimulation (TMS) (Jin et al. 2006), have also been suggested to help with negative symptoms of schizophrenia. However, few of these have been subjected to carefully controlled trials. Those that have, including mirtazapine (Berk et al. 2009), have not consistently shown benefit in treating negative symptoms.

Glutamate-specific agents may have a role to play in treating negative and positive symptoms of schizophrenia. NMDA antagonists such as phencyclidine and ketamine produce not only positive psychotic symptoms but also negative symptoms and cognitive symptoms. Thus, drugs that modulate glutamate activity are under investigation for the treatment of cognitive and negative symptoms (Webber and Marder 2008). Among the more promising agents identified by MATRICS are allosteric modulators of AMPA receptors (Ampakines). One Ampakine, CX-516, has shown mixed results in treating cognitive symptoms of schizophrenia (Goff et al. 2008). Another type of glutamate agent is one that directly acts on NMDA receptors, including the glycine cosite of the receptor. Agents such as D-cycloserine and glycine have been evaluated for treating cognitive symptoms in schizophrenia. Neither has been all that effective. That being said, glutamate-specific agents continue to be evaluated in the treatment of schizophrenia.

It seems unlikely that we will discover antipsychotics that are profoundly and equally effective at treating both the positive and negative symptoms of schizophrenia. Our understanding of the pathophysiology of schizophrenia, limited as it might be, argues against the likelihood of monotherapies being effective for all symptoms of the disorder. Thus, it appears probable that the treatment of schizophrenia will increasingly depend on a combination of agents that target specific positive and negative symptoms and cognitive symptoms of schizophrenia.

Alternatives to Antipsychotic Therapy

There are currently no reliable, safe, effective drug therapies for schizophrenia and other psychotic disorders that can replace dopamine-blocking antipsychotics. ECT can reverse psychotic excitements and catatonic stupor but has no real value in preventing future episodes of psychosis. Lithium can ameliorate the symptoms of schizophrenia or suppress episodic violence in schizophrenic patients, but it almost never is an adequate drug therapy by itself.

Carbamazepine also ameliorates symptoms in some patients with treatment-resistant psychosis when added to a neuroleptic, as a double-blind Israeli study showed (Klein et al. 1984), but it is not by itself an adequate therapy for schizophrenia. Later studies of lithium and anticonvulsants in the adjunctive treatment of schizophrenia have often not supported the earlier trials (Citrome 2009). A trial by Casey and colleagues (2003) found that valproate add-on to risperidone or olanzapine was significantly more effective than placebo add-on in patients with schizophrenia. However, the data on adjunctive use of valproate in schizophrenia appear to be strongest for alleviating aggressive symptoms rather than treating positive or negative symptoms (Schwarz et al. 2008). Diazepam alone has been reported by both Canadian and German groups to rapidly control psychotic symptoms in small numbers of paranoid schizophrenic patients at dosages between 70 and 400 mg/day (the German group used 50-mg tablets). Sedation was not a problem, allegedly, after the first day, and improvement continued for 4 weeks. Neither study reported follow-up data. In one study, high-dose diazepam aggravated schizoaffective symptoms. The findings from these small, brief studies are intriguing, but they do not offer a real and useful pharmacological alternative to the first-generation antipsychotics.

There have been at least seven reports on the use of alprazolam in patients with schizophrenia who are being treated with neuroleptics. Two of the studies involved patients with clear panic attacks as well as chronic psychosis. Both small studies found alprazolam to be useful in suppressing episodes of panic. Several other small studies, mainly in inpatients, found the addition of alprazolam to be beneficial in some patients. The original hypothesis was that alprazolam would be particularly useful in treating negative symptoms, but the studies showed effects of alprazolam on both positive and negative symptoms in some patients. The only large placebo-controlled study involving schizophrenic outpatients yielded completely negative findings (Csernansky et al. 1988); neither diazepam nor alprazolam was more effective than placebo over the course of this 8-week trial. The data from the diverse studies are inconclusive, but a reasonable presumption is that alprazolam might be helpful as an adjunct to neuroleptic treatment in patients with panic attacks or other significant anxiety symptoms.

Propranolol was studied for many years in the treatment of acute and chronic schizophrenia at very high dosages (600–2,000 mg/day) given alone or with a neuroleptic drug. Although Yorkston et al. (1978) reported efficacy in controlled studies, other investigators found equivocal results, with only occasional patients experiencing any benefit. Since two early deaths occurred with this treatment—one death from a silent bleeding peptic ulcer and one sudden death of unknown etiology—this use was not generally recommended. However, subsequent clinical studies of dosages up to 400 mg/day in organically impaired psychiatric patients with impulsive violence or aggression suggested that propranolol might be useful in such patients in controlling temper outbursts, although it did not affect other underlying behavioral organic deficits. If such therapy is attempted, the relevant articles should be reviewed and the dosage should be increased slowly, with blood pressure and pulse monitoring before each dose until the patient is well stabilized at a constant, effective dose. Propranolol has been reported to increase chlorpromazine blood levels and may do so for other antipsychotics as well.

It is possible that carbamazepine, valproate, and lithium also offer more promise in the treatment of disturbed behavior in patients with brain damage, dementia, or mental retardation than do the first-generation antipsychotics. Low doses of valproate and SGAs are helpful adjuncts in dementia. However, no antipsychotics or anticonvulsants have proven consistently effective in treating behavioral or psychotic symptoms in dementia, and none have been approved for this indication.

Antipsychotic Drugs Newly Released or in Development

There are a number of antipsychotics under development in the United States. Of these, the two drugs farthest along are bifeprunox and asenapine. Bifeprunox is a partial dopamine agonist similar to aripiprazole. Like aripiprazole, it is expected to have a relatively good side-effect profile, including a lower proclivity for weight gain, no risk of prolactin level increases, and a relative lack of negative effects on lipids or glucose levels. There are little or no data to suggest that bifeprunox has better efficacy than other second-generation agents. In one multi-center registration trial, bifeprunox 20 mg/day was similar in efficacy to risperidone and superior to placebo in a 6-week study (Casey et al. 2008). In addition, bifeprunox was less likely to increase prolactin levels or weight than was risperidone. However, the FDA rejected the new drug application for bifeprunox in 2007, citing a lack of data supporting efficacy relative to other agents. Work continues with bifeprunox, but it is unclear whether the drug will be subsequently approved or not. Asenapine was approved in 2009 and is a more traditional $D_2/5\text{-}HT_2$-type SGA. Additionally, it may have some selective effects on ionotropic glutamate receptors. Like asenapine, bifeprunox is also being evaluated in the treatment of bipolar disorder.

A number of other antipsychotic agents are available for prescription use in one or more European countries. Some have been available in Europe for years but have never been released in the United States. A few failed to pass the FDA's carcinogenicity screen; we believe this is true of sulpiride, amisulpride, and penfluridol. Fluspirilene, a long-acting injectable drug, is held in suspension by a chemical that is not approved by the FDA.

Another SGA long available in Europe and Japan is zotepine. Zotepine is a $D_2/5\text{-}HT_2$ antagonist that also has significant effects on other serotonin receptors, including $5\text{-}HT_6$ and $5\text{-}HT_7$. In addition, zotepine is a norepinephrine reuptake inhibitor. It has a tricyclics chemical structure and appears to be a reasonable antidepressant. Zotepine appears to be effective in some cases of treatment-resistant schizophrenia, and EPS are quite uncommon with the drug. However, zotepine has two big drawbacks: weight gain and sedation. At least a third of all patients gain a significant amount of weight at dosages of 75–450 mg/day. In addition, many patients have difficulty tolerating the somnolence associated with the drug. As a result, zotepine is not likely to be introduced into the U.S. market.

An active metabolite of clozapine, n-desmethylclozapine (norclozapine) is being actively investigated for the treatment of schizophrenia (Natesan et al. 2007). Norclozapine is a partial agonist at the D_2 receptor and also is a muscarine receptor agonist. Thus, it is being evaluated in treating the cognitive symptoms of schizophrenia. There is some suggestion that norclozapine may be better tolerated and safer than clozapine, but large-scale studies have not been completed to date.

Sulpiride is clearly a second-generation ("atypical") antipsychotic in that it differs from the older antipsychotics in its pharmacology. However, it causes pseudoparkinsonism, akathisia, galactorrhea, and tardive dyskinesia to such a degree that its advantages over other neuroleptics more readily available in the

United States are unclear. Several drugs available in Europe are clinically and pharmacologically related to sulpiride. One of these, metoclopramide (Reglan), is marketed in the United States for gastrointestinal diseases but is probably effective in treating psychosis and certainly can cause typical neurological side effects and tardive dyskinesia. Amisulpiride has shown antipsychotic as well as antidepressant benefits. Its efficacy appears at least as good in the treatment of schizophrenia as other SGAs. Most sulpiride-like drugs are good antiemetics and speed peristalsis, including stomach emptying, making them useful in dyspepsia.

The reason for discussing these drugs in an American psychopharmacology manual is that current FDA and customs policy, influenced by pressures from patients with AIDS, have allowed 3-month supplies of drugs that are not available in the United States to be imported for individual patients with treatment-resistant conditions. It is not clear that any of these drugs are so different and so superior (as was clearly the case with clomipramine in the treatment of OCD) as to impel many psychiatrists to arrange to bring one or more of these drugs to the United States; however, in special situations it might be worth doing. Since 9/11, some patients have at times found importation to be delayed.

Bibliography

Adler L, Peselow E, Rotrosen J, et al: Vitamin E treatment of tardive dyskinesia. Am J Psychiatry 150:1405–1407, 1993

Allison DB, Mentore JL, Heo M, et al: Antipsychotic-induced weight gain: a comprehensive research synthesis. Am J Psychiatry 156:1686–1696, 1999

Alvir JM, Lieberman JA, Safferman AZ, et al: Clozapine-induced agranulocytosis. N Engl J Med 329:162–167, 1993

Aman MG, Arnold LE, McDougle CJ, et al: Acute and long-term safety and tolerability of risperidone in children with autism. J Child Adolesc Psychopharmacol 15:869–884, 2005

American Diabetes Association, American Psychiatric Association, American Association of Clinical Endocrinologists, et al: Consensus development conference on antipsychotic drugs and obesity and diabetes. Diabetes Care 27:596–601, 2004

American Psychiatric Association: Diagnostic and Statistical Manual of Mental Disorders, 2nd Edition. Washington, DC, American Psychiatric Association, 1968

American Psychiatric Association: Diagnostic and Statistical Manual of Mental Disorders, 3rd Edition, Revised. Washington, DC, American Psychiatric Association, 1987

American Psychiatric Association: Diagnostic and Statistical Manual of Mental Disorders, 4th Edition. Washington, DC, American Psychiatric Association, 1994

American Psychiatric Association: Diagnostic and Statistical Manual of Mental Disorders, 4th Edition, Text Revision. Washington, DC, American Psychiatric Association, 2000

Andreescu C, Mulsant BH, Peasley-Miklus C, et al; STOP-PD Study Group: Persisting low use of antipsychotics in the treatment of major depressive disorder with psychotic features. J Clin Psychiatry. 68:194–200, 2007

Ayd F: Lorazepam update: 1977–1985. International Drug Therapy Newsletter 20:33–36, 1985

Azorin JM, Spiegel R, Remington G, et al: A double-blind comparative study of clozapine and risperidone in the management of severe chronic schizophrenia. Am J Psychiatry 158:1305–1313, 2001

Baldessarini R, Viguera A: Neuroleptic withdrawal in schizophrenic patients. Arch Gen Psychiatry 52:189–192, 1995

Baldessarini RJ, Cole JO, Davis JM, et al: Tardive Dyskinesia (Task Force Report No 18). Washington, DC, American Psychiatric Association, 1980

Baldessarini RJ, Cohen BM, Teicher MH: Pharmacological treatment, in Schizophrenia: Treatment of Acute Psychotic Episodes. Edited by Levy ST, Ninan PT. Washington, DC, American Psychiatric Press, 1990, pp 61–118

Baldwin DS, Montgomery SA: First clinical experience with olanzapine (LY 170053): results of an open-label safety and dose-ranging study in patients with schizophrenia. Int Clin Psychopharmacol 10:239–244, 1995

Baptista T, Uzcátegui E, Rangel N, et al: Metformin plus sibutramine for olanzapine-associated weight gain and metabolic dysfunction in schizophrenia: a 12-week double-blind, placebo-controlled pilot study. Psychiatry Res 159:250–253, 2008

Barbee JG, Conrad EJ, Jamhour NJ.: The effectiveness of olanzapine, risperidone, quetiapine, and ziprasidone as augmentation agents in treatment-resistant major depressive disorder. J Clin Psychiatry 65:975–981, 2004

Beckmann H, Haas S: High dose diazepam in schizophrenia. Psychopharmacology (Berl) 71:79–82, 1980

Benedetti F, Sforzini L, Colombo C, et al: Low-dose clozapine in acute and continuation treatment of severe borderline personality disorder. J Clin Psychiatry 59:103–107, 1998

Benvenga MJ, Leander JD: Olanzapine, an atypical antipsychotic, increases rates of punished responding in pigeons. Psychopharmacology (Berl) 119:133–138, 1995

Berk M, Ichim L, Brook S: Olanzapine compared to lithium in mania: a double-blind randomized controlled trial. Int Clin Psychopharmacol 14:339–343, 1999

Berk M, Ichim C, Brook S: Efficacy of mirtazapine add-on therapy to haloperidol in the treatment of negative symptoms of schizophrenia: a double-blind, randomized, placebo-controlled study. Int Clin Psychopharmacol 16:87–92, 2001

Berk M, Gama CS, Sundram S, et al: Mirtazapine add-on therapy in the treatment of schizophrenia with atypical antipsychotics: a double-blind, randomised, placebo-controlled clinical trial. Hum Psychopharmacol 24:233–238, 2009

Berman RM, Fava M, Thase ME, et al: Aripiprazole augmentation in major depressive disorder: a double-blind, placebo-controlled study in patients with inadequate response to antidepressants. CNS Spectr 14(4):197-206, 2009

Bishop M, Simpson G, Dunnett C, et al: Efficacy of loxapine in the treatment of paranoid schizophrenia. Psychopharmacology (Berl) 51:107–114, 1977

Bitter I, Dossenbach MR, Brook S, et al, Olanzapine HGCK Study Group: Olanzapine versus clozapine in treatment-resistant or treatment-intolerant schizophrenia. Prog Neuropsychopharmacol Biol Psychiatry 28:173–180, 2004

Blackwell B: Patient compliance with drug therapy. N Engl J Med 289:249–252, 1973

Bodkin JA, Cohen BM, Salomon MS, et al: Treatment of negative symptoms in schizophrenia and schizoaffective disorder by selegiline augmentation of antipsychotic medication: a pilot study examining the role of dopamine. J Nerv Ment Dis 184:295–301, 1996

Bodkin JA, Siris SG, Bermanzohn PC, et al: Double-blind, placebo-controlled, multicenter trial of selegiline augmentation of antipsychotic medication to treat negative symptoms in outpatients with schizophrenia. Am J Psychiatry 162(2):388–390, 2005

Bogenschutz MP, George Nurnberg H: Olanzapine versus placebo in the treatment of borderline personality disorder. J Clin Psychiatry. 65:104–109, 2004

Boyer P, Lecrubier Y, Puech AJ, et al: Treatment of negative symptoms in schizophrenia with amisulpride. Br J Psychiatry 166:68–72, 1995

Brown W, Laughren T: Low serum prolactin and early relapse following neuroleptic withdrawal. Am J Psychiatry 138:237–239, 1981

Carpenter WT Jr: Serotonin-dopamine antagonists and treatment of negative symptoms. J Clin Psychopharmacol 15 (1, suppl 1):30S–35S, 1995

Carpenter WT Jr, Heinrichs DW: Early intervention, time-limited, targeted pharmacotherapy of schizophrenia. Schizophr Bull 9:533–542, 1983

Carpenter WT Jr, Hanlon TE, Heinrichs DW, et al: Continuous vs targeted medication in schizophrenic outpatients: outcome results. Am J Psychiatry 147:1138–1148, 1990

Carson WH, Stock E, Saha AR, et al: Meta-analysis of the efficacy of aripiprazole in schizophrenia. Eur Psychiatry 17 (suppl 1):105, 2002

Casey DE: Implications of the CATIE trial on treatment: extrapyramidal symptoms. CNS Spectr 11(7, suppl 7):25–31, 2006

Casey DE, Daniel DG, Wassef AA, et al: Effect of divalproex combined with olanzapine or risperidone in patients with an acute exacerbation of schizophrenia. Neuropsychopharmacology 28:182–192, 2003

Casey DE, Sands EE, Heisterberg J, et al: Efficacy and safety of bifeprunox in patients with an acute exacerbation of schizophrenia: results from a randomized, double-blind, placebo-controlled, multicenter, dose-finding study. Psychopharmacology (Berlin) 200:317–331, 2008

Chengappa KN, Ebeling T, Kang JS, et al: Clozapine reduces severe self-mutilation and aggression in psychotic patients with borderline personality disorder. J Clin Psychiatry 60:477–484, 1999

Chouinard G, Jones B, Remington G, et al: A Canadian multicenter placebo-controlled study of fixed doses of risperidone and haloperidol in the treatment of chronic schizophrenic patients. J Clin Psychopharmacol 13:25–40, 1993

Citrome L: Maintenance treatment with olanzapine reduces relapse in people with bipolar I disorder who have responded to acute olanzapine treatment. Evid Based Ment Health 9(3):73, 2006

Citrome L: Adjunctive lithium and anticonvulsants for the treatment of schizophrenia: what is the evidence? Expert Rev Neurother 9:55–71, 2009

Cohen BM: The clinical utility of plasma neuroleptic levels, in Guidelines for the Use of Psychotropic Drugs. Edited by Stancer H. New York, Spectrum Publications, 1984, pp 245–260

Cole JO: Antipsychotic drugs: is more better? McLean Hospital Journal 7:61–87, 1982

Cole JO, Gardos G: Alternatives to neuroleptic drug therapy. McLean Hospital Journal 10:112–127, 1985

Cole JO, Yonkers KA: Non-benzodiazepine anxiolytics, in The American Psychiatric Press Textbook of Psychopharmacology. Edited by Schatzberg AF, Nemeroff CB. Washington, DC, American Psychiatric Press, 1995, pp 231–244

Cole JO, Gardos G, Gelernter J, et al: Supersensitivity psychosis. McLean Hospital Journal 9:46–72, 1984

Cole JO, Gardos G, Boling LA, et al: Early dyskinesia-vulnerability. Psychopharmacology (Berl) 107:503–510, 1992

Comaty JE, Janicak PG: Depot neuroleptics. Psychiatr Ann 17:491–496, 1987

Cornelius JR, Soloff PH, Perel JM, et al: Continuation pharmacotherapy of borderline personality disorder with haloperidol and phenelzine. Am J Psychiatry 150:1843–1848, 1993

Creese I: Dopamine and antipsychotic medications, in Psychiatry Update: The American Psychiatric Association Annual Review, Vol 4. Edited by Hales RE, Frances AJ. Washington, DC, American Psychiatric Press, 1985, pp 17–36

Csernansky JG, Riney SJ, Lombrozo L, et al: Double-blind comparison of alprazolam, diazepam, and placebo for the treatment of negative schizophrenic symptoms. Arch Gen Psychiatry 45:655–659, 1988

Dando TM, Keating GM: Quetiapine: a review of its use in acute mania and depression associated with bipolar disorder. Drugs 65(17):2533–2551, 2005

Davis JM: Overview: maintenance therapy in psychiatry, I: schizophrenia. Am J Psychiatry 132:1237–1245, 1975

Davis JM, Chen N, Glick ID: A meta-analysis of the efficacy of second-generation antipsychotics. Arch Gen Psychiatry 60:553–564, 2003

Davis RJ, Cummings JL: Clinical variants of tardive dyskinesia. Neuropsychiatry Neuropsychol Behav Neurol 1:31–38, 1988

De Deyn PP, Rabheru K, Rasmussen A, et al: A randomized trial of risperidone, placebo, and haloperidol for behavioral symptoms of dementia. Neurology 53:946–955, 1999 [see comments]

De Deyn PP, Carrasco MM, Deberdt W, et al: Olanzapine versus placebo in the treatment of psychosis with or without associated behavioral disturbances in patients with Alzheimer's disease. Int J Geriatr Psychiatry 19(2):115–126, 2004

Delay J, Deniker P, Harl J: Utilization thérapeutique psychiatrique d'une phénothiazine d'action centrale élective. Ann Med Psychol (Paris) 110:112–117, 1952

Delva N, Letemendia F: Lithium treatment in schizophrenic and schizoaffective disorders. Br J Psychiatry 141:387–400, 1982

Dennis K, Le Grange D, Bremer J: Olanzapine use in adolescent anorexia nervosa. Eat Weight Disord 11(2):e53–e56, 2006

Dixon L, Weiden P, Frances AJ, et al: Alprazolam intolerance in stable schizophrenic outpatients. Psychopharmacol Bull 25:213–214, 1989

Donaldson SR, Gelenberg AJ, Baldessarini RJ: The pharmacological treatment of schizophrenia: a progress report. Schizophr Bull 9:504–527, 1983

Douyon R, Angrist B, Peselow E, et al: Neuroleptic augmentation with alprazolam: clinical effects and pharmacokinetic correlates. Am J Psychiatry 146:231–234, 1989

Endicott J, Paulsson B, Gustafsson U, et al: Quetiapine monotherapy in the treatment of depressive episodes of bipolar I and II disorder: improvements in quality of life and quality of sleep. J Affect Disord 111:306–319, 2008

Ferrerri MM, Loze JY, Rouillon F, et al: Clozapine treatment of a borderline personality disorder with severe self-mutilating behaviours. Eur Psychiatry 19(3):177–178, 2004

Finnerty RJ, Goldberg HL, Nathan L, et al: Haloperidol in neurotic outpatients. Dis Nerv Syst 37:621–624, 1976

Fluvoxamine for obsessive-compulsive disorder. Med Lett Drugs Ther 37:13–14, 1995

Fluvoxamine gains approval for obsessive-compulsive disorder. Am J Health Syst Pharm 52:355, 1995

Frankenburg FR, Zanarini MC: Clozapine treatment of borderline patients: a preliminary study. Compr Psychiatry 34:402–405, 1993

Friedman JI, Adler DN, Temporini HD, et al: Guanfacine treatment of cognitive impairment in schizophrenia. Neuropsychopharmacology 25:402–409, 2001

Frye MA, Kettler TA, Altshuler LL, et al: Clozapine in bipolar disorder: treatment implications for other atypical antipsychotics. J Affect Disord 48:91–104, 1998

Galbrecht CR, Klett CJ: Predicting response to phenothiazines: the right drug for the right patient. J Nerv Ment Dis 147:173–183, 1968

Gao K, Gajwani P, Elhaj O,et al: Typical and atypical antipsychotics in bipolar depression. J Clin Psychiatry 66:1376–1385, 2005

Gao K, Muzina D, Gajwani P, et al: Efficacy of typical and atypical antipsychotics for primary and comorbid anxiety symptoms or disorders: a review. J Clin Psychiatry 67:1327–1340, 2006

Garakani A, Martinez JM, Marcus S, et al: A randomized, double-blind, and placebo-controlled trial of quetiapine augmentation of fluoxetine in major depressive disorder. Int Clin Psychopharmacol 23:269-275, 2008

Gardos G, Casey D: Tardive Dyskinesia and Affective Disorders. Washington, DC, American Psychiatric Press, 1984

Gardos G, Cole J: The evaluation and treatment of neuroleptic-induced movement disorders. Harv Rev Psychiatry 3:130–139, 1995

Gardos G, Perenyi A, Cole J: Polypharmacy revisited. McLean Hospital Journal 5:178–195, 1980

Garza-Trevino ES, Hollister LE, Overall JE, et al: Efficacy of combinations of intramuscular antipsychotics and sedative-hypnotics for control of psychotic agitation. Am J Psychiatry 146:1598–1601, 1989

Gelenberg AJ (ed): Risperidone and mania. Biological Therapies in Psychiatry Newsletter 17:45, 1994

Gelenberg AJ, Mandel MR: Catatonic reactions to high-potency neuroleptic drugs. Arch Gen Psychiatry 34:947–950, 1977

Gerson SL: G-CSF and the management of clozapine-induced agranulocytosis. J Clin Psychiatry 55 (suppl B):139–142, 1994

Ghaemi SN, Katzow JJ: The use of quetiapine for treatment-resistant bipolar disorder: a case series. Ann Clin Psychiatry 11:137–140, 1999

Gilbert PL, Harris MJ, McAdams LA, et al: Neuroleptic withdrawal in schizophrenic patients: a review of the literature. Arch Gen Psychiatry 52:173–188, 1995

Glazer WM, Kane JM: Depot neuroleptic therapy: an underutilized treatment option. J Clin Psychiatry 53:426–433, 1992

Goff DC, Posever T, Herz L, et al: An exploratory haloperidol-controlled dose-finding study of ziprasidone in hospitalized patients with schizophrenia or schizoaffective disorder. J Clin Psychopharmacol 18:296–304, 1998

Goff DC, Sullivan LM, McEvoy JP, et al: A comparison of ten-year cardiac risk estimates in schizophrenia patients from the CATIE study and matched controls. Schizophr Res 80:45–53, 2005

Goff DC, Lamberti JS, Leon AC, et al: A placebo-controlled add-on trial of the Ampakine, CX516, for cognitive deficits in schizophrenia. Neuropsychopharmacology 33:465–472, 2008

Gray R: Quetiapine: a new atypical antipsychotic for the treatment of schizophrenia. Ment Health Care 1(5):163–164, 1998

Gray JA, Roth BL: Molecular targets for treating cognitive dysfunction in schizophrenia. Schizophr Bull 33:1100–1119, 2007

Green AI, Garaone SV, Brown WA: Prolactin shift after neuroleptic withdrawal. Psychiatry Res 32:213–219, 1990

Green AI, Tohen M, Patel JK, et al: Clozapine in the treatment of refractory psychotic mania. Am J Psychiatry 157:982–986, 2000

Green MF: Stimulating the development of drug treatments to improve cognition in schizophrenia. Annu Rev Clin Psychol 3:159–180, 2007

Greendyke R, Schuster D, Wooten J: Propranolol in the treatment of assaultive patients with organic brain disease. J Clin Psychopharmacol 4:282–285, 1984

Gründer G, Hippius H, Carlsson A: The 'atypicality' of antipsychotics: a concept re-examined and re-defined. Nat Rev Drug Discov 8(3):197-202, 2009

Hamner MB, Faldowski RA, Ulmer HG, et al: Adjunctive risperidone treatment in posttraumatic stress disorder: a preliminary controlled trial of effects on comorbid psychotic symptoms. Int Clin Psychopharmacol 18:1–8, 2003

Hardoy MC, Hardoy MJ, Carta MG, et al: Gabapentin as a promising treatment for antipsychotic-induced movement disorders in schizoaffective and bipolar patients. J Affect Disord 54:315–317, 1999

Hasan S, Buckley P: Novel antipsychotics and the neuroleptic malignant syndrome: a review and critique. Am J Psychiatry 155:1113–1116, 1998

Hayes P, Schulz C: The use of beta-adrenergic blocking drugs in anxiety disorders and schizophrenia. Pharmacotherapy 3:101–117, 1983

Herrmann N, Mamdani M, Lanctot KL: Atypical antipsychotics and risk of cerebrovascular accidents. Am J Psychiatry 161:1113–1115, 2004

Herz M, Szymanski H, Simon J: Intermittent medication for stable schizophrenic outpatients. Am J Psychiatry 139:918–922, 1982

Herz M, Glazer W, Mosbert M, et al: Intermittent vs maintenance medication in schizophrenia. Arch Gen Psychiatry 48:333–339, 1991

Hilger E, Barnas C, Kasper S: Quetiapine in the treatment of borderline personality disorder. World J Biol Psychiatry 4:42–44, 2003

Hillebrand JJ, van Elburg AA, Kas MJ, et al: Olanzapine reduces physical activity in rats exposed to activity-based anorexia: possible implications for treatment of anorexia nervosa? Biol Psychiatry 58:651–657, 2005

Hirschfeld RM, Keck PE Jr, Kramer M, et al: Rapid antimanic effect of risperidone monotherapy: a three-week multicenter, double-blind, placebo-controlled trial. Am J Psychiatry 161:1057–1065, 2004

Hirschfeld RM, Weisler RH, Raines SR, et al, for the BOLDER Study Group: Quetiapine in the treatment of anxiety in patients with bipolar I or II depression: a secondary analysis from a randomized, double-blind, placebo-controlled study. J Clin Psychiatry 67:355–362, 2006

Hogarty GE: Treatment and course of schizophrenia. Schizophr Bull 3:587–599, 1977

Hogarty GE, Ulrich RJ: Temporal effects of drugs and placebo in delaying relapse in schizophrenic outpatients. Arch Gen Psychiatry 34:297–301, 1977

Hogarty GE, Kornblith SJ, Greenwald D, et al: Personal therapy: a disorder-relevant psychotherapy for schizophrenia. Schizophr Bull 21:379–393, 1995

Hoge EA, Worthington JJ 3rd, Kaufman RE, et al: Aripiprazole as augmentation treatment of refractory generalized anxiety disorder and panic disorder. CNS Spectr 13:522–527, 2008

Hollander E, Baldini Rossi N, Sood E, et al: Risperidone augmentation in treatment-resistant obsessive-compulsive disorder: a double-blind, placebo-controlled study. Int J Neuropsychopharmacol 6:397–401, 2003

Hu RJ: What is the optimal dosing for atypical antipsychotics?: a practical guide based on available evidence. Primary Psychiatry 16:43–49, 2009

Hyttel J, Arnt J, Costall B, et al: Pharmacological profile of the atypical neuroleptic sertindole. Clin Neuropharmacol 15 (suppl 1, pt A):267A–268A, 1992a

Hyttel J, Nielsen JB, Nowak G: The acute effect of sertindole in brain 5-HT$_2$, D$_2$ and alpha-1 receptors (ex vivo radioreceptor binding studies). J Neural Transm Gen Sect 89:61–69, 1992b

Inoue A, Seto M, Sugita S, et al: Differential effects on D$_2$ dopamine receptor and prolactin gene expression by haloperidol and aripiprazole in the rat pituitary. Brain Res Mol Brain Res 55:285–292, 1998

Jandl M, Bittner R, Sack A, et al: Changes in negative symptoms and EEG in schizophrenic patients after repetitive transcranial magnetic stimulation (rtMS): an open-label pilot study. J Neural Transm 112:955–967, 2005

Jefferson J, Greist J: Haloperidol and lithium: their combined use and the issue of their compatibility, in Haloperidol Update, 1958–1980. Edited by Ayd F. Baltimore, MD, Ayd Medical Communications, 1980

Jeste DV, Caligiuri M, Paulsen J, et al: Risk of tardive dyskinesia in older patients: a prospective longitudinal study of 266 outpatients. Arch Gen Psychiatry 52:756–765, 1995

Jin Y, Potkin SG, Kemp AS, et al: Therapeutic effects of individualized alpha frequency transcranial magnetic stimulation (alphaTMS) on the negative symptoms of schizophrenia. Schizophr Bull 32:556–561, 2006

Jockers-Scherubl MC, Bauer A, Godemann F, et al: Negative symptoms of schizophrenia are improved by the addition of paroxetine to neuroleptics: a double-blind placebo-controlled study. Int Clin Psychopharmacol 20:27–31, 2005

Jones PB, Barnes TR, Davies L, et al: Randomized controlled trial of the effect on quality of life of second- vs first-generation antipsychotic drugs in schizophrenia: Cost Utility of the Latest Antipsychotic Drugs in Schizophrenia Study (CUtLASS 1). Arch Gen Psychiatry 63:1079–1087, 2006

Kane JM, Woerner M, Weinhold P, et al: A prospective study of tardive dyskinesia: preliminary results. J Clin Psychopharmacol 2:345–349, 1982

Kane JM, Rifkin A, Woerner M, et al: Low dose neuroleptic treatment of outpatient schizophrenics. Arch Gen Psychiatry 40:893–896, 1983

Kane JM, Honigfeld G, Singer J, et al: Clozapine for the treatment-resistant schizophrenic: a double-blind comparison with chlorpromazine. Arch Gen Psychiatry 45:789–796, 1988

Kane JM, Davis JM, Schooler N, et al: A multidose study of haloperidol decanoate in the maintenance treatment of schizophrenia. Am J Psychiatry 159:554–560, 2002

Kane J, Canas F, Kramer M, et al: Treatment of schizophrenia with paliperidone extended-release tablets: a 6-week placebo-controlled trial. Schizophr Res 90:147–161, 2007

Kane JM, Lauriello J, Laska E, et al: Long-term efficacy and safety of iloperidone: results from 3 clinical trials for the treatment of schizophrenia. J Clin Psychopharmacol 28(2, suppl 1):S29–S35, 2008

Kapur S, Zipursky RB, Remington G: Clinical and theoretical implications of 5-HT$_2$ and D$_2$ receptor occupancy of clozapine, risperidone, and olanzapine in schizophrenia. Am J Psychiatry 156:286–293, 1999

Karagianis JL, Phillips LC, Hogan KP, et al: Clozapine-associated neuroleptic malignant syndrome: two new cases and a review of the literature. Ann Pharmacother 33:623–630, 1999

Katz IR, Jeste DV, Mintzer JE, et al: Comparison of risperidone and placebo for psychosis and behavioral disturbances associated with dementia: a randomized, double-blind trial. Risperidone Study Group. J Clin Psychiatry 60:107–115, 1999

Keck PE Jr, Caroff SM, McElroy SL: Neuroleptic malignant syndrome and malignant hyperthermia: end of a controversy? J Neuropsychiatry Clin Neurosci 7:135–144, 1995

Keck PE Jr, Buffenstein A, Ferguson J, et al: Ziprasidone 40 and 120 mg/day in the acute exacerbation of schizophrenia and schizoaffective disorder: a 4-week placebo-controlled trial. Psychopharmacology (Berl) 140:173–184, 1998

Keck PE Jr, Marcus R, Tourkodimitris S: A placebo-controlled, double-blind study of the efficacy and safety of aripiprazole in patients with acute bipolar mania. Am J Psychiatry 160:1651–1658, 2003a

Keck PE Jr, Versiani M, Potkin S, et al, Ziprasidone in Mania Study Group: Ziprasidone in the treatment of acute bipolar mania: a three-week, placebo-controlled, double-blind, randomized trial. Am J Psychiatry 160:741–748, 2003b

Keepers GA, Clappison VJ, Casey DE: Initial anticholinergic prophylaxis for neuroleptic-induced extrapyramidal syndromes. Arch Gen Psychiatry 40:1113–1117, 1983

Khouzam HR, Donnelly NJ: Remission of self-mutilation in a patient with borderline personality during risperidone therapy. J Nerv Ment Dis 185:348–349, 1997

Klein DF: False suffocation alarms, spontaneous panics and related conditions: an integrative hypothesis. Arch Gen Psychiatry 50:306–317, 1993

Klein E, Bental E, Lerer B, et al: Carbamazepine and haloperidol vs placebo and haloperidol in excited psychosis. Arch Gen Psychiatry 41:165–172, 1984

Koenigsberg HW, Reynolds D, Goodman M, et al: Risperidone in the treatment of schizotypal personality disorders. J Clin Psychiatry 64:628–634, 2003

Kontaxakis VP, Ferentinos PP, Havaki-Kontaxaki BJ, et al: Randomized controlled augmentation trials in clozapine-resistant schizophrenic patients: a critical review. Eur Psychiatry 20:409–415, 2005

Koran LM, Ringold AL, Elliott MA: Olanzapine augmentation for treatment-resistant obsessive-compulsive disorder. J Clin Psychiatry 61:514–517, 2000

Kordon A, Wahl K, Koch N, et al: Quetiapine addition to serotonin reuptake inhibitors in patients with severe obsessive compulsive disorder: a double-blind, randomized, placebo-controlled study. J Clin Psychopharmacol 28:550–554, 2008

Lawler CP, Prioleau C, Mailman RB, et al: Interactions of the novel antipsychotic aripiprazole (OPC-14597) with dopamine and serotonin receptor subtypes. Neuropsychopharmacology 20:612–627, 1999

Lee PE, Gill SS, Freedman M, et al: Atypical antipsychotic drugs in the treatment of behavioural and psychological symptoms of dementia: systematic review. BMJ 329(7457):75, 2004 [Epub]

Leucht S, Arbter D, Engel RR, et al: How effective are second-generation antipsychotic drugs? A meta-analysis of placebo-controlled trials. Mol Psychiatry 14:429–447, 2009a

Leucht S, Komossa K, Rummel-Kluge C, et al: A meta-analysis of head-to-head comparisons of second-generation antipsychotics in the treatment of schizophrenia. Am J Psychiatry 166:152–163, 2009b

Leucht S, Corves C, Arbter D, et al: Second-generation versus first-generation antipsychotic drugs for schizophrenia: a meta-analysis. Lancet 373(9657):31–41, 2009c

Levenson J: Neuroleptic malignant syndrome. Am J Psychiatry 142:1137–1145, 1985

Lieberman J, Kane J, Johns C: Clozapine guidelines for clinical management. J Clin Psychopharmacol 50:329–338, 1989

Lieberman JA, Tollefson G, Tohen M, et al; HGDH Study Group: Comparative efficacy and safety of atypical and conventional antipsychotic drugs in first-episode psychosis: a randomized, double-blind trial of olanzapine versus haloperidol. Am J Psychiatry 160:1396–1404, 2003

Lieberman JA, Stroup TS, McEvoy JP, et al, Clinical Antipsychotic Trials of Intervention Effectiveness (CATIE) Investigators: Effectiveness of antipsychotic drugs in patients with chronic schizophrenia. N Engl J Med 353(12):1209–1223, 2005

Lindenmayer JP: New pharmacotherapeutic modalities for negative symptoms in psychosis. Acta Psychiatr Scand Suppl 388:15–19, 1995

Linehan MM, McDavid JD, Brown MZ, et al: Olanzapine plus dialectical behavior therapy for women with high irritability who meet criteria for borderline personality disorder: a double-blind, placebo-controlled pilot study. J Clin Psychiatry 69:999–1005, 2008

Lingjaerde O: Benzodiazepines in the treatment of schizophrenia, in The Benzodiazepines: From Molecular Biology to Clinical Practice. Edited by Costa E. New York, Raven, 1983, pp 369–381

Lipinski JF, Zubenko G, Cohen BM, et al: Propranolol in the treatment of neuroleptic-induced akathisia. Am J Psychiatry 141:412–415, 1984

Liu HC, Chang WH, Wei FC, et al: Monitoring of plasma clozapine levels and its metabolites in refractory schizophrenic patients. Ther Drug Monit 18: 200–207, 1996

Luby E: Reserpine-like drugs—clinical efficacy, in Psychopharmacology: A Review of Progress, 1957–1967. Edited by Efron D. Washington, DC, U.S. Government Printing Office, 1968, pp 1077–1082

Mahmood T, Devlin M, Silverstone T: Clozapine in the management of bipolar and schizoaffective manic episodes resistant to standard treatment. Aust N Z J Psychiatry 31:424–426, 1997

Mandalos GE, Szarek BL: New-onset panic attacks in a patient treated with olanzapine (letter). J Clin Psychopharmacol 19:191, 1999

Marcus RN, McQuade RD, Carson WH, et al: The efficacy and safety of aripiprazole as adjunctive therapy in major depressive disorder: a second multicenter, randomized, double-blind, placebo-controlled study. J Clin Psychopharmacol 28:156-165, 2008

Marder SR, Van Putten T: Who should receive clozapine? Arch Gen Psychiatry 45:865–867, 1988

Marder SR, Hubbard JW, Van Putten T, et al: Pharmacokinetics of long-acting injectable neuroleptic drugs: clinical implications. Psychopharmacology (Berl) 98:433–439, 1989

Marder SR, Kramer M, Ford L, et al: Efficacy and safety of paliperidone extended-release tablets: results of a 6-week, randomized, placebo-controlled study. Biol Psychiatry 62:1363–1370, 2007

Markowitz JS, Brown CS, Moore TR: Atypical antipsychotics, Part 1: pharmacology, pharmacokinetics, and efficacy. Ann Pharmacother 33:73–85, 1999 [see comments]

Mason AS, Granacher RP: Clinical Handbook of Antipsychotic Drug Therapy. New York, Brunner/Mazel, 1978

May PRA: Treatment of Schizophrenia: A Comparative Study of Five Treatment Methods. New York, Science House, 1968

McDougle CJ, Scahill L, Aman MG, et al: Risperidone for the core symptom domains of autism: results from the study by the autism network of the research units on pediatric psychopharmacology. Am J Psychiatry 162:1142–1148, 2005

McEvoy JP, Hogarty GE, Steingard S: Optimal dose of neuroleptic in acute schizophrenia: a controlled study of the neuroleptic threshold and higher haloperidol dose. Arch Gen Psychiatry 48:739–745, 1991

McEvoy JP, Lieberman JA, Stroup TS, et al, CATIE Investigators: Effectiveness of clozapine versus olanzapine, quetiapine, and risperidone in patients with chronic schizophrenia who did not respond to prior atypical antipsychotic treatment. Am J Psychiatry 163:600–610, 2006

Meltzer HY: Treatment-resistant schizophrenia—the role of clozapine. Curr Med Res Opin 14(1):1–20, 1997

Meltzer HY, Bastani B, Kwon KY, et al: A prospective study of clozapine in treatment-resistant schizophrenic patients, I: preliminary report. Psychopharmacology (Berl) 99(suppl):S68–S72, 1989

Meltzer HY, Alphs L, Green AI, et al, International Suicide Prevention Trial Study Group: Clozapine treatment for suicidality in schizophrenia: International Suicide Prevention Trial (InterSePT). Arch Gen Psychiatry 60:82–91, 2003

Meltzer HY, Chen Y, Jayathilake K: Effect of risperidone and olanzapine on measures associated with the insulin resistance syndrome (abstract). Neuropsychopharmacology 30 (suppl 1):S138, 2005

Menaster M: Use of olanzapine in anorexia nervosa. J Clin Psychiatry 66:654–655, author reply 655–656, 2005

Meyer JM, Nasrallah HA, McEvoy JP, et al: The Clinical Antipsychotic Trials of Intervention Effectiveness (CATIE) Schizophrenia Trial: clinical comparison of subgroups with and without the metabolic syndrome. Schizophr Res 80(1):9–18, 2005

Miller DD, McEvoy JP, Davis SM, et al: Clinical correlates of tardive dyskinesia in schizophrenia: baseline data from the CATIE schizophrenia trial. Schizophr Res 80:33–43, 2005

Mondraty N, Birmingham CL, Touyz S, et al: Randomized controlled trial of olanzapine in the treatment of cognitions in anorexia nervosa. Australas Psychiatry 13(1):72–75, 2005

Monnelly EP, Ciraulo DA: Risperidone effects on irritable aggression in posttraumatic stress disorder. J Clin Psychopharmacol 19:377–378, 1999

Monnelly EP, Ciraulo DA, Knapp C, et al: Low-dose risperidone as adjunctive therapy for irritable aggression in posttraumatic stress disorder. J Clin Psychopharmacol 23:193–196, 2003

Moore NA, Tye NC, Axton MS, et al: The behavioral pharmacology of olanzapine, a novel "atypical" antipsychotic agent. J Pharmacol Exp Ther 262:545–551, 1992

Morrison JA, Cottingham EM, Barton BA: Metformin for weight loss in pediatric patients taking psychotropic drugs. Am J Psychiatry 159(4):655–657, 2002

Moss LE, Neppe VM, Drevets WC: Buspirone in the treatment of tardive dyskinesia. J Clin Psychopharmacol 13:203–209, 1992

Mottard JP, de la Sablonniere JF: Olanzapine-induced obsessive-compulsive disorder. Am J Psychiatry 156:799–800, 1999

Mouaffak F, Tranulis C, Gourevitch R, et al: Augmentation strategies of clozapine with antipsychotics in the treatment of ultraresistant schizophrenia. Clin Neuropharmacol 29(1):28–33, 2006

Natesan S, Reckless GE, Barlow KB, et al: Evaluation of N-desmethylclozapine as a potential antipsychotic—preclinical studies. Neuropsychopharmacology 32:1540–1549, 2007

Nemeroff CB: Use of atypical antipsychotics in refractory depression and anxiety. J Clin Psychiatry 66 (suppl 8):13–21, 2005

Nickel MK, Muehlbacher M, Nickel C, et al: Aripiprazole in the treatment of patients with borderline personality disorder: a double-blind, placebo-controlled study. Am J Psychiatry 163:833–838, 2006

Nose M, Cipriani A, Biancosino B, et al: Efficacy of pharmacotherapy against core traits of borderline personality disorder: meta-analysis of randomized controlled trials. Int Clin Psychopharmacol 21(6):345–353, 2006

Nuttall GA, Eckerman KM, Jacob KA, et al: Does low-dose droperidol administration increase the risk of drug-induced QT prolongation and torsade de pointes in the general surgical population? Anesthesiology 107:531–536, 2007

Owen RR, Cole JO: Molindone hydrochloride: a review of laboratory and clinical findings. J Clin Psychopharmacol 9:268–276, 1989

Owen RR, Beake BJ, Marby D, et al: Response to clozapine in chronic psychotic patients. Psychopharmacol Bull 25:253–256, 1989

Pantelis C, Yücel M, Wood SJ, et al: Early and late neurodevelopmental disturbances in schizophrenia and their functional consequences. Aust N Z J Psychiatry 37:399–406, 2003

Papakostas GI, Petersen TJ, Nierenberg AA, et al: Ziprasidone augmentation of selective serotonin reuptake inhibitors (SSRIs) for SSRI-resistant major depressive disorder. J Clin Psychiatry 65:217–221, 2004

Papakostas GI, Petersen TJ, Kinrys G, et al: Aripiprazole augmentation of selective serotonin reuptake inhibitors for treatment-resistant major depressive disorder. J Clin Psychiatry 66(10):1326–1330, 2005

Patkar AA, Peindl K, Mago R, et al: An open-label, rater-blinded, augmentation study of aripiprazole in treatment-resistant depression. Prim Care Companion J Clin Psychiatry 8:82–87, 2006

Perkins DO, Gu H, Boteva K, et al: Relationship between duration of untreated psychosis and outcome in first-episode schizophrenia: a critical review and meta-analysis. Am J Psychiatry 162:1785–1804, 2005

Perrella C, Carrus D, Costa E, Schifano F: Quetiapine for the treatment of borderline personality disorder; an open-label study. Prog Neuropsychopharmacol Biol Psychiatry 31:158–163, 2007

Phillips KA, McElroy SL, Keck PE, et al: A comparison of delusional and nondelusional body dysmorphic disorder in 100 cases. Psychopharmacol Bull 30:179–186, 1994

Pini S, Abelli M, Cassano GB: The role of quetiapine in the treatment of bipolar disorder. Expert Opin Pharmacother 7(7):929–940, 2006

Pisciotta AV: Agranulocytosis induced by certain phenothiazine derivatives. JAMA 208:1862–1868, 1969

Pivac N, Kozaric-Kovacic D, Muck-Seler D: Olanzapine versus fluphenazine in an open trial in patients with psychotic combat-related posttraumatic stress disorder. Psychopharmacology (Berl) 175:451–456, 2004

Potenza MN, Wasylink S, Longhurst JG, et al: Olanzapine augmentation of fluoxetine in the treatment of refractory obsessive-compulsive disorder (letter). J Clin Psychopharmacol 18:423–424, 1998

Potkin SG, Cohen M, Panagides J: Efficacy and tolerability of asenapine in acute schizophrenia: a placebo- and risperidone-controlled trial. J Clin Psychiatry 68:1492–1500, 2007

Potkin SG, Litman RE, Torres R, et al: Efficacy of iloperidone in the treatment of schizophrenia: initial phase 3 studies. J Clin Psychopharmacol 28(2, suppl 1):S4-S11, 2008

Powers PS, Bannon Y, Eubanks R, et al: Quetiapine in anorexia nervosa patients: an open label outpatient pilot study. Int J Eat Disord 40:21–26, 2007

Rainer MK: Risperidone long-acting injection: a review of its long term safety and efficacy. NeuroPsychiatr Dis Treat 4:919–927, 2008

Ram A, Cao Q, Keck PE Jr, et al: Structural changes in dopamine D_2 receptor gene in a patient with neuroleptic malignant syndrome. Am J Med Genet 60:228–280, 1995

Rapaport MH, Gharabawi GM, Canuso CM, et al: Effects of risperidone augmentation in patients with treatment-resistant depression: results of open-label treatment followed by double-blind continuation. Neuropsychopharmacology 31:2505–2513, 2006

Reaven GM, Lieberman JA, Sethuraman G, et al: In search of moderators and mediators of hyperglycemia with atypical antipsychotic treatment. J Psychiatr Res 43:997–1002, 2009

Remington G, Kapur S: D_2 and 5-HT_2 receptor effects of antipsychotics: bridging basic and clinical findings using PET. J Clin Psychiatry 60 (suppl 10):15–19, 1999

Robertson M, Trimble M: Major tranquilizers used as antidepressants—a review. J Affect Disord 4:173–193, 1982

Rocca P, Marchiaro L, Cocuzza E, et al: Treatment of borderline personality disorder with risperidone. J Clin Psychiatry 63:241–244, 2002

Rothschild AJ, Williamson DJ, Tohen MF, et al: A double-blind, randomized study of olanzapine and olanzapine/fluoxetine combination for major depression with psychotic features. J Clin Psychopharmacol 24:365–373, 2004

Roy-Byrne P, Gerner R, Liston E, et al: ECT for acute mania: a forgotten treatment modality. J Psychiatr Treat Eval 3:83–86, 1981

Sachs GS, Lafer B, Truman CJ, et al: Lithium monotherapy: miracle, myth, and misunderstanding. Psychiatr Ann 24:299–306, 1994

Sachs G, Chengappa KN, Suppes T, et al: Quetiapine with lithium or divalproex for the treatment of bipolar mania: a randomized, double-blind, placebo-controlled study. Bipolar Disord 6:213–223, 2004

Salam S, Kilzieh N: Lorazepam treatment of psychogenic catatonia. J Clin Psychiatry 49 (12, suppl):16–21, 1988

Saltz B, Kane J, Woerner J, et al: Prospective study of tardive dyskinesia in the elderly. Psychopharmacol Bull 25:52–56, 1989

Salzman C: The use of ECT in the treatment of schizophrenia. Am J Psychiatry 137:1032–1041, 1980

Schneider LS, Tariot PN, Dagerman KS, et al; CATIE-AD Study Group: Effectiveness of atypical antipsychotic drugs in patients with Alzheimer's disease. N Engl J Med 355(15):1525–1538, 2006

Schulz SC, Zanarini MC, Bateman A, et al: Olanzapine for the treatment of borderline personality disorder: variable dose 12-week randomised double-blind placebo-controlled study. Br J Psychiatry 193:485-492, 2008

Schwarz C, Volz A, Li C, et al: Valproate for schizophrenia. Cochrane Database Syst Rev, Issue 2. Art No: CD004028 (DOI: 10.1002/14651858.CD004028.pub3), 2008

Seeman P, Tallerico T: Rapid release of antipsychotic drugs from dopamine D_2 receptors: an explanation for low receptor occupancy and early clinical relapse upon withdrawal of clozapine or quetiapine. Am J Psychiatry 156:876–884, 1999

Sernyak MJ, Woods WS: Chronic neuroleptic use in manic-depressive illness. Psychopharmacol Bull 29:375–381, 1993

Shelton RC: Treatment options for refractory depression J Clin Psychiatry 60 (suppl 4):57–61, 1999

Shelton RC, Tollefson GD, Tohen M, et al: A novel augmentation strategy for treating resistant major depression. Am J Psychiatry 158:131–134, 2001

Silver H, Geraisy N: No difference in effect of biperiden and amantadine on negative symptoms in medicated chronic schizophrenic patients. Biol Psychiatry 38:413–415, 1995

Silver J, Yudofsky S: Propranolol for aggression: literature review and clinical guidelines. Int Drug Ther Newsl 20:9–12, 1985

Simpson GM, Glick ID, Weiden PJ, et al: Randomized, controlled, double-blind multicenter comparison of the efficacy and tolerability of ziprasidone and olanzapine in acutely ill inpatients with schizophrenia or schizoaffective disorder. Am J Psychiatry 161:1837–1847, 2004

Siris SG, Morgan V, Fagerstrom R, et al: Adjunctive imipramine in the treatment of postpsychotic depression: a controlled trial. Arch Gen Psychiatry 42:533–539, 1987

Skarsfeldt T: Comparison of short-term administration of sertindole, clozapine and haloperidol on the inactivation of midbrain dopamine neurons in the rat. Eur J Pharmacol 254:291–294, 1994

Soler J, Pascual JC, Campins J, et al: Double-blind, placebo-controlled study of dialectical behavior therapy plus olanzapine for borderline personality disorder. Am J Psychiatry 162:1221–1224, 2005

Soloff PH, Cornelius J, George A, et al: Efficacy of phenelzine and haloperidol in borderline personality disorder. Arch Gen Psychiatry 50:377–385, 1993

Soloff PH, Lis JA, Kelly T, et al: Risk factors for suicidal behavior in borderline personality disorder. Am J Psychiatry 151:1316–1323, 1994

Spina E, De Domenico P, Ruello C, et al: Adjunctive fluoxetine in the treatment of negative symptoms in chronic schizophrenic patients. Int Clin Psychopharmacol 9:281–285, 1994

Stanilla JK, Simpson GM: Drugs to treat extrapyramidal side effects, in The American Psychiatric Press Textbook of Psychopharmacology. Edited by Schatzberg AF, Nemeroff CB. Washington, DC, American Psychiatric Press, 1995, pp 281–299

States JH, St Dennis CD: Chronic sleep disruption and the reexperiencing cluster of posttraumatic stress disorder symptoms are improved by olanzapine: brief review of the literature and a case-based series. Prim Care Companion J Clin Psychiatry 5(2):74–79, 2003

Stoppe G, Brandt CA, Staedt JH: Behavioural problems associated with dementia: the role of newer antipsychotics. Drugs Aging 14:41–54, 1999

Stroup TS, Lieberman JA, McEvoy JP, et al, CATIE Investigators: Effectiveness of olanzapine, quetiapine, risperidone, and ziprasidone in patients with chronic schizophrenia following discontinuation of a previous atypical antipsychotic. Am J Psychiatry 163:611–622, 2006

Sultzer DL, Davis SM, Tariot PN, et al; CATIE-AD Study Group: Clinical symptom responses to atypical antipsychotic medications in Alzheimer's disease: phase 1 outcomes from the CATIE-AD effectiveness trial. Am J Psychiatry 165:844-854, 2008

Sun SX, Liu GG, Christensen DB, et al: Review and analysis of hospitalization costs associated with antipsychotic nonadherence in the treatment of schizophrenia in the United States. Curr Med Res Opin 23:2305-2312, 2007

Suppes T, Baldessarini RJ, Faedda GL, et al: Discontinuing maintenance treatment in bipolar manic-depression: risks and implications. Harv Rev Psychiatry 1:131–144, 1993

Suppes T, Webb A, Paul B, et al: Clinical outcome in a randomized 1-year trial of clozapine versus treatment as usual for patients with treatment-resistant illness and a history of mania. Am J Psychiatry 156:1164–1169, 1999

Suzuki T, Misawa J: Sertindole antagonizes morphine-, cocaine-, and methamphetamine-induced place preference in the rat. Life Sci 57:1277–1284, 1995

Szigethy EM, Schulz SC: Risperidone in comorbid borderline personality disorder and dysthymia (letter). J Clin Psychopharmacol 17:326–327, 1997

Taylor DM, Fischetti C, Sparshatt A, et al: Risperidone long-acting injection: a prospective 3-year analysis of its use in clinical practice. J Clin Psychiatry 70:196–200, 2009a

Taylor D, Fischetti C, Sparshatt A, et al: Risperidone long-acting injection: a 6-year mirror-image study of healthcare resource use. Acta Psychiatr Scand 120:97–101, 2009b

Teicher MH, Glod CA, Aaronson ST, et al: Open assessment of the safety and efficacy of thioridazine in the treatment of patients with borderline personality disorder. Psychopharmacol Bull 25:535–549, 1989

Thase ME, Macfadden W, Weisler RH, et al; BOLDER II Study Group: Efficacy of quetiapine monotherapy in bipolar I and II depression: a double-blind, placebo-controlled study (the BOLDER II study). J Clin Psychopharmacol 26:600–609, 2006 (Erratum in: J Clin Psychopharmacol 27:51, 2007)

Thase ME, Corya SA, Osuntokun O, et al: A randomized, double-blind comparison of olanzapine/fluoxetine combination, olanzapine, and fluoxetine in treatment-resistant major depressive disorder. J Clin Psychiatry 68:224-236, 2007

Tohen M, Chengappa KN, Suppes T, et al: Relapse prevention in bipolar I disorder: 18-month comparison of olanzapine plus mood stabiliser v mood stabiliser alone. Br J Psychiatry 184:337–345, 2004

Tohen M, Calabrese JR, Sachs GS, et al: Randomized, placebo-controlled trial of olanzapine as maintenance therapy in patients with bipolar I disorder responding to acute treatment with olanzapine. Am J Psychiatry. 163:247–256, 2006

Tollefson GD, Sanger TM, Lu Y, et al: Depressive signs and symptoms in schizophrenia: a prospective blinded trial of olanzapine and haloperidol. Arch Gen Psychiatry 55:250–258, 1998 [erratum: Arch Gen Psychiatry 55:1052, 1998]

Tollefson GD, Birkett MA, Kiesler GM, et al, Lilly Resistant Schizophrenia Study Group: Double-blind comparison of olanzapine versus clozapine in schizophrenic patients clinically eligible for treatment with clozapine. Biol Psychiatry 49:52–63, 2001

Tran PV, Dellva MA, Tollefson GD, et al: Oral olanzapine versus oral haloperidol in the maintenance treatment of schizophrenia and related psychoses. Br J Psychiatry 172:499–505, 1998

Tuason V, Escobar J, Garvey M, et al: Loxapine vs chlorpromazine in paranoid schizophrenia. J Clin Psychiatry 45:158–163, 1984

Tzeng TB, Stamm G, Chu SY: Sensitive method for the assay of sertindole in plasma by high-performance liquid chromatography and fluorimetric detection. J Chromatogr B Biomed Appl 661:299–306, 1994

Van der Zwaag C, McGee M, McEvoy JP, et al: Response of patients with treatment-refractory schizophrenia to clozapine within three serum level ranges. Am J Psychiatry 153:1579–1584, 1996

Van Putten T: Why do schizophrenic patients refuse to take their drugs? Arch Gen Psychiatry 31:67–72, 1978

Vieta E, Herraiz M, Fernandez A, et al: Efficacy and safety of risperidone in the treatment of schizoaffective disorder: initial results from a large, multicenter surveillance study. Group for the Study of Risperidone in Affective Disorders. J Clin Psychiatry 62:623–630, 2001

Vulink NC, Denys D, Fluitman SB, et al: Quetiapine augments the effect of citalopram in non-refractory obsessive-compulsive disorder: a randomized, double-blind, placebo-controlled study of 76 patients. J Clin Psychiatry 70:1001–1008, 2009

Webber MA, Marder SR: Better pharmacotherapy for schizophrenia: what does the future hold? Current Psychiatry Rep 10:352–358, 2008

Weiss EL, Potenza MN, McDougle CJ, et al: Olanzapine addition in obsessive-compulsive disorder refractory to selective serotonin reuptake inhibitors: an open-label case series. J Clin Psychiatry 60:524–527, 1999

White E, Cheung P, Silverstone T: Depot antipsychotics in bipolar affective disorder. Int Clin Psychopharmacol 8:119–122, 1993

Wijkstra J, Lijmer J, Balk F, et al: Pharmacological treatment for psychotic depression. Cochrane Database Syst Rev, Issue 4, Art No: CD004044 (DOI: 10.1002/14651858.CD004044.pub2), 2005

Wojcik J: Antiparkinson drug use. Biological Therapies in Psychiatry Newsletter 2:5–7, 1979

Wolfgang SA: Olanzapine in whole, not half, tablets for psychosis from Alzheimer's dementia. Am J Health Syst Pharm 56:2245–2246, 1999

Wolkowitz OM, Breier A, Doran A, et al: Alprazolam augmentation of the antipsychotic effects of fluphenazine in schizophrenic patients: preliminary results. Arch Gen Psychiatry 45:664–671, 1988

Wu RR, Zhao JP, Guo XF, et al: Metformin addition attenuates olanzapine-induced weight gain in drug-naive first-episode schizophrenia patients: a double-blind, placebo-controlled study. Am J Psychiatry 165:352–358, 2008

Yorkston N, Zaki S, Havard C: Some practical aspects of using propranolol in the treatment of schizophrenia, in Propranolol and Schizophrenia. Edited by Roberts E, Amacher P. New York, Alan R Liss, 1978, pp 83–97

Zanarini MC, Frankenburg FR: Olanzapine treatment of female borderline personality disorder patients: a double-blind, placebo-controlled pilot study. J Clin Psychiatry. 62:849–854, 2001

Zanarini MC, Frankenburg FR, Parachini EA: A preliminary, randomized trial of fluoxetine, olanzapine, and the olanzapine-fluoxetine combination in women with borderline personality disorder. J Clin Psychiatry 65:903–907, 2004

Zoccali R, Muscatello MR, Cedro C, et al: The effect of mirtazapine augmentation of clozapine in the treatment of negative symptoms of schizophrenia: a double-blind, placebo-controlled study. Int Clin Psychopharmacol 19(2):71–76, 2004

5

Mood Stabilizers

The term *mood stabilizer* was first applied to the lithium salts when it became clear that they were effective not only in alleviating mania but also as a prophylaxis against both manic and depressive cycles. Since the introduction of lithium to the United States in 1969 there have been very few drugs approved as "mood stabilizers." However, in recent years new drugs, such as lamotrigine, olanzapine, and aripiprazole, have been approved for the prevention of mania and depression in bipolar disorder. In addition, many medications have been approved for the acute treatment of mania, and the first drugs for the acute treatment of bipolar depression have now also been approved. It is somewhat less clear that any of the anticonvulsants currently used in treating bipolar affective disorder are as deserving of the term *mood stabilizer* as is lithium. However, the second-generation antipsychotics (SGAs) with clear benefits in the acute treatment and prevention of both mania and depression do appear deserving of such designation.

A derivative of valproic acid, divalproex sodium, was approved by the U.S. Food and Drug Administration (FDA) for the treatment of acute mania in 1994. Since that time, it has surpassed lithium in the treatment of bipolar disorder in the United States. Divalproex sodium offers the advantages over lithium of a superior therapeutic index and less toxicity. Although divalproex sodium clearly alleviates manic symptoms, the efficacy in preventing manic episodes with this drug is less well established than with lithium. Still, it appears to prevent them and depressive episodes in clinical practice. Valproate may also have a wider range of efficacy in subtypes of bipolar disorder that are less responsive to lithium, including rapid cycling and mixed states.

The anticonvulsant lamotrigine became only the second drug approved for use in the maintenance treatment of bipolar disorder. While results from initial studies of lamotrigine in the treatment of acute mania were disappointing, findings from subsequent studies of lamotrigine in delaying the time to onset of a new mood episode were quite convincing. Lithium is more robust in preventing mania than in preventing depression, but the converse is true for lamotrigine. Since most patients with bipolar disorder live in the depressed phase of the illness, lamotrigine is a welcome option for clinicians treating bipolar patients.

Carbamazepine has been used for many years in the treatment of bipolar disorder, despite the lack of an FDA-approved indication for this purpose. An extended-release formulation of carbamazepine (Equetro) was first approved in the United States for the treatment of mania in 2004. In recent years, carbamazepine has become a third-line agent after lithium and valproate. The less preferred status of carbamazepine has been due in part to its complex pharmacokinetic interactions and lower therapeutic index, which make it somewhat more difficult to use in combination with many medications. In addition, the studies supporting its utility in bipolar disorder had, until recently, been much smaller and less rigorous than the studies that were completed with divalproex sodium and lithium. A related, newer compound, oxcarbazepine, does not appear to induce liver enzymes quite as much as carbamazepine does and may be better tolerated. As of this writing, it is not being actively studied in large-scale monotherapy trials but is being used by practitioners.

A variety of other anticonvulsants have been or are being studied in bipolar disorder. These include gabapentin, pregabalin, topiramate, tiagabine, ethosuximide, zonisamide, and levetiracetam. None of these drugs have convincing controlled data supporting their use as a monotherapy in any phase of the bipolar disorder at the time of this writing. Nonetheless, drugs like topiramate have shown benefits in counteracting weight gain associated with traditional mood stabilizers such as lithium or divalproate.

The SGAs have played a growing role in the treatment of bipolar disorder and are now among the most common agents used in its treatment. Olanzapine, which had been approved for the treatment of acute mania in 2000, became the first antipsychotic also approved in the maintenance treatment of bipolar I disorder. Like lithium, it probably does a better job preventing mania than it does preventing depression. At this time, all of the SGAs, with the exception of clozapine, are approved in the treatment of mania. The popularity of the SGAs stems in no small part from their rapid onset of action relative to other treatments for bipolar disorder and their versatility in the treatment of both poles as well as maintenance treatment.

While there have been literally thousands of controlled studies of antidepressant drugs in the treatment of unipolar depression in the past 50 years, only a handful of studies have ever been completed on the treatment of bipolar depression. The general assumption has been that an antidepressant should be effective whether treating bipolar or unipolar depression. As we know from our clinical experience, however, this assumption appears to be wrong. Bipolar depressions may not respond to, or may be worsened by, standard antidepressants.

In this chapter, we consider the range of potential mood stabilizers currently used in clinical practice. In addition, more investigational agents, such as newer anticonvulsants, calcium channel blockers, and omega-3 fatty acids, are considered. (See Table 5–1 for a listing of mood stabilizers and their formulations and strengths.)

General Treatment Approaches

Acute Mania

In some respects, the treatment of acute mania is among the least problematic components of treating bipolar disorder. Patients with bipolar disorder spend much less time in mania, hypomania, or mixed states than they do in depression. In addition, there are many effective treatments for mania but few for maintenance treatment or treatment of bipolar depression. There are four classes of medications effective in the treatment of acute mania; first-generation antipsychotics, SGAs, anticonvulsants, and lithium. The pharmacotherapy of mania often requires combinations of these agents.

Table 5–1. Mood stabilizers: names, formulations, and strengths

Generic name	Brand name	Formulations and strengths
lithium carbonate[a]	Eskalith*	Capsule: 150, 300, 600 mg
	Lithobid (slow release)	Tablet: 300 mg
	Eskalith-CR* (controlled release)	Tablet: 450 mg[b]
lithium citrate	Generic[c]	Syrup: 8 mEq/5 mL[d] (480-mL bottle)
carbamazepine[a]	Tegretol	Tablets: 200 mg
		Chewable tablet: 100, 200 mg
		Suspension: 100 mg/5 mL (450-mL bottle)
	Tegretol-XR (sustained release)	Tablets: 100, 200, 400 mg
	Carbatrol (sustained release)	Capsules: 100, 200, 300 mg
valproic acid[a]	Depakene	Capsule: 250 mg
		Syrup: 250 mg/5 mL (480-mL bottle)
valproate sodium	Depacon	Injection: 100 mg/mL (5-mL vial)
divalproex sodium[a]	Depakote	Enteric-coated tablets: 125, 250, 500 mg
		Capsule, sprinkle: 125 mg
	Depakote ER (sustained release)	Tablets: 250, 500 mg
lamotrigine[a]	Lamictal	Chewable tablets: 2, 5, 25 mg
		Tablets: 25, 100, 150, 200 mg
gabapentin[a]	Neurontin	Capsules: 100, 300, 400 mg
		Tablets: 100, 300, 400, 600, 800 mg
		Oral solution: 250 mg/5 mL

Table 5–1. Mood stabilizers: names, formulations, and strengths *(continued)*

Generic name	Brand name	Formulations and strengths
oxcarbazepine[a]	Trileptal	Tablets: 150, 300, 600 mg Suspension: 300 mg/5 mL
topiramate[a]	Topamax	Tablets: 25, 50, 100, 200 mg Capsules, sprinkle: 15, 25 mg
tiagabine	Gabitril	Tablets: 2, 4, 12, 16 mg

[a]Available in generic form.
[b]Scored tablets.
[c]Cibalith-S: brand discontinued.
[d]Equivalent to 300 mg lithium carbonate.
*Brand taken off the market; available in generic.

Currently, the SGAs are among the most used agents in acute mania. The advantages over other classes of agents include a more rapid onset of action than lithium or the anticonvulsants, less EPS than the first-generation antipsychotics, and greater evidence of efficacy in the subsequent maintenance treatment and treatment of bipolar depression than other classes of agents. Monotherapy trials with quetiapine, olanzapine, risperidone, ziprasidone, and aripiprazole have consistently shown benefit over placebo in the treatment of acute mania, and all are FDA approved for this indication. In one meta-analysis, the SGAs averaged a 53% reponse rate on the Young Mania Rating Scale compared with 30% for placebo (Perlis et al. 2006). The addition of most SGAs to a mood stabilizer such as lithium or divalproex also has shown superiority over the addition of placebo (Scherk et al. 2007). Thus, for patients not responding to an SGA alone, the addition of a mood stabilizer appears to be a useful strategy.

First-generation antipsychotics probably work as well as SGAs in the treatment of acute mania. Thorazine was the second drug approved in the United States for the treatment of acute mania in 1974. Unlike in the CATIE trial, there have been no comparisons of first-generation drugs and SGAs in terms of the efficacy in the treatment of mania. Clearly, cost would be a benefit of the first-generation antipsychotics. The concerns about EPS, particularly in a population of bipolar patients, may be a factor in first-generation drugs, being used less frequently at this time than are the SGAs.

The classic mood stabilizers—lithium, divalproex, and carbamazepine—clearly are beneficial both in monotherapy and as combination agents in the treatment of acute mania. Their primary limitation is the time it takes for these agents to be effective. Whereas benefits from antipsychotics are often seen in the first days of treatment, it often takes 1 week or longer to see the antimanic benefits of lithium, divalproex, and carbamazepine. This delay of action is due in no small part to the need to titrate up the dose of these agents. In the current environment, where the need for rapid stabilization is required to reduce the number of hospital days, delays can be quite expensive. Beyond this, of course, patients in acute mania may be suffering tremendously, and interventions that can rapidly limit the manic episode are obviously desirable.

Thus, given the available data, it may make sense to start the treatment of acute mania with an SGA or possibly a first-generation antipsychotic. Patients who are unresponsive to a therapeutic dose of an antipsychotic after 3–7 days often respond to the addition of a mood stabilizer. Benzodiazepines, which are discussed later in this chapter, might also be reasonable adjunctive agents to start with to target sleep, anxiety, and agitation in an acutely manic patient.

Acute Bipolar Depression

Depression is the predominant mood state in bipolar disorder. In patients with bipolar I disorder who were followed over 13 years, the patients spent about 32% of the lives in a depressed state versus 9% in mania and 6% mixed or cycling (Judd et al. 2003). In patients with bipolar II disorder, the disparity between poles is even more dramatic; about 1% is spent in hypomania versus 50% in the depressed state. Unfortunately, the depressed state is also the more difficult pole to treat. While we have many good medications to limit mania and hypomania, we have very few proven strategies for bipolar depression.

The long-standing belief that standard antidepressants work in bipolar depression has been increasingly challenged. Sachs and colleagues (2007) have completed among the most rigorous studies to date evaluating antidepressant efficacy in bipolar patients. As part of the Systematic Treatment Enhancement Program for Bipolar Disorder (STEP-BD) program, patients with bipolar disorder who were taking a standard mood stabilizer and experiencing a major depressive episode were randomly assigned to either adjunctive bupropion, paroxetine, or placebo. Durable recovery, defined as at least 8 weeks of consecutive euthymia, was slightly more likely in the placebo group (27%) than in the antidepressant group (23%). On the other hand, switches into mania were no more likely while taking the antidepressant than while taking the placebo. Likewise, in a prospective evaluation of switch rates when venlafaxine, bupropion, or sertraline were added to a standard mood stabilizer, Altshuler and colleagues (2006) found a relatively low rate of switching into mania and achievement of efficacy (as defined by a reduction in symptoms by ≥50%) about 50% of the time with each of the antidepressants. Venlafaxine was more likely than the other antidepressants to induce a switch into mania. This finding is consistent with earlier data suggesting the tricyclic antidepressants were somewhat more likely to induce switching than other classes of medications. In a follow-up study of acute responders to antidepressants, Altshuler and colleagues (2009) found that the vast majority of acute responders to antidepressants (69%) maintained response at 1 year follow-up. The switch rate was no higher than that seen with mood stabilizers alone.

As of this writing, only two medications have been approved for the treatment of bipolar depression. The first was the combination of fluoxetine and olanzapine (Symbyax). Tohen and colleagues (2003b) found that, relative to placebo, the combination of fluoxetine and olanzapine was superior in improving depressive symptoms at all time points over an 8-week trial. In addition, the combination was superior to olanzapine alone. The second drug to be approved for bipolar depression was quetiapine. Two pivotal, placebo-controlled trials have confirmed the efficacy of quetiapine monotherapy at dosages of 300 and 600 mg/day The higher dosage was somewhat more efficacious than 300 mg/day, but more side effects were seen with the higher dosage. Quetiapine remains the only monotherapy approved for bipolar depression to date.

Several other medications have some support for an efficacy claim in bipolar depression, but the data are not overwhelming. For example, lamotrigine appeared efficacious in the treatment of bipolar depression in one placebo-controlled trial (Calabrese et al. 1999b). However, four subsequent trials failed to show benefit. In very small trials, both modafinil and pramipexole have shown benefit in the treatment of bipolar depression. Lithium has long been used in bipolar depression but has not been particularly effective as an acute monotherapy.

Given the available data, patients with bipolar depression should first be taking a mood stabilizer. Patients who cycle into depression despite taking adequate doses of one mood stabilizer should be considered for another. For example, a bipolar patient taking lithium who has a depressive episode might benefit from addition of an SGA such as quetiapine. Likewise, a patient who is already receiving maintenance treatment with olanzapine and cycles into a depressive episode might be expected to benefit from the addition of lithium or lamotrigine. Failure to respond to two mood-stabilizing agents for an acute depressive episode, which is quite common, might prompt consideration of a third agent, such as an antidepressant, modafinil, pramipexole, or yet another mood stabilizer. All too many patients with bipolar depression do not get adequate relief from three or more psychotropic agents. The tendency is to continue adding more agents in an increasingly desperate attempt to provide relief for a suffering patient. Unfortunately, we have very few empirical data to guide our decision beyond the combination of two agents. Ultimately, finding the optimal regimen for a bipolar patient may be a time-consuming trial-

and-error process. However, many patients do find a regimen that, while not perfect, offers substantial benefit.

Maintenance Therapy

As with recurrent depression, each subsequent episode of mania or depression may predispose the patient to yet other recurrences and are associated with greater disability and a poorer prognosis. Since bipolar disorder, by definition, is a recurrent illness, maintenance treatment, with the goal of preventing or reducing the number of subsequent cycles, is a standard part of treatment. A mood stabilizer has long been considered the cornerstone of maintenance therapy. While many agents are used in maintenance therapy, only a handful have convincing evidence supporting their use.

Lithium was the first maintenance medication approved for bipolar disorder (in 1974). In multiple randomized controlled trials done since then, lithium has been consistently effective as a maintenance therapy (see section "Lithium"). However, it is more effective in preventing mania than depression. In addition, many patients still relapse while taking the drug. For example, Geddes and colleagues (2004) found that although the relapse rate did drop in bipolar patients when lithium was used, 40% of the patients still relapsed. Furthermore lithium is difficult to tolerate for many patients, and the dropout rate is high.

Lamotrigine was the second drug approved, in 2003, for the maintenance treatment of bipolar disorder. Unlike the other approved maintenance treatments, lamotrigine appears to have greater efficacy in preventing depression recurrence than in preventing mania. It also distinguishes itself from other maintenance treatments in not being associated with much weight gain or sedation. Lamotrigine's primary disadvantages are its slow titration schedule and its risk of rash (see section "Lamotrigine" later in this chapter).

The SGAs have become increasingly used in maintenance treatment of bipolar disorder. Olanzapine was approved as a maintenance treatment for bipolar disorder in 2004, followed by aripiprazole in 2005 and quetiapine in 2008. Like lithium, the SGAs are probably more effective in preventing mania than depression. Advantages of SGAs over other approved maintenance treatments include rapid and easy titration, relative safety in overdose, and demonstrated benefits of these agents in treating mania and, in the case of olanzapine and quetiapine, depressive symptoms as well. Unfortunately, adverse events associated with SGAs, such as weight gain, metabolic effects, and sedation, often limit adherence and present long-term problems.

Other mood stabilizers, such as divalproex and carbamazepine, are still commonly used as maintenance treatments but do not have as consistent evidence supporting their use as do the FDA-approved maintenance treatments. That being said, many patients find the approved treatments to be ineffective, and clinicians may find divalproex or carbamazepine reasonable alternatives.

Given the data, it makes sense to start maintenance treatment in bipolar patients with a monotherapy, understanding that single agents may well prove to be insufficient. We still think lithium is as good a choice as any to start with. Lamotrigine may be the best tolerated of the approved maintenance treatments and may be a better choice in patients whose primary difficulty is depression recurrence. Among the SGAs, aripiprazole may have some long-term advantages over other SGAs in terms of weight gain and sedation. When a monotherapy fails to prevent a recurrence, combinations of agents are used, but these are not well studied. Ketter (2008) reported that combining an SGA with a standard mood stabilizer such as lithium may improve the outcome of maintenance treatment. This makes good sense, and, clinically, such combinations are common. Unfortunately, few data exist on combination maintenance treatments to help choose one combination over another.

Rapid-Cycling Bipolar Disorder

Rapid-cycling bipolar disorder is characterized in DSM-IV-TR as having four or more cycles per year. The prevalence of rapid cycling in bipolar patients ranges from 14% to 50%, with 20% of STEP-BD patients meeting criteria for rapid cycling at entry. It is unclear whether rapid cycling constitutes a transitory phenomenon or a persistent subtype of bipolar disorder. In most patients rapid cycling appears to be transitory, but some patients have persistent rapid cycling. As with other forms of the illness, depression tends to be the predominant mood state in rapid cycling.

While the pathophysiology of rapid cycling is not fully understood, a number of agents are thought to potentially promote rapid cycling in bipolar patients. These include antidepressants, stimulants, steroids, and possibly sympathomimetics and caffeine. Other potential triggers include shift work, sleep disruption, stresses, substance abuse, hypothyroidism, and other hormonal abnormalities.

The first step in treatment is to identify possible triggers and eliminate or minimize these as feasible. For example, antidepressants should be tapered, as opposed to suddenly discontinued, to minimize discontinuation effects and prevent sudden worsening of mood instability. Thyroid status should be evaluated and treated if necessary. Attempts should be made to control the intake of illicit substances and alcohol.

After potential precipitating factors have been dealt with, the next step in the treatment of bipolar disorder is to apply pharmacotherapy. One of the features of rapid-cycling bipolar disorder has been a greater resistance to lithium. However, the response to lithium does seem to improve substantially if offending agents such as antidepressants are removed and thyroid status is stabilized. Still, successful treatment with lithium often manifests with a sharp reduction in hypomanic and manic cycles but a continuation of depressive cycles. Many studies suggest that rapid-cycling patients who do not respond to lithium are often responsive to divalproex. As with lithium response, divalproex often proves much more successful in reducing manic cycles than depressive episodes. Lamotrigine would seem like a logical choice to add on or substitute for another mood stabilizer, as its primary efficacy is seen in preventing depressive cycles. However, the track record for lamotrigine in the treatment of rapid cycling has also been mixed. Lamotrigine appears to be more successful in treating rapid cycling in bipolar II patients than in bipolar I patients. The SGAs, including clozapine, have shown somewhat more consistent benefits in treating rapid-cycling bipolar disorder than have other agents. Controlled studies with olanzapine-fluoxetine combination, olanzapine alone, aripiprazole , and quetiapine have all suggested probable efficacy in reducing both depressive and manic episodes in patients with rapid-cycling bipolar disorder. Nonetheless, many patients are poorly responsive to SGAs.

The successful treatment of rapid cycling, then, involves identifying and mitigating triggers and using combinations of agents, since monotherapy response often proves to be less than adequate. SGAs appear to often be helpful in controlling rapid cycling, and so we often start there. The addition of lamotrigine or divalproex in patients with rapid-cycling bipolar disorder who are taking another mood stabilizer is often helpful. Clozapine should be considered in patients whose disorder is refractory to standard SGA–mood stabilizer combinations.

Mixed States

Mixed states in bipolar disorder can represent a formidable diagnostic and treatment challenge. The DSM-IV-TR criteria for mixed states, which require simultaneously meeting criteria for both major depression and mania for at least 7 days, are rarely seen in clinical practice. Rather, mixed states typically manifest with some combination of depressive and manic features but not necessarily all the features specified in the DSM-IV-TR criteria. In addition to the combination of manic/hypomanic and depressive features, there are often other associated symptoms, including psychosis, severe anxiety, agitation, and lability of mood. At least 30% of acute episodes of bipolar disorder have mixed features. Mixed states may represent a transition from one pole to another, the late stage of a manic episode, or a consistent hybrid of symptoms seen in some patients.

Relatively few studies have looked at treatment response specifically for mixed states (Krüger et al. 2005). Rather, treatment studies of mania often include patients with mixed states, but these patients represent a minority of the studied population. In the few studies to date that target mixed states specifically, the results are inconclusive. However, divalproex has perhaps been more consistently effective in treating mixed states than has lithium. In fact, in some cross-over studies, patients with mixed states that had not responded to lithium appeared to do much better while taking divalproex. In addition, elevated depressive symptoms in mixed states might predict better response to valproate than to lithium. Carbamazepine may also be useful in treating mixed states. However, there may be greater evidence of the prophylactic benefit of carbamazepine in preventing mixed states than in acute treatment. Lamotrigine has proven to be useful in patients with treatment-refractory bipolar disorder, including in some small open-label studies in mixed states. However the necessity of a slow titration limits the utility of lamotrigine in treating any acute states.

There are perhaps more data on the utility of SGAs in the treatment of mixed states than for other agents. There are at least four double-blind studies of olanzapine that have included patients with mixed states. Baker et al. (2003)

analyzed the response specifically in those patients with mixed features and found that olanzapine, relative to placebo, improved both depressive and manic symptoms in mixed states within the first week of treatment. However, the improvement in depressive symptoms might have been driven by an improvement in symptoms such as insomnia and paranoia rather than an improvement in mood. There is at least one double-blind study examining the efficacy of quetiapine, ziprasidone, and clozapine, and the data suggest some efficacy for all of these agents in lessening both manic and depressed symptoms in patients in mixed states.

From the limited available data, the use of an SGA or divalproex as an initial monotherapy for mixed states seems reasonable. Given the complexity of symptoms in mixed states, it is unlikely that monotherapies will provide sufficient relief. The combination of divalproex and an SGA should be considered when monotherapy is ineffective. The addition of lamotrigine or lithium might be considered if the combination of an SGA and valproate is ineffective. Antidepressants should generally be avoided, but benzodiazepines are often helpful in targeting sleep, anxiety, and agitation.

In summary, mixed states are challenging to treat. The empirical data are not sufficient to provide clear guidelines. However, there is evidence that certain strategies may help more than others and these should be utilized first.

Lithium

History and Indications

Lithium, usually as the carbonate and occasionally as the citrate salt, is still widely used in American psychiatry, However, the use of valproate for the treatment of mood disorders now surpasses that of lithium. Lithium is approved by the FDA for the treatment of acute mania and as maintenance therapy to prevent or diminish the intensity of "subsequent episodes in those manic-depressive patients with a history of mania." As discussed below, lithium is often used in patients with a variety of recurrent episodic illnesses, with or without prominent affective features. It is also used adjunctively in patients with mood lability, with impulsive or episodic violence or anger, or even with premenstrual dysphoria, alcoholism, borderline personality disorder (BPD), or chronic schizophrenia. Further, it is used as a potentiating agent in a variety of treatment-resistant disorders.

Lithium therapy: overview

Efficacy	Bipolar mania and prophylaxis (FDA indicated) Depression augmentation
Side effects	Tremor Polyuria Polydipsia Weight gain Cognitive slowing Hypothyroidism ↓ Renal function Dermatological side effects Memory problems
Safety in overdose	Frequently lethal in blood levels above 3.0 mEq/L and toxic above 1.5 mEq/L. Maintain fluid/electrolyte balance. Gastric lavage; mannitol diuresis vs. hemodialysis for higher blood levels.
Dosage and administration	Start at 300 mg bid or tid and increase total daily dose by up to 300 mg, as needed and tolerated, to blood level of 0.6–1.2 mEq/L for bipolar mania and 0.4–0.8 mEq/L for augmentation.
Discontinuation	Sudden discontinuation associated with ↑ risk of relapse. Taper over 3 months for bipolar mania if feasible.
Drug interactions	Antipsychotics: may ↑ lithium toxicity Bupropion: may ↑ seizure risk Carbamazepine: neurotoxicity (rare) Diuretics: ↑ lithium levels Iodide salts: ↑ hypothyroidism Neuromuscular blockers: respiratory depression NSAIDs: ↑ lithium levels SSRIs: serotonin syndrome (rare) Theophylline: ↓ lithium levels Urinary alkalinizers: ↓ lithium levels Verapamil: ↑ or ↓ lithium levels

Note.   FDA=U.S. Food and Drug Administration; NSAID = nonsteroidal anti-inflammatory drug; SSRI = selective serotonin reuptake inhibitor.

The use of lithium salts in psychiatry was initiated by John Cade, an Australian state hospital superintendent, in 1949, and it proved to be an effective, though somewhat toxic, treatment. The addition of serum level monitoring made the treatment safe and provided the first general use of blood level monitoring for a psychiatric drug. The use of lithium in psychiatry increased worldwide, although the United States was slow to participate because of an earlier disastrous experience in that country with the unmonitored use of lithium chloride as a salt substitute, which had led to severe toxic reactions, some of which were fatal. Schou (1978) was the first to report compelling evidence that lithium carbonate dramatically reduced the incidence and duration of serious affective episodes in bipolar patients. Since that time, a large number of controlled, double-blind studies have confirmed that lithium is clearly effective in reducing recurrences in both bipolar and unipolar affective disorders, as well as being more effective than placebo in treating acute mania.

Pharmacological Effects

Much has been learned in the past 30 years about the possible mechanism of lithium in the treatment of bipolar disorder. However, we are still some way from defining the key factors of lithium's efficacy.

It has become clearer that the pharmacology of lithium is tremendously complex. Lithium may affect different parts of the brain differently at different times. It is evident that lithium's antibipolar effects are probably the result of complex actions on at least three systems. Lithium appears to modulate the balance between excitatory and inhibitory effects of various neurotransmitters such as serotonin (5-hydroxytryptamine; 5-HT), norepinephrine, glutamate, GABA (γ-aminobutyric acid), and dopamine. Lithium also effects neural plasticity through its effects on glycogen synthetase kinase–3β, cyclic AMP–dependent kinase, and protein kinase C. Finally, lithium adjusts signaling activity via effects on second-messenger activity (Jope 1999).

Lithium appears to enhance serotonergic transmission in a number of ways. For example, lithium appears to increase synthesis of serotonin by increasing tryptophan reuptake in synaptosomes after even short-term use. With long-term use (2–3 weeks), lithium appears to enhance the release of 5-HT from neurons in the parietal cortex and the hippocampus. Furthermore, the chronic administration of lithium appears to cause a downregulation in serotonin$_{1A}$ (5-HT$_{1A}$), serotonin$_{1B}$, and serotonin$_2$ (5-HT$_2$) receptor subtypes (Massot et al. 1999). Lithium also affects a number of other monoamine neurotransmitters. Initially, lithium appears to increase the rate of synthesis of norepinephrine in some parts of the brain. It reduces the excretion of norepinephrine in patients with mania but increases the excretion of norepinephrine metabolites in patients with depression. These effects are consistent with lithium's beneficial actions in both mania and depression. Likewise, lithium appears to block postsynaptic dopamine receptors' supersensitivity, in keeping with the clinical data that lithium is effective in controlling mania even when psychotic features are present.

In recent years, the effect of lithium on second-messenger systems has been of particular interest. Because lithium affects a variety of neurotransmitters, some investigators have speculated that the principal action of the drug may be on the postsynaptic signal that a number of neurotransmitters generate. The so-called G proteins have been of particular interest in lithium research because they function as signal transducers for a number of receptor types. G proteins appear to be quite important in coordinating a balance among various neurotransmitters in the brain. Some preliminary evidence suggests that lithium may have a direct or indirect effect on G proteins that mediates their actions.

The role of the phosphatidylinositol (PI) system, another second-messenger system, in the actions of lithium remains unclear. Lithium appears to inhibit a number of enzymes in the PI system, including inositol monophosphatase. It is believed that the PI system affects the receptor activity of many neurotransmitter systems, including the serotonergic, cholinergic, and noradrenergic systems. The role of the PI second-messenger system in lithium's actions is the subject of continued investigation.

Clinical Indications

Lithium use can be divided into four main clinical areas:

1. To control rapidly acute, overt psychopathology as in mania or agitation.
2. To attempt to modify milder, ongoing or frequent but episodic clinical symptoms such as chronic depression or episodic irritability.
3. To establish a prophylactic maintenance regimen to avert future mood episodes.

4. To enhance the effect of antidepressants in patients with major depressive episodes (see Chapters 3 and 9 in this manual).

Acute Mania

There is no final, conclusive statement possible about the use of lithium as a sole or primary drug treatment for acute mania. The initial approval of lithium in the treatment of acute mania was based on three small double-blind studies completed before 1971. A later study addressing the question of lithium for acute mania (Lambert and Venaud 1992) found that half of 36 acutely manic patients who completed a 3-week trial responded to lithium and that this was about twice the rate seen with placebo. These results were similar to those found in a larger, multicenter-based study comparing lithium, valproate, and placebo in the treatment of acute mania (Bowden et al. 1994). In that study, both lithium and valproate were twice as likely as placebo to produce a marked reduction in manic symptoms over a 3-week period.

Lithium alone is clearly more effective than placebo and is probably as effective as an antipsychotic in treating patients with less severe mania. It is probably less effective and slower acting than an antipsychotic in disturbed, psychotic manic, schizoaffective, or very hyperactive patients.

Given the delayed onset of action of lithium (7–14 days), most clinicians do not initiate treatment with lithium alone in acute mania. It is common practice to begin by administering patients an antipsychotic, on the assumption that it will produce the most rapid control of psychopathology or aid in patient management. Many clinicians then add lithium—either on the first day of drug therapy or after the mania has begun to respond to antipsychotics—to stabilize the patient on both drugs. When the patient is clearly much improved, some clinicians gradually taper the antipsychotic over several months so that the patient will be taking lithium alone at the end of the episode. In patients whose hospitalizations are brief, both medications will be in use at discharge, and the antipsychotic will be tapered when the patient is back in the community. Some early studies on antipsychotic use indicated that more than 50% of the patients were still taking antipsychotics at 6-month follow-up. Currently, most patients that have an SGA started for acute mania likely continue it as a maintenance therapy.

An alternative strategy that has long been popular is to initiate treatment of the acutely manic patient with both lithium and a benzodiazepine such as lorazepam or clonazepam (Lenox et al. 1992). This strategy allows the clinician to immediately address the insomnia and hyperactivity without the potentially toxic effects of an antipsychotic. However, using only a benzodiazepine with lithium may not be ideal in the treatment of the acutely psychotic manic patient. In such patients, triple therapy—a benzodiazepine, an antipsychotic, and lithium—allows smaller doses of the first two agents to be used for the acute episode while lithium is initiated for long-term treatment.

The problem of severe neurotoxicity, reported mainly with the combined use of haloperidol or another high-potency antipsychotic and lithium, deserves comment here. In the 1970s there was considerable concern about the possibility of serious drug interactions between lithium and haloperidol, a concern based almost exclusively on anecdotal reports. When the possible interaction was reviewed more recently, no significant interaction between lithium and neuroleptics was detected beyond merely additive adverse effects (Kessel et al. 1992). Neurotoxicity, including delirium and other mental status changes, may occur with lithium alone even at therapeutic dosages in elderly and organically compromised patients. More recent experience suggests that patients who developed neurotoxicity on the combination either were lithium toxic (often at toxic levels) or had a neuroleptic malignant syndrome. In general, the combination of antipsychotics and lithium appears to be safe and efficacious.

Bipolar Maintenance Treatment

The evidence that lithium is effective in the prophylaxis of recurrent bipolar episodes is far more substantial than the evidence of lithium's efficacy in treating acute mania. Until olanzapine received a similar approval, lithium was the only drug with an FDA-approved indication for the maintenance treatment of bipolar disorder. At least 10 double-blind studies suggest that the relapse rate for bipolar patients is two to three times higher with placebo than with lithium. Among the best lithium studies have been those completed recently using lithium as an active control in the lamotrigine maintenance studies (Goodwin et al. 2004). These studies confirmed the utility of lithium in the maintenance treatment of bipolar disorder. In addition, lithium is clearly effective in preventing suicide attempts and completions in bipolar patients (Baldessarini et al. 2006). However, the rapid discontinuation of lithium in some of the earlier trials probably affected the relapse rates. The prophylactic effects of lithium appear more pronounced in preventing manic than depressive recurrences, but both are positively affected. However, only half, or perhaps fewer than half, of lithium-treated patients have complete suppression of all episodes, even with excellent medication compliance. Furthermore, at least some of the patients who have manic recurrences while taking maintenance lithium are blamed for noncompliance unjustifiably: the noncompliance is probably secondary to a recurrence of mania rather than vice versa. In addition, some patients respond to lithium with suppression of mania but with continuing episodes of depression; others show only a partial reduction in severity in both phases.

We have seen a number of patients who had been taking lithium for several years and had poor responses but who continued to have episodes of mania and depression; they were judged to be lithium nonresponders, but their condition was clearly even worse when lithium therapy was abandoned as ineffective. Patients with rapid-cycling and mixed-state types of bipolar disorder generally do less well while taking lithium than do patients with less frequent or purely manic episodes. However, even some of the former can have the severity of their episodes ameliorated. In addition, patients who tend to develop severe stage III manic episodes with psychotic disorganization do more poorly with lithium treatment alone.

In initiating maintenance "prophylactic" lithium therapy, both the patient and (when available) a spouse or a significant other need careful instruction about the purposes and requirements of lithium therapy, including its side effects and complications. There is evidence that continuing involvement of bipolar patients and their spouses in couples groups, or of single patients in lithium support groups, is helpful in maintaining drug compliance and in helping patients deal with past, current, and future problems.

Many bipolar patients, when contemplating maintenance lithium therapy, ask, "Will I have to take lithium forever?" There are two issues in this area. One is whether patients ever stop having recurrent manic and depressive episodes once several episodes have occurred, and the other is whether abruptly stopping lithium will trigger an affective episode that might not have otherwise occurred. The evidence from placebo substitution and lithium discontinuation studies involving patients whose condition was already stabilized successfully with lithium maintenance is that relapses occur with considerable frequency: about half the patients relapsed within 6 months. In other, uncontrolled studies, which involved small series of patients, patients relapsed floridly within a few days. We suspect that the latter consequence is unusual but may actually occur with some patients; it may account for some of the florid relapses seen in patients taking maintenance lithium who experiment with stopping (or forget to take) their medication for a few days. In our experience, however, stopping lithium abruptly for 2 or 3 days in patients who have developed uncomfortable symptoms of lithium toxicity has never led to a florid relapse.

The area of lithium discontinuation is not well understood, but most clinicians assume that essentially all bipolar patients whose condition is stable on lithium need to continue the medication indefinitely. Data confirm that abrupt discontinuation of lithium after long-term treatment significantly increases the rate and speed of relapse (Faedda et al. 1993). More gradual discontinuation of lithium in bipolar patients over several months appears to mitigate this risk substantially (Suppes et al. 1993). Discontinuation of lithium can be associated with increased risk for suicide (Tondo et al. 2001).

One wonders, however, whether withdrawal from lithium could be worth a trial for patients who have really stabilized both their illness and their life circumstances for several years and in whom there is some evidence that prior episodes were precipitated by stressors that are no longer present. Such trials of withdrawal from lithium need to be discussed in detail with patients and their families, with all parties taking into account that about 90% of patients with mania will have a recurrence at some time. Given the occasional rapid relapses observed with sudden discontinuation, slowly tapering the drug in monthly 300-mg decrements would be indicated. Post and colleagues (1992) reported that some patients who discontinued their lithium did not experience a response when readministered lithium for a recurrence of the disorder. These data suggest that it may be prudent to err on the side of continuing lithium maintenance for longer rather than shorter periods. However, a later prospective, naturalistic study demonstrated that patients with a recurrence of mania who had previously had a response to lithium generally appear to have a response to rechallenge with the drug (Coryell et al. 1998).

Schizophrenia Spectrum Illnesses

There is reasonable evidence that lithium, at serum levels in the range of 0.8–1.1 mEq/L, is useful in combination with an antipsychotic in treating patients with schizoaffective disorder. As many as 70% of these patients benefit from the addition of lithium to a regimen of antipsychotics. In the few controlled studies in which lithium was added to an antipsychotic in schizophrenic patients with or without manic symptoms, lithium was often more effective, on average, than placebo. However, monotherapy with lithium appears much less efficacious than treatment with an antipsychotic alone in the treatment of schizophrenia. In some chronically impaired schizophrenic patients with no more than the usual amount of affective overlay, lithium produces useful but limited additional improvement when added to an antipsychotic regimen. This effect occurs often enough to make a trial of lithium easily justifiable for any patient with treatment-resistant schizophrenia or schizoaffective disorder, although perhaps only one in five will show clinical improvement. Also, for a subgroup of chronically schizophrenic patients with brief, episodic angry outbursts, lithium appears to act by decreasing impulsive anger rather than by reducing the level of psychosis. However, in patients with chronic, treatment-resistant psychotic illness, drug treatments are often added and continued for months or years, even if no obvious clinical response or only a trivial improvement has occurred, in the hope that the extra drugs might be helping. There seems little justification for continuing such a use of lithium for longer than 6 months if no clinical benefit is apparent.

Depressive Disorders

Some depressive episodes improve with lithium alone. In fact, a number of controlled studies suggest that lithium may be as effective as tricyclic antidepressants (TCAs) in the treatment of major depression. The response time, however, often lags behind that of standard antidepressants. For recurrent unipolar depression, maintenance treatment with lithium appears to be as effective as long-term treatment with imipramine in preventing recurrences (Prien et al. 1984). A number of studies also suggest that adding lithium to a TCA, a selective serotonin reuptake inhibitor (SSRI), or a monoamine oxidase inhibitor (MAOI) in a patient who has not responded to the antidepressant after 3–6 weeks may lead to a clear favorable response (see Chapter 3: "Antidepressants" and Chapter 9: "Augmentation Strategies for Treatment-Resistant Disorders").

In recurrent unipolar depression, the evidence from large-scale studies is mixed on the exact prophylactic potential of lithium; some studies showed lithium and imipramine to be equally effective, whereas other studies showed imipramine to be superior to lithium and both drugs to be superior to placebo. The combination of imipramine and lithium was not superior to imipramine alone. Thus, clinicians may choose to use lithium alone to prevent recurrence of depression in bipolar patients.

Just as lithium is known to have anti-suicide properties in patients with bipolar disorder, emerging evidence also suggests that lithium is an equally effective prophylaxis in patients with unipolar depression. Guzzetta and colleagues (2007) evaluated suicide attempts and risks in patients with recurrent major depressive disorder who had participated in long-term trials in which lithium was used. The investigators estimated that the risk of completed suicides and suicide attempts was 90% greater when the patients were not treated with adjunctive lithium than when they were taking the drug.

Lithium is among the best studied augmenters of antidepressant response. While most studies of lithium augmentation involved augmentation of TCAs, lithium has proved useful in the augmentation of a variety of antidepressants (Bschor and Bauer 2006). One of the larger randomized, albeit open, trials of lithium augmentation was in the STAR*D (Sequenced Treatment Alternatives for Resistant Depression) trial. In that study, patients who had experienced two previous failed trials were randomly assigned to lithium or triiodothyronine (T_3; Cytomel) augmentation. Approximately 16% of patients achieved remission when lithium was added versus 25% of patients who were randomly assigned to T_3 augmentation (Nierenberg et al. 2006a). The difference was not statistically significant, but lithium was more poorly tolerated than the T_3. While it is clear that lithium is an effective augmenter of antidepressants, there are far more choices for augmentation now than there were 20 years ago, and lithium's popularity in resistant depression has waned.

Rage and Irritability

There is a reasonable clinical literature, mainly but not exclusively uncontrolled, that supports the proposition that some patients with episodic, uncontrolled outbursts of violent rage have a response to lithium. The drug certainly is not always effective in such cases, but these predominantly nonpsychotic behavior disorders often present such appalling clinical problems that any drug with a chance of helping substantially deserves a trial. We concur with Tupin's (1975) classic position that in populations such as violent prisoners, lithium controls outbursts of rage that are nontriggered or are triggered instantaneously by minor stimuli, but that lithium does not affect premeditated aggressive behavior. The drug is helpful in some patients with organic disorders or mental retardation who display episodic angry outbursts. Lithium has also shown some utility in the treatment of children with episodic aggressive outbursts and in mitigating the self-destructive behavior of some patients with BPD. It should be noted that there have been a few case reports of lithium's causing increased aggressive behavior in patients with temporal lobe spike activity on the electroencephalogram (EEG). The use of anticonvulsants and antipsychotics has largely supplanted lithium use in the management of hostility, impulse control, and aggression in a variety of disorders (Goedhard et al. 2006).

Side Effects

Neuromuscular and Central Nervous System

Among the most common side effects in lithium therapy is tremor, principally noticed in the fingers (Table 5–2). It resembles intentional, coffee-induced, or familial tremor in frequency, being faster than pseudoparkinsonian tremor. When tremor is severe enough to affect handwriting, the writing is usually jagged and irregular, but not micrographic as in parkinsonism. Tremor sometimes is worse at peak lithium blood level and can be ameliorated by dosage rearrangement. Dosage reduction can often be used to bring the blood level low enough to make tremor either absent or mild and inconspicuous. If there is good reason to maintain a serum lithium level that causes a disturbing degree of tremor, propranolol at dosages ranging from 10 to 160 mg/day can be used to reduce the tremor.

Some patients taking lithium also develop cogwheeling and mild signs of parkinsonism, and naturally occurring parkinsonism can be aggravated. With toxic lithium levels, gross tremulousness and ataxia with dysarthria occur: the patient appears to have gross neurological disorder and, often, to be confused or, less often, to be delirious at the same time. Seizures occur rarely with severe lithium toxicity.

Some patients taking lithium complain of slowed mentation and forgetfulness and, on testing, show a memory deficit. In fact, pooled data on side effects of lithium therapy suggest that memory problems are perhaps the leading cause of noncompliance and the third most common side effect overall

Table 5–2.   Toxicology of mood stabilizers

System	Drug						
	lithium	valproate	CBZ	gabapentin	lamotrigine	topiramate	tiagabine
CNS	Tremor Ataxia Cognitive slowing	Sedation Tremor Ataxia	Sedation Dizziness Ataxia	Somnolence Dizziness Ataxia	Dizziness Ataxia Somnolence	Dizziness Ataxia Speech problems Cognitive slowing	Dizziness Somnolence Difficulty concentrating
GI	Dyspepsia Weight gain Diarrhea	Dyspepsia LFT increases Weight gain Hepatic failure (rare) Pancreatitis	Dyspepsia LFT increases	Dyspepsia (rare)	Nausea Vomiting	Nausea Dyspepsia Abdominal pain	Nausea Abdominal pain
Dermatological	Rash Hair loss Acne	Rash Hair loss	Rash	Pruritus (rare)	Rash Acne	Rash (rare) Pruritis (rare)	Rash (rare) Alopecia
Renal/ Urogenital	NDI Nephropathy	Minimal	SIADH	None	Vaginitis Urinary tract infection	Dysmenorrhea Metabolic acidosis[a]	None

Table 5–2.   Toxicology of mood stabilizers (*continued*)

System	lithium	valproate	CBZ	gabapentin	lamotrigine	topiramate	tiagabine
Drug							
Cardiac	T wave changes Sinoatrial block	Minimal	Arrhythmia	None	Palpitations (rare) Hypotension (rare)	BP changes (rare)	Hypertension Palpitations
Hematological	Leukocytosis	Thrombocytopenia Coagulation defect	Thrombocytopenia Aplastic anemia (rare)	Leukopenia (rare)	None	Leukopenia	None
Endocrine	Hypothyroidism	Minimal	Lower levels of T_3, T_4	None	Hypothyroidism (rare)	Weight decrease	Goiter (rare)

Note.   BP = blood pressure; CBZ = carbamazepine; CNS = central nervous system; GI = gastrointestinal; LFT = liver function test; NDI = nephrogenic diabetes insipidus; SIADH = syndrome of inappropriate antidiuretic hormone; T_3 = triiodothyronine; T_4 = thyroxine.
[a]Secondary to hyperchloremia.

(Goodwin and Jamison 1990). Although such patients are often suspected or accused of "using" such symptoms to avoid necessary lithium therapy, our impression is that these complaints are real and constitute a basis for lowering the dosage or trying another therapy.

Some patients worry that they may become less creative while taking lithium. Schou (1979), a pioneer in lithium therapy, however, has asserted that 75% of patients note no change or an improvement in their creativity with lithium therapy. The bipolar patients who have the most prominent neuropsychological effects of lithium tend to be younger, depressed patients with higher lithium serum levels (Kocsis et al. 1993). Thus, patients who complain that lithium is affecting their cognition or creativity might do well at a somewhat lower dosage.

In addition, some patients may experience drowsiness and fatigue, which may further exacerbate the feeling of being slowed down.

With all the above neurological symptoms, stopping lithium will lead to a disappearance of the side effects, but the symptoms and signs may persist for 2–5 days, longer than one would expect it to take to clear the offending lithium from the body.

Gastrointestinal

Chronic nausea and watery diarrhea can occur together or separately as signs of lithium toxicity. Episodic nausea occurring only after each dose may be due to local gastric irritation and may be relieved by taking lithium with food. Shifting to a different lithium preparation may also be helpful. For example, in cases of upper gastrointestinal (GI) distress, sustained-release preparations may be beneficial. In contrast, patients with diarrhea who are on sustained-release preparations may benefit from a switch to the shorter-release forms.

Weight Gain and Endocrine

Some patients gain weight progressively while taking lithium, and this side effect is second only to cognitive side effects as a reason that patients stop taking the medication. The mechanisms underlying this side effect are unclear. However, lithium appears to have an insulin-like action that may result in relative hypoglycemia (Jefferson et al. 1987). This hypoglycemia may in turn promote eating and subsequent weight gain. A few patients have overt edema and/or lose several pounds rapidly when lithium is stopped. More commonly, increased appetite with resulting weight gain is the problem, and attempting to control weight with dietary regulation is often very difficult for the patient. Weight gain is greater in patients who are overweight to begin with and is probably greater in patients with polydipsia, perhaps because they drink caloric fluids.

Most patients show a transitory decrease in thyroid levels early in lithium therapy, and a very few show goiter with normal thyroid studies except for elevated thyroid-stimulating hormone (TSH) levels. Some clinicians add thyroid supplements at this point. However, we recommend using exogenous thyroid primarily in patients with marked goiter or in those with associated anergia.

Up to 20% of patients, more commonly women, develop clinical hypothyroidism on lithium therapy, and 30% develop elevated TSH levels (Jefferson et al. 1987).

In our clinic, we will typically obtain a TSH level before initiating lithium and then repeat it at 6 months and annually thereafter.

Renal

Lithium causes polyuria with secondary polydipsia to a noticeable degree in some (perhaps roughly one out of five) patients. In a few patients this effect may extend to severe renal diabetes insipidus, with urine volume up to 8 L/day and difficulty in concentrating urine and maintaining adequate lithium serum levels. This range of renal effects is due to a decrease in the resorption of fluid from the distal tubules of the kidney. It can be treated, obviously, by lowering the dose of lithium or stopping the drug. In most, but not all, cases the renal effect wears off in days or weeks after lithium is stopped.

An alternative strategy with patients in whom lithium is clearly necessary and the polyuria is distressing is to add a loop or thiazide diuretic. It is well documented that hydrochlorothiazide at a dosage of 50 mg/day decreases lithium clearance by about 50% and therefore increases lithium plasma levels. Thus, one can rationally add 50 mg/day of hydrochlorothiazide and then reduce the lithium dosage by 50% and carefully restabilize the desired lithium level. This maneuver is sometimes effective, as it is in naturally occurring nephrogenic diabetes insipidus, and can be used in milder but troublesome cases of polyuria. At the time of our first edition, amiloride (Midamor) had recently been reported to decrease lithium-induced polyuria without, allegedly, affecting either potassium excretion or lithium serum levels. However, we had seen some patients who showed increased lithium levels when amiloride was added. If this strategy is tried, one should check lithium levels carefully while assessing amiloride's effectiveness in improving renal resorption of fluid and decreasing urine volume. The prohibition in the *Physicians' Desk Reference* (PDR) against combining lithium with diuretics, particularly of the thiazide type, is much overstated. It is true that harm can occur if a patient is stabilized on lithium at a clinically useful blood level (e.g., 0.8 mEq/L) and a thiazide diuretic is added in ignorance: the lithium level can double and the patient may suddenly develop signs of lithium toxicity. This increase can also occur with other drugs, most notably nonsteroidal anti-inflammatory drugs such as ibuprofen, naproxen, and indomethacin. However, we see no problem in starting lithium therapy in a patient already stabilized on a thiazide diuretic; even patients undergoing dialysis have been successfully treated with lithium. Renal impairment before lithium therapy means the clinician should raise the dosage very slowly and cautiously, monitoring serum levels carefully.

A different and potentially more serious renal problem is interstitial nephritis, first reported by Danish workers in 1977. It is characterized by renal scarring and destruction. Currently, the problem no longer seems as threatening as it did initially. Major renal impairment manifested by seriously decreased creatinine clearance appears to be quite rare. In a review, Gitlin (1993) suggested that up to 5% of lithium-treated patients developed some renal insufficiency but that these changes were generally not clinically significant ones. In a later review, polyuria secondary to lithium-induced decreases in renal tubular function appeared to be progressive in many patients, whereas changes in glomerular function were not (Gitlin 1999). Patients exposed to multiple periods of lithium toxicity may be at greater risk for developing renal insufficiency. Some patients with chronic affective disorders who have never taken lithium show renal pathology, and not all kidney dysfunction in patients taking lithium is necessarily caused by this drug.

Still, it is worth checking kidney function every 6–12 months in patients on maintenance lithium. The "best" way would be to measure creatinine clearance periodically, but logistic problems and doubts about patient reliability in 24-hour urine collection have caused this procedure to be generally disfavored. Serum creatinine itself offers a reasonable indicator of kidney function, because creatinine production is a function of muscle mass and is not affected by diet.

We typically obtain a serum creatinine level before initiating lithium and repeat it annually thereafter or as clinically indicated. Lithium serum level at constant intake is also a function of glomerular filtration. Watching both measures periodically should allow detection of early changes in glomerular function. Some practitioners check the patients' reactive ability to concentrate their urine. If the lithium dosage requirement gradually decreases and serum creatinine is persistently elevated (above 1.6 mg/100 mL), a nephrology consultation is indicated. Even if renal impairment appears to exist, the decision whether to stop lithium therapy should be based on the total picture. Patients who obtain major benefits from maintenance lithium and have either a mild renal deficit or a kidney problem that may not be lithium related can continue taking lithium, but more frequent monitoring of kidney function is required.

Cardiovascular

Lithium can produce a variety of benign effects on the electrocardiogram (ECG), including T wave flattening and inversion. A few cases have been reported in which a "sick sinus node" syndrome has been brought on by lithium. This complication is very rare and probably not predictable unless the condition antedates the lithium therapy. Some patients have developed problems with sinus node conduction after concurrent use of antiarrhythmic drugs (Jefferson et al. 1987). Baseline ECGs are desirable in older patients or patients with a history of any cardiac dysfunction. Some caution should also be exercised in using lithium in patients with particularly low heart rates at baseline.

Dermatological

A wide variety of diverse rashes from lithium have been described. Acne is perhaps the most common dermatological effect of lithium use and has been reported to be helped by topical retinoic acid. Aggravation of preexisting or dormant psoriasis is well documented, and a dry, noninflamed papular eruption is relatively common with maintenance lithium. Both zinc sulfate and tetracycline have been tried as treatments for rashes, with variable success. Other rashes—of an itchy, presumably allergic nature, less typical with lithium—can occur and often disappear if the specific lithium brand being used is changed. Presumably these are allergic reactions to some ingredient in the capsule or tablet other than the lithium itself. Alopecia can occur in patients taking lithium, but the hair often regrows, either with or without lithium.

Preparations

Lithium is available in the United States in several formulations (Table 5–1). The standard and least expensive form is the carbonate in 300-mg capsules or scored tablets. Sustained-release preparations of the carbonate are also available, as is a liquid preparation of lithium citrate; one teaspoonful of the last has the equivalent in ion content of 300 mg of the carbonate (8 mEq). Other preparations, including the sulfate, and other dosage strengths are used in Europe. Despite more than 50 years of clinical experience with lithium, it is not entirely clear whether any of the formulations have definite superiority for any purpose, aside from relieving GI side effects. Lithium citrate is obviously useful in patients who dislike or cannot swallow pills.

The sustained-release preparations result in lower peak serum lithium levels after ingestion and probably result in the release of less lithium ion in the stomach and more in the small intestine. If lithium irritation of the stomach mucosa is causing nausea after each dose, the sustained-release preparation may reduce gastric irritation. If diarrhea is a problem (and is not due to an elevated serum lithium level), the citrate may cause even faster absorption in the upper GI tract and may reduce the diarrhea. However, we have seen patients who have diarrhea with standard lithium carbonate whose diarrhea lessened when they took sustained-release lithium. The basic problem is that it is still unclear which lithium side effects are related to peak serum level and which are related to steady-state serum level. Clinically, any side effect that mainly occurs 1–2 hours after each oral dose of the standard preparation might be improved by the sustained-release form. For example, nausea may be caused by gastric irritation from lithium or by an elevated serum level. The former causes transient nausea after each dose, whereas the latter causes persistent nausea.

There was a belief that sustained-release lithium would, in general, have fewer side effects and might, in particular, have less effect on the concentrating ability of the renal tubules, leading to less polyuria and polydipsia. So far, this belief does not seem to be the case, and it may even be that massing the total daily dose of lithium at bedtime may cause fewer renal effects. One major European center (Copenhagen) has routinely been using once-a-day lithium dosing for many years, suggesting that this dosage scheme is feasible and effective.

Dosage and Administration

Lithium dosage is titrated to achieve both therapeutic response and adequate plasma levels. The general presumption is that levels of about 0.7–1.0 mEq/L are appropriate for maintenance therapy or the treatment of conditions other than manic or psychotic excitement, whereas levels up to 1.5 mEq/L are sometimes needed in treating acute mania. Levels should be obtained about 12 hours after the last dose, at which time the vagaries of absorption after drug ingestion are well past and a relative steady state has been achieved (see the subsection on blood levels in the section "Tricyclic and Tetracyclic Antidepressants" in Chapter 3: "Antidepressants"). These "ideal" levels are, of course, not carved in stone and must be interpreted in the clinical context. Someone who has marked tremor, oversedation, vomiting, and ataxia at a level of 0.8 mEq/L either cannot tolerate that level or has some other medical condition causing the symptoms; lithium intolerance is the more likely possibility. Other patients receiving maintenance therapy appear to have averted affective episodes for years at levels as low as 0.4–0.6 mEq/L, and patients with daily symptoms such as irritability and anger report clinical improvement at very low plasma levels. It is very hard to prove that these are or are not "real" drug responses. It is our belief that many patients can be successfully maintained at relatively low plasma levels, particularly when the lithium is combined with another agent. Occasionally, for a patient whose mania is still uncontrolled despite a level of 1.5 mEq/L for several days and who has no side effects, a higher level can be cautiously tried.

Expedient establishment of high, adequate plasma levels of lithium (e.g., 0.8–1.2 mEq/L) is desired for acute mania. An initial regimen of 300 mg bid to qid is indicated in healthy adolescent or adult patients; plasma levels should initially be obtained every 3 or 4 days to ensure early detection of toxic lithium levels. The dosage should be titrated up (or down) as necessary to achieve a level of approximately 1.0 mEq/L. In patients older than 60 or those with possible renal impairment, the lower starting dose is indicated. In some elderly patients, we initiate lithium at 150 mg bid. Several articles have described techniques for predicting the optimal dosage of lithium from a loading dose followed by several determinations of levels over the next 24 hours. These techniques can be used, but they do not seem to us to offer benefit over clinical titration. Response in acutely manic states may require 7–14 days, even with adequate plasma levels. As plasma levels stabilize, the frequency of testing may be decreased—to two times a week initially, and eventually to once a week, as both plasma levels and the clinical condition level out. If inadequate clinical response occurs within 4 weeks, it is safe to assume that lithium monotherapy will not be effective for the acute episode. At this point, or earlier, adding a second mood stabilizer should be considered.

With patients who are in remission and are being stabilized with lithium to avert future affective episodes, one can begin at even lower dosages (one or two 300-mg doses per day); weekly plasma levels are often sufficient during dosage adjustment. Again, the goal is to find a well-tolerated plasma level as close to 0.8 mEq/L as possible. It seems reasonable that higher plasma levels should be associated with better prophylaxis. In one major collaborative study sponsored by the National Institute of Mental Health (NIMH), patients whose lithium was maintained at 0.8 mEq/L and above had consistently fewer recurrences than patients stabilized at lower levels (0.6 mEq/L or below) but had more side effects. The efficacy data in this study generated considerable controversy, because when patients were initially randomized to low-plasma-level groups, the dose may have been decreased so rapidly as to enhance the likelihood of relapse. Once a patient on maintenance lithium is stabilized adequately with weekly plasma levels for a few weeks, monthly levels are sufficient, and after 6–12 months of stability, testing the levels every 6 months or as clinically indicated may suffice.

Once a patient has a stable daily dosage, it can be spread over the day in any suitable regimen. Usually, twice a day—morning and bedtime—is convenient and well tolerated, and doses are less likely to be forgotten or overlooked. It has been suggested, but not proved, that once-a-day dosing enhances compliance and may be associated with less polyuria. We have found that once-a-day dosing at bedtime is often effective, but some patients feel drugged or dazed in the morning. Gastric irritation after each dose is the major reason for use of divided doses. Smaller, more frequent doses are common (and logistically easy) among hospitalized patients, but the patients are sometimes inadvertently discharged on these regimens when a simpler regimen would suffice and might be taken more reliably after the patient returns home.

For other target symptoms, when the situation is less urgent, an initial dosage of 300 mg bid seems adequate. Some patients who end up benefiting from lithium have presented with histories of marked lithium intolerance that appears to have been caused by overaggressive initial dosing. In these less acute situations, a plasma level of 0.5–0.8 mEq/L is probably adequate, and less frequent plasma level monitoring may be needed. It is also important to remember that one is treating the patient, not the plasma level, and that both clinical status and adverse effects need frequent and careful monitoring. Some patients report clear symptom relief at levels around 0.5 mEq/L; it seems unwarranted to push them to higher levels unless they break through with symptoms at lower levels. Similarly, keeping a patient chronically nauseated, mentally dulled, and grossly tremulous just to maintain an "adequate" plasma level is counterproductive in almost all situations. In general, we advise aiming for lower levels (<0.6 mEq/L) in elderly patients.

For patients with chronic disorders manifesting overt, current target psychopathology—depression, schizophrenia, and cyclothymia—a trial of about 4 weeks at adequate blood levels (or the highest tolerated levels) is usually sufficient to determine whether lithium will be clinically useful.

If a patient has responded in the past to lithium but has stopped the drug for weeks or months, and if there is no reason to believe that kidney function has changed in the interim, it is clinically reasonable to place the patient immediately back on the drug at the prior dosage without retitrating. However, some patients require gradual dose escalation to allow optimal dosing. Frequent blood level monitoring should be reinstituted.

Use in Pregnancy

Lithium is the only psychoactive, nonanticonvulsant drug that is thought to be associated with a specific birth defect, Ebstein's anomaly. This serious cardiac abnormality is not common in children born to mothers taking lithium (between 0.1% and 0.7%), but the defect is at least 20 times more common in these children than in the population at large. These estimates are much lower than were earlier estimates, and some reviews have called into question whether there is a valid association of Ebstein's anomaly and lithium use (Giles and Bannigan 2006). The risk of a major birth defect needs to be discussed with female patients taking lithium who either are planning to become pregnant or are already pregnant, because the risk appears to exist primarily with first-trimester use (see Chapter 12: "Pharmacotherapy in Special Situations"). The general risk of a major birth defect appears to be two to three times greater with lithium use than in the general population (Cohen et al. 1994). Echocardiography and fetal ultrasound can be used after the sixteenth week of pregnancy to check for the presence of cardiac abnormalities.

Table 5–3.   Anticonvulsant dosages in bipolar illness

Medication	Usual dosage range	Serum level (μg/mL)
valproate	15–60 mg/kg/day	50–125
carbamazepine	200–1,600 mg/day	6–10
lamotrigine	50–200 mg/day	NA
gabapentin	900–3,600 mg/day	NA
oxcarbazepine	600–2,400 mg/day	NA

Note.   NA = not applicable.

Another risk of lithium use, particularly in the third trimester, is large-gestational-weight infants. Higher birth weights have been reported for some time in mothers exposed to lithium. The long-term significance of these higher birth weights in infants is not established, but higher birth weight is not necessarily associated with poorer health outcomes.

Lithium Information Center

A lithium information center exists at the Madison Institute of Medicine in Madison, Wisconsin (telephone 608-827-2470; fax 608-827-2479; www.miminc.org/aboutlithinfoctr.html). The staff is most helpful in conducting focused literature searches for a small fee and can provide interested clinicians with answers to a wide variety of questions about lithium problems encountered in their practice.

Anticonvulsants

In the past two decades, increasing attention has been paid to the use of anticonvulsant medications in psychiatry, mainly to promote mood stabilization (Table 5–3). The application of these agents stems from a number of observations on the psychiatric sequelae of temporal lobe epilepsy, including hallucinations, angry outbursts, religiosity, and so forth. These observations spurred on the use of phenytoin in the 1950s in psychiatric patients—with, at best, equivocal results (although a controlled trial found phenytoin to be effective in the treatment of mania; Mishory et al. 2000). In more recent years, several groups have further suggested that psychiatric symptoms could emanate from limbic seizures and that kindling phenomena could play a major role in the development of psychoses and psychiatric disorders. Understandably, then, a number of reports have emerged that other anticonvulsant agents (e.g., carbamazepine and valproic acid), which act preferentially on temporal lobe or limbic systems, are effective in patients with bipolar disorder, particularly in acute mania. Three compounds, valproic acid, carbamazepine, and lamotrigine, have received the lion's share of attention (for chemical structures of the thymoleptic anticonvulsants, see Figure 5–1), although several of the available anticonvulsants could eventually prove useful in treating mood disorders.

Valproate

In contrast to almost all other drugs used in psychiatry, valproic acid has no rings. (Carbamazepine is tricyclic; valproic acid could be said to be acyclic.) The drug is available in this country in the following forms: immediate-release valproic acid (Depakene) and sodium valproate (Depakene syrup); delayed-release divalproex sodium (Depakote and Depakote Sprinkle), containing equal molar of valproic acid and sodium valproate; an extended-release formulation of divalproex (Depakote-ER), approved for migraines and bipolar mania; and an injectable form (Depacon). The amide of valproic acid (valpromide [Dépamide]) is used in Europe. All these preparations convert to valproic acid in the plasma.

Valproate may be the most convenient general term to encompass all these formulations. Valproate is FDA approved in epilepsy for use in simple and complex absence attacks, partial seizures, and migraine prophylaxis. Valproate was given FDA approval for the treatment of acute mania in 1994, followed by approval for Depakote ER in 2005. Valproate is still among the most commonly used drugs in the treatment of bipolar disorder in American psychiatry. Valproate also continues to be employed in treating many other kinds of symptoms, including aggression, agitation, and impulsivity in patients with a variety of disorders.

Clinical Indications

Early work in the late 1960s by Lambert in France identified valproate as effective in a wide range of patients with mania and schizoaffective mania when added to a wide variety of other drugs. Lambert's group reported on more than 100 patients but did not describe the patients in detail. In their study, which

Figure 5–1.   Chemical structures of thymoleptic anticonvulsants.

involved mainly patients with treatment-resistant schizoaffective disorder with mania, moderate improvement was reported in more than half of the patients. In those patients with acute mania without prior drug therapy, 10 of 14 improved. These results agree with the findings of a study of valproate by Pope and colleagues (1991) at McLean Hospital and with other local clinical experience. In Pope et al.'s study, there was a 54% improvement in a standard mania rating score in the valproate group, compared with only a 5% improvement in this score in the placebo group. Interestingly, the antimanic effects of valproate were often observed in the first few days of treatment.

Since the Pope study, a number of double-blind studies have been completed attesting to the efficacy of valproate in treating acute mania. The largest, a double-blind, placebo-controlled study of 179 patients, found that lithium and valproate were equivalent in effectiveness in treating acute mania and twice as effective as placebo (Bowden and McElroy 1995). In addition, there is evidence that a loading dose strategy, typically using about 20 mg/kg/day of

Lamotrigine

Topiramate

Tiagabine

Oxcarbazepine

Figure 5–1. Chemical structures of thymoleptic anticonvulsants *(continued)*.

valproate, may reduce the onset of action to 5 days or less (Keck et al. 1993a; McElroy et al. 1993). Using a 30 mg/kg loading dose to start, with a reduction to 20 mg/kg after a few days, has also been suggested. The current data suggest that valproate is at least as well studied and as effective as lithium in the treat-

Valproate therapy: overview	
Efficacy	Acute mania (FDA approved) Bipolar prophylaxis (may be effective) Mixed, rapid-cycling bipolar Seizure disorders (FDA approved)
Side effects	Weight gain Sedation GI upset
Safety in overdose	Serious effects notable mostly at 20 times normal serum level. Symptoms include nausea, vomiting, CNS depression, and seizures. Manage with gastric lavage, forced emesis, and assisted ventilation.
Dosage and administration	Start IR formulation at 15 mg/kg/day and ER formulation at 25 mg/kg/day in divided doses, up to a maximum of 60 mg/kg. Achieve serum levels of 50–100 µg/mL.
Discontinuation	Rapid discontinuation increases the risk of rapid relapse in bipolar disorder. Otherwise, discontinuation symptoms are uncommon.
Drug interactions	Drugs that ↑ valproate serum levels include: cimetidine erythromycin phenothiazines fluoxetine aspirin ibuprofen Drugs that ↓ valproate serum levels include: rifampin carbamazepine phenobarbital ethosuximide

Note.   CNS=central nervous system; ER=extended-release; FDA = U.S. Food and Drug Administration; GI = gastrointestinal; IR=immediate-release.

ment of acute mania. However, both lithium and valproate appear to be slower acting than the atypical antipsychotics in the treatment of acute mania.

Valproate may be particularly useful in patients with mixed-state or rapid-cycling types of bipolar disorder. Freeman et al. (1992) found that valproate showed good efficacy relative to lithium in the acute and long-term management of mixed states. Bowden et al. (Bowden and Singh 2005; Bowden et al. 1994) noted that valproate was more effective than lithium in treating bipolar patients with mixed states and irritable features and was also effective in treating bipolar patients with rapid cycling. A number of other small open-label studies suggested that valproate may be quite useful in treating mixed and manic states but somewhat less useful in preventing depressive episodes in bipolar patients with rapid cycling. Patients with a history of EEG abnormalities in conjunction with bipolar disorder appear to be good candidates for valproate treatment. Other predictors of response to valproate include lack of psychotic episodes in patients with concurrent BPD (Calabrese et al. 1993). A double-blind, placebo-controlled study has also reported significant effects for valproate in Cluster B patients (Hollander et al. 2001).

A number of open-label studies have suggested that valproate is an effective prophylactic agent in the treatment of bipolar disorder. Most of these studies suggested that valproate may be somewhat more effective in preventing manic than depressive episodes. In a double-blind longitudinal study, Lambert and Venaud (1992) found that valproate was better tolerated than, and as effective as, lithium in preventing subsequent bipolar episodes over a 2-year period. A large multicenter study involving more than 300 patients failed, however, to demonstrate the efficacy of valproate over placebo in the prevention of mania (Bowden et al. 2000). A priori selection of primary outcome measures appeared to interfere with demonstrating the effectiveness of divalproex in the prophylaxis of mania. However, clinical experience with the drug still suggests that it is effective in the maintenance treatment of bipolar disorder.

The efficacy of valproate in treating acute unipolar or bipolar depression is largely untested. As of this seventh edition, there are still no controlled studies of valproate in treating unipolar depression. Several uncontrolled studies and case reports suggested that valproate may have modest antidepressant efficacy in bipolar depression. We have reported that valproate may be useful in the treatment of agitation associated with major depression (DeBattista et al. 2005). There are also case reports suggesting that valproate may have a role in treating refractory major depression. Bowden, Calabrese, and colleagues' (2000) maintenance study suggested that divalproex prevented depressive episodes better than placebo in bipolar patients even though it failed to show similar effects in mania. Low-dose valproate has been successfully used to treat cyclothymia (Jacobsen 1993).

Some case reports and open-label studies have suggested that valproate may be useful in treating panic disorder, particularly when the disorder is complicated by substance abuse and there is concern about using a benzodiazepine (Baetz and Bowen 1998; Keck et al. 1993b; Ontiveros and Fontaine 1992; Woodman and Noyes 1994). We have generally not found valproate to be that useful in treating anxiety disorders.

A study compared 4 weeks of valproate with placebo as an add-on to risperidone or olanzapine in decompensating schizophrenic patients. Valproate add-on was significantly more effective than placebo in reducing positive symptoms (Casey et al. 2001). There is also some evidence that valproate might speed response to antipsychotics in schizophrenia.

Valproate has been used for many years in the treatment of agitation. A number of open-label trials have reported that valproic acid is effective in treating agitation associated with dementia and brain injury (Herrmann 1998; Hilty et al. 1998; Kunik et al. 1998; Lott et al. 1995). We have found that agitated dementia patients often respond to dosages as low as 125 mg/day, although higher dosages are often tolerated and sometimes needed in these patients. Controlled trials have suggested that low-dose valproate is often ineffective but that higher doses are often associated with high rates of discontinuation secondary to side effects (Lonergan et al. 2004). Our group has also been interested in the use of divalproex sodium as an adjunctive agent in the treatment of agitation associated with depression (DeBattista et al. 2005). In a 4-week open trial, we found that an average dose of about 750 mg of divalproex significantly diminished agitation in depressed patients.

Valproate is also increasingly being used to control aggression, particularly in patients with brain injuries. Several open studies reported that valproate helps control impulsivity, explosive outbursts, physical aggression, and self-destructiveness in patients with brain injuries or mental retardation (Geracioti 1994; Ruedrich et al. 1999; Wroblewski et al. 1997). Some evidence suggests that valproate may attenuate disruptive behavior in aggressive adolescents (Donovan et al. 1997). A recent double-blind, placebo-controlled trial of valproate in patients with intermittent explosive personality failed to find significant differences between drug and placebo, although both groups improved. However, in juvenile offenders, the drug appeared to decrease aggressive outbursts (Steiner et al. 2003). In addition, adolescents who are at risk for developing bipolar disorder and who also have problems with aggression tend to be less so while taking valproate (Saxena et al. 2006).

Valproate has been studied in the treatment of the impulsivity, affective instability, and self-destructiveness of BPD. Borderline personality symptoms are sometimes thought to overlap with those of bipolar II disorder, and it makes some sense to apply valproate to the treatment of BPD patients. Most studies have been small and uncontrolled (Hirschman et al. 1997; Stein et al. 1995; Wilcox 1995). However, in a more recent, larger trial, valproate did appear to be significantly more effective than placebo in patients with Cluster B personality disorders. Valproate does appear to be an important adjunctive agent for controlling some symptoms in many BPD patients. It has the advantage of being less toxic than lithium and most other anticonvulsants in this population with self-destructive behavior. As indicated earlier, the drug appears to reduce positive symptoms in relapsing patients with schizophrenia (Casey et al. 2001).

Dosage and Administration

The plasma half-life of valproate is on the order of 10–15 hours. A drug such as carbamazepine, phenobarbital, or phenytoin, given concurrently, will induce hepatic enzymes and shorten valproate's half-life by speeding its metabolism. In contrast to carbamazepine, valproate is a modest hepatic enzyme inhibitor. Once an adequate blood level has been attained, it is likely to remain adequate if intake remains constant. Blood levels should be taken about 12 hours after the last dose.

The usual starting dose of valproate in the immediate-release (IR) formulation is 15 mg/kg/day in two divided doses. Thus, the average 75-kg male might be started on 500 mg bid. In less acute settings, we tend to recommend a starting dose of 250–500 mg the first day, and that dose, if tolerated, is titrated upward. Some clinicians employ a once-a-day dosing of valproate for the IR formulation in an effort to enhance compliance. Given the pharmacokinetics of IR valproate, bid dosing is probably ideal. In addition, the large peaks in plasma levels with once-a-day dosing often produce GI side effects, and this strategy tends to be poorly tolerated. Still, attaining high levels of this highly bound, hydrophilic agent could allow more effective delivery into the central nervous system (CNS). The extended-release formula of divalproex sodium (Depakote ER) was approved for use in the treatment of acute mania or mixed episodes in bipolar disorder. The ER form is not bioequivalent to the immediate-release form—it appears to produce a serum level that is 10%–20% lower than with Depakote—which suggests some need for increasing the dose (by about one-third) when converting patients to the ER formulation. The ER formulation may be somewhat less associated with side effects such as weight gain. Preliminary studies have indicated that switching from the delayed-release Depakote DR to the even-slower release ER formulation of Depakote in bipolar patients was well tolerated and maintained stability. The dosage can be increased each week by 10 mg/kg/day until an adequate therapeutic level is achieved, or to a maximum dosage of 60 mg/kg/day.

As described earlier, loading doses in the range of 20 mg/kg seem to speed the onset of action in treating acute mania. Intravenous loading of divalproex sodium also appears to help stabilize mixed states and rapid cycling but may have little effect on bipolar depression (Grunze et al. 1999a). Patients with mania tolerate medication side effects better than those with depression. Thus, loading strategies are generally avoided in the latter.

In manic patients, levels greater than 45 µg/mL seem to be required for antimanic effect, and levels up to 100 µg/mL are well tolerated. Sometimes, levels as high as 125 µg/mL are required for optimal efficacy of valproate in the treatment of acute mania. Most data suggest that blood levels should probably be between 85 µg/ml and 125 µg/ml in the treatment of patients with mania or mixed states. Higher levels appear to be associated with side effects, including thrombocytopenia, weight gain, and sedation (Bowden and Singh 2005). In beginning valproate therapy, the enteric-coated divalproex sodium is generally less likely to cause GI distress than are the other formulations. Initial dosages of 250 mg bid are common; the higher daily dosage should be reserved for actively manic patients. Valproic acid plasma levels should be obtained every few days until a level greater than 50 µg/mL is reached. There is some suggestion that clinicians should push the dose to achieve levels greater than 75 µg/mL in patients who are not responding. There is considerable variability in levels obtained depending on the time since last dose. Over time blood levels should be collected in a similar relationship to last dose. As with other drugs with which dosage is titrated to reach a specified blood level, the final daily dosage could vary widely, anywhere from 750 to 3,000 mg/day. Some improvement may be evident within 4 days and should be seen within 2 weeks of attaining a therapeutic blood level. If improvement has not occurred, higher doses and levels can be tried for another 2 weeks, but side effects may prove limiting. Sedation and GI distress are the likeliest limiting side effects early in therapy, but only sedation is common, and valproate seems generally better tolerated than lithium carbonate.

When a patient acutely improves while taking valproate, one assumes that the drug can be continued as a maintenance therapy at the same dosage and level, watching for any toxicity. This may, in fact, be a wise course. However, many patients undergoing a trial of valproate are already taking various other drugs (e.g., lithium, a neuroleptic, carbamazepine, antidepressants, clonazepam). Once valproate is working, the other drugs can be gradually withdrawn one at a time to determine whether they are needed. Some may prove unnecessary, but tapering and stopping others may invite a relapse. Only one-third of patients experience adequate response to monotherapy, so combination treatment is now the rule rather than the exception. Valproic acid levels can be monitored weekly until stable and presumably adequate levels are achieved, then monthly or less often during prolonged maintenance therapy. The level should be rechecked if new side effects occur or if the clinical condition worsens.

Side Effects

When valproate was initially introduced, as an anti-epileptic, a major concern was the risk of severe, sometimes fatal, hepatotoxicity (Table 5–2). Fatal cases have all been in neonates receiving multiple anticonvulsants, particularly barbiturates. Children younger than 2 years appear at greatest risk for severe hepatotoxicity. The risk of hepatotoxicity makes the task of monitoring psychiatric patients taking valproate a risk-benefit conundrum. One could order liver function tests every month or so because no one is sure whether severe hepatocellular toxicity will occur. On the other hand, the available data support the position that frequent liver function tests are unnecessary and that patients and/or relatives should be told of the remote risk and informed about early symptoms of liver disease (e.g., anorexia, jaundice, nausea, lethargy). We recommend liver function tests every 6–12 months at most. If liver function tests are done, minor elevations of hepatic enzyme levels up to three times the normal limit should not necessarily lead to stopping the drug. Balancing the apparent clinical benefit to the patient with the abnormality of the liver function tests is reasonable. The better the patient's response, the more one persists in giving valproate in the face of progressively abnormal liver function tests.

Pancreatitis can occur with Depakote after varying lengths of exposure. We have had one case of pancreatitis that occurred after the patient had been taking the drug for more than 1 year. The patient presented with abdominal pain and had elevated serum amylase levels. The reaction abated with drug cessation. The side effect is rare but does occur at a high enough incidence for the clinician to consider.

Weight gain is the most common reason patients discontinue valproate. As many as half of the patients who use valproate chronically experience significant weight gain. Maintaining an adequate diet and exercise regimen is clearly necessary for patients taking valproate. Despite their best efforts, however, many patients find it difficult to control their weight. We have found that the addition of topiramate at dosages of 50–200 mg/day has been an effective anorexiant for many patients and may help with mood stabilization.

Thrombocytopenia and platelet dysfunction have been reported in patients taking valproate. Warning patients to report easy bruising or bleeding is indicated. Platelet levels can be checked periodically, but generally, counts above 75,000/cc do not require anything other than monitoring.

Sedation is among the most common side effects of valproate therapy. As with other medications, shifting more of the dose closer to bedtime will mitigate daytime sedation.

GI upset, the second most common side effect of valproate after weight gain, can take the form of nausea, cramps, emesis, and diarrhea and is dose related. Enteric-coated tablets or divalproex sprinkle capsules help, as do histamine$_2$ blockers (e.g., famotidine [Pepcid] at 20 mg bid). Tremor and ataxia can also occur.

Another side effect, alopecia, is thought to be due to valproate's interference with zinc and selenium deposition. Some clinicians instruct patients to take multivitamins fortified with these two metals; Centrum Silver is a vitamin supplement commonly used for this purpose. If significant alopecia occurs, the valproate should be discontinued. Hair regrowth may take several months.

Coma and death are rare when valproate is taken with suicidal intent. The drug can be removed by hemodialysis. There is also one report that valproate coma was reversed by naloxone.

Another, more recent concern has been the observation that valproic acid may be associated with the development of polycystic ovaries in women. A study of 238 epileptic women found that 43% of patients taking valproic acid had polycystic ovaries and 17% had elevated testosterone levels (Isojarvi et al. 1993). Among the women who started valproic acid before age 20, 80% had polycystic ovaries. Since over 50% of women on valproic acid were also obese, and because obesity is associated with polycystic ovaries, it is unclear whether valproic acid's effects on the high rate of polycystic ovaries are a direct result of the drug or an indirect effect of contributing to obesity. However, in STEP-BD, women with polycystic ovarian syndrome (PCOS) who discontinued their valproate appeared to have significant improvement in PCOS symptoms despite the fact that there was no significant change in weight (Joffe et al. 2006). This suggests that there may be a direct contribution of valproate to PCOS independent of obesity. In addition, some forms of epilepsy appear to be associated with polycystic ovaries, independent of anticonvulsant use. Independent replication of valproate as a cause of polycystic ovaries has not been reported despite hundreds of thousands of patients having been treated. Two recent small surveys suggest rates of about 8%–10% in women treated with the drug, which are slightly higher than the rates (4%–7%) in the general population (Joffe and Cohen 2004). Some child psychiatrists have suggested caution in treating adolescent female bipolar patients with valproate, given the available data on polycystic ovaries (Eberle 1998). Some studies involving women with bipolar disorder who were taking divalproex also have not shown an association with polycystic ovary disease (Rasgon et al. 2004). There has been, however, a suggestion of a relationship to increased testosterone levels in women with bipolar disorder (Rasgon et al. 2004). Most recently, women who were treated with valproate demonstrated significantly more common ovulatory polycystic ovary syndrome and dysfunction than did women treated with lamotrigine (Morrell et al. 2008). It is best to monitor females who are taking valproate for the development of weight gain, hirsutism, menstrual irregularities, and acne.

Drug Interactions

Serious drug interactions are uncommon with valproate. However, the metabolism of valproate is approximately 25% dependent on the cytochrome P450 system. A number of drugs that competitively inhibit various enzymes of the cytochrome P450 system—including cimetidine, the SSRIs, and erythromycin—may be associated with an increase in valproate levels (Table 5–4). Additionally, many nonsteroidal anti-inflammatory agents, including aspirin, may increase free valproate levels. Other drugs, such as carbamazepine and rifampin, have been associated with reducing valproate levels.

Valproate has been associated with an increase in the serum levels of a variety of drugs, including carbamazepine, warfarin, and tolbutamide. These interactions are generally not clinically significant but may require reduced doses of the concurrent medications. Valproate can double the levels of concurrent lamotrigine and increase the risk of rashes. When these two agents are used together, lamotrigine doses are increased very gradually. In rare cases, valproate therapy has been associated with hyperammonemia, with or without encephalopathy, which may occur despite normal hepatic function tests. Concomitant administration of topiramate and valproate may raise this risk. In the package insert, a precaution is issued of the associated risk of hyperammonemia with topiramate use. Moreover, valproate is contraindicated in patients with known urea cycle disorder (e.g., ornithine transcarbamylase deficiency).

Use in Pregnancy

When valproate is taken during the first trimester of pregnancy, neural tube defects can occur (e.g., spina bifida, anencephaly). Thus, valproate should generally be discontinued before anticipated pregnancies. However, if it is necessary to continue valproate because of the significant risk of a disruptive relapse of bipolar illness during pregnancy, the patient should be started on folate, 1 mg/day, early in the pregnancy and an ultrasound should be ordered at 18–20 weeks to assess for fetal abnormalities. During the last 6 weeks of the pregnancy, vitamin K should also be prescribed to decrease the risk of excessive bleeding. Given the risk of relapse in the postpartum period, valproate should generally be restarted after delivery to reduce the risk of relapse.

Reports of lower IQ in children exposed in utero to valproate continue to be published (Vinten et al. 2005; Meador et al. 2009) and are very troubling, and we currently recommend avoiding use of the drug during pregnancy whenever possible.

Table 5–4. Drug interactions of anticonvulsant mood stabilizers

Anticonvulsant	Drugs that may ↑ anticonvulsant levels	Drugs that may ↓ anticonvulsant levels	Drugs whose blood levels ↓ with concurrent anticonvulsant use
valproate	aspirin cimetidine clarithromycin erythromycin fluvoxamine fluoxetine ibuprofen phenothiazines topiramate troleandomycin	carbamazepine ethosuximide oxcarbazepine phenobarbital phenytoin primidone rifampin	zonisamide Clinically significant metabolic induction by other drugs with valproate not reported
carbamazepine	cimetidine ciprofloxacin clarithromycin diltiazem doxycycline erythromycin fluconazole fluoxetine fluvoxamine grapefruit juice isoniazid itraconazole ketoconazole	felbamate phenobarbital rifampin	atypical antipsychotics benzodiazepines doxycycline ethosuximide fentanyl glucocorticoids methadone neuroleptics oral contraceptives phenytoin protease inhibitors TCAs (?) theophylline

Table 5–4. Drug interactions of anticonvulsant mood stabilizers *(continued)*

Anticonvulsant	Drugs that may ↑ anticonvulsant levels	Drugs that may ↓ anticonvulsant levels	Drugs whose blood levels ↓ with concurrent anticonvulsant use
carbamazepine *(continued)*	nefazodone norfloxacin prednisolone propoxyphene protease inhibitors (e.g., ritonavir, indinavir) TCAs troleandomycin valproate verapamil warfarin		
lamotrigine	valproate	carbamazepine ethosuximide oral contraceptives oxcarbazepine phenobarbital phenytoin primidone	valproate
oxcarbazepine			ethinyl estradiol levonorgestrel
topiramate			oral contraceptives

Note.   TCAs = tricyclic antidepressants; ↑ = increase; ↓ = decrease.

Carbamazepine

Carbamazepine was originally synthesized in 1957 and introduced into the European market in the early 1960s as a treatment for epilepsy, particularly epilepsy involving the temporal lobes. Subsequently, it became widely used as a treatment for "tic douloureux"—trigeminal neuralgia. Its use for bipolar disorder stems from the early 1970s when Japanese researchers reported it was effective in many patients with manic-depressive illness, including patients whose condition was refractory to lithium. In 1980, Ballenger and Post reported that carbamazepine was effective in a double-blind crossover trial in patients with acute bipolar disorder. Since that time, many other controlled studies have documented the utility of carbamazepine for acute mania. Kishimoto et al. (1983) reported that it was also effective in maintenance therapy, and a number of controlled studies have subsequently confirmed this finding. However, carbamazepine had never been FDA approved for the treatment of any aspect of bipolar disorder until an extended-release (ER) form of the drug (Equetro) was approved in 2005 for the treatment of acute mania. We tend to regard carbamazepine as a less good initial choice than either valproate, lithium, or an atypical in the treatment of bipolar disorder because of the propensity for pharmacokinetic interactions with carbamazepine.

Carbamazepine has drug-interaction and side-effect profiles that make it more cumbersome to use, and, though well studied, it is still less well studied than either lithium or valproate at this time. Still, there are many patients who do well with carbamazepine who do not have an adequate response to valproate or lithium, and the combination of carbamazepine and another mood stabilizer or atypical antipsychotic is often helpful.

Clinical Indications

There are now multiple controlled studies of carbamazepine in the treatment of acute mania and additional controlled studies on its use as a mood stabilizer in the maintenance treatment of bipolar disorder. The FDA approval of Equetro for the treatment of acute mania and mixed states was based on data from three controlled trials (Owen 2006; Weisler et al. 2006). Many of the earlier studies have been compromised by concurrent neuroleptic or other drug use. Enough clinical evidence exists to justify using carbamazepine in patients with bipolar disorder with a reasonable expectation that a proportion of them—about 50%—will show clear clinical benefit. However, some pa-

Carbamazepine therapy: overview

Efficacy	Acute mania (FDA approved for Equetro only) Mixed, rapid-cycling bipolar (not FDA approved) Seizure disorders (FDA approved)
Side effects	Sedation Dizziness Fatigue and nausea Ataxia
Safety in overdose	Serious symptoms may occur at 10–20 times normal serum levels. Symptoms include nausea, vomiting, CNS depression, respiratory depression, and seizures. Management includes gastric lavage, forced emesis, assisted ventilation.
Dosage and administration	For the XR form: 200 mg bid, to therapeutic range of 800–1,200 mg/day. Follow serum levels to 6–10 µg/mL.
Discontinuation	Carbamazepine has not been associated with a withdrawal syndrome with rapid discontinuation. However, as with other mood stabilizers, rapid discontinuation is associated with an increased risk of rapid relapse. In bipolar patients, decrease dose over 6 months. In nonbipolar patients, dose may be decreased by 25% every 3 days.
Drug interactions	Drugs that may ↑ carbamazepine levels include: cimetidine, ciprofloxacin, diltiazem, fluoxetine, fluvoxamine, doxycycline, erythromycin, fluconazole, grapefruit juice, INH (isoniazid), ketoconazole, macrolide antibiotics (erythromycin, clarithromycin, troleandomycin), nefazodone, norfloxacin, prednisolone, propoxyphene, protease inhibitors (e.g., ritonavir), TCAs, valproate, verapamil, and warfarin Drugs whose blood levels are ↓ by coadministration with carbamazepine include: atypical antipsychotics, benzodiazepines, doxycycline, ethosuximide, fentanyl, glucocorticoids, haloperidol, methadone, oral contraceptives, phenothiazines, phenytoin, sertraline, TCAs, and theophylline

Note. CNS=central nervous system; FDA = U.S. Food and Drug Administration; TCAs = tricyclic antidepressants; XR = extended-release.

tients who derive benefit from carbamazepine have residual symptoms. The drug may work more rapidly than lithium but less rapidly than antipsychotics in acute mania.

Some patients who have a response to carbamazepine improve or stabilize with the drug alone; others do better with carbamazepine plus another mood stabilizer or antipsychotic (see Chapter 9: "Augmentation Strategies for Treatment-Resistant Disorders"). The major problem in assessing the clinical value of a drug like carbamazepine, which is used mainly in treating seriously symptomatic psychiatric patients in whom more standard treatments have failed, is that all other medications are rarely discontinued before the carbamazepine is added. Later, if the patient does well, other preexisting drugs may or may not be tapered and stopped. Clinically, it is often hard to be sure when carbamazepine itself is really working and when prior therapy may finally have begun to work.

Some evidence suggests that carbamazepine works better than lithium in producing stability in rapid-cycling bipolar patients—those with four or more affective episodes a year. Even though there is some preliminary evidence of carbamazepine's superiority to lithium in rapid cycling, it is clear that this bipolar subtype is difficult to treat with any agent. In one major study, patients without rapid-cycling bipolar illness were much more likely to respond to carbamazepine alone than were patients with rapid-cycling bipolar illness (Okuma 1993). Likewise, carbamazepine may be more effective than lithium in the maintenance treatment of patients with mixed episodes or rapid cycling (Greil et al. 1998). Some evidence suggests that carbamazepine is preferentially effective in more severe, paranoid, and angry manic patients than in euphoric, overactive, overtalkative, or overfriendly manic patients. Other potential indications for the drug include continuous-cycling bipolar illness, in which there are no periods of euthymia between bipolar episodes. Overall, the data on predictors of carbamazepine response have been mixed.

Carbamazepine has not been well studied in the treatment of major depression. Several small studies suggested that carbamazepine may be useful in the treatment of bipolar depression, particularly when lithium is added to the regimen. In general, carbamazepine does not appear to be nearly as effective in acute depression as in acute mania. Likewise, some case reports suggest that carbamazepine is effective in the treatment of panic disorder, but there are much better antipanic drugs than carbamazepine, and the only controlled trial yielded negative findings.

A complicating factor in adding carbamazepine to an antipsychotic is that carbamazepine induces liver enzymes and speeds metabolism of some other drugs. Haloperidol levels are clearly lowered substantially. Likewise, carbamazepine is known to induce the metabolism of a number of atypical agents, including olanzapine, risperidone, and clozapine. Levels of other antipsychotics can be checked before and 2–4 weeks after carbamazepine is added to see whether they have changed. Worsening in some patients (and improvement in others) could be attributed to lowering of the neuroleptic blood level rather than to the direct effects of carbamazepine. Similarly, carbamazepine may lower TCA and other antidepressant plasma levels, making such combinations difficult.

Pilot studies of carbamazepine show some promise for this drug in treating violent nonpsychotic patients and patients undergoing alcohol or benzodiazepine withdrawal.

An intriguing study by Cowdry and Gardner (1988) involved patients with BPD who had histories of frequent impulsive acts. In this small but double-blind study, carbamazepine was notable for substantially decreasing impulsivity. The patients' therapists all judged the patients to be much better. The patients, however, did not feel the drug was very effective. In the same study, the patients felt better—but were much more impulsive—while taking alprazolam. Thus, there may be a role for carbamazepine in treating patients with BPD. However, valproate also appears to be helpful in treating patients with BPD and may be easier to use.

Other psychiatric disorders may also be characterized by impulsivity, aggressive outbursts, and affective instability. Patients with posttraumatic stress disorder (PTSD) sometimes have these difficulties, and a number of open-label studies suggest that carbamazepine is useful in treating some of these patients. Carbamazepine has demonstrated utility in the treatment of agitation and violent outbursts associated with dementia. It is possible that carbamazepine is helpful in nephrogenic diabetes insipidus, because it increases vasopressin release. Unfortunately, carbamazepine's ability to effect such an increase is blocked by lithium, making carbamazepine ineffective in lithium-induced polyuria and polydipsia. Carbamazepine can, but rarely does, cause hyponatremia and water intoxication.

Dosage and Administration

Blood levels of carbamazepine should be monitored at least weekly throughout the first 8 weeks of treatment, because the drug induces liver enzymes, which then speed the drug's own metabolism. The blood level established at 3 weeks may decrease by one-third at 6 weeks, even when the carbamazepine dosage is held constant. Starting with 100 mg (one-half tablet) at bedtime is suggested to see whether the patient is oversedated. If the drug is well tolerated, it should be given at a dosage of 100 mg bid on the second day, followed by 200 mg bid for the next few days. A sustained-release form of carbamazepine, Tegretol-XR, is often taken once a day. Serum levels should be obtained twice a week in the first 2 weeks, when possible—always about 12 hours after the last dose.

The dose should be adjusted to maintain a serum level of 4–12 µg/mL. Higher levels are not generally more effective and are often difficult to attain because of hepatic induction. We generally aim for levels in the range of 6–10 µg/mL. Adjusting levels upward means more risk of side effects. The most common signs of excessive carbamazepine blood levels are diplopia, malcoordination, and sedation. Tolerance will also often develop. Moving all or most of the daily dose to bedtime may help mitigate problems with sedation.

Carbamazepine ER (Equetro) is usually started at 400 mg/day in divided doses, and the dosage is then increased by 200 mg/day to a target dosage of around 600–1,200 mg/day. In the pooled bipolar trials, the mean dosage was 707 mg/day. The maximum studied dosage is 1,600 mg/day.

Side Effects

The major concern with the clinical use of carbamazepine is the threat of agranulocytosis or aplastic anemia, both potentially lethal conditions. As is usual with very rare, serious adverse drug reactions, estimates of incidence vary widely, in this cases from 1 in 10,000 patients treated to a more recently estimated 1 in 125,000. There is a growing consensus that frequent monitoring of blood counts is of limited value for patients on carbamazepine therapy. Aplastic anemia, thrombocytopenia, and agranulocytosis occur so rapidly that a daily blood count would be required to detect them. Thus, some experts have taken the position that regular blood counts are unnecessary and that warning the patient and/or significant others to watch for overt symptoms of bone marrow suppression (e.g., fever, bruising, bleeding, sore throat, petechiae) is more cost-effective.

Clinical practice with respect to chlorpromazine, with which agranulocytosis may be more frequent than with carbamazepine, has long been to avoid regular blood counts. With clozapine, with which the rate of agranulocytosis is perhaps 1%–2%, weekly counts have been demanded by the FDA. Obviously, no compelling recommendation is possible with respect to carbamazepine. One compromise would be to get a complete blood count with every carbamazepine blood level.

Once patients have started taking carbamazepine, a surprising number of them show a relative leukopenia, with or without a drop in erythrocytes, during the first few weeks. Approximately 7% of adult patients and 12% of children develop leukopenias while taking carbamazepine (Sobotka et al. 1990). Patients who run low white blood cell counts (WBCs) at baseline appear to be at particular risk for developing significant leukopenias. Drops in WBC (in cells/mm^3) to the low 3,500s are not uncommon. If the differential is normal (more than 1,000 polymorphonuclear leukocytes) and the patient seems to be benefiting from the treatment, carbamazepine can be continued. However, high-risk patients should be monitored frequently in the first 3 months of therapy. After observing a WBC under 3,000 cells/mm^3, the clinician will almost certainly feel a need to get counts more frequently. The availability of consultation with a friendly, interested, helpful hematologist is an asset to clinicians working with drugs such as carbamazepine and clozapine.

The most common side effects of carbamazepine are sedation, fatigue, nausea, and dizziness. At higher doses, ataxia, diplopia, muscle incoordination, and nystagmus may be evident. Overdose of carbamazepine may result in stupor progressing to coma and death.

Carbamazepine also can occasionally cause elevations in liver enzymes, but serious hepatotoxicity is quite rare. γ-Glutamyl transferase (GGT), an index of hepatic activity, is frequently increased (up to 100%) and is typically not a cause for concern unless the level is more than three times the normal level. Carbamazepine shares with TCAs the ability to slow cardiac conduction. Rashes with carbamazepine are probably a bit more common than with other psychiatric drugs; one review estimated a 5% incidence during the initiation of carbamazepine therapy.

Drug Interactions

Carbamazepine can influence the metabolism of a variety of drugs (Table 5–4), a feature that complicates its clinical use. Quite frequently, it is difficult to assess the effect of carbamazepine on concurrent drug therapy.

Carbamazepine is metabolized mostly by the cytochrome P450 3A3/4 enzyme and can be increased by drugs that inhibit this enzyme, including erythromycin, ketoconazole, fluvoxamine, fluoxetine, and calcium channel blockers. Serum carbamazepine levels should be monitored closely with concurrent use of these medications.

In turn, carbamazepine induces the hepatic metabolism of many drugs that are metabolized via the cytochrome P450 enzyme 3A3/4, including steroids, oral contraceptives, TCAs, sertraline, benzodiazepines, and calcium channel blockers. This interaction reduces the serum levels of these drugs and may decrease their efficacy. For some drugs, such as the TCAs, blood levels can be monitored. For most other drugs, monitoring serum levels is not helpful. There is little information about carbamazepine's effects on SSRI levels. There have been cases of oral contraceptive failure with concurrent carbamazepine use, and patients may need higher doses of benzodiazepines or antipsychotics if carbamazepine is used concurrently.

There have been some reports of CNS toxicity associated with the combination of carbamazepine and lamotrigine (Besag et al. 1998). Symptoms have included dizziness and diplopia and appear to be related to changes in the serum level of lamotrigine. Adding lamotrigine to carbamazepine appears to be more problematic than vice versa.

The use of clozapine in combination with carbamazepine is probably ill-advised. Although it is unclear whether the combination substantially increases the risks of leukopenias, other options should be exercised before carbamazepine and clozapine are used together.

Use in Pregnancy

In the past, carbamazepine was believed to be the safest of the anticonvulsants and the mood stabilizers for use during pregnancy. However, it has become evident that carbamazepine is associated with the occurrence of fetal abnormalities of the type seen with hydantoin: an increased incidence of craniofacial defects, fingernail hypoplasia, neural tube defects, and developmental delay. Therefore, carbamazepine should be discontinued, if possible, during the first trimester of pregnancy. As with divalproex sodium, folate supplements may reduce the risk of some of the neural tube effects of carbamazepine.

Carbamazepine does enter the breast milk, and the serum concentrations in the infant may be as high as 15% of the maternal serum level (Brent and Wisner

1998). Although it is unclear what effect this serum level has on a developing infant, breast-feeding should be discouraged unless no reasonable alternative exists.

Lamotrigine

Lamotrigine (Lamictal) had been used for a number of years in Europe before being introduced in the United States. Lamotrigine has an FDA-approved indication for the treatment of partial complex and generalized seizures. In the early 1990s, lamotrigine began to be investigated as a treatment for bipolar disorder when epileptic patients reported an improvement in their general sense of well-being independent of seizure control. While early controlled trials focusing on acute mania failed to show benefit, subsequent trials in the maintenance treatment of bipolar disorder demonstrated that lamotrigine delays the time to a next depressive or manic episode. These trials led to lamotrigine's FDA approval in 2003 as only the second drug, after lithium, indicated for the maintenance treatment of bipolar I disorder to delay the time to occurrence of mood episodes.

Lamotrigine has a variety of pharmacodynamic effects that may explain its mood-stabilizing properties. For example, in addition to decreasing glutamate release, lamotrigine also appears to modulate the reuptake of serotonin and generally blocks the reuptake of monoamines, including dopamine (Xie and Hagan 1998). Despite the evidence that lamotrigine has a profile that may confer antidepressant effects in addition to anticycling effects, the switch rate appears very low in bipolar patients treated with lamotrigine. In fact, the pivotal maintenance trials of lamotrigine in bipolar disorder did not suggest any higher rate of switching than with placebo.

Clinical Indications

Lamotrigine is indicated to delay the onset of new mood episodes in the maintenance treatment of bipolar disorder. Two pivotal studies were completed, involving more that 500 bipolar I patients, that provided evidence of the efficacy of lamotrigine in maintenance treatment. The first started with patients who were hypomanic or manic, whereas the second started with patients in the depressed phase of the illness. Once the patients' acute mood symptoms had resolved, they were randomized to receive either lamotrigine or placebo for 12 months. What these studies demonstrated was that patients receiving the lamotrigine did better longer than the patients receiving placebo. The time to a new episode of depression or mania was delayed in the lamotrigine-treated patients—sometimes as much as twofold—relative to placebo, and this delay was most pronounced for depressive episodes.

Lamotrigine may be useful in other aspects of bipolar disorder. For example, several open-label trials suggested that lamotrigine is effective as an add-on or as monotherapy in patients who had no response to traditional trials of lithium, often in combination with other mood stabilizers (Calabrese et al. 1999a, 1999b; Fogelson and Sternbach 1997; Koek and Yerevanian 1998; Kotler and Matar 1998; Kusumakar and Yatham 1997a, 1997b). Case studies suggest that lamotrigine may be effective in treating rapid cycling and mixed presentations of bipolar disorder (Fatemi et al. 1997; Kusumakar and Yatham 1997a).

In a larger open trial (N=75) involving bipolar patients, Calabrese and colleagues (1999b) found that 48% of patients in a depressive episode had marked improvement in symptoms, while 20% had moderate improvement. In patients in a hypomanic or manic state, 81% had marked improvement while taking lamotrigine. However, in controlled studies (whose results are not yet published), lamotrigine has not proved effective for the treatment of mania.

There is some evidence that lamotrigine may also be effective in the treatment of bipolar depression. In a study by Calabrese and colleagues (1999b), 175 patients with bipolar depression were randomized to either 200 mg of lamotrigine, 50 mg of lamotrigine, or placebo for 7 weeks. Despite the promise of this early trial, four subsequent studies of lamotrigine monotherapy in the treatment of depression failed to show benefit. However, there may be benefit of adding lamotrigine to lithium in bipolar depressed patients. Van der Loos and colleagues (2009) added lamotrigine or placebo to lithium in patients with bipolar depression and found that lamotrigine was superior to placebo in reducing overall Montgomery-Åsberg Depression Rating Scale scores as well as in achieving a 50% reduction in symptoms. Thus, adjunctive lamotrigine would appear to be one additional option in the treatment of bipolar depression.

Lamotrigine has been compared with OFC (Symbyax) in the treatment of bipolar depression. In one trial, lamotrigine monotherapy did not appear as effective as OFC in improving acute bipolar depression (Brown et al. 2006). On the other hand, it was much better tolerated than OFC. In addition, augmenting mood stabilizer–antidepressant combinations with lamotrigine also appeared to be of some benefit relative to adding either risperidone or inositol in one STEP-BD analysis of refractory bipolar depression (Nierenberg et al. 2006b). Finally, as reported earlier in this chapter, lamotrigine is also effective in delaying recurrence of depression and mania in bipolar patients. Thus, lamotrigine became the second drug approved, in 2003, for the maintenance treatment of bipolar disorder. In addition, lamotrigine is not associated with a significant switch to mania or hypomania.

In a crossover study of patients with refractory (mainly) rapid cycling, lamotrigine (52% response rate), but not gabapentin (26% response rate), was more effective than placebo (23% response rate) in reducing symptoms (Frye et al. 2000).

Preliminary evidence suggests that, in addition to its potential use in treating bipolar disorder, lamotrigine may have a role in treating related conditions. Case reports suggest that lamotrigine may be effective in cyclothymia, resistant unipolar depression, schizoaffective disorder (Erfurth et al. 1998a, 1998b), and even BPD (Pinto and Akiskal 1998).

Side Effects

Lamotrigine, when dosed conservatively, appears to be generally well tolerated by most patients. In fact, compared with other available approved maintenance treatments in bipolar disorder, lamotrigine is the least likely to be associated with weight gain (Sachs et al. 2006) or cognitive side effects. However, a black box warning in the PDR indicates that lamotrigine is associated with an increased risk of rash in up to 10% of patients. More concerning is the risk of serious skin reactions, which occur in 1 in 1,000 adults and 1 in 100 children. These serious rashes, which include Stevens-Johnson syndrome, may be fatal. Our general recommendation is that patients be well informed about the risk of rashes. We provide patients with a list of antigen precautions. For example, in the first 3 months of treatment, we recommend avoiding new food or new deodorants, detergents, cosmetics, fabric softeners, and so forth. Also, patients should be advised to avoid excessive sun exposure early in treatment. Furthermore, anyone with a rash accompanied by systemic symptoms such as fever or discomfort in the mouth, eye, or bladder should be instructed to discontinue the lamotrigine and go into the emergency room for evaluation. Patients without systemic symptoms should be advised to see a dermatologist immediately. The risk of rash appears to be increased when the dose of lamotrigine is titrated too rapidly or when lamotrigine is added to valproate, which doubles the serum level of lamotrigine. In addition, patients who develop a rash while taking lamotrigine may well have a recurrence of the rash when rechallenged with the drug (Buzan and Dubovsky 1998).

Common side effects include (in order of frequency) dizziness, headache, double vision, unsteadiness, sedation, and uncomplicated rash. These symptoms occur in over 10% of treated patients, appear to be dose related, and may improve over time. There have been reports that lamotrigine may, perhaps because of its serotonergic properties, decrease libido and delay orgasm in both men and women. It is unclear if any of the antidotes regarding SSRIs reported in Chapter 3 ("Antidepressants") will help with lamotrigine-induced sexual dysfunction. Weight gain appears less common with lamotrigine than with lithium or valproate.

Overdoses can be serious and have been associated with the ingestion of 5 g or more of lamotrigine at one time. Symptoms of overdose can include delirium, periorbital edema, generalized erythema, hepatitis, and renal failure (Briassoulis et al. 1998; Mylonakis et al. 1999). The management of overdose includes gastric lavage and supportive care.

Dosage and Administration

Lamotrigine is typically started at 25 mg/day for the first week, and the dosage is typically increased by 25–50 mg every 2 weeks. If the patient is currently taking valproate, the lamotrigine should be started at 12.5 mg/day and increased to 25 mg/day by the end of the third week. Thereafter, the dosage should be increased by no more than 12.5–25 mg every 2 weeks. Most of the bipolar disorder studies have had a target dosage of around 200 mg/day. We have certainly seen bipolar and unipolar patients who appear to do well with dosages of 50–100 mg/day . However, maximum dosages for lamotrigine may be as high as 500 mg/day.

No clear association between serum levels of lamotrigine and response exists. Thus, routine monitoring of serum levels is not advised. However, in one small case series involving lamotrigine in treating schizoaffective disorder, serum levels greater than 10 mg/L were associated with a greater response than were lower levels.

Like all mood stabilizers, lamotrigine should be gradually tapered rather than abruptly discontinued if possible. Although no discontinuation syndromes have been reported to date with lamotrigine, seizures are occasionally reported with the abrupt discontinuation of any anticonvulsant.

Drug Interactions

As noted earlier, the primary interactions with lamotrigine are a doubling of serum levels with the addition of valproate and a reduction of at least 25% of serum levels in conjunction with carbamazepine. Likewise, phenobarbital and primidone decrease serum levels of lamotrigine by about 40%. Thus, higher doses of lamotrigine may be needed with carbamazepine, primidone, and phenobarbital, while the dose of lamotrigine should be cut in half with concurrent valproate. In addition lamotrigine appears to reduce serum levels of valproate by about 25%.

Valproate appears to increase lamotrigine levels; hence, the more conservative dosing strategy when a patient is taking it. One report indicated that sertraline can substantially increase lamotrigine levels and lead to lamotrigine toxicity (Kaufman and Gerner 1998). Sertraline's inhibition of lamotrigine glucuronidation was suspected, and lamotrigine levels were increased by 25% with just 25 mg of sertraline. At this time, it is advisable to adjust the starting and maintenance doses of lamotrigine downward with concurrent use of sertraline.

Alcohol theoretically can exacerbate the sedation associated with lamotrigine. Interactions with over-the-counter drugs are not known.

Use in Pregnancy

Lamotrigine is a category C teratogen. Animal studies suggest the possibility of fetal abnormalities, but human studies do not exist. As with other agents, the known risks of discontinuing the drug for a pregnant patient should be assessed along with the unknown risk of continuing taking it. At this time, most patients would be advised to discontinue the drug before conception if possible.

Other Anticonvulsants

Several other anticonvulsants have become available in recent years that, as with valproate, carbamazepine, and lamotrigine, are being explored in treating bipolar disorder and other psychiatric conditions (Table 5–5). Gabapentin has been well studied in bipolar disorder and generally has been an ineffective albeit benign treatment. In addition, preliminary studies have been done on oxcarbazepine, topiramate, and tiagabine in the treatment of bipolar disorder, with variable results. In contrast, almost no data exist on the psychiatric benefits

Table 5–5. New anticonvulsants

	pregabalin (Lyrica)	oxcarbazepine (Trileptal)	gabapentin (Neurontin)	lamotrigine (Lamictal)	topiramate (Topamax)	tiagabine (Gabitril)
Serum plasma level, ng/mL	NA	NA	NA	NA	NA	1–234
Adult dosage, mg/day	150–600 300–450 mg/day given in divided doses (for fibromyalgia) 150–300 mg/day given in divided doses (for neuropathic pain)	600–2,400	900–2,400 (for seizure maintenance treatment)	300–500 (for seizure maintenance treatment) 200 (for bipolar disorder monotherapy) 100 (concurrently with valproate for bipolar disorder) 400 (concurrently with carbamazepine or other enzyme-inducing drugs [and not taking valproate] for bipolar disorder)	200–400 (for seizure maintenance treatment) 100 mg/day given in two divided doses (for migraine prophylaxis)	4–32
Protein binding	—	40% bound	Minimally bound (<3%)	55% bound	20% bound	96% bound
Half-life, hours	—	2–9	5–7	25–32	20–30	7–9
Metabolic pathway		Hepatic CYP 3A enzyme	Drug not appreciably metabolized hepatically	Glucuronidation/ conjugation	20% metabolized hepatically	Oxidation/ glucuronidation

Table 5–5. New anticonvulsants *(continued)*

	pregabalin (Lyrica)	oxcarbazepine (Trileptal)	gabapentin (Neurontin)	lamotrigine (Lamictal)	topiramate (Topamax)	tiagabine (Gabitril)
Routes of elimination	—	Renal (95%); fecal (5%)	Renal	Renal	Renal	Urinary (25%); fecal (63%)
Common drug interactions	No significant drug interactions are known; antacids decrease absorption and bioavailability of pregabalin	Induces metabolism of CYP 3A3/4–dependent drugs (weaker than carbamazepine); decreases levels of phenobarbital, phenytoin, sex steroids, haloperidol, valproic acid, calcium channel blockers, and others (see Table 5–4)	No significant drug interactions are known; antacids decrease bioavailability of gabapentin by 20%; cimetidine decreases renal clearance by 13%	Valproate doubles serum levels; carbamazepine decreases serum levels by 50%; phenytoin decreases serum levels by 50%	Phenobarbital decreases serum levels by 40%; carbamazepine decreases topiramate levels by 50%–60%; valproate decreases topiramate levels by 15%; phenytoin decreases topiramate levels by 48%	Carbamazepine decreases tiagabine levels; phenytoin decreases tiagabine levels; tiagabine decreases valproate levels

Table 5–5. New anticonvulsants (*continued*)

	pregabalin (Lyrica)	oxcarbazepine (Trileptal)	gabapentin (Neurontin)	lamotrigine (Lamictal)	topiramate (Topamax)	tiagabine (Gabitril)
Common adverse effects	Somnolence, dizziness, ataxia, fatigue	Dizziness, drowsiness, ataxia, weight gain	Somnolence, dizziness, fatigue, ataxia	Rash: 1 of 10 (serious rashes, such as Stevens-Johnson syndrome: 1 of 1,000), dizziness, ataxia, nausea, vomiting	Psychomotor slowing, decreased concentration, somnolence, fatigue, anorexia, kidney stone formation	Dizziness, depression, asthenia, nervousness, tremors, somnolence, cognitive deficits
Indication (FDA approved)	Partial seizures Postherpetic neuralgia Fibromyalgia Neuropathic pain associated with diabetic neuropathy	Partial complex seizures	Partial seizures Postherpetic neuralgia	Partial seizures Maintenance treatment of bipolar I disorder	Epilepsy Prophylaxis of migraine headaches	Epilepsy

Note. CYP = cytochrome P450; FDA = U.S. Food and Drug Administration; NA = not applicable.
Source. Adapted for the most part from 2002 black book.

of anticonvulsants such as ethosuximide, levetiracetam, and zonisamide at the time of this writing.

Gabapentin and Pregabalin

Gabapentin (Neurontin) was released in the United States in 1994 as an adjunctive treatment for focal seizures. In animal models, gabapentin appeared to have anxiolytic properties and, as with other anticonvulsants, began to be examined in the treatment of bipolar disorder. The mechanism of action for gabapentin was once thought to be via increasing GABA levels in the brain, but the mode by which it accomplishes this increase, if it does so, is still not elucidated. Gabapentin does seem to affect calcium channels, and this may be important in its anticonvulsant and analgesic properties. Gabapentin, and its chemical cousin pregabalin, have been more promising in the treatment of anxiety disorders than in the treatment of mood disorders. Both pregabalin and gabapentin are known to bind to the α_2-δ subunit of a voltage-gated calcium channel in the brain and spinal cord. The result is to reduce the flow of calcium into the axon during depolarization and thus reduce neurotransmitter release from that neuron. Pregabalin has been approved in the treatment of epilepsy, fibromyalgia, and neuropathic pain and is under review for the treatment of generalized anxiety disorder (GAD). The studies showing benefit of pregabalin in GAD appear compelling, and pregabalin might ultimately be approved for this anxiety disorder. Pregabalin's advantage is that it has more predictable absorption and, thus, blood levels than does gabapentin.

Clinical indications.   As with all the anticonvulsants used in psychiatry except divalproex sodium and lamotrigine, the only FDA-approved indication for gabapentin and pregabalin had been adjunct treatment of patients with complex partial seizures. Both drugs are approved for use in pain conditions.

Soon after its release, however, reports began to emerge that gabapentin might be useful for a variety of psychiatric and nonpsychiatric conditions. Much of the psychiatric investigation of gabapentin over the past 7 years has focused on its role in the treatment of bipolar disorder. The very benign side-effect and drug-interaction profiles of gabapentin made it a potentially attractive alternative to other mood stabilizers. However, much of the data on gabapentin in bipolar disorder is anecdotal, and more rigorous studies suggested that gabapentin has modest mood-stabilizing effects.

A number of open-label studies, most of which are small, suggest a modest role for gabapentin in bipolar disorder. These studies suggest that gabapentin, typically in dosages of 900–2,700 mg/day, may help with bipolar depression, mixed states, mania, and hypomania (Letterman and Markowitz 1999).

Data from double-blind studies are much more limited. One study at NIMH (Frye et al. 2000) examined the efficacy of gabapentin in a small group of patients with treatment-resistant bipolar disorder; over 6 weeks, 26% of the patients taking gabapentin, compared with 23% of the patients receiving placebo, had a response. Unfortunately, more definite controlled studies of gabapentin as an add-on to lithium or valproic acid done by Parke-Davis showed that gabapentin was no more effective than placebo (Pande et al. 2000). Upward adjustment of the lithium dose in the placebo group may have obscured an effect for the drug.

What one can draw from the gabapentin studies to date is that the mood-stabilizing effects of gabapentin are modest to negligible. Gabapentin may help somewhat with the depressive and manic phases of bipolar disorder, and it tends to be well tolerated. However, the use of gabapentin as a monotherapy for the treatment of mania or rapid cycling does not appear to be justified.

The role of gabapentin in treating anxiety disorders may be greater than its role in treating bipolar disorder. Case reports and double-blind studies support a possible role for gabapentin in anxiety disorders, particularly social phobia and panic disorder. In a randomized, controlled trial, Pande and colleagues (1999) found that gabapentin, at dosages of 900–3,600 mg/day, was superior to placebo in the treatment of 69 patients with social phobia. However, the difference in response to gabapentin relative to placebo, though statistically significant, was not dramatic. Still, gabapentin appears to be a well-tolerated option for some patients with social anxiety disorder. Gabapentin may also prove to be a useful add-on for patients getting only a partial response to antidepressants in the treatment of social phobia.

In contrast, pregabalin is fairly well studied in anxiety disorders but, on the basis of the experience of gabapentin, is not being actively studied in bipolar disorder. Pregabalin at dosages ranging from 300 to 600 mg/day appear to be as effective as a benzodiazepine in the treatment of GAD but without the risk of dependence (Frampton and Foster 2006). Pregabalin is also being investigated in other anxiety disorders such as social anxiety disorder.

Another psychiatric use of gabapentin may be in the treatment of neuroleptic-induced movement disorders. Hardoy et al. (1999) found that 14 of 16 patients with various mood disorders who had tardive dyskinesia improved with the addition of gabapentin at dosages above 900 mg/day. Blepharospasms and oral mandibular dyskinesias appeared to improve with the addition of gabapentin.

Finally, small case series suggest that gabapentin might help mitigate symptoms of withdrawal from cocaine and alcohol (Chatterjee and Ringold 1999; Letterman and Markowitz 1999; Myrick et al. 1998).

Gabapentin and pregabalin are now commonly used in the treatment of neuropathic pain conditions. A number of studies, including several double-blind studies, attest to the efficacy of gabapentin in improving pain associated with trigeminal neuralgia (Carrazana and Schacter 1998), postherpetic neuralgia (Coleman and Stadel 1999; Rowbotham 1998), and diabetic neuropathy (Backonja et al. 1998; Gorson et al. 1999; Morello et al. 1999). It has also been suggested that gabapentin is helpful in migraine prophylaxis (D'Andrea et al. 1999; Lampl et al. 1999).

In 2007, pregabalin became the first drug approved for the treatment of fibromyalgia (duloxetine was subsequently approved). Studies of pregabalin in the treatment of fibromyalgia suggest that the drug improves pain, sleep, and anxiety but not depressed mood in these patients (Häuser et al. 2009).

Side effects.   Gabapentin and pregabalin are generally well tolerated. The most common side effects of both gabapentin and pregabalin leading to discontinuation of the drug are somnolence and dizziness. The extent of these symptoms can be mitigated by administering a larger percentage of the drug at night.

Other possible adverse effects associated with both gabapentin and pregabalin include ataxia, tremor, nausea, double vision, and headache. Pregabalin may be associated with more weight gain than gabapentin. It is our experience that these side effects tend to be dose related, mild, and manageable. If possible, a lower dose should be attempted before the drug is discontinued. The headache often responds to nonsteroidal anti-inflammatory drugs and tends to improve with time. Patients can gain weight while taking gabapentin, but, apparently, weight gain is much less than with most other potential mood stabilizers. Sexual side effects appear to be uncommon.

Neither gabapentin nor pregabalin is appreciably metabolized by the liver, and both are excreted largely unchanged. Thus, both drugs can be used by patients with advanced liver disease.

No completed suicides have been reported to date with gabapentin or pregabalin doses alone. Overdoses have not typically been associated with significant adverse effects other than somnolence.

Drug interactions. No serious drug interactions have been reported with gabapentin or pregabalin. Neither gabapentin nor pregabalin appears to inhibit cytochrome P450 enzymes to any degree and does not appear to alter the kinetics of lithium or additional anticonvulsants. Antacids can reduce the bioavailability of gabapentin and pregabalin by 20%, so these agents should not be taken simultaneously with gabapentin. Alcohol and other CNS depressants, theoretically, can increase the somnolence and cognitive effects associated with gabapentin and pregabalin.

Use in pregnancy. Gabapentin and pregabalin are category C drugs, and their teratogenic effects in pregnancy have not been well studied. In rats exposed to much higher relative doses than are typically used in patients, gabapentin appeared to inhibit bone ossification in fetal pups. Neural tube defects do not appear to be common. As with all anticonvulsants, the risks of discontinuing the gabapentin have to be weighed against the largely unknown risk of continuing to take the drug during pregnancy. When possible, the gabapentin should be discontinued before conception or in the first trimester in most patients until additional data are available on the safety of the drug in pregnancy.

Dosage and administration. Gabapentin is usually started at 300 mg at night. If tolerated, the dose can be increased to 300 mg bid the next day. For some anxiety conditions, we start at 300 mg bid or tid. If the patient complains of excessive somnolence or dizziness, most of the dose can be given at night to a maximum dose of 1,200 mg taken at one time. Doses higher than 1,200 mg at one time are not well absorbed. To maximize compliance, we suggest sticking with bid dosing up to 1,200 mg bid. Thereafter, tid dosing will be necessary up to dosages of 3,600 mg/day. Some patients do quite well at dosages in the range of 900 to 2,400 mg/day. For patients being treated for pain, the dosage is often titrated up to as high as 3,600 mg/day.

Pregabalin is usually started at a dosage of 75 mg twice daily, and the dosage is increased to a maximum of 450 mg/day in divided doses (bid or tid regimen). After a week, the dosage may be increased to 150 mg twice daily. The target dosage of 300–450 mg/day is the same for GAD as it is for epilepsy and fibromyalgia. Dosages up to 600 mg/day have been studied but are not necessarily more effective than lower dosages. Patients with postherpetic neuralgia and neuropathic pain associated with diabetes often benefit from 150–300 mg/day.

Topiramate

Topiramate was FDA approved in 1998 and has the unique property among potential mood stabilizers of being associated with weight loss rather than weight gain in 20%–50% of patients on the drug. A few preliminary reports suggest that topiramate may have mood-stabilizing effects as an adjunctive therapy in bipolar disorder, cyclothymia, and schizoaffective disorder (Gordon and Price 1999; Stephen et al. 1998). Unfortunately, none of the four double-blind trials conducted showed any benefit of topiramate in the treatment of mania, mixed states, or any other aspect of bipolar disorder (Kushner et al. 2006). Open trials and case series have suggested that the addition of topiramate to a standard mood stabilizer might help in the treatment of rapid cycling and co-morbid alcohol abuse and comorbid aggression in bipolar patients. Topiramate may also help with substance abuse problems independent of bipolar disorder.

Perhaps the most common use of topiramate in current clinical practice is as an anorexiant to mitigate weight gain associated with other mood-stabilizing agents such as olanzapine. In one prospective study, the addition of topiramate to olanzapine for 1 year seems to have mitigated the expected weight gain from olanzapine (Vieta et al. 2004). Another controlled trial has suggested that patients with bipolar disorder and concurrent binge eating disorder benefit from the addition of topiramate to lithium (Kotwal et al. 2006). Even in nonpsychiatric patients, topiramate seems to promote weight loss in many patients. Weight loss of up to 25 kg in 6 months has been reported in patients who started topiramate in addition to their mood stabilizer. In our experience, 50 mg/day is often an optimal dosage of topiramate to help with weight loss.

The most common side effects of topiramate are somnolence, paresthesias, dizziness, vision problems, anorexia, and cognitive problems. The cognitive side effects are the most troublesome, with some patients reporting dullness or memory problems. These effects generally occur at dosages greater than 100 mg/day, but we have seen them persist in an older patient even with dosage reduction to 25 mg/day. The side effects of the drug will remit in such cases with cessation.

Discontinuation of topiramate occurs most commonly secondary to psychomotor slowing, memory problems, fatigue, and sedation. There is an increased risk of kidney stone formation with topiramate, particularly when the patient is on a ketogenic diet and/or taking a carbonic anhydrase inhibitor. Patients should be instructed to drink plenty of water.

Hyperchloremic metabolic acidosis is also a theoretical side effect that we have not observed. The risk of developing this condition may be enhanced by concomitant use of carbonic anhydrase inhibitors (e.g., acetazolamide), renal disease, diarrhea, and so forth. Monitoring of serum bicarbonate during topiramate treatment is recommended.

Drugs with which topiramate interacts include carbamazepine and valproate, which reduce topiramate blood levels by 50% and 15%, respectively. Conversely, topiramate can lower valproate levels by about 15%. Alcohol appears to potentiate the somnolence and ataxia associated with topiramate.

Topiramate is usually initiated at a dosage of 12.5–25 mg/day, and the dosage is usually increased by 25 mg per week. Dosages as low as 50 mg/day have anecdotally been added to standard mood stabilizers or olanzapine to counteract weight gain associated with these agents. We have found this to be a helpful strategy at 50–150 mg/day. For mood effects, the average dosages have been 100–200 mg/day given in divided doses. The usual maximum dosage of topiramate is 400 mg/day.

Tiagabine

Tiagabine was FDA approved for the treatment of epilepsy in 1998 and appears to have GABA reuptake blocking properties. It may have anxiolytic properties in animal models. However, phase III trials conducted by Cephalon in GAD patients failed to show benefit of tiagabine in this population. In one small case series, the addition of tiagabine appeared to help three patients with treatment-resistant bipolar disorder (Kaufman and Gerner 1998). In another open study of acute mania, tiagabine was rapidly loaded and was found to be ineffective and poorly tolerated (Grunze et al. 1999b). In this small series, one patient had a seizure that was probably related to the higher starting dose of tiagabine. Likewise, in an open case series of tiagabine in refractory bipolar disorder, tiagabine was poorly tolerated and not particularly effective (Suppes et al. 2002). At this time, there does not appear to be much evidence supporting the utility of tiagabine in either acute treatment of manic symptoms or maintenance treatment of bipolar disorder (Young et al. 2006a, 2006b). In addition, the tolerability of tiagabine has been problematic. Common side effects of tiagabine include dose-related somnolence, dizziness, syncope, and nausea. Tiagabine is usually started at a dosage of 4 mg/day, and the dosage is increased by 4–8 mg per week. The maximum dosage of tiagabine is 56 mg/day given in two to four divided doses.

Oxcarbazepine

Oxcarbazepine (Trileptal) is chemically related to carbamazepine and was introduced in the United States in 2000. Oxcarbazepine has been used in Europe for many years, and its use in treating bipolar disorder dates at least to the early 1980s. However, few studies have examined the efficacy of oxcarbazepine in bipolar disorder. Controlled studies in pediatric bipolar populations have not found oxcarbazepine particularly efficacious (MacMillan et al. 2006; Wagner et al. 2006). The few small studies and case reports available suggest that oxcarbazepine is effective as an add-on therapy in the treatment of acute mania and perhaps other aspects of bipolar disorder (Emrich 1990; Pratoomsri et al. 2006). Randomized comparison trials of oxcarbazepine added to lithium suggest that oxcarbazepine is about as effective as valproate add-on (Suppes et al. 2007) and may be better tolerated than carbamazepine (Juruena et al. 2009). However, limited placebo-controlled studies have not demonstrated clear efficacy of oxcarbazepine in bipolar disorder (Vieta et al. 2008). We have used oxcarbazepine in treating bipolar patients who could not tolerate carbamazepine or with whom we were concerned about drug interactions. As with carbamazepine, we have sometimes used oxcarbazepine to treat agitation.

The primary advantages of oxcarbazepine over its chemical analog, carbamazepine, may be that it is better tolerated, does not tend to autoinduce its own metabolism, and has somewhat less significant drug interactions. Importantly, oxcarbazepine has not had the tendency to induce blood dyscrasias, such as aplastic anemia, that are occasionally reported with carbamazepine.

Oxcarbazepine is often a milder inducer of the cytochrome 3A3/4 enzyme compared with carbamazepine. Still, oxcarbazepine can render oral contraceptives less effective and reduce serum levels of valproate, phenytoin, and other drugs. Thus, it is important to advise patients who are taking oral contraceptives that they may need to switch to a higher-potency oral contraceptive or to supplement the pill with a barrier method.

The major disadvantage of oxcarbazepine is cost. Generic carbamazepine is inexpensive. Oxcarbazepine is not. Oxcarbazepine is usually started at around 300 mg bid, and the dosage is increased gradually up to 2,400 mg/day. In the clinical trials of oxcarbazepine in bipolar disorder, the average dosage in most studies was 600–1,200 mg/day. Our experience is that the dosages of oxcarbazepine required to treat psychiatric symptoms are about 50% higher than those for carbamazepine.

Levetiracetam, Zonisamide, and Ethosuximide

With the sudden availability of many anticonvulsants on the market, there has been an interest in the potential role of these newer agents in bipolar and other psychiatric disorders. Levetiracetam is a rather benign anticonvulsant with a good side-effect profile. At the highest doses, some patients experience somnolence and fatigue, but levetiracetam appears to be fairly weight neutral and has not been associated with much in the way of cognitive or sexual side effects. Dosages of 500 mg bid to 1,500 mg bid have been said to be effective in a few case reports and a small open study in the treatment of mania and depression with few side effects (Post et al. 2005). However, there is no convincing evidence of the drug's utility in bipolar disorder at this time, and our limited clinical experience with the drug has not been consistent with robust benefits. Likewise, zonisamide at dosages of 100–600 mg/day has been reported to improve manic and depressive symptoms as an adjunctive treatment (Ghaemi et al. 2006b, 2008). In addition, zonisamide, like topiramate, may have utility as an adjunctive treatment to control weight gain in bipolar patients (Wang et al. 2008). We have also found that zonisamide 200–400 mg/day, like topiramate, can facilitate weight loss in bipolar patients. However, zonisamide has also been associated with worsening mood symptoms in some patients (McElroy et al. 2005). In fact, a placebo-controlled trial demonstrating the efficacy of zonisamide in bipolar disorder has yet to be published as of this writing. Ethosuximide might also have a role as an anorexiant, but its role in bipolar disorder has not been evaluated. None of these anticonvulsants can be justified as a monotherapy in the treatment of any phase of bipolar disorder at this time, but they may have a role as an adjunctive treatment in some bipolar patients.

Antipsychotics

Antipsychotic drugs have long been recognized as important agents in treating acute mania (see Chapter 4: "Antipsychotic Drugs"). Chlorpromazine was the second drug approved for acute mania after lithium. Since all the standard mood stabilizers (lithium, valproate, carbamazepine) require monitoring, have slow onsets of action, and are not as helpful during the depressed phase of the illness, the atypical antipsychotics are becoming more commonly used as "mood stabilizers." In fact, much of the use of atypical antipsychotics is already in the treatment of mood disorders. Olanzapine has more FDA indications in the treatment of bipolar disorder than does lithium. Olanzapine has long been approved for acute mania and was more recently approved for use in the maintenance treatment of bipolar and the acute treatment of bipolar depression (in combination with fluoxetine). Compared with lithium and carbamazepine, antipsychotics tend to work more rapidly in controlling the excitement, agitation, thought disorder, and psychosis that may accompany acute mania. However, even in contexts in which psychotic symptoms are not present, the antipsychotics work at least as well as lithium in acute mania and perhaps even better. Like olanzapine, the other SGAs are also proving to be more versatile than agents such as lithium and valproate in treating different aspects of bipolar disorder.

Olanzapine was FDA approved for the treatment of acute mania in 2000 and, in 2003, for maintenance therapy. For several years, there were case reports suggesting that olanzapine is effective in mixed states (Ketter et al. 1998; Zullino and Baumann 1999), bipolar depression (Weisler et al. 1997), and acute mania (Ravindran et al. 1997). A pivotal double-blind study of 139 manic bipolar patients indicated that 48% of patients responded to olanzapine, whereas only half that number responded to placebo (Tohen et al. 1999). Olanzapine was well tolerated in these patients. There are now multiple positive trials of olanzapine in acute mania. There are two comparison trials with valproate in acute mania (Tohen et al. 2003a; Zajecka et al. 2002). In both, olanzapine produced better efficacy, although in only the larger study (Tohen et al. 2003a) did the difference reach statistical significance. Olanzapine appeared to produce more side effects. Sporadic reports suggest that olanzapine may induce hypomania or mania in some patients (Lindenmayer and Klebanov 1998; Reeves et al. 1998). However, it has become evident that olanzapine and other atypicals probably do not result in switching to mania commonly and have a role to play in the long-term maintenance of bipolar disorder. Olanzapine alone also appears to do better than placebo in treating bipolar depression, but the combination with fluoxetine is even more effective (Tohen et al. 2003b). However, the combination of olanzapine and an SSRI is more effective than olanzapine alone (see Chapter 9, "Augmentation Strategies for Treatment-Resistant Disorders").

Virtually all of the current atypical antipsychotic agents except clozapine have had at least two double-blind studies (e.g., Keck et al. 2003a, 2003b) that indicated the drugs were effective in the treatment of acute mania. Quetiapine, ziprasidone, risperidone, and aripiprazole are all approved for the treatment of acute mania. While olanzapine appears to be effective in delaying the time to a new mood episode in bipolar I patients, some patients will not tolerate chronic treatment with olanzapine. Weight gain or metabolic concerns will be an issue for some patients. Aripiprazole has also demonstrated efficacy in the maintenance treatment of bipolar disorder and is an alternative to olanzapine for some patients. In addition the atypicals have proved helpful in the treatment of acute bipolar depression.

Olanzapine was first approved in combination with fluoxetine for the treatment of bipolar depression, and in 2006, quetiapine also obtained approval as a monotherapy for the treatment of acute bipolar depression. More recently, the OFC combination was approved for the treatment of resistant unipolar depression (see Chapter 3, "Antidepressants"). Both ziprasidone and aripiprazole continue to be explored in the treatment of bipolar depression, and it would not be particularly surprising if both of these drugs prove equal to quetiapine and olanzapine in this regard. Likewise, virtually all of the atypicals are being investigated in the maintenance treatment of bipolar disorder. It is evident that the atypical antipsychotics will play an increasingly large role in the treatment of bipolar disorder relative to the anticonvulsants or other classes of agents.

Although clozapine is without pivotal trials in bipolar disorder, it should be considered in the treatment of some bipolar patients. Clozapine appears to be effective in the treatment of patients with more refractory bipolar disorder, including the rapid-cycling subtype and bipolar disorder accompanied by psychosis (Green et al. 2000; Kimmel et al. 1994; Suppes et al. 1994). The toxicity of clozapine relegates it to use as a third-line treatment when standard agents have failed.

Among the new SGAs, asenapine was approved in 2009 for the treatment of acute mania and mixed states in adults with bipolar I disorder (see Chapter 4, "Antipsychotics"). Two 3-week randomized, placebo-controlled studies indicated superiority of asenapine over placebo (Citrome 2009). There is no evidence of asenapine's having superior efficacy relative to other SGAs. However, it does cause less weight gain than do clozapine and quetiapine. Iloperidone should also be useful in the treatment of bipolar disorder; however, there are no published data on this potential application.

Benzodiazepines

Several benzodiazepines, chiefly clonazepam and lorazepam, have been reported to be useful in the treatment of acute mania. It was initially believed that clonazepam might have antimanic properties unique among the benzodiazepines. However, it has become increasingly clear that this is probably not the case. All the benzodiazepines appear to have a role in treating the hyperkinesis, agitation, and insomnia associated with acute mania. Chouinard and associates in Montreal had done much of the key work with clonazepam in mania (see, e.g., Chouinard et al. 1983). Reports suggested that clonazepam might be useful as an adjunct to lithium or neuroleptics in the treatment of acute mania. However, Bradwejn and colleagues (1990) found that clonazepam did not appear to be efficacious in the treatment of acute mania and was inferior to lorazepam in this regard. Salzman and colleagues (1991) reported that lorazepam 2 mg im was as effective in reducing aggression and agitation in psychotic patients as haloperidol 5 mg im. Lorazepam's effects appeared to be independent of its sedative properties. Lorazepam was better tolerated than was haloperidol. No evidence up to this time has supported the use of a benzodiazepine alone for the maintenance treatment of bipolar disorder. The one study that used clonazepam alone for prophylaxis was stopped early because all the enrolled subjects had relapsed within 3 months while taking the medication.

Experience with clonazepam in the treatment of acute mania has been that it tends to lead to sedated manic patients whose mania is unchanged when the sedation wears off. We have not been impressed with the antimanic versus sedating properties of clonazepam. When a bipolar patient requires an agent for sleep, anxiety, or catatonia, clonazepam or the other benzodiazepines should be considered. Clonazepam was among the most expensive benzodiazepines, and its only advantage over agents like lorazepam may be its long half-life.

The dosages of clonazepam typically employed are 1–6 mg/day, although much higher dosages were used in the original studies. Lorazepam dosages are similar, ranging from 1.5 to 8 mg/day.

The side effects of clonazepam and lorazepam are those of all current benzodiazepines: sedation, ataxia, and malcoordination. With any sedative drug, in rare cases patients become disinhibited and agitated. Patients with a history of attention-deficit/hyperactivity disorder in childhood may be at particular risk for sedative-induced angry agitation. We have seen occasional bipolar patients who reported feeling more angry after taking clonazepam. No prospective data on this potential side effect are available.

Calcium Channel Blockers

The calcium channel blockers, which include verapamil, nifedipine, diltiazem, and a number of newer agents, are used primarily in the treatment of hypertension, angina, and supraventricular arrhythmias. Dysregulation of intracellular calcium may be involved in some affective disorders, and this notion prompted Dubovsky and colleagues to begin studying the efficacy of calcium channel blockers in treating bipolar patients (Dubovsky et al. 1982). Since then, a number of studies have suggested that calcium channel blockers may have antimanic properties. Most of these studies were uncontrolled and small, and interpretation of their findings was complicated by other drug use.

There is no evidence that patients whose condition is resistant to lithium or the anticonvulsants are any more likely to respond to the calcium channel antagonists. On the contrary, patients who are unresponsive to the standard agents appear likely to be unresponsive to calcium channel agents as well. There may, however, be instances in which the calcium channel blockers are worth considering in the treatment of a bipolar patient. For example, bipolar patients with cardiovascular problems (such as supraventricular arrhythmias and hypertension) that may be helped by a calcium channel blocker might be assessed for antimanic effect while taking these drugs to determine whether they could be substituted for standard mood-stabilizing agents. Likewise, a calcium channel blocker may be worth trying with a pregnant bipolar patient, because the teratogenic risk of this category of drugs appears to be substantially lower than that of any of the standard agents. The most common side effects of the calcium channel blockers are dizziness, headache, and nausea.

More serious side effects, which are rare, include malignant arrhythmias, hepatotoxicity, and severe hypotension and syncope. The calcium channel blockers can produce orthostasis in elderly patients and may have an additive hypotensive effect when used with other antihypertensive drugs. At high doses, anergy and somnolence are sometimes reported.

Dosing for the calcium channel blockers in treating bipolar illness is not well defined. Most investigators have used the typical doses used for cardiovascular indications. Verapamil has been the most studied agent in its class. The usual starting dosage in treating hypertension is 80 mg bid or tid, up to a maximum dosage of 480 mg/day. An alternative strategy is to start with a half or a full 240-mg slow-release tablet and titrate the dosage upward to the maximum dosage as tolerated. It is important to monitor blood pressure and pulse regularly as the dose is being titrated. Given the risk of arrhythmias, a baseline ECG is also advised. Blood levels have never been correlated with efficacy or toxicity for any indication of a calcium channel antagonist. Some investigators believe that the novel biochemical profile of nimodipine and other dihydropyridines may confer greater brain penetrance and more efficacy in the treatment of bipolar disorder. Controlled trials are currently under way.

Although combining the standard mood stabilizers is supported by the literature in difficult cases of bipolar illness, there is no substantial evidence that adding a calcium channel blocker to lithium or other agents is advantageous. In fact, there are reports of enhanced neurotoxicity when verapamil was added to lithium and carbamazepine. In general, it appears prudent to avoid these combinations until we better understand the risks and benefits.

Omega-3 Fatty Acids

Omega-3 and omega-6 fatty acids are the building blocks of fats in the same way that amino acids are the building blocks of proteins. A number of reports over the past 13 years suggest that affective illness may be associated with deficiencies of some omega-3 fatty acids. For example, there appears to be some correlation between a higher ratio of arachidonic acid to eicosapentaenoic acid (EPA) in more severely depressed patients than in less severely depressed patients. Other studies have suggested that there may be lower levels of omega-3 fatty acids in the membranes of red blood cells in depressed patients than in healthy control subjects. Furthermore, there is limited evidence suggesting that omega-3 fatty acids may impact signal transduction in a manner analogous to the way lithium affects it. The lower rates of depression in some Asian countries may be due to greater amounts of fish consumed in regular diets. A double-blind study reported that adding supplemental omega-3 fatty acids to the drug regimens of bipolar patients improved their outcomes (Stoll et al. 1999). In this study, 30 bipolar patients were randomized to either 9.6 g/day of omega-3 supplements or olive oil (as a control) for 4 months. They continued taking standard mood stabilizers. The patients treated with omega-3 experienced longer remission and more complete resolution of symptoms than the placebo-treated patients.

Since the Stoll study, there have been several controlled trials of omega-3 fatty acids in the treatment of depression and bipolar disorder. The data supporting the efficacy of omega-3 fatty acids in the treatment of bipolar disorder have been mixed. For example, two other controlled trials of omega fatty acids (up to 6 g/day of EPA) in bipolar disorder failed to show benefit (Keck et al. 2006; Post et al. 2003). However, in perhaps the most rigorous controlled trial to date, Frangou and colleagues (2006) found that the addition of both 1 and 2 g/day of EPA to a standard mood stabilizer was superior to adjunctive placebo in reducing Hamilton Depression Rating Scale scores and global impression of illness scores in bipolar patients. The EPA did not show benefit in improving manic symptoms, and 2 g/day was no more effective than 1 g/day.

In unipolar depression, the data on omega-3 fatty acids are also unclear. For example, some studies of omega-3 fatty acids in perinatal depression (Freeman et al. 2006) and pediatric depression (Nemets et al. 2006) have suggested benefits, whereas other controlled studies have failed to show any advantage of supplementing omega-3 fatty acids in adult depressed patients (Marangell et al. 2003). Most studies have used 1–6 mg/day of EPA, while others have used DHA. A few reports mentioned use of the combination of EPA and DHA.

The role of omega-3 fatty acid supplements in the treatment of affective illness remains uncertain. Studies thus far suggest a more reliable effect of omega-3 fatty acids in some forms of unipolar depression than in bipolar maintenance. In addition, the data to date are more indicative of a benefit in treating depressive symptoms in bipolar disorder than in treating or preventing manic symptoms. However, the correct dose, duration of treatment, and form of omega-3 fatty acids remain to be established. Since these fatty acids are fairly benign and may have other health benefits, some clinicians are supplementing the mood-stabilizing or antidepressant regimens with omega-3 fatty acids. The most commonly reported side effects are belching and a fishy aftertaste. Given the available data that suggests that omega-3 fatty acids may be beneficial in some patients and have few side effects, the American Psychiatric Association (APA) has endorsed the use of EPA/DHA in patients with mood, impulse-control and psychotic disorders. Th APA recommends at least 1 g/day of EPA/DHA.

Bibliography

Abou-Saleh MT: Who responds to prophylactic lithium therapy? Br J Psychiatry (suppl 21):20–26, 1993

Abraham G, Delva N, Waldron J, et al: Lithium treatment: a comparison of once- and twice-daily dosing. Acta Psychiatr Scand 85:65–69, 1992

Altesman R, Cole JO: Lithium therapy: a practical review, in Psychopharmacology Update. Edited by Cole JO. Lexington, MA, Collamore Press, 1980, pp 3–18

Altshuler LL, Suppes T, Black DO, et al: Lower switch rate in depressed patients with bipolar II than bipolar I disorder treated adjunctively with second-generation antidepressants. Am J Psychiatry 163:313–315, 2006

Altshuler LL, Post RM, Hellemann G, et al: Impact of antidepressant continuation after acute positive or partial treatment response for bipolar depression: a blinded, randomized study. J Clin Psychiatry 70:450–457, 2009

Ayd F: Carbamazepine for aggression, schizophrenia and nonaffective syndromes. Int Drug Ther Newsl 19:9–12, 1984

Backonja M, Beydoun A, Edwards KR, et al: Gabapentin for the symptomatic treatment of painful neuropathy in patients with diabetes mellitus: a randomized controlled trial. JAMA 280:1831–1836, 1998 [see comments]

Baetz M, Bowen RC: Efficiency of divalproex sodium in patients with panic disorder and mood instability who have not responded to conventional therapy. Can J Psychiatry 43:73–77, 1998

Bahk WM, Shin YC, Woo JM, et al: Topiramate and divalproex in combination with risperidone for acute mania: a randomized open-label study. Prog Neuropsychopharmacol Biol Psychiatry 29:115–121, 2005

Baker RW, Milton DR, Stauffer VL, et al: Placebo-controlled trials do not find association of olanzapine with exacerbation of bipolar mania. J Affect Disord 73:147–153, 2003

Baldessarini RJ, Tondo L: Lithium and suicidal risk. Bipolar Disord 10:114–115, 2008

Baldessarini RJ, Tondo L: Suicidal risks during treatment of bipolar disorder patients with lithium versus anticonvulsants. Pharmacopsychiatry 42:72–75, 2009

Baldessarini RJ, Pompili M, Tondo L: Suicide in bipolar disorder: risks and management. CNS Spectr 11:465–471, 2006

Ballenger JC, Post RM: Carbamazepine (Tegretol) in manic-depressive illness: a new treatment. Am J Psychiatry 137:782–790, 1980

Barzman DH, Delbello MP: Topiramate for co-occurring bipolar disorder and disruptive behavior disorders. Am J Psychiatry 163:1451–1452, 2006

Benedetti A, Lattanzi L, Pini S, et al: Oxcarbazepine as add-on treatment in patients with bipolar manic, mixed or depressive episode. J Affect Disord 79(1–3):273–277, 2004

Besag FM, Berry DJ, Pool F, et al: Carbamazepine toxicity with lamotrigine: pharmacokinetic or pharmacodynamic interaction? Epilepsia 39:183–187, 1998

Biederman J, Lerner Y, Belmaker R: Combination of lithium carbonate and haloperidol in schizoaffective disorder. Arch Gen Psychiatry 36:327–333, 1979

Bowden CL: Predictors of response to divalproex and lithium. J Clin Psychiatry 56 (3, suppl):25–30, 1995

Bowden CL, McElroy SL: History of the development of valproate for treatment of bipolar disorder. J Clin Psychiatry 56 (3, suppl):3–5, 1995

Bowden CL, Singh V: Valproate in bipolar disorder: 2000 onwards. Acta Psychiatr Scand Suppl 426:13–20, 2005

Bowden CL, Brugger AM, Swann AC, et al: Efficacy of divalproex vs lithium and placebo in the treatment of mania. The Depakote Mania Study Group. JAMA 271:918–924, 1994 [erratum: JAMA 271:1830, 1994]

Bowden CL, Calabrese JK, McElroy SL, et al: A randomized placebo-controlled 12-month trial of divalproex and lithium in bipolar I disorder. Arch Gen Psychiatry 57:481–489, 2000

Bradwejn J, Shriqui C, Koszycki D, et al: Double-blind comparison of the effects of clonazepam and lorazepam in acute mania. J Clin Psychopharmacol 10:403–408, 1990

Brent NB, Wisner KL: Fluoxetine and carbamazepine concentrations in a nursing mother/infant pair. Clin Pediatr (Phil) 37:41–44, 1998

Briassoulis G, Kalabalikis P, Tamiolaki M, et al: Lamotrigine childhood overdose. Pediatr Neurol 19:239–242, 1998

Brown EB, McElroy SL, Keck PE Jr, et al: A 7-week, randomized, double-blind trial of olanzapine/fluoxetine combination versus lamotrigine in the treatment of bipolar I depression. J Clin Psychiatry 67:1025–1033, 2006

Bschor T, Bauer M: Efficacy and mechanisms of action of lithium augmentation in refractory major depression. Curr Pharm Des 12(23):2985–2992, 2006

Buzan RD, Dubovsky SL: Recurrence of lamotrigine-associated rash with rechallenge (letter). J Clin Psychiatry 59:87, 1998

Cade JF: Lithium salts in treatment of psychotic excitement. Med J Aust 36:349–352, 1949

Calabrese JR, Delucchi GA: Spectrum of efficacy of valproate in 55 patients with rapid-cycling bipolar disorder. Am J Psychiatry 147:431–434, 1990

Calabrese JR, Markovitz PJ, Kimmel SE, et al: Spectrum of efficacy of valproate in 78 rapid-cycling bipolar patients. J Clin Psychopharmacol 12 (1, suppl):53S–56S, 1992

Calabrese JR, Woyshville MJ, Kimmel SE, et al: Predictors of valproate response in bipolar rapid cycling. J Clin Psychopharmacol 13:280–283, 1993

Calabrese JR, Bowden CL, McElroy SL, et al: Spectrum of activity of lamotrigine in treatment-refractory bipolar disorder. Am J Psychiatry 156:1019–1023, 1999a

Calabrese JR, Bowden CL, Sachs GS, et al: A double-blind placebo-controlled study of lamotrigine monotherapy in outpatients with bipolar I depression. Lamictal 602 Study Group. J Clin Psychiatry 60:79–88, 1999b

Calvert NW, Burch SP, Fu AZ, et al: The cost-effectiveness of lamotrigine in the maintenance treatment of adults with bipolar I disorder. J Manag Care Pharm 12:322–330, 2006

Carrazana EJ, Schachter SC: Alternative uses of lamotrigine and gabapentin in the treatment of trigeminal neuralgia (letter; comment). Neurology 50:1192, 1998

Casey DE, Tracy KA, Daniel D, et al: Divalproex sodium enhances antipsychotic-induced improvement in schizophrenia, in Abstracts of the 40th Annual Meeting of the American College of Neuropsychopharmacology, Waikoloa, HI, 2001, p 281

Chatterjee CR, Ringold AL: A case report of reduction in alcohol craving and protection against alcohol withdrawal by gabapentin (letter). J Clin Psychiatry 60:617, 1999

Chen CK, Shiah IS, Yeh CB, et al: Combination treatment of clozapine and topiramate in resistant rapid-cycling bipolar disorder. Clin Neuropharmacol 28(3):136–138, 2005

Chouinard G, Young S, Annable L: Antimanic effects of clonazepam. Biol Psychiatry 18:451–466, 1983

Citrome L: Asenapine for schizophrenia and bipolar disorder: a review of the efficacy and safety profile for this newly approved sublingually absorbed second-generation antipsychotic. Int J Clin Pract 63:1762–1784, 2009

Cohen LS, Friedman JM, Jefferson JW, et al: A reevaluation of risk of in utero exposure to lithium. JAMA 271:146–150, 1994 [erratum: JAMA 271:1485, 1994]

Coleman E, Stadel BV: Gabapentin for postherpetic neuralgia (letter; comment). JAMA 282:134–135, 1999

Conway CR, Chibnall JT, Nelson LA, et al: An open-label trial of adjunctive oxcarbazepine for bipolar disorder. J Clin Psychopharmacol 26:95–97, 2006

Coryell W, Solomon D, Leon AC, et al: Lithium discontinuation and subsequent effectiveness. Am J Psychiatry 155:895–898, 1998 [see comments]

Cowdry R, Gardner D: Pharmacotherapy of borderline personality disorder: alprazolam, carbamazepine, trifluoperazine, and tranylcypromine. Arch Gen Psychiatry 45:111–119, 1988

Daban C, Martinez-Aran A, Torrent C, et al: Cognitive functioning in bipolar patients receiving lamotrigine: preliminary results. J Clin Psychopharmacol 26:178–181, 2006

D'Andrea G, Granella F, Cadaldini M, et al: Effectiveness of lamotrigine in the prophylaxis of migraine with aura: an open pilot study. Cephalalgia 19:64–66, 1999

Davanzo P, Nikore V, Yehya N, et al: Oxcarbazepine treatment of juvenile-onset bipolar disorder. J Child Adolesc Psychopharmacol 14:344–345, 2004

Deandrea D, Walker D, Mehlmauer M, et al: Dermatological reactions to lithium: a critical review of the literature. J Clin Psychopharmacol 2:199–204, 1982

DeBattista C, Solomon A, Arnow B, et al: The efficacy of divalproex sodium in the treatment of agitation associated with major depression. J Clin Psychopharmacol 25:476–479, 2005

Deicken RF: Verapamil treatment of bipolar depression (letter). J Clin Psychopharmacol 10:148–149, 1990

Deltito JA: The effect of valproate on bipolar spectrum temperamental disorders. J Clin Psychiatry 54:300–304, 1993

Delva N, Letemendia F: Lithium treatment in schizophrenia and schizoaffective disorders. Br J Psychiatry 141:387–400, 1982

Denicoff KD, Meglathery SB, Post RM, et al: Efficacy of carbamazepine compared with other agents: a clinical practice survey. J Clin Psychiatry 55:70–76, 1994

Di Costanzo E, Schifano F: Lithium alone or in combination with carbamazepine for the treatment of rapid-cycling bipolar affective disorder. Acta Psychiatr Scand 83:456–459, 1991

Dilsaver SC, Swann AC, Shoaib AM, et al: The manic syndrome: factors which may predict a patient's response to lithium, carbamazepine and valproate. J Psychiatry Neurosci 18:61–66, 1993

Donovan SJ, Susser ES, Nunes EV, et al: Divalproex treatment of disruptive adolescents: a report of 10 cases. J Clin Psychiatry 58:12–15, 1997

Dubovsky SL, Franks RD, Lifschitz M, et al: Effectiveness of verapamil in the treatment of manic patients. Am J Psychiatry 139:502–504, 1982

Dwight MM, Keck P Jr, Stanton S, et al: Antidepressant activity and mania associated with risperidone treatment of schizoaffective disorder (letter). Lancet 344:554–555, 1994

Eberle AJ: Valproate and polycystic ovaries (letter). J Am Acad Child Adolesc Psychiatry 37:1009, 1998 [see comments]

Emrich HM: Studies with oxcarbazepine (Trileptal) in acute mania. Int Clin Psychopharmacol 5(suppl):83–88, 1990

Erfurth A, Kammerer C, Grunze H, et al: An open label study of gabapentin in the treatment of acute mania. J Psychiatr Res 32:261–264, 1998a

Erfurth A, Walden J, Grunze H: Lamotrigine in the treatment of schizoaffective disorder. Neuropsychobiology 38:204–205, 1998b

Evans RW, Gualtieri CT: Carbamazepine: a neuropsychological and psychiatric profile. Clin Neuropharmacol 8:221–241, 1985

Faedda GL, Tondo DD, Baldessarini RJ: Outcome after rapid vs gradual discontinuation of lithium treatment of bipolar disorders. Arch Gen Psychiatry 50:448–455, 1993

Fatemi SH, Rapport DJ, Calabrese JR, et al: Lamotrigine in rapid-cycling bipolar disorder. J Clin Psychiatry 58:522–527, 1997

Fogelson DL, Sternbach H: Lamotrigine treatment of refractory bipolar disorder. J Clin Psychiatry 58:271–273, 1997

Frampton JE, Foster RH: Pregabalin: in the treatment of generalised anxiety disorder. CNS Drugs 20(8):685–693 [discussion 694–695], 2006

Frangou S, Lewis M, McCrone P: Efficacy of ethyl-eicosapentaenoic acid in bipolar depression: randomised double-blind placebo-controlled study. Br J Psychiatry 188:46–50, 2006

Frankenburg FR, Tohen M, Cohen BM, et al: Long-term response to carbamazepine: a retrospective review. J Clin Psychopharmacol 8:130–132, 1988

Freeman MP, Hibbeln JR, Wisner KL, et al: Randomized dose-ranging pilot trial of omega-3 fatty acids for postpartum depression. Acta Psychiatr Scand 113:31–35, 2006

Freeman TW, Clothier JL, Pazzaglia P, et al: A double-blind comparison of valproate and lithium in the treatment of acute mania. Am J Psychiatry 149:108–111, 1992

Frye MA, Ketter TA, Kimbrell TA, et al: A placebo-controlled study of lamotrigine and gabapentin monotherapy in refractory mood disorders. J Clin Psychopharmacol 20:607–614, 2000

Geddes JR, Burgess S, Hawton K, et al: Long-term lithium therapy for bipolar disorder: systematic review and meta-analysis of randomized controlled trials. Am J Psychiatry 161:217–222, 2004

Gelenberg AJ, Carroll JA, Baudhuin MG, et al: The meaning of serum lithium levels in maintenance therapy of mood disorders: a review of the literature. J Clin Psychiatry 50 (suppl 12):17–22, 1989a

Gelenberg AJ, Kane JM, Keller MB, et al: Comparison of standard and low serum levels of lithium for maintenance treatment of bipolar disorder. N Engl J Med 321:1489–1493, 1989b

Geracioti TD Jr: Valproic acid treatment of episodic explosiveness related to brain injury (letter). J Clin Psychiatry 55:416–417, 1994

Gerner RH, Stanton A: Algorithm for patient management of acute manic states: lithium, valproate, or carbamazepine? J Clin Psychopharmacol 12 (1, suppl):57S–63S, 1992

Ghaemi SN, Schrauwen E, Klugman J, et al: Long-term lamotrigine plus lithium for bipolar disorder: One year outcome. J Psychiatr Pract 12(5):300–305, 2006a

Ghaemi SN, Zablotsky B, Filkowski MM, et al: An open prospective study of zonisamide in acute bipolar depression. J Clin Psychopharmacol 26(4):385–388, 2006b

Ghaemi SN, Shirzadi AA, Klugman J, et al: Is adjunctive open-label zonisamide effective for bipolar disorder? J Affect Disord 105:311–314, 2008

Giles JJ, Bannigan JG: Teratogenic and developmental effects of lithium. Curr Pharm Des 12:1531–1541, 2006

Gitlin MJ: Lithium-induced renal insufficiency. J Clin Psychopharmacol 13:276–279, 1993

Gitlin M: Lithium and the kidney: an updated review. Drug Saf 20:231–243, 1999

Gobbi G, Gaudreau PO, Leblanc N: Efficacy of topiramate, valproate, and their combination on aggression/agitation behavior in patients with psychosis. J Clin Psychopharmacol 26:467–473, 2006

Goedhard LE, Stolker JJ, Heerdink ER, et al: Pharmacotherapy for the treatment of aggressive behavior in general adult psychiatry: A systematic review. J Clin Psychiatry 67:1013–1024, 2006

Goodnick PJ: Verapamil prophylaxis in pregnant women with bipolar disorder (letter). Am J Psychiatry 150:1560, 1993

Goodwin FK, Jamison KR: Manic-Depressive Illness. New York, Oxford University Press, 1990

Goodwin GM: Recurrence of mania after lithium withdrawal. Implications for the use of lithium in the treatment of bipolar affective disorder (editorial). Br J Psychiatry 164:149–152, 1994

Goodwin GM, Bowden CL, Calabrese JR, et al: A pooled analysis of 2 placebo-controlled 18-month trials of lamotrigine and lithium maintenance in bipolar I disorder. J Clin Psychiatry 65:432–441, 2004

Gordon A, Price LH: Mood stabilization and weight loss with topiramate (letter). Am J Psychiatry 156:968–969, 1999

Gorson KC, Schott C, Herman R, et al: Gabapentin in the treatment of painful diabetic neuropathy: a placebo controlled, double blind, crossover trial (letter). J Neurol Neurosurg Psychiatry 66:251–252, 1999

Green AI, Tohen M, Patel JK, et al: Clozapine in the treatment of refractory psychotic mania. Am J Psychiatry 157:982–986, 2000

Greil W, Kleindienst N, Erazo N, et al: Differential response to lithium and carbamazepine in the prophylaxis of bipolar disorder. J Clin Psychopharmacol 18:455–460, 1998

Grunze H, Erfurth A, Amann B, et al: Intravenous valproate loading in acutely manic and depressed bipolar I patients. J Clin Psychopharmacol 19:303–309, 1999a

Grunze H, Erfurth A, Marcuse A, et al: Tiagabine appears not to be efficacious in the treatment of acute mania. J Clin Psychiatry 60:759–762, 1999b

Guscott R, Taylor L: Lithium prophylaxis in recurrent affective illness: efficacy, effectiveness and efficiency. Br J Psychiatry 164:741–746, 1994

Guzzetta F, Tondo L, Centorrino F, et al: Lithium treatment reduces suicide risk in recurrent major depressive disorder. J Clin Psychiatry 68:380–383, 2007

Hardoy MC, Hardoy MJ, Carta MG, et al: Gabapentin as a promising treatment for antipsychotic-induced movement disorders in schizoaffective and bipolar patients. J Affect Disord 54:315–317, 1999

Häuser W, Bernardy K, Uçeyler N, et al: Treatment of fibromyalgia syndrome with gabapentin and pregabalin: a meta-analysis of randomized controlled trials. Pain 145:69–81, 2009

Herrmann N: Valproic acid treatment of agitation in dementia. Can J Psychiatry 43:69–72, 1998

Hilty DM, Rodriguez GD, Hales RE: Intravenous valproate for rapid stabilization of agitation in neuropsychiatric disorders (letter). J Neuropsychiatry Clin Neurosci 10:365–366, 1998

Himmelhoch JM, Poust RI, Mallinger AG: Adjustment of lithium dose during lithium-chlorothiazide therapy. Clin Pharmacol Ther 22:225–227, 1977

Hirschman S, Dolberg OT, Stern L, et al: The use of valproic acid in the treatment of borderline personality disorder [in Hebrew]. Harefuah 133:205–208, 1997

Hollander E, Allen A, Lopez RP, et al: A preliminary double-blind, placebo-controlled trial of divalproex sodium in borderline personality disorder. J Clin Psychiatry 62(3):199–203, 2001

Huguelet P, Morand-Collomb S: Effect of topiramate augmentation on two patients suffering from schizophrenia or bipolar disorder with comorbid alcohol abuse. Pharmacol Res 52(5):392–394, 2005

Isojarvi JI, Laatikainen TJ, Pakarinen AJ, et al: Polycystic ovaries and hyperandrogenism in women taking valproate for epilepsy. N Engl J Med 329:1383–1388, 1993

Jacobsen FM: Low-dose valproate: a new treatment for cyclothymia, mild rapid cycling disorders, and premenstrual syndrome. J Clin Psychiatry 54:229–234, 1993

Jefferson JW, Greist JH, Ackerman DL, et al: Lithium Encyclopedia for Clinical Practice, 2nd Edition. Washington, DC, American Psychiatric Press, 1987

Joffe H, Cohen LS: Presentation at the 157rd annual meeting of the American Psychiatric Association, New York City, May 1–6, 2004

Joffe H, Cohen LS, Suppes T, et al: Longitudinal follow-up of reproductive and metabolic features of valproate-associated polycystic ovarian syndrome features: a preliminary report. Biol Psychiatry 60:1378–1381, 2006

Joffe R, Post R, Roy-Byrne P, et al: Hematological effects of carbamazepine in patients with affective illness. Am J Psychiatry 142:1196–1199, 1985

Jones KL, Lacro RV, Johnson KA, et al: Pattern of malformations in the children of women treated with carbamazepine during pregnancy. N Engl J Med 320:1661–1666, 1989

Jope RS: Anti-bipolar therapy: mechanism of action of lithium. Mol Psychiatry 4:117–128, 1999

Judd LL, Schettler PJ, Akiskal HS, et al: Long-term symptomatic status of bipolar I vs. bipolar II disorders. Int J Neuropsychopharmacol 6:127–137, 2003

Juruena MF, Ottoni GL, Machado-Vieira R, et al: Bipolar I and II disorder residual symptoms: oxcarbazepine and carbamazepine as add-on treatment to lithium in a double-blind, randomized trial. Prog Neuropsychopharmacol Biol Psychiatry 33:94–99, 2009

Kaufman KR, Gerner R: Lamotrigine toxicity secondary to sertraline. Seizure 7:163–165, 1998

Keck P Jr, McElroy SL, Vuckovic A, et al: Combined valproate and carbamazepine treatment of bipolar disorder. J Neuropsychiatry Clin Neurosci 4:319–322, 1992

Keck P Jr, McElroy SL, Tugrul KC, et al: Valproate oral loading in the treatment of acute mania. J Clin Psychiatry 54:305–308, 1993a

Keck PE Jr, Taylor VE, Tugrul KC, et al: Valproate treatment of panic disorder and lactate-induced panic attacks. Biol Psychiatry 33:542–546, 1993b

Keck PE Jr, Marcus R, Tourkodimitris S, et al: A placebo-controlled, double-blind study of the efficacy and safety of aripiprazole in patients with acute bipolar mania. Am J Psychiatry 160:1651–1658, 2003a

Keck PE Jr, Versiani M, Potkins S, et al: Ziprasidone in the treatment of acute bipolar mania: a three-week, placebo-controlled, double-blind, randomized trial. Am J Psychiatry 160:741–748, 2003b

Keck PE Jr, Mintz J, McElroy SL, et al: Double-blind, randomized, placebo-controlled trials of ethyl-eicosapentanoate in the treatment of bipolar depression and rapid cycling bipolar disorder. Biol Psychiatry 60:1020–1022, 2006

Kenna HA, Jiang B, Rasgon NL: Reproductive and metabolic abnormalities associated with bipolar disorder and its treatment. Harv Rev Psychiatry 17:138–146, 2009

Kessel JB, Verghese C, Simpson GM: Neurotoxicity related to lithium and neuroleptic combinations? A retrospective review. J Psychiatry Neurosci 17:28–30, 1992

Ketter TA: Monotherapy versus combined treatment with second-generation antipsychotics in bipolar disorder. J Clin Psychiatry 69 (suppl 5):9–15, 2008

Ketter TA, Pazzaglia PJ, Post RM: Synergy of carbamazepine and valproic acid in affective illness: case report and review of the literature. J Clin Psychopharmacol 12:276–281, 1992

Ketter TA, Winsberg ME, DeGolia SG, et al: Rapid efficacy of olanzapine augmentation in nonpsychotic bipolar mixed states. J Clin Psychiatry 59:83–85, 1998

Kimmel SE, Calabrese JR, Woyshville MJ, et al: Clozapine in treatment-refractory mood disorders. J Clin Psychiatry 55:91–93, 1994

Kishimoto A, Ogura C, Hazama H, et al: Long-term prophylactic effects of carbamazepine in affective disorder. Br J Psychiatry 143:327–331, 1983

Kocsis JH, Shaw ED, Stokes PE, et al: Neuropsychologic effects of lithium discontinuation. J Clin Psychopharmacol 13:268–275, 1993

Koek RJ, Yerevanian BI: Is lamotrigine effective for treatment-refractory mania? (letter). Pharmacopsychiatry 31:35, 1998

Kotler M, Matar MA: Lamotrigine in the treatment of resistant bipolar disorder. Clin Neuropharmacol 21:65–67, 1998

Kotwal R, Guerdjikova A, McElroy SL, et al: Lithium augmentation of topiramate for bipolar disorder with comorbid binge eating disorder and obesity. Hum Psychopharmacol 21:425–431, 2006

Krüger S, Trevor Young L, Bräunig P: Pharmacotherapy of bipolar mixed states. Bipolar Disord 7:205–215, 2005

Kunik ME, Puryear L, Orengo CA, et al: The efficacy and tolerability of divalproex sodium in elderly demented patients with behavioral disturbances. Int J Geriatr Psychiatry 13:29–34, 1998

Kushner SF, Khan A, Lane R, et al: Topiramate monotherapy in the management of acute mania: results of four double-blind placebo-controlled trials. Bipolar Disord 8:15–27, 2006

Kusumakar V, Yatham LN: Lamotrigine treatment of rapid cycling bipolar disorder (letter; comment). Am J Psychiatry 154:1171–1172, 1997a

Kusumakar V, Yatham LN: An open study of lamotrigine in refractory bipolar depression. Psychiatry Res 72:145–148, 1997b

Lambert PA, Venaud G: A comparative study of valpromide versus lithium in the treatment of affective disorders. Nervure 5(2):57–65, 1992

Lampl C, Buzath A, Klinger D, et al: Lamotrigine in the prophylactic treatment of migraine aura—a pilot study. Cephalalgia 19:58–63, 1999

Lenox RH, Watson DG: Lithium and the brain: a psychopharmacological strategy to a molecular basis for manic depressive illness. Clin Chem 40:309–314, 1994

Lenox RH, Newhouse PA, Creelman WL, et al: Adjunctive treatment of manic agitation with lorazepam vs. haloperidol: a double-blind study. J Clin Psychiatry 53:47–52, 1992

Letterman L, Markowitz JS: Gabapentin: a review of published experience in the treatment of bipolar disorder and other psychiatric conditions. Pharmacotherapy 19:565–572, 1999

Li PP, Young LT, Tam YK, et al: Effects of chronic lithium and carbamazepine treatment on G-protein subunit expression in rat cerebral cortex. Biol Psychiatry 34:162–170, 1993

Lin YH, Liu CY, Hsiao MC: Management of atypical antipsychotic-induced weight gain in schizophrenic patients with topiramate. Psychiatry Clin Neurosci 59:613–615, 2005

Lindenmayer JP, Klebanov R: Olanzapine-induced manic-like syndrome. J Clin Psychiatry 59:318–319, 1998

Lipinski JF, Pope HD Jr: Possible synergistic action between carbamazepine and lithium carbonate in the treatment of three acutely manic patients. Am J Psychiatry 139:948–949, 1982

Lonergan ET, Cameron M, Luxenberg J: Valproic acid for agitation in dementia. Cochrane Database Syst Rev 2:CD003945, 2004

Lott AD, McElroy SL, Keys MA: Valproate in the treatment of behavioral agitation in elderly patients with dementia. J Neuropsychiatry Clin Neurosci 7:314–319, 1995

MacMillan CM, Korndorfer SR, Rao S, et al: A comparison of divalproex and oxcarbazepine in aggressive youth with bipolar disorder. J Psychiatr Pract 12(4):214–222, 2006

Marangell LB, Martinez JM, Zboyan HA, et al: A double-blind, placebo-controlled study of the omega-3 fatty acid docosahexaenoic acid in the treatment of major depression. Am J Psychiatry 160:996–998, 2003

Marcotte D: Use of topiramate, a new antiepileptic, as a mood stabilizer. J Affect Disord 50:245–251, 1998

Marcus WL: Lithium: a review of its pharmacokinetics, health effects, and toxicology. J Environ Pathol Toxicol Oncol 13:73–79, 1994

Massot O, Rousselle JC, Fillion MP, et al: 5-HT$_{1B}$ receptors: a novel target for lithium: possible involvement in mood disorders. Neuropsychopharmacology 21:530–541, 1999

McCoy L, Votolato NA, Schwarzkopf SB, et al: Clinical correlates of valproate augmentation in refractory bipolar disorder. Ann Clin Psychiatry 5:29–33, 1993

McElroy SL, Keck P Jr: Treatment guidelines for valproate in bipolar and schizoaffective disorders. Can J Psychiatry 38 (3, suppl 2):S62–S66, 1993

McElroy SL, Keck PE Jr, Pope HG Jr: Sodium valproate: its use in primary psychiatric disorders. J Clin Psychopharmacol 7:16–24, 1987

McElroy SL, Keck PE Jr, Tugrul KC, et al: Valproate as a loading treatment in acute mania. Neuropsychobiology 27:146–149, 1993

McElroy SL, Suppes T, Keck PE Jr, et al: Open-label adjunctive zonisamide in the treatment of bipolar disorders: a prospective trial. J Clin Psychiatry 66:617–624, 2005

Meador KJ, Baker GA, Browning N, et al; NEAD Study Group: Cognitive function at 3 years of age after fetal exposure to antiepileptic drugs. N Engl J Med 360:1597–1605, 2009

Mishory A, Yaroslavsky Y, Bersudsky Y, et al: Phenytoin as an antimanic anticonvulsant: a controlled study. Am J Psychiatry 157:463–465, 2000

Mitchell P, Withers K, Jacobs G, et al: Combining lithium and sodium valproate for bipolar disorder. Aust N Z J Psychiatry 28:141–143, 1994

Modell J, Lenox R, Weiner S: Inpatient clinical trial of lorazepam for the management of manic agitation. J Clin Psychopharmacol 5:109–113, 1985

Morello CM, Leckband SG, Stoner CP, et al: Randomized double-blind study comparing the efficacy of gabapentin with amitriptyline on diabetic peripheral neuropathy pain. Arch Intern Med 159:1931–1937, 1999

Mork A, Geisler A, Hollund P: Effects of lithium on second-messenger systems in the brain. Pharmacol Toxicol 1:4–17, 1992

Morrell MJ, Hayes FJ, Sluss PM, et al: Hyperandrogenism, ovulatory dysfunction, and polycystic ovary syndrome with valproate versus lamotrigine. Ann Neurol 64:200–211, 2008

Murray JB: Lithium maintenance therapy for bipolar I patients: possible refractoriness to reinstitution after discontinuation. Psychol Rep 74:355–361, 1994

Mylonakis E, Vittorio CC, Hollik DA, et al: Lamotrigine overdose presenting as anticonvulsant hypersensitivity syndrome. Ann Pharmacotherapy 33:557–559, 1999

Myrick H, Malcolm R, Brady KT: Gabapentin treatment of alcohol withdrawal (letter). Am J Psychiatry 155:1632, 1998

Nemets H, Nemets B, Apter A, et al: Omega-3 treatment of childhood depression: a controlled, double-blind pilot study. Am J Psychiatry 163:1098–1100, 2006

Nierenberg AA, Fava M, Trivedi MH, et al: A comparison of lithium and T3 augmentation following two failed medication treatments for depression: a STAR*D report. Am J Psychiatry 163:1519–1530, 2006a

Nierenberg AA, Ostacher MJ, Calabrese JR, et al: Treatment-resistant bipolar depression: a STEP-BD equipoise randomized effectiveness trial of antidepressant augmentation with lamotrigine, inositol, or risperidone. Am J Psychiatry 163:210–216, 2006b

Nilsson A, Axelsson R: Lithium discontinuers, II: therapeutic outcome. Acta Psychiatr Scand 84:78–82, 1991

Okuma T: Effects of carbamazepine and lithium on affective disorders. Neuropsychobiology 27:138–145, 1993

Okuma T, Yamashita I, Takahashi R, et al: Comparison of the antimanic efficacy of carbamazepine and lithium carbonate by double-blind controlled study. Pharmacopsychiatry 23:143–150, 1990

Ontiveros A, Fontaine R: Sodium valproate and clonazepam for treatment-resistant panic disorder. J Psychiatry Neurosci 17:78–80, 1992

Owen RT: Extended-release carbamazepine for acute bipolar mania: a review. Drugs Today (Barc) 42(5):283–289, 2006

Pande AC, Davidson JR, Jefferson JW, et al: Treatment of social phobia with gabapentin: a placebo-controlled study. J Clin Psychopharmacol 19:341–348, 1999

Pande AC, Crockatt JG, Janney CA, et al: Gabapentin in bipolar disorder: a placebo-controlled trial of adjunctive therapy. Gabapentin Bipolar Disorder Study Group. Bipolar Disord 2(3, pt 2):249–255, 2000

Pazzaglia PJ, Post RM: Contingent tolerance and response to carbamazepine: a case study in a patient with trigeminal neuralgia and bipolar disorder. J Neuropsychiatry Clin Neurosci 4:76–81, 1992

Pazzaglia P, Post R, Ketter T, et al: Preliminary controlled trial of nimodipine in ultra-rapid cycling affective dysregulation. Psychiatry Res 49:257–272, 1993

Perlis RH, Baker RW, Zarate CA Jr, et al: Olanzapine versus risperidone in the treatment of manic or mixed States in bipolar I disorder: a randomized, double-blind trial. J Clin Psychiatry 67:1747–1753, 2006

Pinto OC, Akiskal HS: Lamotrigine as a promising approach to borderline personality: an open case series without concurrent DSM-IV major mood disorder. J Affect Disord 51:333–343, 1998

Pope HG Jr, McElroy SL, Keck P, et al: Valproate in the treatment of acute mania: a placebo-controlled study. Arch Gen Psychiatry 48:62–68, 1991

Post RM, Rubinow DR, Ballenger JC: Conditioning and sensitisation in the longitudinal course of affective illness. Br J Psychiatry 149:191–201, 1986

Post RM, Uhde T, Roy-Byrne P, et al: Correlates of antimanic response to carbamazepine. Psychiatry Res 21:71–83, 1987

Post RM, Weiss SR, Chuang DM: Mechanisms of action of anticonvulsants in affective disorders: comparisons with lithium. J Clin Psychopharmacol 12 (1, suppl):23S–35S, 1992

Post RM, Leverich GS, Altshuler LL, et al: An overview of recent findings of the Stanley Foundation Bipolar Network (Part I). Bipolar Disord 5:310–319, 2003

Post RM, Altshuler LL, Frye MA, et al: Preliminary observations on the effectiveness of levetiracetam in the open adjunctive treatment of refractory bipolar disorder. J Clin Psychiatry 66:370–374, 2005

Pratoomsri W, Yatham LN, Sohn CH, et al: Oxcarbazepine add-on in the treatment of refractory bipolar disorder. Bipolar Disord 7 (suppl 5):37–42, 2005

Pratoomsri W, Yatham LN, Bond DJ, et al: Oxcarbazepine in the treatment of bipolar disorder: a review. Can J Psychiatry 51:540–545, 2006

Prettyman R: Lithium neurotoxicity at subtherapeutic serum levels (letter; comment). Br J Psychiatry 164:123, 1994

Price LH, Heninger GR: Lithium in the treatment of mood disorders. N Engl J Med 331:591–598, 1994

Prien RF, Caffey EM Jr: Long-term maintenance drug therapy in recurrent affective illness: current status and issues. Dis Nerv Syst 38:981–992, 1977

Prien R, Kupfer D, Mansky P, et al: Drug therapy in the prevention of recurrences in unipolar and bipolar affective disorders. Arch Gen Psychiatry 41:1096–1104, 1984

Rasgon N: The relationship between polycystic ovary syndrome and antiepileptic drugs: a review of the evidence. J Clin Psychopharmacol 24:322–334, 2004

Rasgon NL, Altshuler LL, Fairbanks L, et al: Reproductive function and risk for PCOS in women treated for bipolar disorder. Bipolar Disord 7:246–259, 2005

Ravindran AV, Jones BW, al-Zaid K, et al: Effective treatment of mania with olanzapine. J Psychiatry Neurosci 22:345–346, 1997

Reeves RR, McBride WA, Brannon GE: Olanzapine-induced mania. J Am Osteopath Assoc 98:549–550, 1998

Rowbotham M, Harden N, Stacey B, et al: Gabapentin for the treatment of postherpetic neuralgia: a randomized controlled trial. JAMA 280:1837–1842, 1998 [see comments]

Ruedrich S, Swales T, Fossaceca C, et al: Effect of divalproex sodium on aggression and self-injurious behaviour in adults with intellectual disability: a retrospective review. J Intellect Disabil Res 43:105–111, 1999

Sachs G, Rosenbaum J, Jones L: Adjunctive clonazepam for maintenance treatment of bipolar affective disorder. J Clin Psychopharmacol 10:42–47, 1990a

Sachs GS, Weilburg JB, Rosenbaum JF: Clonazepam vs neuroleptics as adjuncts to lithium maintenance. Psychopharmacol Bull 26:137–143, 1990b

Sachs G, Bowden C, Calabrese JR, et al: Effects of lamotrigine and lithium on body weight during maintenance treatment of bipolar I disorder. Bipolar Disord 8(2):175–181, 2006

Sachs GS, Nierenberg AA, Calabrese JR, et al: Effectiveness of adjunctive antidepressant treatment for bipolar depression. N Engl J Med 356:1711–1722, 2007

Salzman C, Solomon D, Miyawaki E, et al: Parenteral lorazepam versus parenteral haloperidol for the control of psychotic disruptive behavior. J Clin Psychopharmacol 52:177–180, 1991

Saxena K, Howe M, Simeonova D, et al: Divalproex sodium reduces overall aggression in youth at high risk for bipolar disorder. J Child Adolesc Psychopharmacol 16:252–259, 2006

Schatzberg AF, DeBattista C: Phenomenology and treatment of agitation. J Clin Psychiatry 60:17–20, 1999

Schatzberg AF, DeBattista CB, DeGolia S: Valproate in the treatment of agitation associated with depression. Psychiatr Ann 26:1–4, 1996

Scherk H, Pajonk FG, Leucht S: Second-generation antipsychotic agents in the treatment of acute mania: a systematic review and meta-analysis of randomized controlled trials. Arch Gen Psychiatry 64:442–455, 2007

Schou M: The range of clinical uses of lithium, in Lithium in Medical Practice. Edited by Johnson FN, Johnson S. Baltimore, MD, University Park Press, 1978

Schou M: Artistic productivity and lithium prophylaxis in manic-depressive illness. Br J Psychiatry 135:97–103, 1979

Schou M: Lithium treatment during pregnancy, delivery, and lactation: an update. J Clin Psychiatry 51:410–413, 1990

Sheard JH, Marini JL, Bridges CI, et al: The effect of lithium on impulsive aggressive behavior in man. Am J Psychiatry 133:1409–1413, 1976

Silvers KM, Woolley CC, Hamilton FC, et al: Randomised double-blind placebo-controlled trial of fish oil in the treatment of depression. Prostaglandins Leukot Essent Fatty Acids 72(3):211–218, 2005

Simhandl C, Denk E, Thau K: The comparative efficacy of carbamazepine low and high serum levels and lithium carbonate in the prophylaxis of affective disorders. J Affect Disord 28:221–231, 1993

Small JG, Klapper MH, Milstein V, et al: Carbamazepine compared with lithium in the treatment of mania. Arch Gen Psychiatry 48:915–921, 1991

Sobotka JL, Alexander B, Cook BL: A review of carbamazepine's hematologic reactions and monitoring recommendations. DICP 24:1214–1219, 1990

Stein DJ, Simeon D, Frenkel M, et al: An open trial of valproate in borderline personality disorder. J Clin Psychiatry 56:506–510, 1995

Steiner H, Petersen ML, Saxena K, et al: Divalproex sodium for the treatment of conduct disorder: a randomized controlled clinical trial. J Clin Psychiatry 64:1183–1191, 2003

Stephen LJ, Sills GJ, Brodie MJ: Lamotrigine and topiramate may be a useful combination (letter). Lancet 351:958–959, 1998

Stoll AL, Severus WE, Freeman MP, et al: Omega 3 fatty acids in bipolar disorder: a preliminary double-blind, placebo-controlled trial. Arch Gen Psychiatry 56:407–412, 1999

Stromgren LS: The combination of lithium and carbamazepine in treatment and prevention of manic-depressive disorder: a review and a case report. Compr Psychiatry 31:261–265, 1990

Suppes T, Baldessarini RJ, Faedda GL, et al: Risk of recurrence following discontinuation of lithium treatment in bipolar disorder. Arch Gen Psychiatry 48:1082–1088, 1991

Suppes T, Baldessarini RJ, Faedda GL, et al: Discontinuation of maintenance treatment in bipolar disorder; risks and implication. Harv Rev Psychiatry 1:131–144, 1993

Suppes T, Phillips KA, Judd CR: Clozapine treatment of nonpsychotic rapid cycling bipolar disorder: a report of three cases. Biol Psychiatry 36:338–340, 1994

Suppes T, Chisholm KA, Dhavale D, et al: Tiagabine in treatment refractory bipolar disorder: a clinical case series. Bipolar Disord 4:283–289, 2002

Suppes T, Kelly DI, Hynan LS, et al: Comparison of two anticonvulsants in a randomized, single-blind treatment of hypomanic symptoms in patients with bipolar disorder. Aust N Z J Psychiatry 41:397–402, 2007

Teratogenic effects of carbamazepine (letter). N Engl J Med 321:1480–1481, 1989

Tilkian AG, Schroder JS, Kao JJ, et al: The cardiovascular effects of lithium in man. Am J Med 61:665–670, 1976

Tohen M, Castillo J, Cole JO, et al: Thrombocytopenia associated with carbamazepine: a case series. J Clin Psychiatry 52:496–498, 1991 [see comments]

Tohen M, Castillo J, Pope HG Jr, et al: Concomitant use of valproate and carbamazepine in bipolar and schizoaffective disorders. J Clin Psychopharmacol 14:67–70, 1994

Tohen M, Sanger TM, McElroy SL, et al: Olanzapine versus placebo in the treatment of acute mania. Olanzapine HGEH Study Group. Am J Psychiatry 156:702–709, 1999

Tohen M, Ketter TA, Zarate CA, et al: Olanzapine versus divalproex sodium for the treatment of acute mania and maintenance of remission: a 47-week study. Am J Psychiatry 160:1263–1271, 2003a

Tohen M, Vieta E, Calabrese J, et al: Efficacy of olanzapine and olanzapine-fluoxetine combination in the treatment of bipolar I depression. Arch Gen Psychiatry 60:1079–1088, 2003b

Tondo L, Hennen J, Baldessarini RJ: Lower suicide risk with long-term lithium treatment in major affective illness. a meta-analysis. Acta Psychiatr Scand 104:163–172, 2001

Tupin J: Management of violent patients, in Manual of Psychiatric Therapeutics. Edited by Shader RI. Boston, MA, Little, Brown, 1975, pp 125–133

Uhde T, Post R, Ballenger J, et al: Carbamazepine in the treatment of neuropsychiatric disorders, in Anticonvulsants in Affective Disorders (Excerpta Medica International Congress Series, No 626). Edited by Emrich H, Okuma T, Muller A. Amsterdam, Excerpta Medica, 1984, pp 111–131

Valproate and carbamazepine join lithium as primary treatments for bipolar disorder [news]. Am J Health Syst Pharm 52:358, 361, 1995

Valproate and mood disorders: perspectives. J Clin Psychopharmacol 12:1S–68S, 1992

Valproate for bipolar disorder. Med Lett Drugs Ther 36:74–75, 1994

van der Loos ML, Mulder PG, Hartong EG, et al; LamLit Study Group: Efficacy and safety of lamotrigine as add-on treatment to lithium in bipolar depression: a multicenter, double-blind, placebo-controlled trial. J Clin Psychiatry 70:223–231, 2009

Vendsborg PB, Bech P, Rafaelson OJ: Lithium treatment and weight gain. Acta Psychiatr Scand 53:139–147, 1976

Vieta E, Sanchez-Moreno J, Goikolea JM, et al: Effects on weight and outcome of long-term olanzapine-topiramate combination treatment in bipolar disorder. J Clin Psychopharmacol 24:374–378, 2004

Vieta E, Cruz N, García-Campayo J, et al: A double-blind, randomized, placebo-controlled prophylaxis trial of oxcarbazepine as adjunctive treatment to lithium in the long-term treatment of bipolar I and II disorder. Int J Neuropsychopharmacol 11:445–452, 2008

Vinten J, Adab N, Kini A, et al: Neuropsychological effects of exposure to anticonvulsant medication in utero. Neurology 64:949–954, 2005

Wagner KD, Kowatch RA, Emslie GJ, et al: A double-blind, randomized, placebo-controlled trial of oxcarbazepine in the treatment of bipolar disorder in children and adolescents. Am J Psychiatry 163:1179–1186, 2006 [erratum: Am J Psychiatry 163:1843, 2006]

Wang PW, Yang YS, Chandler RA, et al: Adjunctive zonisamide for weight loss in euthymic bipolar disorder patients: a pilot study. J Psychiatr Res 42:451–457, 2008

Weisler RH, Ahearn EP, Davidson JR, et al: Adjunctive use of olanzapine in mood disorders: five case reports. Ann Clin Psychiatry 9:259–262, 1997

Weisler RH, Hirschfeld R, Cutler AJ, et al, SPD417 Study Group: Extended-release carbamazepine capsules as monotherapy in bipolar disorder: pooled results from two randomised, double-blind, placebo-controlled trials. CNS Drugs 20:219–231, 2006

Wilcox JA: Divalproex sodium as a treatment for borderline personality disorder. Ann Clin Psychiatry 7:33–37, 1995

Williams AL, Katz D, Ali A, et al: Do essential fatty acids have a role in the treatment of depression? J Affect Disord 93(1–3):117–123, 2006

Woodman CL, Noyes R Jr: Panic disorder: treatment with valproate. J Clin Psychiatry 55:134–136, 1994

Wright BA, Jarrett DB: Lithium and calcium-channel blockers: possible neurotoxicity (letter). Biol Psychiatry 30:635–636, 1991

Wroblewski BA, Joseph AB, Kupfer J, et al: Effectiveness of valproic acid on destructive and aggressive behaviours in patients with acquired brain injury. Brain Inj 11:37–47, 1997

Xie X, Hagan RM: Cellular and molecular actions of lamotrigine: possible mechanisms of efficacy in bipolar disorder. Neuropsychobiology 38:119–130, 1998

Young AH, Geddes JR, Macritchie K, et al: Tiagabine in the maintenance treatment of bipolar disorders. Cochrane Database Syst Rev 3:CD005173, 2006a

Young AH, Geddes JR, Macritchie K, et al: Tiagabine in the treatment of acute affective episodes in bipolar disorder: efficacy and acceptability. Cochrane Database Syst Rev 3:CD004694, 2006b

Zajecka JM, Weisler R, Sachs G, et al: A comparison of the efficacy, safety, and tolerability of divalproex sodium and olanzapine in the treatment of bipolar disorder. J Clin Psychiatry 63:1148–1155, 2002

Zarate C Jr, Tohen M, Banov MD, et al: Is clozapine a mood stabilizer? J Clin Psychiatry 56:108–112, 1995

Zullino D, Baumann P: Olanzapine for mixed episodes of bipolar disorder (letter). J Psychopharmacol 13:198, 1999

6

Antianxiety Agents

Anxiolytic agents—usually defined in the past as chiefly the benzodiaze-pines—are among the most commonly used psychotropic drugs. The vast majority of prescriptions for these medications are issued by primary care physicians. Psychiatrists write less than 20% of the prescriptions for anxiolytics in this country, reflecting, in part, the fact that most anxious patients never see psychiatrists. Moreover, anxiolytics are prescribed for a wide variety of patients who do not have a primary anxiety disorder—namely, patients who present to primary care physicians with somatic complaints or true somatic disease.

Antianxiety agents may be divided into many subclasses, of which the benzodiazepines are the most frequently prescribed. Several of the subclasses of anxiolytics (e.g., benzodiazepines) include agents that were originally marketed primarily as hypnotics (e.g., flurazepam). In this manual, we have separated the pharmacological treatments of anxiety from those of insomnia. The distinction, however, is rather artificial, because almost any sedative or antianxiety drug can be used at a low dose in the daytime for anxiety and at a similar or higher dose for difficulty in sleeping. While newer hypnotics like eszopiclone have somewhat more selective properties for sedation rather than anxiety, even eszopiclone has some anxiolytic properties. This reflects common pharmacological effects on benzodiazepine binding sites on γ-aminobutyric acid A (GABA-A) receptors. On the other hand, it is not clear that the sleep agent rozerem, a melatonin agonist, has any utility in the treatment of anxiety.

The first major anxiolytic group, the *barbiturates*, were developed as sedative-hypnotic and antiepileptic agents and were first introduced in the early 1900s. These drugs are also discussed in the chapter on hypnotics (see Chapter 7: "Hypnotics"). Meprobamate, a *carbamate* derivative, was introduced almost 60 years later as a sedative-anxiolytic agent. Although use of the two classes— barbiturates and carbamates—has waned dramatically in recent decades, they are still used on occasion.

Benzodiazepines, introduced in the early 1960s, dramatically changed the pharmacological approach to anxiety. First developed as muscle relaxants, their anxiolytic-hypnotic properties, wider safety margin in overdose, and potential to elicit physical dependence quickly became apparent. Buspirone, a serotonin$_{1A}$ (5-HT$_{1A}$) agonist with some mixed dopaminergic effects, was released in the United States in 1987 for use in anxiety. Its use by psychiatrists in the treatment of anxiety and related conditions was less than its use in primary care and nursing home settings (see "Buspirone" section in this chapter; Cole and Yonkers 1995).

Increasingly, anticonvulsants are being used in the treatment of anxiety states. Agents such as gabapentin and pregabalin may be alternatives or adjuncts to the more commonly used antidepressants and benzodiazepines in treating some anxiety disorders.

Less widely used pharmacological approaches to anxiety include antihistamines and autonomic agents (e.g., β-blockers). The former have primarily a general sedative action; the latter, which are more commonly used than antihistamines, act by blocking peripheral or central noradrenergic activity and many of the manifestations of anxiety (e.g., tremor, palpitations, sweating). Several of the phenothiazines also have indications in anxiety, although in the United States they have become less widely used in recent years for this purpose; the second-generation antipsychotics (SGAs) also appear to have anti-anxiety effects. There is evidence, for example, that quetiapine is efficacious in the treatment of generalized anxiety disorder (GAD) and that drugs such as risperidone may augment the anti-obsessive properties of selective serotonin reuptake inhibitors (SSRIs). Nonetheless, the safety concerns about the

SGAs render them second- or third-line agents in the management of anxiety disorders.

Many antidepressants (mainly SSRIs and serotonin-norepinephrine reuptake inhibitors (SNRIs) such as venlafaxine) have taken center stage in the treatment of the whole range of anxiety disorders but not in the treatment of insomnia. However, mirtazapine and trazodone are commonly used as hypnotic agents. Clomipramine is the only tricyclic antidepressant (TCA) shown to be consistently effective in the treatment of obsessive-compulsive disorder (OCD). However, all the SSRIs are also presumably effective treatments for OCD (see "Obsessive-Compulsive Disorder" section later in this chapter). The SSRIs and related or unrelated newer drugs (e.g., gabapentin, venlafaxine) may already have become the primary drugs used by psychiatrists for the treatment of specific anxiety disorders, whereas benzodiazepines may still be the first drugs prescribed by primary care physicians.

In addition to this major shift in the patterns of treatment of anxiety disorders, there has been a major upsurge of interest in cognitive-behavioral therapy (CBT), whose efficacy has been shown in well-designed studies, mainly done by psychologists. Specific or semispecific programs have been designed to address the symptoms and treatment requirements of individual anxiety disorders. Almost all these programs, however, have elements of desensitization, exposure, and cognitive restructuring and include having the patient demonstrate new learning in real-life situations.

As a very general overview, benzodiazepines often work fastest in relieving symptoms, antidepressants (SSRIs and newer agents) take several weeks, and CBT may take 2 months or longer. There is some evidence that patients who show improvement while participating in CBT programs maintain the improvement longer after treatment is stopped than do patients who show improvement while receiving drug therapies (Barlow et al. 2000). Recent studies point to D-cycloserine, a glutamatergic agent, augmenting the effects of behavior therapy in several types of anxiety disorders (Hofmann et al. 2006; Norberg et al. 2008; Ressler et al. 2004). The mechanism is through enhancing fear extinction, and effectiveness was first demonstrated in patients with acrophobia (Ressler et al. 2004).

We begin the chapter by discussing the use of benzodiazepines in treating general and panic anxiety. We then address the use of antidepressants in treating other anxiety disorders, such as posttraumatic stress disorder (PTSD), social phobia, and OCD, and body dysmorphic disorder. Finally, we discuss the use of other classes of medication for anxiety and other conditions, such as catatonia, a syndrome uniquely responsive to sedative drugs and electroconvulsive therapy (ECT).

Since the SSRIs have already been considered in some detail in Chapter 3 ("Antidepressants"), we give them less detailed attention here. Several of the SSRIs and venlafaxine have been approved by the U.S. Food and Drug Administration (FDA) for one or more specific anxiety diagnoses, including paroxetine for GAD, PTSD, OCD, panic disorder, premenstrual dysphoric disorder (PMDD) (controlled-release form only), and social phobia; fluoxetine for OCD, bulimia, panic disorder, and PMDD; sertraline for OCD, panic disorder, PMDD, social anxiety disorder, and PTSD; escitalopram for GAD; venlafaxine (extended-release form) for GAD and social anxiety disorder; duloxetine for GAD; and fluvoxamine for social anxiety disorder and OCD. It is our position that until studies clearly show differences in efficacy between these drugs in the treatment of specific anxiety disorders, all SSRIs and perhaps most SNRIs are probably reasonably effective across most anxiety disorders. Their use in such conditions may require adjustments, but these apply to the specific disorder and the whole class of SSRIs. For example, use very low dosages (particularly initially) in patients with panic disorder with agoraphobia; use higher dosages and wait even longer for clinical response in patients with OCD.

Benzodiazepines

Indications

In addition to anxiety, benzodiazepines are indicated for muscle tension, insomnia, status epilepticus (diazepam), myoclonic epilepsy (clonazepam), preoperative anesthesia, and alcohol withdrawal. One benzodiazepine, the triazolobenzodiazepine alprazolam, is also indicated for anxiety associated with depression (as is lorazepam), and some studies have shown that alprazolam also parallels imipramine and phenelzine in having both antipanic and antidepressant properties (see Chapter 3: "Antidepressants"). Clonazepam is also approved in the treatment of panic disorder, and it is likely that all benzodiazepines are effective in the treatment of panic if given at high enough doses.

Likewise, all currently available benzodiazepines are useful in treating both chronic anxiety and anxiety secondary to life stresses or medical conditions. The definition of GAD in DSM-IV-TR (American Psychiatric Associ-

Benzodiazepines (e.g., diazepam, clonazepam, alprazolam): overview	
Efficacy	Generalized anxiety (FDA approved) Panic disorder (FDA approved for alprazolam, clonazepam) Insomnia (FDA approved) Seizure disorder (FDA approved for clonazepam) Muscle relaxation Anesthesia
Side effects	Sedation Lethargy Dependence/Withdrawal
Safety in overdose	Safe in overdose up to 30 times the normal daily dose. Usual symptoms of overdose include sedation, drowsiness, ataxia, and slurred speech. May result in respiratory depression in combination with other CNS depressants. Management includes gastric lavage, forced emesis, and assisted ventilation.
Dosage and administration	Varies by benzodiazepine and indication; see Table 6–1.
Discontinuation	Taper by no more than 25% of total dose per week after long-term administration. Withdrawal includes insomnia, agitation, anxiety, and, rarely, seizures.
Drug interactions	Additive CNS depression with ethanol, barbiturates, and other CNS depressants Drugs that ↑ triazolo-benzodiazepine levels include: cytochrome P450 3A4 inhibitors, ketoconazole, fluconazole, nefazodone Drugs that ↓ triazolo-benzodiazepine levels include: carbamazepine

Note. CNS = central nervous system; FDA = U.S. Food and Drug Administration.

ation 2000) is probably too restrictive to cover all the forms of anxiety for which benzodiazepines can be helpful. It is even likely that there are "double anxiety" disorders, analogous to the concept of double depression; some patients have lifelong mild to moderate anxiety symptoms with episodic periods of worsening during which they seek therapy.

Panic disorder with or without agoraphobia is a chronic, fluctuating condition; some patients experience episodes of illness (like depressive episodes), whereas other patients have mild, infrequent attacks during some life phases and incapacitating symptoms at other times. Alprazolam is the only benzodiazepine officially deemed effective and well studied in the treatment of panic disorder with or without agoraphobia, although other benzodiazepines may also be effective.

Both panic and GAD are conditions often accompanying other disorders, such as major depression, PTSD, and borderline personality disorder, as well as other specific anxiety disorders (e.g., social phobia).

It is likely that patients seen in primary care settings may show even more complex mixtures of milder anxiety and depressive symptoms than patients seen by psychiatrists. The old-fashioned wastebasket diagnosis of mixed anxiety and depression may still deserve recognition because of the prevalence of such a presentation, even though recent diagnostic systems (DSM-III-R [American Psychiatric Association 1987] and DSM-IV [American Psychiatric Association 1994]) have not fully endorsed the condition. Such disorders could explain why antidepressants and antianxiety agents often work in the same types of patients (Rickels and Schweizer 1995).

Clonazepam has been reported to speed response in patients with major depression treated with fluoxetine (Smith et al. 1998) and in panic disorder patients treated with sertraline (Goddard et al. 2001). The drug appeared to have a calming effect and to offset any anxiogenic effect associated with initiation of the SSRI. The benzodiazepine was used for brief periods (about 3 weeks) at doses of 0.5–1.5 mg hs and was then discontinued. Such uses are discussed in Chapter 9 ("Augmentation Strategies for Treatment-Resistant Disorders").

Pharmacological Effects

In recent years there has been considerable attention to the mode of action of benzodiazepines, spurred on by the identification of specific benzodiazepine sites on the GABA-A receptor. This receptor complex appears to mediate the anxiolytic, sedative, and anticonvulsant actions of the benzodiazepines. The location of specific receptors may be related to the relative anticonvulsant, anxiolytic, or sedative properties of the various benzodiazepines.

It has been hypothesized that it may be possible to develop increasingly specific agents that act as site-specific agonists or partial agonists to produce anxiolysis without sedation or sedation without much muscle relaxation. These approaches are being explored. Thus far, drugs more specifically binding to the benzodiazepine α_1 site (e.g., zolpidem) do not seem particularly unique but appear to have more potent sedative than muscle-relaxing properties. Partial agonists or drugs with more specific binding could substantially reduce the risk for tolerance, dependence, and withdrawal effects. Unfortunately, neither partial agonists nor more uniquely binding drugs appear so far to be different from available benzodiazepines.

The triazolobenzodiazepine alprazolam appears to also have effects on noradrenergic systems, causing downregulation of postsynaptic β-adrenergic receptors in reserpine-treated mice and increasing the activity of the N protein in humans (the protein that couples the postsynaptic receptor to the intraneuronal energy system). These effects may help to explain the drug's antipanic and moderate antidepressant effects beyond the effects mediated by the benzodiazepine-GABA receptor complex.

Subclasses

The anxiolytic benzodiazepines are commonly divided into three subclasses on the basis of structure: 2-keto (chlordiazepoxide, clonazepam, clorazepate, diazepam, halazepam, prazepam, and the hypnotic flurazepam); 3-hydroxy (lorazepam, oxazepam, and the hypnotic temazepam); and triazolo (alprazolam, adinazolam, estazolam, and the hypnotic triazolam) (see Figure 6–1 and Table 6–1).

The pharmacokinetic properties (i.e., half-lives) vary among these classes, in part reflecting differences in their modes of drug metabolism, as summarized in Table 6–2. The 2-keto drugs and their active metabolites are oxidized in the liver, and because this process is relatively slow, these compounds have relatively long half-lives. For example, the half-life of diazepam is approximately 40 hours. One active metabolite (desmethyldiazepam) has an even longer half-life (about 60 hours). Moreover, because desmethyldiazepam is further metabolized to oxazepam, which is also active as an anxiolytic (Table 6–1), diazepam imparts long-range sedative and anxiolytic effects. The half-life of clonazepam is approximately 40 hours. Many of the marketed 2-keto drugs are prodrugs—they are themselves inactive but eventually form active metabolites. Thus, prazepam, clorazepate, and halazepam are mere precursors to desmethyldiazepam, as is diazepam. Differences among these specific 2-keto compounds revolve around the rates of absorption and the specific active metabolites formed.

Table 6–1. Benzodiazepines: names, formulations and strengths, and anxiolytic dosage range

Generic name	Brand name[a]	Formulations and strengths	Anxiolytic dosage range (mg/day)[b]
2-Keto			
chlordiazepoxide	Librium	Capsules: 5, 10, 25 mg	15–40
clorazepate	Tranxene	Tablets: 3.75, 7.5, 15 mg	15–40
diazepam	Valium	Tablets: 2, 5, 10 mg	5–40
		Oral solution: 5 mg/5 mL (30-mL)	
		Injection: 5 mg/mL (2-mL prefilled syringe; 2-mL ampule; 1-mL, 2-mL, 10-mL vials)	
clonazepam	Klonopin	Tablets: 0.5, 1, 2 mg	
		Wafers: 0.125, 0.25, 0.5, 1, 2 mg	
3-Hydroxy			
lorazepam	Ativan	Tablets: 0.5, 1, 2 mg	1–6
		Oral solution: 2 mg/mL (30-mL)	
		Injection: 2 mg/mL, 4 mg/mL (both in 1-mL prefilled syringe and single-dose vial and 10-mL multidose vial)	1–2
oxazepam	Serax	Capsules: 10, 15, 30 mg	15–120
Triazolo			
alprazolam	Xanax	Tablets: 0.25, 0.5, 1, 2 mg	1–4
		Disintegrating tablets: 0.25, 0.5, 1, 2 mg	
		Oral solution: 1 mg/mL (30-mL)	
alprazolam XR	Xanax XR	1, 2, 3 mg	

[a]The benzodiazepines shown are available in generic form.
[b]Approximate dosage ranges. Some patients will require higher dosages; others may respond to dosages below the range.

Figure 6–1. Chemical structures of anxiolytic benzodiazepines.

In contrast, the 3-hydroxy compounds are metabolized via direct conjugation with a glucuronide radical, a process that is more rapid than oxidation and does not involve the formation of active metabolites. The two major examples of this subclass are oxazepam and lorazepam, which have considerably shorter half-lives (9 and 14 hours, respectively) than do their 2-keto counterparts. Similarly, the hypnotic temazepam has a half-life (8 hours) that is much shorter than flurazepam's.

The triazolo compounds are also oxidized; however, they appear to have more limited active metabolites and thus relatively shorter half-lives. The half-

Table 6–2. Benzodiazepines: absorption and pharmacokinetics

Generic name	Oral absorption	Major active components	Approximate half-life (hours)[a]
2-Keto			
chlordiazepoxide	Intermediate	chlordiazepoxide	20
		desmethylchlordiazepoxide	30
		demoxepam	Unknown
		desmethyldiazepam	60
clorazepate	Fast	desmethyldiazepam	60
diazepam	Fast	diazepam	40
		desmethyldiazepam	60
		methyloxazepam	10
halazepam	Intermediate	desmethyldiazepam	60
prazepam	Slow	desmethyldiazepam	60
3-Hydroxy			
lorazepam	Intermediate	lorazepam	14
oxazepam	Slow to intermediate	oxazepam	9
Triazolo			
alprazolam	Intermediate	alprazolam	14
alprazolam XR			

[a]Based on ranges of half-lives reported in young, psychiatrically and physically healthy volunteers.

life of alprazolam is about 14 hours; adinazolam, 2 hours; and *N*-desmethyl-adinazolam (adinazolam's active metabolite), 4 hours; the half-life of the hypnotic triazolam is 3–4 hours.

The pharmacokinetic properties of benzodiazepines that are oxidized in the liver may be affected by other medications. Of particular note, nefazodone, fluoxetine, fluvoxamine, sertraline, cimetidine (Tagamet), and contraceptive pills inhibit the liver oxidative enzyme cytochrome P450 3A3/4 and thus slow the degradation of the 2-keto and triazolo compounds. Clinicians should keep this in mind in treating anxious patients who are also taking these drugs. Fluoxetine's effects on alprazolam metabolism have not appeared to be clinically meaningful.

Other differences among benzodiazepines revolve around their rates of absorption and distribution. For example, although prazepam and clorazepate are similar in structure and both are prodrugs of desmethyldiazepam, the two differ in terms of the metabolic processes required for absorption and, thus, in the rates at which they appear in blood (Table 6–2). Clorazepate and diazepam are rapidly absorbed and produce peaks in plasma levels more quickly than does prazepam, whose absorption is mediated via slower processes. Halazepam's conversion to desmethyldiazepam is even slower. The lipophilic and hydrophilic properties of these drugs also vary, resulting in pronounced differences in how quickly they work and for how long. Drugs that are more lipophilic (e.g., diazepam) enter the brain more quickly, "turning on" the effect promptly, but "turning off" the effect more quickly as well as they disappear into body fat. Less lipophilic compounds (e.g., lorazepam) produce clinical effects more slowly but may provide more sustained relief. These properties are largely independent of pharmacokinetics. Some drugs with long half-lives (e.g., diazepam) can also be highly lipophilic, providing rapid relief but for shorter periods than one might predict from half-life data alone. In contrast, lorazepam is less lipophilic and turns on and off more slowly, potentially providing more sustained effects, despite its shorter half-life compared with diazepam. In short, traditional half-life pharmacokinetics can be misleading and tell only a part of the story of how drugs work.

In addition, investigators have begun to pay more attention to relative receptor affinity, a property that may play a more important role than was previously thought in determining the duration of action. High-potency benzodiazepines, such as lorazepam and alprazolam, may have such high receptor affinity that withdrawal symptoms may be far more intense than might be expected from inspecting other variables such as half-lives. Interestingly, oxazepam, which is similar in lipid solubility and half-life to lorazepam, appears to produce fewer withdrawal symptoms. This position has been most eloquently stated by Lader (1982) in the United Kingdom. Unfortunately, there are few data to confirm or refute this assertion.

Although several of the benzodiazepines are available for parenteral use (see Table 6–1), there is wide variability in the absorption properties of these compounds when given intramuscularly. For example, lorazepam is relatively rapidly absorbed when given intramuscularly. In contrast, chlordiazepoxide and diazepam are slowly absorbed. Lorazepam has become increasingly popular as an adjunctive treatment for agitation in acutely psychotic patients and also often relieves catatonic and depressive stupor. Oral concentrate forms of some benzodiazepines, such as diazepam, lorazepam, and alprazolam, are available in the United States. In addition, lorazepam and clonazepam tablets are given sublingually in some emergency room situations to promote rapid absorption of the drug from the oral mucosa. Clonazepam is available as a rapidly disintegrating sublingual wafer, and some anxious patients or patients with panic find the sublingual wafer quite helpful. In some studies alprazolam given by nasal spray at the onset of panic attacks proved effective in aborting them. An American pharmaceutical company acquired the rights to intranasal alprazolam (Panistat) in 2001. However, to our knowledge, the drug has not been further developed. A number of attempts to develop alternative delivery through nasal or buccal administration have failed to demonstrate efficacy. Abuse concerns are likely to be an issue with the development of any intranasal or rapidly absorbed benzodiazepine.

Dosage and Administration

The efficacy of benzodiazepines in treating patients with symptomatic anxiety or diagnosable anxiety disorders has been established in many double-blind, random-assignment comparisons with placebo. When treating a GAD patient, the clinician might begin with a benzodiazepine (e.g., diazepam at approximately 2 mg tid, with increases as needed to a maximum regular daily dose of 40 mg). A modal dosage of diazepam for GAD is 15–20 mg/day. Chlordiazepoxide has a much wider dosage range: the recommended starting dosage is

5–10 mg po tid, with a maximum of 60 mg/day for anxiety. The dosage of chlordiazepoxide for acute alcohol withdrawal is much higher: 50–200 mg/day. Generally, clinicians prescribe chlordiazepoxide 25 mg every 1–2 hours until symptomatic relief or sedation occurs, up to a maximum dosage of 200 mg/day. For lorazepam, the starting dosage is 0.5 mg tid, with titration upward as needed to 6 mg/day. Higher daily doses are approved but are frequently associated with intense sedation. Dosage ranges for the anxiolytic benzodiazepines are listed in Table 6–1.

Clonazepam is generally started at 0.5–1 mg/day. Dosages up to 4 mg/day are sometimes needed to control panic attacks, but most patients do well with 1–2 mg/day. Clonazepam wafers can also be given in doses as small as 0.125 mg to treat an acute panic attack. The ideal dosing regimen, however, prevents panic attacks and circumvents the need to use sublingual wafers. Clonazepam, like other benzodiazepines, works much faster than antidepressants. We will often treat a panic disorder for the first 4–6 weeks with a benzodiazepine such as clonazepam while simultaneously starting an antidepressant. Studies have suggested that the addition of clonazepam to an SSRI speeds up treatment effects in panic disorder (Pollack et al. 2003).

The use of alprazolam in panic disorder patients often requires higher dosages than those used in GAD. Currently, alprazolam is approved in dosages up to 10 mg/day, but generally 4–5 mg/day or less is used. In our early studies on depression, we used the much higher dosage regimen, but we have been impressed that patients generally do not require more than 4 mg/day for a response, and some are even oversedated at 2–3 mg/day. Because of concern about dependence, this drug should be used at the lowest effective dose possible. There is evidence from controlled, fixed-dose studies that blood levels of alprazolam in the range of 20–40 ng/mL are optimal for improvement in patients with panic disorder. At higher plasma levels (40–60 ng/mL), some additional patients may improve, but sedative-type side effects and ataxia increase (Greenblatt et al. 1993). Alprazolam is available in an extended-release formulation (XR) for qd or bid dosing (Glue et al. 2006). The XR form generally allows for once-a-day dosing and may mitigate some of the withdrawal associated with missed doses. However, alprazolam XR can still result in withdrawal symptoms. Several biotechnology start-up companies are attempting to develop more rapidly absorbed or even longer-acting formulations.

The starting dosage of alprazolam in both GAD and panic disorder should be 1.5 mg/day or less, given in divided doses, with a gradual increase in dosage as tolerated by the patient. In treating patients with panic disorder, alprazolam dosage may be increased, to block not only panic attacks but anticipatory anxiety as well. This often requires higher dosages (4–5 mg/day) in the first 6 or more weeks. Over time, however, as patients overcome their anticipatory anxiety, the dosage can be reduced to 2–3 mg/day for continued blocking of panic attacks. Although alprazolam was thought to have unique antipanic properties, subsequent reports have indicated that lorazepam, clonazepam, and diazepam may all be effective in ameliorating or preventing panic symptoms. Clonazepam is used at dosages of 1–3 mg/day.

Although TCAs, monoamine oxidase inhibitors (MAOIs), and SSRIs are all probably as effective as alprazolam or clonazepam in treating patients with panic disorder with agoraphobia, only the benzodiazepines provide rapid relief; the other drug groups take at least 4–6 weeks, compared with 1 week or less for alprazolam. With the more conventional antidepressants, more patients drop out early in treatment because of side effects, and there is a general belief that some panic patients are even more sensitive to antidepressant drug side effects than are depressed patients. In patients who have occasional bouts of moderate anxiety occurring only every few days or weeks, benzodiazepines may be preferable to maintenance antidepressants, since they work as prn medication. Diazepam's ability to act rapidly without prolonged sedation makes it particularly useful in such situations with patients not prone to drug abuse. Other benzodiazepines can also be used in this manner, of course. Oxazepam's slow absorption rate raises concern about its utility as a prn medication. However, patient acceptance of oxazepam is fairly good, and its low abuse liability makes it a reasonable choice for some patients.

In patients with long histories of a particular kind of panic disorder with agoraphobia, 6-month and 18-month courses of alprazolam therapy were studied in terms of relapse/recurrence rates after the alprazolam was tapered and stopped; the longer period was found to be associated with symptomatic relief (Ballenger et al. 1993).

One major area of debate revolves around how long to use these drugs for patients with significant anxiety. For patients whose anxiety is very acute and related to specific stressors, use of these agents should be directed at reduction of acute symptoms, and thus prolonged use beyond 1–2 weeks is generally not required or advised. In patients whose anxiety symptoms are of several months' or greater duration, we recommend treatment for 4–6 weeks at doses that provide relief, then reduction of dosage to the minimum needed for maintenance for the next few months, followed by discontinuation when possible. Patients who meet DSM-IV-TR criteria for GAD have by definition an even more chronic condition and require even longer treatment (e.g., 4–6 months or longer) before discontinuation is attempted. For these patients, SSRIs may be the preferred agent to use first. Unfortunately, psychiatrists often first see patients with histories compatible with GAD only after they have received benzodiazepines for years from other physicians; there are many such patients who obtain relief from these drugs but who relapse when the drugs are stopped. Further, because many patients seem to do well on reasonable dosages over longer periods, the clinician may be faced with the difficult decision of how long to maintain use of the benzodiazepine. This dilemma is intensified by the observation that tolerance can develop to some effects of benzodiazepines (e.g., hypnosis), suggesting that the apparent relief experienced by patients could reflect a nonspecific psychological effect.

Although tolerance can occur, it is our belief that most patients do not develop tolerance but are still responding. We base this observation on the number of patients we have seen over the years who have functioned well on a given daily dose of benzodiazepine and have not found themselves escalating their total daily intake. Longer-term data from alprazolam studies indicate that panic patients do not escalate their daily dosages but, rather, frequently lower them over time. There does not appear to be a loss of efficacy of alprazolam in patients followed for up to 1 year. It is our impression that animal and human models of tolerance may not be totally applicable to chronic anxiety per se. Rather, such models emphasize self-administration of a drug or drug-induced ataxia produced in "normal" specimens but do not fully take into account the biological and clinical status of the anxious patient. If possible, the clinician should attempt gradually to taper benzodiazepines, using psychotherapy, behavior therapy, or other drug therapies to help patients deal with their anxiety (see "Withdrawal" subsection later in this chapter). Some patients, however, may require continued benzodiazepine therapy. Overlapping an SSRI with the benzodiazepine for several weeks, in the hope that the patient will feel still further relief of symptoms, before tapering the benzodiazepine appears to be a useful strategy. For example, Goddard and colleagues (2001) found that the co-administration of sertraline and clonazepam in patients with panic disorder facilitated early improvement of symptoms when compared with sertraline alone. True longer-term harmful effects of benzodiazepines have not been convincingly described. For example, Lader (1982) reported computed tomography (CT) scan abnormalities in a series of patients who had taken benzodiazepines for a long time. Although these observations could be interpreted as indicating that these drugs produce organic or structural changes in brain tissue (as chronic alcohol use does), an equally acceptable explanation is that some anxious patients who require chronic treatment with benzodiazepines may have neuropsychiatric disorders, as evidenced by CT scan abnormalities. A study by Lucki et al. (1986) of patients on chronic long-term benzodiazepine treatment failed to show significant cognitive impairment on psychometric tests. The most recent controlled study in this area failed to find significant long-term cognitive effects for alprazolam XR in panic patients (Gladsjo et al. 2001). However, some investigators believe such impairment can occur, particularly in elderly patients. Certainly elderly medical patients taking long-acting benzodiazepines (or antidepressants) are at increased risk for falls leading to hip fractures.

How addictive are benzodiazepines? How long does one have to take a benzodiazepine before withdrawal is seen with discontinuation? Studies in animals have indicated that benzodiazepines can reinforce use and can produce physical dependence and tolerance. Available survey and treatment facility data suggest that benzodiazepines are rarely sought after or craved in the sense that heroin and cocaine are. Rather, they are used as part of a polysubstance abuse pattern to modulate the effects of primary drugs of abuse (e.g., cocaine) or as backup drugs when more euphoriant drugs are not available.

Risk factors for benzodiazepine abuse include a history of alcohol or other substance abuse and the presence of a personality disorder. In patients with a history of substance abuse, benzodiazepines should generally not be prescribed routinely. However, in some recreational drug users with anxiety, they can be used, particularly if trials of other agents have failed. In patients with an Axis II disorder, benzodiazepines should be administered only if necessary and for brief periods at low doses. Benzodiazepine dependence is mainly, or at least partially, an iatrogenic problem in that patients receive the medication from physicians originally for legitimate reasons but may then take it for too long or at too large a dosage. Possible length of treatment with these drugs should be thought out in advance of their prescription, and longer-term trials should be monitored carefully.

Given the current medicolegal climate and the existence of experts and medical boards devoted to "pharmacologic Calvinism," physicians planning to recommend that patients, particularly those with a past history of substance abuse, continue taking benzodiazepines for long periods should get outside consultation to help in confirming or changing their treatment plans.

Withdrawal

Should one attempt to gradually discontinue benzodiazepines from patients who have taken them regularly over longer periods? As a rule, this approach is sensible; reduction should be made at a maximum rate of approximately 10% per day. Many patients, however, will require much slower tapering. In their classic study of benzodiazepine withdrawal, Rickels et al. (1983) noted that when benzodiazepines were abruptly discontinued under double-blind conditions, withdrawal symptoms were demonstrated in more patients who had been taking benzodiazepines for more than 8 months (43%) than patients who had been taking them for shorter periods (5%). In a subsequent study, this group reported similar rates of withdrawal symptoms in patients who had been receiving maintenance therapy with clorazepate for 6 months (Rickels et al. 1988). Pecknold et al. (1988) reported that sudden discontinuation after an 8-week trial of alprazolam resulted in symptoms of anxiety in about 35% of panic disorder patients. Some of these patients may have experienced re-emergence of their panic symptoms rather than withdrawal.

Common symptoms of benzodiazepine withdrawal include jitteriness, anxiety, palpitations, clamminess, sweating, nausea, confusion, and heightened sensitivity to light and sound. Seizures represent the most worrisome of withdrawal reactions, but fortunately they are generally rare. No patients in the 1983 study by Rickels et al. experienced seizures. Seizures with abrupt diazepam withdrawal occur about 5–7 days after the drug is stopped and not within 24 hours, reflecting the long half-lives of both diazepam and desmethyldiazepam. With shorter-acting drugs (e.g., lorazepam and alprazolam), withdrawal symptoms emerge more rapidly—within 2–3 days. Thus, with diazepam, physicians cannot be confident that seizures will not occur unless the patient has stopped taking the drug for at least 1 week. Any signs of withdrawal (even at day 5) should be reviewed carefully, and consideration should be given to re-instituting the drug and then withdrawing it more gradually. A few days after discontinuation of benzodiazepines, some patients reexperience their original anxiety symptoms, but in a more severe form (so-called rebound anxiety). (In the case of hypnotics, this takes the form of rebound insomnia.) This syndrome is generally transient, usually lasting 48–72 hours.

As Rickels and Schweizer (1995) suggested, withdrawal symptoms usually occur during benzodiazepine tapering and in approximately the week following cessation and have passed after the patient has been without benzodiazepines for 3 weeks. Symptoms of the preexisting anxiety disorder usually reemerge more rapidly.

It is becoming increasingly clear that many patients stop adhering to withdrawal regimens for benzodiazepines early in the process, well before appreciable withdrawal symptoms could occur (see Rickels et al. 1999 and the entire supplement of the journal in which their article appears for more details). This strongly suggests a psychological belief that the medications are necessary and a strong overreaction to somatic symptoms related to anxiety. Not surprisingly, CBT of the kind used in treating panic disorder with agoraphobia and instituted well before tapering of the benzodiazepines can be very effective in facilitating tapering and allowing the patient to become free of these drugs (Spiegel 1999).

In a follow-up of patients who had been in benzodiazepine tapering trials 2–3 years earlier, Rickels et al. (1999) found patients who were still free of benzodiazepines to be less symptomatic than patients who failed to complete the taper or had returned to benzodiazepine use. These data unfortunately do not unscramble cause and effect.

Factors that make benzodiazepine withdrawal more difficult include higher daily dose, shorter half-life, longer duration of prior benzodiazepine therapy, and more rapid taper. At the patient level, a diagnosis of panic disorder, higher pretaper levels of anxiety or depression, more personality disorder, and concomitant alcohol or substance abuse make tapering more difficult. Successful tapering of benzodiazepines is often demanding of the clinician's time and energy (Rickels et al. 1999). The clinician needs to be available at all hours to provide counseling, support, and reassurance.

Generally the first half of the benzodiazepine dose can be tapered over a 4-week period, but tapering the remaining half of the dose can be a prolonged process. Patients may need to be kept at the 50% dose for several months before further tapering is attempted. However, many patients drop out of tapering attempts very early before any significant withdrawal symptoms occur, mainly for personality reasons. So far, adjunctive therapy with other nonbenzodiazepine drugs—carbamazepine, trazodone, valproate, buspirone, and imipramine—has not been shown to be of help in decreasing withdrawal symptoms, although some of these drugs—imipramine and valproate—may enable some patients to remain free of benzodiazepines for a few weeks.

If a patient is to undertake benzodiazepine withdrawal with any real prospect of success, prewithdrawal symptoms of anxiety and depression need to be actively treated with either pharmacological or psychological therapies.

Panic control treatment (PCT), a type of CBT, is an educational-experiential approach aimed at having patients learn to tolerate somatic symptoms of panic without undue anxiety. A controlled study has shown that use of PCT in combination with a very slow and cautious benzodiazepine taper (0.125 mg of alprazolam every 2 days for patients taking more than 1 mg/day initially, or 0.25 mg every 8 days once the dosage has been reduced to 1 mg/day) is effective. In another study, the taper was even slower. In both studies, PCT plus very slow taper was substantially better than medical management plus slow taper, although the sample sizes were small. Most of the patients whose benzodiazepine use had been successfully tapered with PCT were still free of benzodiazepines 3 years later (Spiegel 1999). Some informal clinical experience suggests that CBT should be continued for at least a few weeks after benzodiazepine taper is completed for better long-term success.

As noted later in this chapter, other forms of CBT are now being successfully used in treating most of the anxiety disorders and may well prove useful in the primary treatment of drug-free patients as well as in assisting benzodiazepine withdrawal.

Side Effects

Compared with many other classes of psychotropic agents, benzodiazepines have relatively favorable side-effect profiles. The most common side effect is sedation, which is in part related to dose and can be managed by reducing it. Other effects include dizziness, weakness, ataxia, anterograde amnesia (particularly with the short-acting benzodiazepines [e.g., triazolam]), decreased motoric performance (e.g., driving), nausea, and slight hypotension. Falls in elderly patients have been reported to be related to the use of longer-acting benzodiazepines as well as to the use of antidepressants (see Chapter 12: "Pharmacotherapy in Special Situations"). In the popular press, there have been reports of severe dyscontrol syndromes in patients taking certain benzodiazepines, particularly triazolam. We personally have not encountered any such syndrome in our clinical practice.

Overdose

Fortunately, these drugs have a relatively wide safety margin, and deaths due to benzodiazepine ingestion alone are rare. Most deaths that have involved these drugs have been associated with concomitant ingestion of other agents (e.g., alcohol or TCAs).

Antidepressants

Since the antidepressants have already been considered in some detail in Chapter 3 ("Antidepressants"), we give them less detailed attention here. Although several of the SSRIs have been FDA approved for one or more specific anxiety diagnoses (e.g., paroxetine for social anxiety, GAD, OCD, panic disorder, PMDD, and PTSD; sertraline for panic disorder, OCD, PMDD, social anxiety disorder, and PTSD), it is our position, as noted earlier, that until studies clearly show differences between these drugs in treating specific anxiety disorders, all SSRIs are probably reasonably effective across the whole range of anxiety disorders. Their use for such conditions may require adjustments, but these apply to the specific disorder and the whole class of SSRIs. (For example, in treating patients with panic with agoraphobia, begin with very low dosages; in treating OCD patients, use higher dosages and wait even longer for clinical response.) Likewise, the SNRIs are probably useful for a range of anxiety disorders. Venlafaxine is approved in the treatment of panic disorder, GAD, and social anxiety disorder, while the manufacturer of duloxetine has sought and received approval only for GAD.

Agoraphobia and Panic

Several antidepressants exert major antianxiety effects. Imipramine was first reported by Klein and various colleagues in the 1960s (Klein 1967) to have potent anxiolytic effects in agoraphobic patients with panic. Clinically, it appears that most, if not all, TCAs and SSRIs exert similar antipanic effects. In addition, the MAOI phenelzine is a potent antipanic agent, as probably are the other MAOIs and trazodone. However, not all antidepressants are as effective in treating panic. Most notably, bupropion does not appear to exert antipanic effects and may be anxiogenic in some patients. The noradrenergic effects of various antidepressants (particularly the TCAs and MAOIs) on the locus coeruleus generally have been invoked to explain their antipanic activity. Whether such a mode of action explains the possible antipanic effects of trazodone is unclear.

The SSRIs appear to prevent or lessen panic attacks. Indeed, paroxetine and sertraline have FDA approval for use in panic disorder. Generally speaking, doses for paroxetine are higher in treating panic than in treating major depression. The starting dosage is 10 mg/day, and the therapeutic dosage range is 40–60 mg/day.

Early on, the general rule of thumb was that panic patients required only low doses of TCAs (e.g., 50 mg/day of imipramine) for a response to occur. Over the years, it became more evident that, as in depression, many panic patients require relatively higher doses of TCAs or MAOIs, although a small proportion are very sensitive to TCAs, tolerating only 10–25 mg/day of imipramine. We recommend, when indicated, using the general dosage regimens of TCAs that are used for depression (see Chapter 3: "Antidepressants").

Klein (1993) proposed that TCAs are effective in panic disorder by affecting a supersensitive threshold for feeling smothered. In a second international collaborative study comparing imipramine with alprazolam and placebo in panic patients, patients with prominent respiratory panic symptoms (e.g., shortness of breath, choking feelings) showed more improvement with imipramine, whereas patients who did not have these symptoms during panic attacks did better with alprazolam. We know of no similar data on SSRIs.

Given the utility of TCAs in the treatment of panic disorder, it is not surprising that the SNRIs also appear effective. In 2005, venlafaxine received an FDA approval for the treatment of panic disorder. Two controlled registration trials of 12 weeks' duration indicate that venlafaxine XR reduces the frequency of panic attacks at dosages ranging from 75 to 225 mg/day. It would be expected that the other SNRIs are also useful in the treatment of panic disorder. However, since all the other SNRIs are more noradrenergic than is venlafaxine, tolerability in panic disorder patients may vary among this class of drugs.

Generalized Anxiety Disorder

Past studies have pointed out that TCAs also exert effects in GAD. In one major study, imipramine was as effective at 4–6 weeks as the benzodiazepine chlordiazepoxide in patients with this disorder. However, in the first 2 weeks, the benzodiazepine was more effective. More recent studies have led to FDA approvals for venlafaxine, duloxetine, and escitalopram in the treatment of GAD. Given the current DSM-IV-TR criteria for GAD as a chronic disorder—one that probably requires long-term treatment—the role of benzodiazepines has been reduced to the short-term relief of symptoms, if clinically necessary, while a longer-term non-dependence-inducing therapeutic program is implemented. Currently, venlafaxine, escitalopram, and paroxetine are FDA approved for use in GAD, but probably all SSRIs are effective, and all the newer drugs are probably more benign than the older TCAs, though we know of no direct comparisons between newer and older antidepressants in treating this condition. CBT approaches are available for the symptoms of GAD. Again, we know of no direct comparisons of specific drugs and specific CBT approaches for GAD, but the use of multimodal approaches is a function of the cost, the patient's response to the initial treatment trial, and the availability of skilled CBT therapists in the geographic area.

Social Anxiety Disorder

Seriously symptomatic patients with social anxiety disorder experience marked anxiety in a range of "social" situations, such as eating in public, signing checks, public speaking, and even being in large groups. The condition, as defined in DSM-IV-TR, may also include more limited fears of performing or speaking in public, often called *performance anxiety.* Performance anxiety is less incapacitating than generalized social phobia but may affect an area vital to a patient's career or interests. There is reasonable evidence that milder degrees of performance anxiety studied in volunteers (e.g., music students) respond to β-blockers given a couple of hours before the performance. Several β-blockers, including propranolol, oxprenolol, alprenolol, and atenolol, have been a bit more effective than placebo in individual controlled studies (see subsection "Noradrenergic Agents" later in this chapter). Likewise, the β-blockers appear to be helpful in managing test anxiety without the cognitive impairing effects of benzodiazepines. A number of open studies have suggested that a single dose of propranolol 10–40 mg before an exam reduces the peripheral symptoms of anxiety and appears to enhance test performance in individuals who may be incapacitated by severe anxiety. Atenolol is cardioselective and does not cross the blood-brain barrier easily, suggesting that β-blockers may act, at least in part, by suppressing tachycardia and tremor. Side effects may include hypotension and bradycardia. Thus, some caution is required in using the β-blockers for test or performance anxiety.

Social phobia has been increasingly well studied over the past few years. This disorder is often comorbid with a variety of other Axis I disorders, such as panic disorder, major depressive disorder, body dysmorphic disorder, and substance abuse. Because social anxiety disorder appears to begin in childhood or adolescence, early identification and treatment may be of special value in preventing the onset of other complicating disorders.

At present, there is good evidence that a variety of drug therapies are more effective than placebo. Paroxetine has been very well studied and has an FDA-approved indication for the treatment of social phobia. Dosages from 20 to 60 mg/day appeared equally effective in one multisite study (Davidson et al. 2004; Westenberg et al. 2004). Other SSRIs are presumably also effective, and several have shown efficacy in smaller double-blind or open studies. In 2008, fluvoxamine maleate received an FDA approval for the treatment of social anxiety disorder based on two trials of 12 weeks' duration. An average dose of fluvoxamine of about 200 mg/day was effective in reducing social anxiety compared with a placebo. Venlafaxine is also approved for the treatment of social anxiety disorder and appears to be at least as effective as the SSRIs. β-Blockers (or at least atenolol) are not much better than placebo in controlled studies in the treatment of generalized social phobia, despite their efficacy in ameliorating performance anxiety.

MAOIs also are effective in social anxiety disorder, with the conventional MAOI phenelzine being the most effective and best studied of this class of antidepressants. Moclobemide, a short-acting, reversible MAOI available in Canada and Europe, appears to be somewhat less effective. Brofaromine, another reversible MAOI, was reported to not separate from placebo in social phobia. Clonazepam has been well studied by Davidson's group (Davidson 2000) and is substantially more effective than placebo. Alprazolam, in other studies, has had a weaker effect.

There are only a few small studies comparing CBT with pharmacotherapy, and these show equivalent efficacy. Interesting reasons have been suggested as to why the "exposure" socially phobic patients receive to anxiety-producing situations in the course of their lives does not extinguish the anxiety; CBT programs have been developed that get around this problem and are quite successful. There is a report of a double-blind, pilot study of D-cycloserine versus placebo in patients with social anxiety receiving behavior therapy (Hofmann et al. 2006). Significant effects were seen for the compound.

One tentative algorithm for treating new patients with generalized social phobia is to begin with a benzodiazepine to reduce initial apprehension; then add an SSRI, stopping the benzodiazepine after the SSRI has begun to work; and then add CBT before phasing out the SSRI.

Duration of treatment for patients with generalized social anxiety has not been well studied. Since the condition is generally chronic, pharmacotherapy of at least a year's duration with evidence that the patient can handle previously feared situations seems reasonable before attempts are made to taper medication. Some patients may require medication indefinitely.

It should be noted that gabapentin—an α_2-δ calcium channel blocker—at dosages averaging about 3,000 mg/day has been shown to be more effective than placebo in treating social anxiety disorder. The reason for its presumed efficacy is unclear. However, an analog pregabalin has been reported in multiple studies of GAD to be effective and is currently under review by the FDA (see below).

For patients who have not responded to SSRIs and CBT, an MAOI trial is obviously the next step. Clomipramine may also be effective in treating social phobia.

On the basis of the available evidence, mild social and/or performance anxiety could be treated first with a β-blocker, and patients with more severe impairment could be given an SSRI before a trial of phenelzine. Clomipramine could be tried in patients adverse to trying MAOIs who have not had a response to SSRIs either because of discontinuation due to side effects or because of lack of improvement. If both clonazepam and alprazolam are effective in treating social phobia, clonazepam should be tried first because of its longer half-life. Benzodiazepines probably rapidly exert an effect on social anxiety; SSRIs or MAOIs may take weeks to obtain a full effect.

Posttraumatic Stress Disorder

Posttraumatic stress disorder is considered an anxiety disorder with a presumed cause: exposure to a markedly traumatic event or series of events. In general, studies show that about 20% of persons exposed to a severe stress develop the disorder. Probably a variety of factors predispose individuals to develop the full syndrome and to need treatment, including preexisting exposure to other stresses, prior psychiatric disorders, and the severity and prolongation of the traumatic experience(s). Group cohesion during major stresses may offer some protection. Most patients with PTSD have one or more comorbid psychiatric disorders; depression, various other anxiety disorders, dissociative disorders, and substance abuse are all relatively common and both increase morbidity and complicate treatment. Further, PTSD syndromes occurring after single adverse events—rape, fire, motor vehicle accident, volcanic eruption—may be different from PTSD seen in combat veterans or in patients who were sexually or physically abused as children.

Although one might assume that PTSD is a close chronological sequela of the bad event (and it sometimes is), some patients may be fine or at least may function well for months or years until some factor—known, hypothetical, or unknown—causes a sudden emergence or reemergence of the typical patterns of symptoms. An episode of PTSD has been estimated to last around 7 years; however, some patients adapt to the memories and symptoms and recover early, whereas others have symptoms that vary in intensity but seem to persist for decades. PTSD was reported in some World War I veterans in studies published as late as the 1980s.

It is generally presumed that patients with PTSD have overactive autonomic nervous systems and that their cortisol responses to stress or dexamethasone are blunted—the opposite of the status in severe depression. Some patients with PTSD feel much better after being given a single dose of an opiate antagonist (nalmefene), whereas others feel much worse (Glover 1993). In one study of PTSD patients, a serotonin agonist, *m*-chlorophenylpiperazine, induced an exacerbation of PTSD symptoms, while yohimbine, an adrenergic agonist, induced panic and flashback symptoms (Southwick et al. 1997). In a similar small study, the pure benzodiazepine antagonist flumazenil relieved symptoms in PTSD patients (Coupland et al. 1997).

Further, most published clinical trials of treatments for PTSD involved outpatients who were not taking any medications and whose illness is presumably less severe than that of patients in their seventh inpatient psychiatric hospital admission whose condition has worsened despite having received prolonged trials of a variety of concomitant medications and, often, psychosocial therapies.

In these days of limited hospital stays, it is no longer an option to withdraw a patient's numerous drug therapies to see whether any are helping or hurting. At least at McLean Hopsital, such readmissions for severe PTSD usually involve women with histories of childhood sexual abuse who meet the criteria for, in addition to PTSD, a number of other psychiatric disorders. These patients often dissociate a lot; have auditory hallucinations, severe insomnia, severe depression, and recurrent substance abuse; and exhibit self-injurious behavior. They are likely to be taking clonazepam, valproic acid, gabapentin, olanzapine, SSRIs, bupropion, clonidine, or lamotrigine, as well as Fioricet for headaches, and despite their medications they still feel terrible. It may be that severe symptoms and self-destructive behavior elicit overprescribing in psychiatrists and that the presence of such patients on psychiatric wards encourages other, more naive patients to emulate an expanding repertoire of symptoms. Although some reported trauma histories sound rather incredible, most seem valid and are likely true.

Given all the above factors, the most widely studied drugs for the treatment of PTSD are the SSRIs. They are often more effective than placebo, though only 40%–50% of patients taking SSRIs for PTSD show major improvement. The older MAOIs and brofaromine, a short-acting reversible MAOI no longer in development, may be more often effective than SSRIs, but these drugs' serious adverse effects in unstable, self-destructive outpatients make it hard to risk prescribing them. Using nefazodone was found to be helpful in several small open studies, and lamotrigine was helpful in one small placebo-controlled study. Uncontrolled studies of moclobemide, fluvoxamine, paroxetine, mirtazapine, venlafaxine, valproate, and carbamazepine have all shown some benefit. Both paroxetine and sertraline were significantly more effective than placebo in PTSD patients, and both now have FDA approval for the disorder. It may be that anticonvulsants are better for rage and instability, whereas antidepressants are better for depression and anxiety. Clonidine and guanfacine are said to suppress nightmares. These have not been well studied (Pearlstein 2000). There is currently a large-scale, multicenter VA study of prazosin—an α_1 antagonist— for nightmares in patients with PTSD. The study was instituted after a number of positive clinical reports (Miller 2008; Thompson et al. 2008).

PTSD patients who experience intrusive sounds and images ("flashbacks") of traumatic events, and "paranoid" ideas (e.g., fear of being attacked when exposed in public places) have found the first-generation antipsychotics (e.g., perphenazine 16 mg/day) helpful, though the psychotic-like symptoms do not completely abate. The SGAs are being investigated in PTSD. A number of open-label studies with quetiapine and at least once randomized controlled trial with olanzapine in the treatment of PTSD suggest benefit. The combination of antidepressants with SGAs in the treatment of PTSD has been useful clinically in some patients but is not well studied. The side effects, including weight gain and metabolic issues, limit the SGAs to adjunctive use or use as second-line agents.

Autonomic drugs—clonidine, guanfacine, propranolol—have been suggested for treating PTSD symptoms without there being any clear evidence of efficacy. Propranolol appeared to block the development of PTSD symptoms when administered to patients seen acutely in the emergency room (Pitman et al. 2005), although its efficacy in later studies has been less impressive (McGhee et al. 2009). Its use was based on observations in rodents that surges of epinephrine in the brain were needed for memory cosolidation of specific events.

One study showed that among recent trauma survivors, acute use of a benzodiazepine for several weeks after the traumatic experience tended to increase the likelihood that PTSD would develop. After PTSD is well established, patients often have severe initial insomnia and severe anxiety and thus almost invariably are prescribed benzodiazepines. There is even suggestive evidence that using alcohol regularly may delay onset of PTSD; thus, the role of sedatives in PTSD is quite unclear.

In patients with severe depression with melancholic features plus PTSD, ECT will occasionally be quite helpful.

In short, for milder or less intractable PTSD, SSRIs are the treatment of choice. In one study of PTSD patients, longer-term treatment with fluvoxamine led to a better outcome, with more improvement in PTSD symptoms after 1 year than had been seen at 6 weeks. Because PTSD in the majority of patients seems to have a prolonged, chronic course, long-term use of any substantially helpful medication seems sensible.

Current expert opinion on psychosocial therapies (Foa 2000; Hembree and Foa 2000) favors exposure therapies (though frequent experiencing of flashbacks is clearly not helpful), perhaps with some cognitive therapy aspects to encourage compliance. Certainly, PTSD patients often have "bad" cognitions: typically that the world is much more dangerous than it really is and that they are much more helpless and inadequate than they really are. Eye movement desensitization and reprocessing (EMDR) therapy—having the patient reexperience traumatic memories while the therapist's fingers are waved back and forth before the patient's eyes and the patient moves his or her eyes from side to side—has been assessed in controlled trials and seems to be a form of exposure therapy. Holding the eyes still does not affect the benefit achieved through EMDR.

All in all, the treatment of PTSD is now in the state that treatment of OCD was before the advent of clomipramine. There is no very effective definitive pharmacotherapy. SSRIs are probably the best studied, relatively effective medications, and here the resemblance to OCD occurs: both PTSD and OCD are long-term conditions, and prolonged drug therapy, at least with the SSRIs, is likely to yield better results over time. A wide variety of other agents are said to be helpful sometimes but are not well studied. In PTSD, memory consolidation and stress arousal systems are probably malfunctioning. Benzodiazepines are, perhaps, contraindicated, but many PTSD patients have already been taking them for quite some time, and there is no evidence that discontinuing them results in long-term improvement to compensate for the probable distress caused by withdrawal.

Behavioral therapies, particularly limited exposure therapies with some cognitive therapy, may be quite helpful, but perhaps more so in patients with more recent trauma.

Obsessive-Compulsive Disorder

When the second edition of this manual was published in 1991, only one drug, clomipramine, had been approved by the FDA for use in treating OCD. By 1996, fluoxetine and paroxetine were approved for use in treating both OCD and depression, and fluvoxamine was approved for use only in OCD. Now there is evidence that essentially all SSRIs are effective for both depression and OCD.

Despite this overlap in indications, the evidence is strong that the way all the SSRIs work in OCD is different from the way they work in depression. Depression tends to respond relatively rapidly—in 2–6 weeks—and most patients improve; there is a substantial placebo response. In OCD, improvement is delayed and may take 6–12 weeks, only half the patients improve, and the placebo response is smaller. The presence of coexisting or comorbid depression in OCD patients does not affect the response of their OCD to serotonergic antidepressants. Generally, OCD patients do better with higher doses of SSRIs (e.g., 40–80 mg of fluoxetine), whereas patients with depression respond to 20 mg. Noradrenergic drugs (desipramine, nortriptyline, and bupropion), which are quite effective in depression, are ineffective in OCD. However, SNRIs such as venlafaxine appear to be helpful.

If one accepts that all currently prescribable SSRIs are effective in OCD, it is hard to make choices among them. All cause a fair amount of sexual dysfunction. Some differences in their degrees of binding to various receptors and their interactions with drug metabolism exist. It is hard to compare efficacies of these drugs, even in meta-analyses, because the kinds of patients being recruited have likely changed over time. In early clomipramine studies, most patients had never had an adequate trial of an effective drug, and drug response rates and placebo rates were around 50% and 5%, respectively. Since then, placebo rates have risen and drug improvement rates have dropped.

The principles of treating patients with any of the SSRIs remain clear: begin with a standard antidepressant dose and increase gradually to three to four times that dose if improvement does not clearly occur. Prepare the patient for at least an 8- to 12-week trial before changing drugs or adding other drugs to the SSRI.

Over the years a variety of drugs have been tried alone or added to clomipramine or one of the SSRIs to elicit or increase a therapeutic effect. So far, none—lithium, buspirone, L-tryptophan, fenfluramine, neuroleptics, clonazepam—has had any regular, substantiated success, though case reports suggest that an occasional patient may improve when one of these drugs is added. Buspirone appeared very effective as an augmenter in open trials but did not separate from placebo in a double-blind study. It should be noted that buspirone *could* elicit a serotonin syndrome when added to an SSRI (although this was not commonly seen) and that L-tryptophan and fenfluramine are no longer available in the United States. In the last few years, as evidence has increased on the overlap of OCD with Tourette's disorder, the newer atypical antipsychotics have been added to SSRIs in patients with OCD, with impressive improvements in symptoms seen in occasional patients. Such a response is perhaps more likely if the patient also has schizotypal features or has a history or family history of tics. At this point, risperidone at dosages up to 3 mg/day seems safest in terms of weight gain and oversedation, but orthostatic hypotension has occurred in older depressed patients when risperidone and an SSRI were combined. So far, ziprasidone has not even been looked at informally in this regard. Conversely, consider, as an illustration that almost any drug or drug class stretches across DSM-IV-defined boundaries, a controlled study showing that fluvoxamine was substantially more effective than placebo in about half of a group of male autistic adults, improving sociability as well as autistic compulsions (McDougle 1997). The bottom line is that about half of patients with OCD are a good deal better while taking an SSRI or clomipramine and about 15%–20% drop out of drug therapy because of side effects. Not an ideal situation.

On the other hand, CBT (Baer and Greist 1997) is about as effective as pharmacotherapy if adequately done; relaxation therapy does not help, but therapies involving in vivo exposure and ritual prevention are typically quite effective. OCD patients with cleanliness or counting rituals do much better than patients with pure mental obsessions and no compulsive behaviors, hoarders, or patients with compulsive slowness. Perhaps all OCD patients should get both CBT and medication. However, therapists capable of doing CBT are mainly at major university centers with specialized OCD programs, so availability of CBT (and cost, sometimes) is a major problem. Early efforts that incorporate computerized programs and books that patients can use to carry out their own CBT with backup from a live professional seem to be effective (Baer and Greist 1997).

With or without CBT, OCD patients should receive, in adequate dose and length, separate trials of at least two of the SSRIs and of clomipramine before going on to more elaborate or complex therapies. For extremely treatment-resistant OCD, either intravenous clomipramine therapy (not available in the United States) or stereotactic psychosurgery (Jenike et al. 1995; Mindus and Jenike 1992), both of which have some reported benefit, could be tried. The FDA approved deep brain stimulation (DBS) in 2009 for resistant OCD. Although the approval of DBS was based on minimal data (26 subjects with resistant OCD), DBS was given a "humanitarian device exemption," given the limited options available to patients with resistant OCD and the debilitating nature of the illness.

If a patient has long-standing OCD symptoms and improves on a drug regimen, long-term maintenance therapy on that regimen seems advisable. Patients who are taken off medications tend to relapse fairly rapidly. With CBT, it is more likely that a series of treatments—say 12 sessions—with marked behavioral improvement will lead to maintained improvement after CBT is stopped, though occasional "booster" sessions may be useful.

Anticonvulsants

A number of anticonvulsants are being used with increased frequency for the treatment of anxiety disorders. Many of these drugs were thought primarily to act on the GABAergic system and would be expected to have anxiolytic properties. They also tend to have utility in the treatment of neuropathic pain. Among these anticonvulsants are gabapentin, tiagabine, and pregabalin. The anticonvulsants probably work slower than benzodiazepines and faster than antidepressants in the treatment of anxiety. Among the advantages of the anticonvulsants relative to benzodiazepines is a lower risk of dependence and withdrawal.

Gabapentin (Neurontin) has been used for many years in the treatment of bipolar disorder, although very little evidence exists as to its efficacy in this disorder. Once thought to be primarily GABAergic, it appears now that it binds to an α_2-δ subunit of calcium channels found in brain, and this is the more relevant mechanism of action. On the other hand, there is more evidence that gabapentin is at least modestly effective in the treatment of social anxiety, including public speaking, generalized anxiety, and panic disorder. Our experience is that gabapentin is much less effective than either benzodiazepines or antidepressants in the treatment of anxiety. However, gabapentin has few side effects or drug interactions and has not been associated with a risk for dependence. Doses as low as 300–400 mg may be helpful in the treatment of social anxiety, but most patients seem to need between 900 and 2,700 mg/day (in divided doses) for the treatment of panic or more serious anxiety. The primary side effects are somnolence and fatigue.

Pregabalin (Lyrica), an analog of GABA that is related to gabapentin, has been extensively studied in the treatment of GAD, fibromyalgia, neuropathic pain, and partial complex seizures. It appears to act even more selectively on the α_2-δ subunit of calcium channels found in brain than does gabapentin. Pregabalin received FDA approval in late 2004 for use in treating neuropathic pain and epilepsy. In 2008, it became the first drug approved for the treatment of fibromyalgia. Even though pregabalin received approval for the treatment of GAD in the European Union in 2006, the FDA has not approved pregabalin for GAD in the United States as of this writing. With the consistent efficacy in clinical trials and the known safety of pregabalin in clinical experience, it is not completely clear what has held up approval of pregabalin for GAD. There was reported concern of the risk-benefit ratio for the drug, given the hepatotoxicity seen in mice, but this has not proven to be a problem postrelease in humans. The drug is under re-review currently by the FDA.

There have been at least seven placebo-controlled trials which suggest that pregabalin is at least as effective as alprazolam and venlafaxine and more effective than placebo in the treatment of GAD. Pregabalin was more rapidly acting than venlafaxine and controlled somatic symptoms as well as did alprazolam (Montgomery 2006). In addition, pregabalin looks about as effective as venlafaxine in treating GAD but is better tolerated and probably more rapidly acting (Montgomery et al. 2006). The starting dosage of pregabalin in the treatment of anxiety is expected to be 150 mg/day, with the dosage increasing to 300 mg/day. Most patients should do fine at 300–400 mg/day, but the dosage can be increased by 150 mg every few days to the maximum of 600 mg/day. Although the studies suggest pregabalin should be a good first-line agent for the treatment of GAD, other promising anxiolytics, such as buspirone, did not live up to their expectations. Still, we expect pregabalin will fill an important niche. We have seen some patients who have either not tolerated or not responded to SSRIs who have done well with pregabalin. Patients requiring immediate relief of anxiety in an emergency setting will still receive benzodiazepines. However, pregabalin will be a more rapidly acting and probably better alternative to the SSRIs for some patients. The most common side effects of pregabalin have been dizziness and somnolence. This drug, like gabapentin, lacks the sexual side effects of most antidepressants.

Tiagabine (Gabitril) is a more potent drug than gabapentin and selectively inhibits GABA reuptake and the GAT1 GABA transporter. Tiagabine has been studied primarily in GAD either as a monotherapy or in combination with SSRIs. In one study, tiagabine was as effective as paroxetine and more effective than placebo in the treatment of GAD. There are anecdotal reports of tiagabine's efficacy as an adjunctive agent in treating PTSD and in treating panic disorder. However, at least two phase III studies of tiagabine in the treatment of GAD failed to meet their primary endpoint. Thus, development of tiagabine for GAD was discontinued. The other difficulty with tiagabine has been tolerability. Tiagabine's risks for seizures, cognitive problems, and sedation have limited its application in treating psychiatric disorders. That being said, we have seen a few patients do well with tiagabine at small dosages (2–4 mg/day) when other strategies were less successful.

Antipsychotics

Antipsychotics have long been used as adjunctive agents in the treatment of anxiety associated with disorders such as schizophrenia and bipolar disorder (Hirschfield et al. 2006; Keck et al. 2006). In addition, early work with agents such as trifluoperazine suggested that antipsychotics might be as effective as benzodiazepines in the treatment of GAD. The SGAs, with their 5-HT$_2$ and 5-HT$_{1A}$ effects, would be expected to have some benefits in anxiety disorders. Indeed, quetiapine does appear to be effective in controlled trials in the treatment of GAD (see Chapter 4: "Antipsychotics"). Additional controlled studies of antipsychotics in anxiety states have involved the adjunctive use of SGAs to augment antidepressant effects in OCD and PTSD. While the data are somewhat conflicting, most of the studies suggest that the SGAs, especially risperidone, olanzapine, and quetiapine, may be useful adjunctive agents in the treatment of refractory OCD and PTSD (Gao et al. 2006). In addition, the SGAs have sometimes been said to be effective in the adjunctive treatment of panic disorder and OCD.

We have seen instances when the SGAs have been well tolerated and effective as monotherapy of anxiety states when other conventional agents were not. Still, as of this writing, there are no adequately controlled studies of atypical antipsychotics in the monotherapy of any anxiety disorder. Until there is, we would recommend using the atypical antipsychotics in the treatment of anxiety only when more established agents have been exhausted.

Noradrenergic Agents

A number of studies have pointed to the potential use of β-blockers (e.g., propranolol) and primarily presynaptic but also postsynaptic α_2 receptor agonists (e.g., clonidine) to ameliorate symptoms of anxiety. Use of these agents stems from the observation that certain symptoms of anxiety (e.g., palpitations, sweating) suggest involvement of the sympathetic nervous system. Investigations were first directed toward the use of β-blockers in anxious musical performers. A number of years later, clonidine was shown by Gold et al. (1978) to be effective in blocking physiological symptoms associated with opioid withdrawal, resulting in its eventual study in patients with anxiety disorders and possibly nicotine withdrawal. This drug exerts α_2 (presynaptic) receptor agonist effects; however, because it is also a postsynaptic α_2 agonist, its pharmacological actions are complex.

Generic and trade names of key noradrenergic agents are summarized in Table 6–3 later in this chapter.

Clinical Indications

β-Blockers (e.g., propranolol) are indicated for hypertension and for prophylaxis against angina, arrhythmias, migraine headaches, and hypertrophic subaortic stenosis. They are often quite useful in relieving akathisia in patients taking antipsychotics, although they are not approved by the FDA for this use (see Chapter 4: "Antipsychotic Drugs"). They are also not approved by the FDA for use in anxiety, although several studies have suggested that propranolol may be useful. These studies, originally conducted in Great Britain, pointed to β-blockers' having particularly potent effects on the somatic manifestations of anxiety (e.g., palpitations, tremors) and less dramatic effects on the psychic component of anxiety. The antitremor properties of these drugs have resulted in their being commonly used in treating patients whose hand tremors developed secondary to lithium carbonate use (see Chapter 5: "Mood Stabilizers").

A number of reports suggested that although β-blockers had some use in generalized anxiety, they were not particularly effective in blocking panic attacks. Indeed, Gorman et al. (1983) reported that propranolol failed to block lactate-induced panic attacks. However, some investigators noted that propranolol might block panic anxiety resulting from isoproterenol (an adrenergic agonist) infusions and thus could still be effective in treating some patients with panic attacks. Pindolol, a mixed β-adrenergic receptor agonist and antagonist with serotonergic properties, has been reported to augment antidepressant response to SSRIs (see Chapter 9: "Augmentation Strategies for Treatment-Resistant Disorders").

As reported earlier in this chapter, β-blockers are widely believed, by medical students, house staff, musicians, and performers, to be useful in allaying anxiety during speaking or performing in public. Such use means that either the several weakly positive controlled studies of the efficacy of β-blockers in such situations are somehow flawed or placebos that have convincing rationales for efficacy can have a powerful effect. Again, open-label data also support the use of β-blockers for treating test anxiety.

Clonidine has an FDA-approved indication for the treatment of hypertension. As noted earlier, clonidine has been widely studied as a means of blocking physiological symptoms of opioid withdrawal (e.g., palpitations, sweating). The drug has also been studied in anxiety and in panic disorder and has been shown to be effective in both, although tolerance to the antianxiety effects frequently develops. It is conceivable that the drug's mixed, partial pre- and postsynaptic receptor agonist properties may enter into the development of tolerance. Clonidine has also been used to test various aspects of the catecholamine hypotheses of affective and anxiety disorders. Studies on nicotine withdrawal have yielded mixed results (Franks et al. 1989; Glassman et al. 1988). Clonidine has also been used to block the tachycardia and excessive salivation seen with clozapine use (see Chapter 4: "Antipsychotic Drugs").

As reported earlier in this chapter, prazosin also has shown utility in the treatment of some anxiety symptoms. In particular, open-label studies have suggested that prazosin may help ameliorate sleep disturbance (nightmares and middle insomnia) in PTSD patients. Some PTSD patients report an increase in general well-being with this α_1-adrenergic agent independent of its effect on sleep. However, a dose-related increase in orthostatic hypotension may limit prazosin's utility in many patients.

Dosage and Administration

Using propranolol as a model, clinicians should begin patients with peripheral symptoms of anxiety or patients with lithium-induced tremor or with familial tremor at 10 mg bid and increase the dosage incrementally to approximately 30–120 mg/day (see Table 6–3). Although the usual maintenance dosage of the drug in patients with hypertension is as high as 240 mg/day, such a dosage is rarely needed for anxious or tremulous patients. Generally, the use of these agents in patients with anxiety disorders should parallel that of the benzodiazepines; trials should be made of having patients stop the drug after a few weeks of treatment.

Many patients with tremors secondary to lithium carbonate treated with a β-blocker show a reemergence of their tremors after discontinuation of the β-blocker, resulting in their continuing to take a β-blocker for a prolonged period. We know of no major untoward effects; however, some patients may become lethargic and even depressed while taking β-blockers, so clinicians need to keep this in mind when treating patients with a major affective disorder (see "Side Effects" section below). This potential effect is a matter of some debate. We have also used propranolol for TCA-induced tremor without affecting the depression in the vast majority of patients.

If propranolol or another β-blocker is to be used as prn medication to decrease the physiological and, perhaps, psychological effects of performance anxiety or other circumscribed, predictable, socially phobic situations, the patient should try the proposed dose (usually 10 or 20 mg) once or twice before using it before a performance to block stage fright to make sure he or she can tolerate the drug comfortably at that dose (Jefferson 1995). Clonidine should be started at a dosage of 0.1 mg bid, and the dosage should be increased by 0.1 mg every 1–2 days to a total daily dose of 0.4–0.6 mg (Table 6–3). Because some studies have indicated that tolerance to this drug develops, clinicians should attempt to limit the duration of exposure whenever possible.

Side Effects

Side effects of the β-blockers include bradycardia, hypotension, weakness, fatigue, clouded sensorium, impotence, gastrointestinal upset, and bronchospasm. For the psychiatrist, a few caveats appear warranted. Clinicians need to remember that these drugs are contraindicated in asthmatic patients because they may produce bronchospasm and in patients with Raynaud's disease because of the risk of increased peripheral vasoconstriction. Pindolol, which acts as a mixed β-adrenergic receptor agonist and antagonist, has less effect on receptors that control bronchial constriction and has been argued to be potentially safe in patients with asthma. However, its marked agonist effects can result in unpleasant stimulation, and we have not found it particularly useful in treating anxious patients. As for the capacity of β-blockers to cause depression, we have not seen patients who have developed true depressive disorders. Rather, we have noted that some patients may feel "washed out" or lethargic. However, clinicians at other institutions have reported cases of propranolol-induced depression with endogenous features that remitted on discontinuation of the drug. One strategy is to switch to a β-blocker that is less lipophilic and that exerts fewer central nervous system (CNS) effects (e.g., atenolol).

This strategy may be particularly useful in men who have experienced decreased sexual potency while taking propranolol. In stopping β-blockers, it is wisest to taper the dose to avoid any rebound phenomena that could result in untoward cardiac or blood pressure effects. Clonidine has a mixed side-effect profile. Its major side effects include dry mouth, sedation or fatigue, and hypotension. These effects are often found unacceptable by anxious patients. In hypertensive patients, scheduling bid dosing (with two-thirds of the dose given at bedtime) has been advocated to deal with its sedating effects. Discontinuation should be gradual to avoid rebound autonomic symptoms or the hypertensive crises that have been reported in hypertensive patients who were suddenly withdrawn from the drug.

Prazosin's primary side effects are dizziness, headaches, sedation, and fatigue. Most patients are able to tolerate the 3–6 mg/day of prazosin that has been used to help sleep disturbance and anxiety in PTSD patients. However, there are case reports of patients benefitting from dosages as high as 20 mg/day or more. Monitoring of blood pressure is important as prazosin doses are increased, since orthostatic hypotension can be a substantial problem in some patients.

Antihistamines

The antihistamine hydroxyzine has indications for the treatment of anxiety and tension associated with psychoneurotic conditions or physical disease states. It is also indicated in the treatment of pruritus due to allergic conditions and for pre- and postoperative sedation. In psychiatric practice, antihistamines are less commonly used in treating anxious patients, reflecting their less potent anxiolytic effect (Table 6–3). Hydroxyzine's major side effects are drowsiness and dry mouth. It does not produce physical dependence; it may produce CNS depression when added to alcohol, narcotic analgesics, CNS depressants, or TCAs. Another antihistamine, diphenhydramine, is commonly used in medicine and psychiatry as a sedative-hypnotic (see Chapter 7: "Hypnotics").

Buspirone

The development of buspirone—a nonbenzodiazepine, generally nonsedating anxiolytic—stirred considerable excitement in psychopharmacological circles two decades or more ago. It represented the first prominent anxiolytic to be introduced since the benzodiazepines. The drug was originally developed as a potential antipsychotic agent. Although found in early clinical trials to have little antipsychotic potency, buspirone was eventually shown to have antiaggression effects in primates and antianxiety effects in humans. The structure of buspirone is shown in Figure 6–2. Buspirone went off patent in 2001 and is now available generically in the United States.

The drug does not bind with high affinity to benzodiazepine and GABA receptors, although it may have an effect on the chloride channel coupled to the benzodiazepine-GABA receptor complex. Buspirone has little antiseizure effect. Its anxiolytic effects were originally postulated to occur via dopaminergic properties, although the drug's central dopaminergic effects were not entirely clear. Later, buspirone was shown to exert its antianxiety effects by acting as a partial agonist of the 5-HT$_{1A}$ receptor. This action is shared by gepirone and ipsapirone, related antianxiety drugs that do not have effects on the dopaminergic system.

Buspirone is an interesting, frustrating drug (Cole and Yonkers 1995) with properties that should make it the drug of choice in treating GAD and related anxiety disorders (e.g., social phobia, mixed anxiety and depression, anxiety in patients with a history of substance abuse). Buspirone is as effective as diazepam and superior to placebo in double-blind trials involving anxious outpatients. The available data from such studies do not show diazepam to be faster acting than buspirone, although most physicians assume that benzodiazepines are faster acting. One small subanalysis showed that patients with a history of benzodiazepine treatment did less well while taking buspirone than patients who had never taken a benzodiazepine. Although the difference was statistically significant, half the patients with a history of benzodiazepine use did improve while taking buspirone.

Most psychiatrists and many physicians assume that buspirone is weaker and slower in onset than are benzodiazepines, and many believe it is never effective in patients who have had a benzodiazepine in the past. These assumptions are simply not true. Buspirone is lacking in benzodiazepine-like effects and will not relieve benzodiazepine withdrawal symptoms. If patients like the sedation they feel after a single dose of benzodiazepine (most do not like it), they will not get that "pause that refreshes" from buspirone. Unfortunately, both buspirone and benzodiazepines take 2–4 weeks to cause a full antianxiety

Figure 6–2. Chemical structure of buspirone.

effect. Psychiatrists rarely see anxiety patients who have never taken a benzodiazepine and therefore never see buspirone-appropriate patients and do not believe that buspirone is effective. Primary care physicians tend to learn from psychiatrists about drugs with complex dosage requirements that take weeks to act. Buspirone therefore is rarely used in adequate dosages—up to 30 mg/day or higher for 4–6 weeks—and is consequently widely believed not to work. Some, but not all, more recent studies show that buspirone is more effective than placebo in patients with depression, with social phobia, and with combined anxiety and alcoholism, at dosages of 30–60 mg/day, which patients do not tolerate as initial dosages. The best part of the buspirone story is therefore seldom reached.

Patients receiving drug therapy for anxiety disorders often do not need years of maintenance medication. Benzodiazepines can pose problems when they are tapered (particularly abruptly) and stopped. Anxious patients find that benzodiazepine withdrawal symptoms resemble the anxiety symptoms that first brought them to the doctor, become upset, and often end up taking diazepam or alprazolam again. If the patient had been taking buspirone instead, no withdrawal symptoms would have occurred; in fact, patients tend to improve a bit more in the first 2 weeks after buspirone is stopped. Buspirone is therefore a much more flexible drug to use in treating anxious patients: it can be tapered and withdrawn easily, and it enables the treating doctor to know readily whether it is still needed—without the patient's having to struggle with physical symptoms of drug withdrawal.

Buspirone should be initiated at a dosage of 5 mg bid, and the dosage should be increased gradually to 30–60 mg/day. Buspirone is not helpful in patients who are just stopping a benzodiazepine. However, if buspirone is added to the benzodiazepine for 2–6 weeks, the patient may feel "more better" because the two antianxiety drugs work by different mechanisms. Even if this effect does not occur, the benzodiazepine can be slowly tapered, often quite smoothly (Udelman and Udelman 1990), and the patient can be stabilized while taking buspirone.

Buspirone is well tolerated by medically ill elderly patients, does not depress respiration in patients with lung disease, and has some utility in patients with organic impulse disorders and in AIDS patients with anxiety. It does not adversely affect coordination or cognition. In short, it ought to be a major improvement over the benzodiazepines. However, its use in psychiatry has been limited to mainly adjunctive treatment.

Side effects of buspirone include headache, nausea, dizziness, and tension, which generally are not major problems. Indeed, the drug appears to have a more desirable side-effect profile than do the benzodiazepines. It does not appear to impair motor coordination, and it shows little untoward interaction with alcohol. It is also not sedating. According to an early report, the drug may exacerbate psychosis in patients with schizoaffective disorder, an effect that reflects complex prodopaminergic properties. This has not been a problem in clinical usage in the United States. High doses have, on the other hand, been reported to improve dyskinesia in patients with severe tardive dyskinesia. As noted in Chapter 11 ("Pharmacotherapy for Substance Use Disorders"), buspirone use also can result in reduced drinking in alcoholic outpatients.

The relative merits and side effects of buspirone versus the antidepressants in treating GAD have not been well studied. Davidson and colleagues (1999) found that venlafaxine XR appeared somewhat more effective in the treatment of GAD than did buspirone. It seems safe to say that buspirone has even fewer discontinuation effects than does venlafaxine or any of the antidepressants.

Barbiturates

Sixty to seventy years ago, the only medications widely used in psychiatric patients for the treatment of anxiety or agitation were barbiturates. Although barbiturates are still widely used in anesthesia and the treatment of epilepsy, use of barbiturates in psychiatry is now exceedingly uncommon. Longer-acting barbiturates, such as phenobarbital or barbital, were widely used for daytime sedation, and shorter-acting barbiturates with presumably more rapid onset of action, such as secobarbital, amobarbital, or pentobarbital, were widely used as hypnotics. (For further discussion of hypnotics, see Chapter 7: "Hypnotics.") Amobarbital in particular was also widely used as a daytime sedative and, in combination with D-amphetamine, as a widely used mixed sedative and stimulant called Dexamyl, no longer available in the United States. Phenobarbital is the only barbiturate that is widely used in general clinical practice currently, and it is used essentially only in the treatment of epilepsy. It has some efficacy as a daytime sedative and possibly as an antianxiety agent in doses of 15–30 mg three or four times a day. It was also used as a long-acting sedative in some detoxification programs (as the "methadone" of the barbiturate group) in withdrawing shorter-acting sedatives or, occasionally, alcohol. However, the small therapeutic index and high abuse potential relative to the benzodiazepines have rendered the oral barbiturates all but obsolete. Still, the barbiturates are widely used in anesthesia and are still occasionally used in hospital settings.

In double-blind, controlled clinical trials comparing phenobarbital with placebo as well as with a benzodiazepine or meprobamate, phenobarbital was generally slightly more effective than placebo and inferior to the newer antianxiety agents. In many such studies, the dose of phenobarbital used was fixed and low, and its efficacy may well have been reduced by the conditions of the trial. However, many patients find the sedative effect of phenobarbital rather dysphoric and unpleasant, and its utility as an antianxiety drug is therefore limited. In patients taking phenobarbital for epilepsy and, more strikingly, in children or even adults with a history of attention-deficit/hyperactivity disorder (ADHD), phenobarbital can in fact aggravate hyperactivity and disorganized behavior. Occasionally, increased hyperactivity and disturbed behavior in some children and adolescents can be traced to antiasthmatic drugs that contain phenobarbital. Meprobamate and benzodiazepines can also exacerbate symptoms of ADHD.

It is quite possible that amobarbital or other relatively shorter-acting barbiturates, unlike phenobarbital, might be as effective as benzodiazepines in the daytime treatment of anxiety. Several have indications for daytime sedation, and of these, butabarbital (Butisol) is occasionally used in such a way. (See Table 6–3 for formulations and strengths and Figure 6–3 for chemical structures of the barbiturates.) No good controlled clinical trials have been done

Compound	R_{5a}	R_{5b}
Amobarbital	ethyl	isopentyl
Aprobarbital	allyl	isopropyl
Butabarbital	ethyl	sec-butyl
Pentobarbital	ethyl	l-methylbutyl
Phenobarbital	ethyl	phenyl
Secobarbital	allyl	l-methylbutyl

Figure 6–3.   General chemical formulas of the barbiturates.

comparing such shorter-acting and possibly less dysphoric and more euphoric barbiturates with benzodiazepines. There is, however, little point in carrying out such trials, because it is clear that the addiction and abuse liability of barbiturates is substantially greater than that of any benzodiazepine, including even alprazolam. Barbiturates like amobarbital also have the disadvantage of a relatively low lethal dose, perhaps 1,000 mg taken in a single overdose. In addition, barbiturates induce enzymes that metabolize other important medications. It is also possible, but not proved, that tolerance to barbiturates develops somewhat more rapidly when they are taken in escalating doses. In a classic study by Isbell et al. (1950), performed at the Addiction Research Center in Lexington, Kentucky, in the 1940s, patients taking very large daily doses of barbiturates managed to complain of going into withdrawal while being so ataxic and malcoordinated that they were falling down when they tried to

Table 6–3. Other antianxiety/daytime sedative agents

Generic name	Brand name	Formulations and strengths	Dosage range (mg/day)
Barbiturates			
amobarbital	Amytal	Powder for injection: 500-mg vial	60–150
butabarbital	Butisol	Tablets: 30, 50 mg	45–120
		Elixir: 30 mg/5 mL (480-mL)	
mephobarbital	Mebaral	Tablets: 32, 50, 100 mg	150–200
pentobarbital	Nembutal	Injection: 50 mg/mL (20-mL, 50-mL vials)	150–200 once (up to 500 mg)
phenobarbital	Various generics	Tablets: 15, 30, 60, 100 mg	30–120
		Tablets: 16.2, 32.4, 64.8, 97.2 mg[a]	
		Elixir: 20 mg/5 mL (480-mL)	
		Injection: 65 mg/mL, 130 mg/mL (1-mL prefilled syringes, single-dose vials)	
Carbamate			
meprobamate	Miltown	Tablets: 200, 400 mg	1,200–1,600
Noradrenergic agents			
clonidine	Catapres	Tablets: 0.1, 0.2, 0.3 mg	0.2–0.6
	Catapres-TTS	Transdermal patch: 0.1, 0.2, 0.3 mg/day	
	Duraclon	Injection: 0.1 mg/mL, 0.5 mg/mL (10-mL vial)	

Table 6–3.   Other antianxiety/daytime sedative agents *(continued)*

Generic name	Brand name	Formulations and strengths	Dosage range (mg/day)
Noradrenergic agents (continued)			
propranolol	Inderal	Tablets: 10, 20, 40, 60, 80, 90 mg	60–160
		Concentrate: 80 mg/mL (30-mL)	
		Oral solution: 20 mg/5 mL, 40 mg/5 mL (500-mL)	
		Injection: 1 mg/mL (1-mL ampule)	
	Inderal LA[b]	Capsules: 60, 80, 120, 160 mg	
Antihistamines			
hydroxyzine HCl	Atarax	Tablets: 10, 25, 50 mg	200–400
		Syrup: 10 mg/5 mL (120-mL, 480-mL)	
	Vistaril	Injection: 25 mg/mL, 50 mg/mL (1-mL single-dose vial, 10-mL multidose vial)	50–100
hydroxyzine pamoate	Vistaril	Capsules: 25, 50, 100 mg	200–400
		Suspension: 25 mg/5 mL (120-mL, 480-mL)	
Other			
buspirone	BuSpar	Tablets: 5, 7.5, 10 mg; Dividose tablets: 15, 30 mg	15–60

Note.   For information regarding antidepressants as anxiolytics, see Chapter 3: "Antidepressants."
[a]16.2 mg equivalent to ¼ grain, 32.4 to ½ grain, and so forth.
[b]Sustained release.

walk and were slurring their speech. This suggests that tolerance to the anti-anxiety and/or euphoriant effects of the barbiturates develops more rapidly than does tolerance to the drugs' effects on psychomotor functions.

Catatonia

Catatonia is generally only recognized when the patient becomes mute and immobilized, though other signs can make the syndromal diagnosis. Catatonia used to be considered a form of schizophrenia, but it is now clear that in most cases a mood disorder diagnosis ends up being made, although it can occur as part of schizophrenia, delirious mania, or toxic disorders. It is given special mention here, in a chapter on antianxiety agents, because it responds very well, usually, to sedative drugs—amobarbital sodium in the 1950s and benzodiazepines in the last few decades—and because catatonia does *not* respond to neuroleptics. Perhaps neuroleptic malignant syndrome (NMS) is, in fact, a variant of catatonia produced by neuroleptics. If sedatives in systematic, high dosages (see below) do not relieve the symptoms rapidly (in minutes or hours), then ECT almost always works early in the condition and can even be used as a maintenance treatment to prevent recurrence (Fink 2001b).

Giving either amobarbital sodium intravenously at a slow rate (50 mg/mL, 1 mL/minute) or 1–2 mg of lorazepam intravenously in the same way slowly, the physician has a chance to carefully titrate the dose of sedation, to watch for the patient's awakening from stupor, and to avoid respiratory depression. Even when the medication is given this way, the procedure should be done only in a medical facility with oxygen and a crash cart and where facilities for intubation and tracheotomy are available. These facilities are almost never needed, but laryngospasm can be a lethal side effect of sodium amobarbital if the patient has an irritated larynx and pharynx. No one knows whether lorazepam is totally free of this risk.

Having given this warning, it is noteworthy that many patients in catatonic stupor will relax, awake, talk, feed, and hydrate themselves and act quite normal for 1–4 hours after an amobarbital injection—one of the most remarkable therapeutic events in psychiatry. In the experience of one of the authors (J.O.C.), most patients in acute stupor, when they were awakened, were nonpsychotic and had no idea why they had been unable to move or talk. Some, of course, were delusional and were presumed to have schizophrenia. Repeated amobarbital infusions, if given twice a day, enabled staff to feed and hydrate catatonic patients but did not seem to produce any lasting change in the recurring stupor. Lorazepam, as a single therapy, often seems to treat the stupor effectively. Fink and associates at Stony Brook begin with lorazepam 3 mg/day in divided doses but increase the dosage in daily or every-other-day steps to as high as 16 mg/day. Patients presenting with catatonia should immediately receive a workup for ECT and, if the trial of lorazepam fails, be given at least six suprathreshold seizures, even if the patient appears much improved after, say, three treatments. A regression after early improvement following two or three seizures is likely if ECT is stopped (Petrides and Fink 1996).

Excited catatonia and delirious mania respond equally well to benzodiazepines followed by ECT if necessary.

Neuroleptic malignant syndrome is claimed to also respond to benzodiazepines. These medications may be less toxic than dantrolene or bromocriptine. Initial cooling of febrile NMS patients is the first order of business, and ECT can be effective if drug therapies fail.

Maintenance treatment for 6 months using whatever treatment worked in the acute treatment of the catatonia is indicated. Lorazepam at a dosage of 2–6 mg/day, as well as augmentation with maintenance ECT (biweekly, monthly, or bimonthly), may be needed. One choice is to pick a regular schedule; an alternative is to restart ECT within 48 hours of any sign of recurrence.

One interdisciplinary caution: Neurologists have been known to use the abnormal interictal EEG seen with patients administered ECT to diagnose encephalitis and stop the needed ECT regimen (Petrides et al. 2001).

Obviously, the Amytal interview can occasionally be useful in those rare cases when a mute catatonic patient has been admitted to an emergency room or a psychiatric unit with no history and no identification and the clinician is unable to discover even what the patient's name and address are, much less what the patient's history or probable psychiatric diagnosis is. In such situations, amobarbital given intravenously can be quite helpful in clarifying the situation. However, it should be administered only after all reasonable medical or pharmacological causes for such a mute or unresponsive state have been ruled out. Lorazepam, given intramuscularly, may well be as useful as amobarbital sodium in relieving such stupor.

Meprobamate

Meprobamate is another agent of historical significance that is rarely used for any condition at this time. Meprobamate occupies an intermediate position between the benzodiazepines and the barbiturates, both pharmacologically and historically. It was first marketed about 1956, having evolved from a chemically related muscle relaxant, mephenesin. Meprobamate, whose structure is shown in Figure 6–4, has muscle relaxant and sedative properties but was initially evaluated as an antianxiety agent. On the basis of a small number of enthusiastic findings from uncontrolled studies on anxiety, it was released to the market at a time when the FDA required only evidence of safety rather than evidence of efficacy as well. It became an instant national success and had widespread publicity in the lay media. Meprobamate has anticonvulsant activity, mainly against absence attacks. Its antianxiety effects in laboratory animals can be blocked by naloxone. However, although not as toxic as barbiturates, meprobamate has proved less safe than the benzodiazepines. Given the number of alternatives currently available, it is increasingly difficult to justify a meprobamate prescription.

After an oral dose, peak blood level occurs in 1–3 hours. It is hydroxylated by the liver, then changed to a glucuronide and excreted through the kidney. Its half-life is 6–17 hours in acute administration and longer after chronic administration. In suicidal overdose, meprobamate tablets form a lump (bezoar) in the patient's stomach, which, if not removed by gastroscopy, can break up and reinduce coma after the patient has appeared to recover.

Meprobamate does not affect benzodiazepine or GABA receptors. It seems to act by potentiating the action of endogenously released adenosine; it blocks reuptake of adenosine, which is itself a sedative. Caffeine is an adenosine antagonist.

Now that the dust has settled, some 50 years later, it is clear that meprobamate is effective as an antianxiety agent in the same sense that diazepam or chlordiazepoxide is effective (Cole and Yonkers 1995), although controlled studies directly comparing the efficacy of meprobamate with that of benzodiazepines are almost nonexistent.

The clinical dosage of meprobamate is on the order of 400 mg three or four times a day, being approximately equivalent to 5 mg of diazepam three or four times a day (Table 6–3).

Figure 6–4.   Chemical structure of meprobamate.

The major side effects are sedation and malcoordination. The drug is relatively safe in overdose—less lethal than intermediate-acting barbiturates like pentobarbital but a good deal less safe than diazepam. The drug produces physical dependence and tolerance in much the same way as do the barbiturates and the benzodiazepines. Significant withdrawal effects, such as convulsions, agitation, and delirium, occur after clinically relatively lower doses of meprobamate—for example, after 3,200 mg, or eight 400-mg tablets a day.

Currently, it is hard to identify any unique advantages of meprobamate as an antianxiety drug (Cole and Yonkers 1995). It is a reasonably effective and satisfactory hypnotic at a dosage of 400–800 mg/day at bedtime. Clinically, we have occasionally seen anxious patients who have a marked subjective intolerance to benzodiazepines, becoming agitated, dysphoric, and restless while taking any of several of them. Some of these patients tolerate meprobamate quite well, perhaps because its action is extremely different from that of benzodiazepines. To our knowledge, no one has evaluated meprobamate in the treatment of conditions such as akathisia or panic disorder, for which some benzodiazepines appear to be effective. The introduction of triplicate prescriptions for benzodiazepines in New York State (essentially placing them in Schedule II) reportedly led to an acute rise in prescriptions for meprobamate, which remained in Schedule IV—an unfortunate consequence of legislative action. The drug is less safe than are the benzodiazepines.

Some older patients have been receiving maintenance meprobamate therapy for many years; it may be clinically sensible for them to continue taking that drug. One study showed that a large number of elderly patients in Florida judged their meprobamate regimen to be quite helpful (Hale et al. 1988).

Deprol, a discontinued meprobamate-containing combination medication, deserves mention here. This combination of benactyzine and meprobamate was marketed for use in depression. Each tablet contained 400 mg of meprobamate and 1 mg of benactyzine hydrochloride. There is essentially no evidence that benactyzine by itself is an effective antidepressant, although the compound is anticholinergic and might conceivably have some antidepressant properties. One trial many years ago involving patients with schizophrenia showed that benactyzine alone increased hallucinatory and psychotic behavior. However, a handful of studies suggested that Deprol was effective in treating some depressions and may perhaps be more effective than either of its ingredients alone. The question remains moot, as the drug is no longer available.

Bibliography

American Psychiatric Association: Diagnostic and Statistical Manual of Mental Disorders, 3rd Edition, Revised. Washington, DC, American Psychiatric Association, 1987

American Psychiatric Association: Diagnostic and Statistical Manual of Mental Disorders, 4th Edition. Washington, DC, American Psychiatric Association, 1994

American Psychiatric Association: Diagnostic and Statistical Manual of Mental Disorders, 4th Edition, Text Revision. Washington, DC, American Psychiatric Association, 2000

Baer L, Greist JH: An interactive computer administered self-assessment and self-help program for behavior therapy. J Clin Psychiatry 58 (12, suppl):23–28, 1997

Ballenger JC, Burrows GD, DuPont RL Jr, et al: Alprazolam in panic disorder and agoraphobia: results from a multicenter trial, I: efficacy in short-term treatment. Arch Gen Psychiatry 45:413–422, 1988

Ballenger JC, Pecknold J, Rickels K, et al: Medication discontinuation in panic disorder. J Clin Psychiatry 54 (10, suppl):15–21, 1993

Barlow DH, Gorman JM, Shear MK, et al: Cognitive-behavioral therapy, imipramine, or their combination for panic disorder: a randomized controlled trial. JAMA 238:2529–2536, 2000

Baxter LR, Thompson JM, Schwartz JM, et al: Trazodone treatment response in obsessive-compulsive disorders correlated with shifts in glucose metabolism in the caudate nuclei. Psychopathology 20:114–122, 1987

Benzodiazepine seizures: an update. Int Drug Ther Newsl 24:5–7, 1989

Bloch MH, Landeros-Weisenberger A, Kelmendi B, et al: A systematic review: antipsychotic augmentation with treatment refractory obsessive-compulsive disorder. Mol Psychiatry 11(7):622–632, 2006 [erratum: Mol Psychiatry 11:795, 2006]

Bogan AM, Koran LM, Chuong HW, et al: Quetiapine augmentation in obsessive-compulsive disorder resistant to serotonin reuptake inhibitors: an open-label study. J Clin Psychiatry 66:73–79, 2005

Braestrup C, Squires RF: Brain specific benzodiazepine receptors. Br J Psychiatry 133:249–260, 1978

Bystritsky A, Ackerman DL, Rosen RM, et al: Augmentation of serotonin reuptake inhibitors in refractory obsessive-compulsive disorder using adjunctive olanzapine: a placebo-controlled trial. J Clin Psychiatry 65:565–568, 2004

Chao IL: Olanzapine augmentation in panic disorder: a case report. Pharmacopsychiatry 37(5):239–240, 2004

Cole JO, Yonkers KA: Non-benzodiazepine anxiolytics, in American Psychiatric Press Textbook of Psychopharmacology. Edited by Schatzberg AF, Nemeroff CB. Washington, DC, American Psychiatric Press, 1995, pp 231–244

Coupland NJ, Lillywhite A, Bell CE, et al: A pilot controlled study of the effects of flumazenil in post-traumatic stress disorder. Biol Psychiatry 41:988–990, 1997

Davidson JRT: Pharmacotherapy of post-traumatic stress disorder: treatment options, long-term follow-up, and predictors of outcome. J Clin Psychiatry 61 (5, suppl):52–56, 2000

Davidson JR, Dupont RL, Hedges D, et al: Efficacy, safety, and tolerability of venlafaxine extended-release and buspirone in outpatients with generalized anxiety disorder. J Clin Psychiatry 60:528–535, 1999

Davidson J, Yaryura-Tobias J, DuPont R, et al: Fluvoxamine-controlled release formulation for the treatment of generalized social anxiety disorder. J Clin Psychopharmacol 24:118–125, 2004

deBeurs E, van Balkom AJ, Lange A, et al: Treatment of panic disorder with agoraphobia: comparison of fluvoxamine, placebo, and psychological panic management combined with exposure and of exposure in vivo alone. Am J Psychiatry 152:683–691, 1995

DeVeaugh-Geiss J, Landau P, Katz R: Preliminary results from a multicenter trial of clomipramine in obsessive-compulsive disorder. Psychopharmacol Bull 25:36–40, 1989

Fink M: Catatonia: syndrome or schizophrenia subtype? Recognition and treatment. J Neural Transm 108:637–644, 2001a

Fink M: Treating neuroleptic malignant syndrome as catatonia. J Clin Psychopharmacol 21:121–122, 2001b

Fluvoxamine for obsessive-compulsive disorder. Med Lett Drugs Ther 37(942):13–14, 1995

Foa EB: Psychosocial treatment of post-traumatic stress disorder. J Clin Psychiatry 61 (5, suppl):43–48, 2000

Frank JB, Kosten TR, Giller EL, et al: A randomized clinical trial of phenelzine and imipramine for PTSD. Am J Psychiatry 145:1289–1291, 1988

Franks P, Harp J, Bell B: Randomized, controlled trial of clonidine for smoking cessation in a primary care setting. JAMA 262:3011–3013, 1989

Freeman CP, Trimble MR, Deakin JF, et al: Fluvoxamine vs clomipramine in the treatment of obsessive-compulsive disorder: a multicenter, randomized, double-blind, parallel group comparison. J Clin Psychiatry 55:301–305, 1994

Friedman MJ: Toward a rational pharmacotherapy for post-traumatic stress disorder: an interim report. Am J Psychiatry 145:281–285, 1988

Friedman MJ: What might the psychobiology of post-traumatic stress disorder teach us about future approaches to pharmacotherapy? J Clin Psychiatry 61 (7, suppl):44–51, 2000

Fyer AJ, Liebowitz MR, Gorman JM, et al: Discontinuation of alprazolam treatment in panic patients. Am J Psychiatry 144:303–308, 1987

Gao K, Muzina D, Gajwani P, et al: Efficacy of typical and atypical antipsychotics for primary and comorbid anxiety symptoms or disorders: a review. J Clin Psychiatry 67:1327–1340, 2006

Gelpin E, Bonne O, Peri T, et al: Treatment of recent trauma survivors with benzodiazepines: a prospective study. J Clin Psychiatry 57:390–394, 1996

Gladsjo JA, Rapaport MH, McKinney R, et al: Absence of neuropsychological deficits in patients receiving long-term treatment with alprazolam-XR for panic disorder. J Clin Psychopharmacol 21:131–138, 2001

Glassman AH, Stetner F, Walsh BT, et al: Heavy smokers, smoking cessation, and clonidine: results of a double-blind, randomized trial. JAMA 259:2863–2866, 1988

Glover H: A preliminary trial of nalmefene for the treatment of emotional numbing in combat veterans with post-traumatic stress disorder. Isr J Psychiatry Relat Sci 30:255–263, 1993

Glue P, Fang A, Gandelman K, et al: Pharmacokinetics of an extended release formulation of alprazolam (Xanax XR) in healthy normal adolescent and adult volunteers. Am J Ther 13:418–422, 2006

Goddard AW, Brouette T, Almai A, et al: Early coadministration of clonazepam with sertraline for panic disorder. Arch Gen Psychiatry 58:681–686, 2001

Gold MS, Redmond DE Jr, Kleber HD: Clonidine in opiate withdrawal. Lancet 1:929–930, 1978

Goldberg HL: Buspirone hydrochloride: a unique new anxiolytic agent: pharmacokinetics, clinical pharmacology, abuse potential, and clinical efficacy. Pharmacotherapy 4:315–324, 1984

Gorman JM, Levy GF, Liebowitz MR, et al: Effect of acute beta-adrenergic blockade on lactate induced panic. Arch Gen Psychiatry 40:1079–1082, 1983

Granville-Grossman KL, Turner P: The effect of propranolol on anxiety. Lancet 1:788–790, 1966

Greenblatt DJ, Shader RI, Abernethy DR: Current status of benzodiazepines [first of two parts]. N Engl J Med 309:354–359, 1983a

Greenblatt DJ, Shader RI, Abernethy DR: Current status of benzodiazepines [second of two parts]. N Engl J Med 309:410–415, 1983b

Greenblatt DJ, von Moltke LL, Harmatz JS, et al: Alprazolam pharmacokinetics, metabolism, and plasma level: clinical implications. J Clin Psychiatry 54 (10, suppl):4–11, 1993

Hale WE, May F, Moore M, et al: Meprobamate use in the elderly: a report from the Dunedin Program. J Am Geriatr Soc 30:1003–1005, 1988

Heimberg RG: Current status of psychotherapeutic interventions for social phobia. J Clin Psychiatry 62 (1, suppl):36–42, 2001

Hembree EA, Foa EB: Posttraumatic stress disorder: psychological factors and psychosocial interventions. J Clin Psychiatry 61 (7, suppl):33–39, 2000

Henry M, Fishman JR, Youngner SJ: Propranolol and the prevention of post-traumatic stress disorder: is it wrong to erase the "sting" of bad memories? Am J Bioeth 7:12–20, 2007

Herman JB, Rosenbaum JF, Brotman AW: The alprazolam to clonazepam switch for the treatment of panic disorder. J Clin Psychopharmacol 7:175–178, 1987

Hirschfeld RM, Weisler RH, Raines SR, et al, for the BOLDER Study Group: Quetiapine in the treatment of anxiety in patients with bipolar I or II depression: a secondary analysis from a randomized, double-blind, placebo-controlled study. J Clin Psychiatry 67:355-362, 2006

Hofmann SG, Pollack MH, Otto MW: Augmentation treatment of psychotherapy for anxiety disorders with D-cycloserine. CNS Drug Rev 12:208–217, 2006

Insel TR (ed): New Findings in Obsessive-Compulsive Disorder. Washington, DC, American Psychiatric Press, 1984

Insel TR, Murphy DL, Cohen RM, et al: Obsessive-compulsive disorder: a double-blind trial of clomipramine and clorgyline. Arch Gen Psychiatry 40:605–612, 1983

Isbell H, Altschul S, Kornetsky C, et al: Chronic barbiturate intoxication: an experimental study. AMA Archives of Neurology and Psychiatry 64:1–28, 1950

Jefferson JW: Social phobia: a pharmacological treatment overview. J Clin Psychiatry 56 (5, suppl):18–24, 1995

Jenike MA, Baer L, Ballantine T, et al: Cingulotomy for refractory obsessive-compulsive disorder. Arch Gen Psychiatry 52:384–392, 1995

Kahn R, McNair D, Covi L, et al: Effects of psychotropic agents in high anxiety subjects. Psychopharmacol Bull 17:97–100, 1981

Kavirajan H: The amobarbital interview revisited: a review of the literature since 1966. Harv Rev Psychiatry 7:153–165, 1999

Keck PE Jr, Strawn JR, McElroy SL: Pharmacologic treatment considerations in co-occurring bipolar and anxiety disorders. J Clin Psychiatry 67(suppl 1):8–15, 2006

Klein DF: Importance of psychiatric diagnosis in prediction of clinical drug effects. Arch Gen Psychiatry 16:118–126, 1967

Klein DF: False suffocation alarms, spontaneous panics, and related conditions: an integrative hypothesis. Arch Gen Psychiatry 50:306–317, 1993

Lader M: Summary and commentary, in Pharmacology of Benzodiazepines. Edited by Usdin E, Skolnick P, Tallman JF, et al. New York, Macmillan, 1982, pp 53–60

Liebowitz MR, Fyer AJ, McGrath P, et al: Clonidine treatment of panic disorder. Psychopharmacol Bull 17:122–123, 1981

Liebowitz MR, Gorman JM, Fyer AJ, et al: Social phobia: review of a neglected anxiety disorder. Arch Gen Psychiatry 42:729–736, 1985

Liebowitz MR, Fyer AJ, Gorman JM, et al: Phenelzine in social phobia. J Clin Psychopharmacol 6:93–98, 1986

Lucki I, Rickels K, Geller AM: Chronic use of benzodiazepines and psychomotor and cognitive test performance. Psychopharmacology (Berl) 88:426–433, 1986

Lydiard RB, Falsetti SA: Treatment options for social phobia. Psychiatr Ann 17:409–423, 1994

Marazziti D, Pfanner C, Dell'Osso B, et al: Augmentation strategy with olanzapine in resistant obsessive compulsive disorder: an Italian long-term open-label study. J Psychopharmacol 19:392–324, 2005

McDougle CJ: Update on pharmacologic management of obsessive-compulsive disorder: agents and augmentation. J Clin Psychiatry 58 (12, suppl):11–22, 1997

McDougle CJ, Naylor ST, Cohen DT, et al: A double-blind placebo-controlled study of fluvoxamine in adults with autistic disorder. Arch Gen Psychiatry 53:1001–1008, 1996

McGhee LL, Maani CV, Garza TH, et al: The effect of propranolol on posttraumatic stress disorder in burned service members. J Burn Care Res 30:92–97, 2009

Meltzer HY, Fleming R, Robertson A: The effect of buspirone on prolactin and growth hormone secretion in man. Arch Gen Psychiatry 40:1099–1102, 1983

Menza M, Harris D: Benzodiazepines and catatonia: an overview. Biol Psychiatry 26:842–846, 1989

Miller LJ: Prazosin for the treatment of posttraumatic stress disorder sleep disturbances. Pharmacotherapy 28:656–666, 2008

Mindus P, Jenike MA: Neurosurgical treatment of malignant obsessive-compulsive disorder. Psychiatr Clin North Am 15:921–938, 1992

Montgomery SA, Tobias K, Zomberg GL, et al: Efficacy and safety of pregabalin in the treatment of generalized anxiety disorder: a 6-week, multicenter, randomized, double-blind, placebo-controlled comparison of pregabalin and venlafaxine. J Clin Psychiatry 67:771–782, 2006

Mooney JJ, Schatzberg AF, Cole JO, et al: Enhanced signal transduction by adenylate cyclase in platelet membranes of patients showing antidepressant responses to alprazolam: preliminary data. J Psychiatr Res 19:65–75, 1985

Nemeroff CB: Use of atypical antipsychotics in refractory depression and anxiety. J Clin Psychiatry 66 (suppl 8):13–21, 2005

Norberg MM, Krystal JH, Tolin DF: A meta-analysis of D-cycloserine and the facilitation of fear extinction and exposure therapy. Biol Psychiatry 63:1118–1126, 2008

Noyes R, Anderson DJ, Clancy J, et al: Diazepam and propranolol in panic disorder and agoraphobia. Arch Gen Psychiatry 41:287–292, 1984

Noyes R Jr, DuPont RL Jr, Pecknold JC, et al: Alprazolam in panic disorder and agoraphobia: results from a multicenter trial, II: patient acceptance, side effects, and safety. Arch Gen Psychiatry 45:423–428, 1988

Nutt DJ: The psychobiology of postraumatic stress disorder. J Clin Psychiatry 61 (5, suppl):24–29, 2000

Pande AC, Davidson JR, Jefferson JJ, et al: Treatment of social phobia with gabapentin: a placebo-controlled study. J Clin Psychopharmacol 19:341–348, 1999

Pearlstein T: Antidepressant treatment of post-traumatic stress disorder. J Clin Psychiatry 61 (7, suppl):40–43, 2000

Pecknold JC, Swinson RP, Kuch K, et al: Alprazolam in panic disorder and agoraphobia: results from a multicenter trial, III: discontinuation effects. Arch Gen Psychiatry 45:429–436, 1988

Petrides G, Fink M: Choosing a dosing strategy for electrical stimulation in ECT. J Clin Psychiatry 57:487–488, 1996

Petrides G, Fink M, Husain MM, et al: ECT readmission rates in psychotic vs nonpsychotic depressed patients: a report from CORE. J ECT 17:244–253, 2001

Pitman RK, Delahanty DL: Conceptually driven pharmacologic approaches to acute trauma. CNS Spectr 10:99–106, 2005

Pivac N, Kozaric-Kovacic D, Muck-Seler D: Olanzapine versus fluphenazine in an open trial in patients with psychotic combat-related post-traumatic stress disorder. Psychopharmacology (Berl) 175:451–456, 2004

Pollack MH, Tesar GE, Rosenbaum JF, et al: Clonazepam in the treatment of panic disorder and agoraphobias: a one-year follow-up. J Clin Psychopharmacol 6:302–304, 1986

Pollack MH, Simon NM, Worthington JJ, et al: Combined paroxetine and clonazepam treatment strategies compared to paroxetine monotherapy for panic disorder. J Psychopharmacol 17:276–282, 2003

Pollack MH, Simon NM, Zalta AK, et al: Olanzapine augmentation of fluoxetine for refractory generalized anxiety disorder: a placebo controlled study. Biol Psychiatry 59:211–215, 2006

Problems associated with alprazolam therapy. Int Drug Ther Newsl 23:29–31, 1988

Ressler KJ, Rothbaum BO, Tannenbaum L, et al: Cognitive enhancers as adjuncts to psychotherapy: use of D-cycloserine in phobic individuals to facilitate extinction of fear. Arch Gen Psychiatry 61:1136–1144, 2004

Riba J, Rodriguez-Fornells A, Strassman RJ, et al: Psychometric assessment of the Hallucinogen Rating Scale. Drug Alcohol Depend 62:215–223, 2001

Rickels K: Alprazolam extended-release in panic disorder. Expert Opin Pharmacother 5:1599–1611, 2004

Rickels K, Schweizer E: Maintenance treatment studies in anxiety disorders: some methodological notes. Psychopharmacol Bull 31:115–123, 1995

Rickels K, Chase WG, Downing RW: Long-term diazepam therapy and clinical outcome. JAMA 250:767–771, 1983

Rickels K, Schweizer E, Csanalosi I, et al: Long-term treatment of anxiety and risk of withdrawal: prospective comparison of clorazepate and buspirone. Arch Gen Psychiatry 45:444–450, 1988

Rickels K, DeMartinis N, Rynn M, et al: Pharmacologic strategies in discontinuing benzodiazepine treatment. J Clin Psychopharmacol 19 (suppl 2):12S–16S, 1999

Ries RK, Roy-Byrne PP, Ward NG, et al: Carbamazepine treatment for benzodiazepine withdrawal. Am J Psychiatry 146:536–537, 1989

Sathananthan GL, Sanghavi I, Phillips N, et al: MJ 9022: correlation between neuroleptic potential and stereotypy. Curr Ther Res Clin Exp 18:701–705, 1975

Schneier FR: Treatment of social phobia with antidepressants. J Clin Psychiatry 62 (1, suppl):43–48, 2001

Schweizer E, Rickels K, Lucki I: Resistance to the antianxiety effect of buspirone in patients with a history of benzodiazepine use (letter). N Engl J Med 314:719–720, 1986

Sheehan DV, Ballenger J, Jacobsen G: Treatment of endogenous anxiety with phobic, hysterical, and hypochondriacal symptoms. Arch Gen Psychiatry 37:51–59, 1980

Smith WT, Londborg PD, Glaudin V, et al: Short-term augmentation of fluoxetine with clonazepam in the treatment of depression: a double-blind study. Am J Psychiatry 155:1339–1345, 1998

Solomon SD, Gerrity ET, Muff AM: Efficacy of treatments for posttraumatic stress disorder: an empirical review. JAMA 268:633–638, 1992

Southwick SM, Krystal JH, Bremmer JD, et al: Noradrenergic and serotonergic function in posttraumatic stress disorder. Arch Gen Psychiatry 54:749–758, 1997

Spiegel DA: Psychological strategies for discontinuing benzodiazepine treatment. J Clin Psychopharmacol 19 (suppl 2):17S-23S, 1999

Strassman RJ: Hallucinogenic drugs in psychiatric research and treatment: perspectives and prospects. J Nerv Ment Dis 183:127–138, 1995

Sutherland SM, Davidson JRT: Pharmacotherapy for posttraumatic stress disorder. Psychiatr Clin North Am 17:409–423, 1994

Swedo SE, Leonard HL, Rapoport JL, et al: A double-blind comparison of clomipramine and desipramine in the treatment of trichotillomania (hair pulling). N Engl J Med 321:497–501, 1989

Tesar GE, Rosenbaum JF: Successful use of clonazepam in patients with treatment-resistant panic disorder. J Nerv Ment Dis 174:447–482, 1986

Thompson CE, Taylor FB, McFall ME, et al: Nonnightmare distressed awakenings in veterans with posttraumatic stress disorder: response to prazosin. J Trauma Stress 21:417–420, 2008

Tyrer PJ, Lader MH: Clinical response to propranolol and diazepam in somatic and psychic anxiety. BMJ 2:14–16, 1974

Tyrer P, Shawcross C: Monoamine oxidase inhibitors in anxiety disorders. J Psychiatr Res 22 (suppl 1):87–98, 1988

Udelman HD, Udelman DL: Concurrent use of buspirone in anxious patients during withdrawal from alprazolam therapy. J Clin Psychiatry 51 (9, suppl):46–50, 1990

Uhlenhuth EH (ed): Benzodiazepine dependence and withdrawal: myths and management. J Clin Psychopharmacol 19 (suppl 2):1S–29S, 1999

van der Kolk BA: The drug treatment of post-traumatic stress disorder. J Affect Disord 13:203–213, 1987

van der Kolk BA, Dreyfuss D, Michaels M, et al: Fluoxetine in posttraumatic stress disorder. J Clin Psychiatry 55:517–522, 1994

Westenberg HG, Stein DJ, Yang H, et al: A double-blind placebo-controlled study of controlled release fluvoxamine for the treatment of generalized social anxiety disorder. J Clin Psychopharmacol 24:49–55, 2004

Zitrin CM, Klein DF, Woerner MG: Treatment of phobias, I: comparison of imipramine hydrochloride and placebo. Arch Gen Psychiatry 40:125–138, 1983

7

Hypnotics

Insomnia

Insomnia is generally defined as a difficulty initiating or maintaining sleep or a poor quality of sleep. Insomnia may be primary or secondary to other conditions such as depression, anxiety, mania, or substance abuse. Primary insomnia appears to be uncommon relative to secondary insomnia. Various population surveys have found self-reported rates of symptoms of insomnia in about a third of adults. About 10% of the U.S. population report having experienced symptoms of chronic insomnia that may have lasted for many years. However a smaller percentage of patients have insomnia with significant daytime impairment. According to the "NIH State of the Science Conference Statement on Manifestations and Management of Chronic Insomnia in Adults Statement" (2005), perhaps 10% of the population has clinically significant insomnia if the criterion of daytime impairment is included in the criteria. Women and older adults appear to be the demographic groups at greatest risk for significant insomnia, but of course transient insomnia can affect anyone.

The chronic use of hypnotics is typically discouraged in the medical literature, and it is assumed that the sleepless public will go to physicians or sleep clinics, where staff will find types of insomnia that respond to behavioral or other nonsedative medical therapies. However, there may be some patients for whom chronic use of a hypnotic is beneficial and not subject to abuse. Certainly conditions such as sleep apnea, narcolepsy, and restless legs syndrome do occur, and they can be treated in a variety of ways. Sleep apnea can be life-threatening. Some insomnia may respond to treatment of the underlying illness (e.g., hyperthyroidism, depression, mania). One U.S. National Institutes of Health (NIH) Consensus Conference spent a great deal of time worrying about the possible adverse effects of hypnotics and suggested that, at most, hypnotics be prescribed for brief periods or be used only every third night. Lasagna (1996), in a cogent editorial documenting the adverse effects of untreated insomnia on auto accidents, job performance, and quality of life, noted that in the United States individuals with insomnia rarely consult physicians and, when they do, rarely mention the insomnia. About 3% of the population regularly takes over-the-counter hypnotics containing sedative antihistamines or sedative antihistamines plus mild analgesics. Sales of both types of sleep aids have been escalating, essentially unstudied, for many years.

We therefore have a situation in which a growing number of prescription hypnotics are available for prescription use but are rather unpopular with some polysomnographers and sleep experts in particular and with physicians in general. One gets the odd impression that many individuals with chronic insomnia make do with diphenhydramine or with wakefulness while more effective hypnotics are withheld from them. While eszopiclone is now approved for chronic use, and zolpidem has been studied for periods of 24 weeks without substantial evidence of tolerance, the perceived risk of dependence tends to limit their extended use as hypnotics even when better alternatives may be lacking.

The availability of ramelteon has altered the discourse on hypnotics somewhat. Ramelteon, a melatonin agonist, does not have the habit-forming potential of traditional hypnotics and is not sedating. On the other hand, ramelteon may not be as effective in addressing the spectrum of sleep difficulties as benzodiazepine and nonbenzodiazepine hypnotics.

When insomnia does lead patients to seek help from a psychiatrist or a sleep disorder specialist, the patients complain, often despairingly, of very poor sleep or total insomnia, but they nevertheless appear, on all-night sleep recordings or from nurses' or relatives' observations, to be sleeping most of the night. Attempts to objectify insomnia in terms of the time it takes for the person to fall asleep or the length of time actually slept have often not proved useful. Further, the psychiatrist is not uncommonly faced with patients who are actually awake all night, particularly those with marked depression and anxiety, whose sleep is so disturbed that they feel exhausted the next day and claim that they "can't function" or, in reality, cannot function.

Primary care physicians often see patients with untreated and undiagnosed insomnia. The presence of two of the treatable sleep disorders can be guessed at by the physician's asking questions of the patient and his or her bed partner. Sleep apnea is likely present when the partner notes the patient stops breathing in the night then snorts and gasps; snoring is also likely. The patient may note daytime sleepiness instead of wakefulness at night. Restless legs syndrome is subjectively obvious to the patient as a discomfort in his or her limbs that is relieved by movement, much like akathisia. The restlessness is worse later in the day and can disturb sleep or can disturb the bed partner, since jerky leg movements at night feel like kicks. Periodic leg movement disorder is diagnosed when the leg movements occur mainly during sleep and may cause awakenings.

Falling asleep during the day can be a symptom of narcolepsy and responds well to older stimulants and to modafinil (Provigil) or armodafinil (Nuvigil).

However, most patients coming to psychiatrists or psychiatric clinics with insomnia will already be taking medication. In these cases, the clinical problems are as follows:

1. Is a diagnosable, special sleep disorder being missed? Is referral to a sleep clinic indicated?
2. Are any of the patient's prescribed or self-administered medications (selective serotonin reuptake inhibitors [SSRIs], bronchodilators, caffeine, cocaine) causing the problem, or is the problem due to a medical condition (i.e., chronic pain, urinary frequency)?
3. Is the insomnia due to an undertreated or recurrent psychiatric condition?
4. If the patient is already taking a hypnotic and it is (or is not) working, should the medication be continued or stopped, and if the medication is stopped, should a new medication be started?

Among psychiatric patients, troublesome insomnia is often one feature of a wider symptom complex, which may also include diurnal rhythm disturbances of activity, mood, and so forth. Depressed patients classically experience early-morning awakening and diurnal variation. Many, however, have marked difficulty falling asleep and staying asleep as well. Patients with pronounced initial insomnia may be separated into those who sleep fitfully and poorly even after falling asleep and those who sleep well even after several hours of initial insomnia. Such patients can sleep from 4:00 A.M. until noon. A few patients with very severe depression complain of almost complete insomnia, reporting that they lie in bed all night without sleeping, often experiencing dysphoric, miserable ruminations.

Other psychiatric conditions are also manifested by sleep disturbances. Patients with anxiety disorders are more likely to have trouble falling asleep. Patients with mania or hypomania may stay up all night, either happily overactive or dysphorically agitated, as may patients with schizophrenia or schizophreniform psychoses. Classically, manic patients do not necessarily complain of experiencing sleeplessness; rather, they may claim that they are not sleeping much and do not seem to miss the usual sleep they get. Patients with dementia may become more confused and agitated toward evening (sundowning) and may also be agitated at night after sleeping all day. Fatigue is often a factor in sundowning. Patients very upset by major stressors—for example, bereavement, rejections, or physical trauma—may have insomnia as part of an acute stress response. Patients with posttraumatic stress disorder (PTSD) are often afraid of falling asleep and thus have initial insomnia.

Insomnia in all the relatively acute psychiatric conditions mentioned above may be fairly straightforward to treat. Insomnia as part of a depressive disorder often responds to a standard antidepressant; in fact, some of the more sedating antidepressants (mirtazapine, amitriptyline, doxepin, trazodone) may be useful hypnotics even in the absence of depression (see "Sedative Antihistamines and Other Nonbenzodiazepine Psychoactive Drugs With Hypnotic Properties" section later in this chapter). For depression with poor sleep, it is sensible to begin with a sedative antidepressant (see Chapter 3: "Antidepressants"), but antidepressants with more stimulant effects, such as bupropion and fluoxetine, usually improve sleep as the depressive syndrome improves. Protriptyline was once reported to be a good treatment for sleep apnea. In a study at McLean Hospital of more than 100 depressed patients taking fluoxetine, we found that insomnia at intake was not associated with a poorer clinical response to fluoxetine, even though fluoxetine can cause insomnia and negatively impact sleep architecture as a side effect. In cases of manic and schizophrenic excitement and in some cases of agitation, the insomnia often responds well to antipsychotic drugs of any class, although one of the sedating second-generation antipsychotics, chlorpromazine, or loxapine may initially be more effective as a hypnotic before the general syndrome ameliorates.

Thus, the best general approach is to treat the psychiatric condition that underlies the insomnia with drugs that are appropriate to that condition rather than first prescribing a benzodiazepine or other hypnotic drug for the insomnia and then treating the depression or psychosis. If a patient should be taking a drug that turns out to aggravate or cause insomnia, short-term use of a hypnotic or a drug like trazodone or mirtazapine may be useful.

In principle, a psychiatrist can run an inpatient ward or treat outpatients without ever prescribing a hypnotic. In practice, however, life often is (or appears to be) more complicated. Other patients, families, and nursing staff members become very upset if patients do not retire to bed and sleep without disturbing them. Often, hypnotics end up being prescribed to reduce the patient's distress and distress in his or her milieu. Such prescribing is often justifiable but can pose problems. First, the hypnotic may not put the patient to sleep, but instead may leave the patient (unpredictably) groggy, confused, and even more agitated. Second, a long-acting hypnotic, such as flurazepam, may leave the patient groggy the next day. Third, once the patient is used to getting a hypnotic (and the doctor is used to prescribing it), the practice may continue for weeks or even months, long after the initial phase of the illness or the stress of hospitalization has passed. When the sleeping pill is finally stopped, rebound insomnia is likely to occur, and hypnotic use is likely to be resumed to control it. (*Rebound insomnia* is a transient worsening of sleep disturbance occurring soon after discontinuation of the hypnotic.) In fact, with short-acting hypnotics such as triazolam (or alcohol), rebound insomnia can occur even 4 hours after the medication is taken. Such an effect can precipitate overuse of the compound: some patients will take additional doses to help them fall back to sleep.

Another problematic situation involves the new patient being admitted to the hospital (or visiting a new psychiatrist) who is thoroughly accustomed to taking 10 mg of zolpidem, 60 mg of flurazepam, or 3 mg of eszopiclone at bedtime (having taken the medication for months or years) but who still complains of poor sleep. As might be expected, the quality of sleep is reportedly much worse if the hypnotic is stopped. Here, two obvious options are available: to taper the hypnotic gradually while treating the major psychiatric disorder or to continue it while dealing with the disorder. The difficulty with the second, interpersonally easier, option is that the hypnotic may never be discontinued. A more complicated version of this scenario is when the patient, at the time he or she comes to the psychiatrist for treatment, is taking several psychoactive drugs of different classes, all of which need to be withdrawn or changed. In this situation, it is common to leave the hypnotic at a stable dose and taper and stop the other drugs first. This method avoids combining, and thus confusing, the effects of stopping the hypnotic with the already potentially complex effects of discontinuing an antidepressant or an antipsychotic.

At present, the only widely approved indications for hypnotics in treating insomnia are 1) brief (3- to 7-day) use or 2) occasional use for transitory insomnia caused by either acute life stressors or major shifts in diurnal rhythm (as in jet lag or in changing from one work shift to another). One hypnotic, eszopiclone (Lunesta), has been approved for more chronic use.

Although it is wise to avoid prolonged hypnotic use, prolonged use of a benzodiazepine hypnotic may be less harmful than is often said and may, in fact, provide some benefit. Sleep loss is widely believed to sometimes precipitate manic or depressive episodes. The available evidence from sleep laboratories suggests that hypnotics improve sleep measurably for only a few weeks, though placebo-controlled studies have shown no diminution in the efficacy of hypnotics for up to 24 weeks, and single-blind studies show efficacy up to a year. So far, no studies have clearly established a treatment duration after which benzodiazepine hypnotics fail to "work." Many confirmed users of hypnotics swear that the hypnotics are always helpful and even vitally necessary for years. Perhaps the initial sedation at peak blood levels provides a familiar, conditioned cue conducive to falling asleep. There is also evidence that benzodiazepines cause the patient to forget episodes of wakefulness; when the patient is no longer taking benzodiazepines, sleep may objectively be no worse, but he or she perceives (recalls) it as being worse. Certainly, some patients who have taken a hypnotic every night for several years continue to complain of poor sleep and daytime fatigue and dysphoria for months after the hypnotic was stopped.

The current evidence is that triazolam, zolpidem, zaleplon, and eszopi-clone continue to be effective (i.e., improve sleep as measured by polysomno-graphic criteria) for 4–5 weeks in placebo-controlled studies and for as long as 6 months in single-blind studies. Studies using other, less formal criteria (subject or observer ratings of sleep) have shown benefit for up to a year. Data are not available beyond that point. Since earlier editions of this manual, sleep experts appear to have become more permissive about the possible benefits of longer-term use of benzodiazepine-like hypnotics (Buysse and Dorsey 2002). However, package inserts still limit the use of such hypnotics to durations of use validated by placebo-controlled studies. The exception to this admonition is eszopiclone, which is approved for both acute and maintenance treatment of insomnia. Patients sometimes interpret such restrictions to mean that seri-ous toxicity has been shown to occur if the hypnotic is taken for longer than specified in the *Physicians' Desk Reference* (PDR). Such an interpretation does not seem to be accurate. Oversedation, poor coordination, and memory prob-lems are more likely to occur very early in treatment. The evidence for serious behavioral or other toxicity (e.g., impaired psychomotor performance early in treatment, auto accidents, falls in the elderly) is mixed and inconclusive (Buysse and Dorsey 2002).

Behavioral Approaches

Sleep hygiene recommendations are often useful to patients with both primary and secondary insomnia (see below). However, insomnia secondary to anoth-er condition is not likely to resolve with improved sleep hygiene alone. Thus, it is important to first identify and then treat the underlying condition.

Sleep Hygiene Recommendations

- Sleep only when sleepy.
- If you can't fall asleep within 20 minutes, get up and do something until you feel sleepy.
- Don't take naps.
- Get up and go to bed the same time every day.
- Refrain from exercise at least 4 hours before bedtime.
- Develop a sleep routine.
- Only use your bed for sleeping or sex.

- Stay away from caffeine, nicotine, and alcohol at least 4 hours before bedtime.
- Do not eat heavy, spicy, or rich foods 4 hours before bedtime.
- Make sure your bed and bedroom are quiet and comfortable.
- Use sunlight to set your biological clock.

Cognitive-behavioral therapy is one of the most consistently effective approaches to the long-term management of primary insomnia (Edinger and Means 2005). The more clinically and scientifically validated (nonpharmacological) approaches to insomnia are as follows:

1. *Stimulus control therapy* (sleep hygiene). The patient learns to associate being in bed only with sleep (or sex) by getting out of bed when he or she does not fall asleep rapidly in order to avoid linking bed and bedroom with miserable sleepless nights.
2. *Sleep restriction therapy.* The patient reduces time in bed progressively (with daytime naps forbidden) until he or she is asleep for 80%–90% of the time he or she is allowed to be in bed.
3. *Continuous positive airway pressure* (for patients with sleep apnea). The patient learns to wear a mask that delivers light, constant positive air pressure to the pharynx and thereby prevents the choking spells from occurring.
4. *Bright light therapy.* A patient who sleeps an adequate amount but at the wrong time of the night or day can have his or her sleep-wake rhythm reset through exposure to a light box.

Obviously, behavioral approaches require patient involvement and cooperation and are best managed by experts in sleep problems.

Pharmacological Approaches

For the past 30 years, the major efforts to develop better hypnotics have focused entirely on chemicals that bind to at least some form of benzodiazepine receptor. These agents are hoped to turn out to be better than, say, temazepam by being faster acting, being less likely to cause a morning hangover, not being "abusable" or "addictive," and not causing any change in polysomnographic sleep records, or, perhaps, causing only an increase in stage 3 and rapid eye movement (REM) sleep.

So far, this semisystematic approach has yielded a plethora of benzodiazepines, one of which, quazepam, may be selective for benzodiazepine$_1$ receptors, and three agents (zolpidem, zaleplon, and eszopiclone) that are active at benzodiazepine receptors but are not chemically benzodiazepines. So far, none of these drugs have been shown to be remarkably different in effect from the older benzodiazepine hypnotics, though zolpidem, eszopiclone, and zaleplon may have some advantages in that they are less likely to cause rebound insomnia, are less likely to exacerbate obstructive airway problems through muscle relaxation, and may show continued efficacy, when given nightly, for much longer.

In the interim, in fact for decades, drugs developed for other purposes end up being used for insomnia, at least by psychiatrists. Trazodone in doses of 50–200 mg hs is used more frequently for insomnia than for its original, U.S. Food and Drug Administration (FDA)–approved indication, depression. Unfortunately, trazodone's use for insomnia began only as the company's patent was expiring, so no systematic or extensive studies of its effects on sleep and insomnia have been done. However, most clinicians agree that it works. Its problems are morning drowsiness and, conceivably though very rarely, priapism. If tolerance to its hypnotic effect occurs, it develops only after months or years. The drug has no known abuse liability and has no clear withdrawal symptoms. Nefazodone, a related agent, also may improve sleep but, in our clinical judgment, is a much weaker hypnotic than trazodone and carries the risk of hepatotoxicity. For this reason, nefazodone is rarely used now as an antidepressant and is almost never used as a hypnotic. Both trazodone and nefazodone have potent antagonist effects for 5-HT$_2$ receptors, an effect shared with other agents such as the antidepressant mirtazapine and second-generation antipsychotics such as olanzapine and quetiapine. Indeed, quetiapine at low dosages of 25–100 mg/day has become a commonly used hypnotic for patients with mood and personality disorders.

A new generation of 5-HT$_2$ antagonists are in current development as hypnotics. Among these, eplivanserin is perhaps farthest along. Eplivanserin, given in a 1 mg or 5 mg dose at bedtime, appears to reduce sleep latency and the number of nocturnal awakenings. Its primary side effect at these doses is dry mouth. It is unclear whether there are advantages over low-dose trazodone.

Among the older tricyclic antidepressants (TCAs), amitriptyline, imipramine, doxepin, and trimipramine, and probably nortriptyline, are good hypnotics, though they are rarely studied as such. Katz et al. (1991), in a report from the

National Institute of Mental Health (NIMH) Collaborative Depression Study, noted that sleep ratings improved strikingly in the first 2 weeks with amitriptyline but that this hypnotic effect did not predict an overall improvement in the depressions being treated. Trimipramine is the best studied and appears to be the only TCA to facilitate sleep but not to affect REM latency or nocturnal penile tumescence. If it did not sometimes cause morning drowsiness, dry mouth, constipation, and weight gain, trimipramine might be the ideal hypnotic at doses of 25–100 mg at bedtime. It is not safe for use by suicidal patients.

Since gabapentin was released for use in seizures, its use has widely spread into treating pain, anxiety, and insomnia. It seems quite safe in doses from 100 mg to 900 mg at bedtime and maybe higher. It is not metabolized by the body and seems quite safe in overdose, since the intestine appears not to be able to absorb more than about 900 mg at any one time. It appears to be free of abuse liability. For this reason, gabapentin is sometimes used in patients with alcohol dependence as an alternative to benzodiazepines. One open study found that in alchoholic patients with sleep disturbance, gabapentin appeared more effective than trazodone as a hypnotic (Karam-Hage et al. 2003). Again, although commonly prescribed by neurologists and psychiatrists in treating insomnia, gabapentin is not approved by the FDA for this indication.

All these nonbenzodiazepines (as well as diphenhydramine and maybe melatonin and valerian) may be nonabusable, relatively safe and effective ways to treat insomnia, but prescribing clinicians would sleep better if someone—perhaps the NIH or, in the case of gabapentin, the drug company—would undertake the studies necessary to document their potential safety and efficacy, if such proves to be the case.

Benzodiazepine Hypnotics

The benzodiazepines are still among the most widely prescribed sedative-hypnotics in the United States today. Although most benzodiazepines have hypnotic properties, as of this writing, only five benzodiazepines have an FDA-approved indication as a hypnotic: flurazepam, temazepam, estazolam, quazepam, and triazolam. Four nonbenzodiazepines, zolpidem, zaleplon, eszopiclone, and ramelteon, are also FDA approved as hypnotics.

The principles for discriminating among these drugs are similar to those described in Chapter 6 ("Antianxiety Agents") for the anxiolytic benzodiazepines: structure, pharmacokinetics, absorption, and distribution (Table 7–1). For example, most of the benzodiazepine hypnotics belong to separate structural subclasses: 2-keto (flurazepam), 3-hydroxy (temazepam), and triazolo (triazolam and estazolam) (Figure 7–1). The metabolism and half-lives of these subclass members parallel those of their anxiolytic counterparts. Flurazepam is oxidized in the liver and, like diazepam, has a relatively long half-life (40 hours). It also forms a long-acting (100 hours) metabolite, desalkylflurazepam, a metabolite shared with quazepam. Temazepam is conjugated with a glucuronide radical in the liver and has a much shorter half-life (8 hours) and no active metabolites. Triazolam and estazolam are oxidized but with no clearly active metabolites; triazolam has an extremely short half-life (3–6 hours) (Table 7–1), while estazolam is more like temazepam. Flurazepam and triazolam have more rapid absorption (peak blood levels at 30 and 20 minutes, respectively) than temazepam, which may not be absorbed for 45–60 minutes. The slower absorption accounts for patients' not falling asleep rapidly after taking this medication. Clinicians should advise patients to take temazepam approximately 1 hour before bedtime to avoid anticipatory discomfort and their resorting to premature repeat dosing.

A benzodiazepine hypnotic, quazepam, was released in the early 1990s. Chemically, it does not fall into any of the three classes described in Chapter 6 ("Antianxiety Agents"). However, the drug's pharmacokinetics are in the same range as those of flurazepam, and it is metabolized to desalkylflurazepam in the body; the drug and its metabolite have half-lives of about 40 hours. Metabolism and elimination are slowed in elderly patients. This pattern suggests that sedation the next morning should be more of a problem than early rebound insomnia. Quazepam's only special feature is that it binds selectively to type 1 benzodiazepine receptors, whereas flurazepam and other older benzodiazepines bind equally to both type 1 and type 2 sites in the brain. There is no evidence that this special binding property is of particular clinical value. Quazepam's active metabolite does bind to both receptor types. Quazepam is a long-acting hypnotic, probably similar to flurazepam in its clinical utility. It is available in 7.5-mg and 15-mg tablets.

The distribution of the sedative benzodiazepines is relatively rapid. Indeed, the acute formation of high peak blood levels is thought to account for patients' falling asleep relatively quickly with these drugs. The decline from peak levels

2-Keto

Flurazepam

3-Hydroxy

Temazepam

Triazolo

Triazolam

Estazolam

Trifluoroethyl

Quazepam

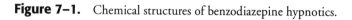

Figure 7–1.   Chemical structures of benzodiazepine hypnotics.

Table 7–1.   Benzodiazepine hypnotics

Generic name	Brand name	Formulation and strengths	Dosage (mg/day)	Absorption	Major active metabolites	Approximate half-life (hrs)
flurazepam[a]	Dalmane	Capsules: 15, 30 mg	15–30	Intermediate	hydroxyethylflurazepam desalkylflurazepam	1 100
temazepam[a]	Restoril	Capsules: 7.5, 15, 22.5, 30 mg	15–30	Intermediate	None	8
quazepam	Doral	Tablets: 7.5, 15 mg	7.5–15	Intermediate	oxoquazepam desalkyloxoquazepam	39 73
triazolam[a]	Halcion	Tablets: 0.125, 0.25 mg	0.125–0.5	Intermediate	—	3
estazolam[a]	ProSom	Tablets: 1, 2 mg	1–4	Intermediate	—	16

[a]Available in generic form.

may account for why patients can awaken often, even when significant drug plasma levels are still apparent. Moreover, the decline from peak levels and the need for peak levels to induce sleep also explain why patients treated with longer-acting benzodiazepines like flurazepam require nightly doses.

Some investigators and clinicians have argued that a non-long-acting compound (e.g., temazepam or zolpidem) offers great advantages over longer-acting agents, because it is largely excreted before the next morning. Although at least one study has pointed to the safe use of triazolam for inducing sleep on transatlantic flights and preventing jet lag, there may be disadvantages associated with very-short-acting hypnotics, particularly rebound insomnia and anterograde amnesia. With some short-acting hypnotics, rebound insomnia occurs within the first 2 nights after discontinuation and can be troublesome for patients. Although acutely apparent with shorter-acting compounds, it may occur 5–7 days after discontinuation of benzodiazepines with longer half-lives and may be misinterpreted as a reemergence of the underlying insomnia rather than as a rebound phenomenon. It seems less likely to occur with zolpidem and zaleplon. When rebound insomnia occurs, clinicians should avoid resumption of the drug. Rather, reassurance and the prescription of antihistamine sedatives (e.g., 50 mg of diphenhydramine), sedating antidepressants (e.g., 50–100 mg of trazodone), or gabapentin (100 or 300 mg hs) for a few days may prove beneficial. When this does not work, reinstituting the benzodiazepine and gradually tapering the dose is an alternative strategy.

The side effects of the sedative-hypnotic benzodiazepines are similar to those of their anxiolytic counterparts. They include sedation, ataxia, anterograde amnesia, slurred speech, and nausea. These side effects are not particularly dangerous, although sedation can be a problem if the individual attempts to drive, to operate heavy machinery, and so forth. There is weak evidence to suggest that the longer-half-life compounds cause clinically important cognitive problems the following day; however, this area has not been well studied. Refined and detailed psychological testing can usually detect impairment of cognitive or psychomotor function the morning after a benzodiazepine hypnotic has been used to induce sleep. The real question is whether this impairment is clinically important; the vast majority of users of hypnotics do not note behavioral impairment the next day unless they note persistent sedation as well. However, as noted earlier, there have been several reports of pronounced anterograde amnesia ("blackouts") in patients treated with triazolam.

Indeed, some healthy individuals who have used triazolam to induce sleep during a transatlantic flight have described not remembering arriving in Europe or what they did the next day. In the few personal accounts from patients and their friends and colleagues of blackouts after taking a benzodiazepine, the individuals appear to have done their usual activities blamelessly during the period they cannot recall. Similar reactions have been observed with other benzodiazepines and with zolpidem and zaleplon. By far, the greater number of published or FDA reports of anterograde amnesia concern triazolam, but it is difficult to tell whether this difference is real or due to the extensive media publicity about triazolam (Bunney et al. 1999).

One possible problem with longer-acting benzodiazepines is illustrated by the case of a patient who had been treated with flurazepam nightly for years but who was shifted to an equivalent dose of temazepam. He developed a clear benzodiazepine withdrawal syndrome; the shorter-acting drug could not adequately replace the longer-acting one for the full 24 hours between doses.

In addition to pharmacologically explainable differences in shifting from one hypnotic to another, some patients claim (vigorously) that, say, lorazepam works beautifully, whereas temazepam in its new formulation does nothing. Beyond this, zolpidem or zaleplon is often rejected or criticized by patients who are used to triazolam or flurazepam; in these cases, these agents may be just different enough in their subjective effects from benzodiazepines to leave the patient worried that the hypnotic "isn't working," even though these same agents do fine as hypnotics in patients with insomnia who have never taken a benzodiazepine. The newer drugs affect mainly sleep latency; they may get the patient to sleep but may not keep him or her sleeping for long enough. Zolpidem, zaleplon, and eszopiclone appear to be different enough from benzodiazepines to be free of rebound insomnia but may not have less danger of abuse than older benzodiazepines (Rush and Griffiths 1996; Rush et al. 1999).

Time (and further studies) will tell, but these newer, not-quite-a-benzodiazepine hypnotics seem effective and well tolerated by both young and old. They deserve the benefit of the doubt as being safer than chloral hydrate or pentobarbital, probably better than the benzodiazepine hypnotics, and probably more effective than the antihistamine over-the-counter Benadryl types of preparations.

Melatonin, the newly advertised, naturally occurring sleep-inducing hormone, and valerian, an old herbal preparation, are discussed at the end of this chapter.

Nonbenzodiazepine Hypnotics

Drugs such as zolpidem, zaleplon, and eszopiclone lack the chemical structure of the benzodiazepines (Figure 7–2). However, these drugs still act on α_1 benzodiazepine sites on the GABA-A receptor. The nonbenzodiazepine hypnotics lack activity at α_2 and peripheral α_3 benzodiazepine sites. Thus, the nonbenzodiazepine hypnotics are not as potent muscle-relaxing and anticonvulsant agents as the benzodiazepines. The specific hypnotic effects of these drugs have distinct advantages in some patients. For example, the muscle-relaxing properties of benzodiazepines may further compromise the airways of patients with sleep apnea. The nonbenzodiazepine hypnotics appear to be less of a problem for obstructive sleep apnea patients. Likewise, we prefer that patients undergoing electroconvulsive therapy (ECT) use a nonbenzodiazepine hypnotic rather than a benzodiazepine hypnotic in the evening prior to ECT because a nonbenzodiazepine is somewhat less likely to raise the seizure threshold.

The nonbenzodiazepines have a reputation of being less addictive than benzodiazepines. It is unclear whether this reputation is deserved. Even though high doses of the nonbenzodiazepines may induce euphoria (Gelenberg 2000), very few cases of dependence have been described in the world literature. In a survey of the scientific literature, only 36 cases of zolpidem dependence and 22 cases of zopiclone (related to eszopiclone) dependence had been described by 2003 (Hajak et al. 2003). More recent surveys suggest that reports of dependence and abuse of these agents may be rising (Victorri-Vigneau et al. 2007). Over half of the patients who end up abusing drugs such as zolpidem have a previous history of abuse, but about 40% were prescribed the drug for sleep, developed a tolerance, and then started taking more and more of the drug. In the literature, dosages of 300 mg/day or more of zolpidem have been reported in some insomnia patients who have become dependent on the drug. While these cases appear to be the exception, it is not clear that the abuse potential of the nonbenzodiazepine hypnotics is substantially lower than that of the benzodiazepines.

At the time of this writing, zolpidem still is among the most common of the hypnotics prescribed in the United States. There are probably more prescriptions written for benzodiazepine hypnotics, but these are available in generic form and less expensive. While all nonbenzodiazepines have short half-lives in healthy subjects (zaleplon, about 1–2 hours; zolpidem, 2–4 hours; eszopi-

Zolpidem   Zaleplon

Eszopiclone

Figure 7–2. Chemical structures of the nonbenzodiazepine hypnotics zolpidem, zaleplon, and eszopiclone.

clone, 4–5 hours), many patients taking these medications, particularly zolpidem and eszopiclone, are able to sleep through the night. Zaleplon is somewhat lighter, and some patients complain of not being able to fall or stay asleep as well as they do with zolpidem. However, zaleplon is the only hypnotic that one could effectively take in the middle of the night and not feel too groggy in the morning.

The most common side effects of the nonbenzodiazepines are drowsiness and dizziness. Other benzodiazepine side effects, such as ataxia, slurred speech, and amnestic symptoms, are less common with the nonbenzodiazepine hypnotics. However, withdrawal symptoms, including insomnia, muscle cramps, and even seizures, have been (rarely) reported.

The nonbenzodiazepine hypnotics should be taken on an empty stomach to induce more rapid onset of sleep. Zolpidem is usually dosed at 5–10 mg at night. Some patients seem to need 20 mg, although there is little evidence that this dose is much more effective than 10 mg. But there is little evidence it presents more of a problem than smaller doses. Zaleplon can be taken in doses of 10–20 mg at night. If the patient wakes up in the middle of the night, a 10-mg dose may be taken. Eszopiclone has usually been initiated at a dose of 1–2 mg to facilitate falling asleep and 3 mg to sustain sleep if 2 mg is inadequate. In the elderly, the recommended dosage is 1–2 mg/day. Unlike most hypnotics, eszopiclone has been studied in the management of insomnia for periods of 12 months with no substantial evidence of tolerance.

Melatonin Receptor Agonist: Ramelteon

While melatonin has been available over the counter for many years as a potential treatment of insomnia and phase-shift disorders, melatonin supplements are not subject to careful and consistent manufacturing. In addition, the efficacy of most melatonin supplements appears to range from modest to minimal. Ramelteon (Rozerem) is a specific melatonin MT_1 and MT_2 receptor agonist that was approved in 2005 as the first FDA-approved hypnotic that is not a controlled substance. Ramelteon appears to act on melatonin receptors in the suprachiasmatic nucleus responsible for sleep-wake cycles. Since it has no effects on the benzodiazepine receptor, it is not associated with abuse potential, rebound insomnia, motor deficits, or exacerbation of problems such as chronic obstructive pulmonary disease or obstructive sleep apnea. In addition, it is not likely to contribute to confusion or memory in geriatric patients in a way that benzodiazepine or nonbenzodiazepine agents can. On the other hand, the primary utility of ramelteon is in reducing sleep latency or the time it takes to fall asleep; it may be of less utility than standard hypnotics in keeping patients asleep. Single-dose and repeated-dose studies have indicated that 8 mg of ramelteon decreases the time to persistent sleep relative to placebo and might increase total sleep time (Erman et al. 2006). Preliminary studies also indicate that ramelteon might be useful in shifting disorders associated with phase delay of the sleep cycle, such as in jet lag, insomnia in the elderly, and insomnia associated with other neuropsychiatric disorders (McGechan and Wellington 2005).

The primary side effects of ramelteon have included headache, somnolence, fatigue, dizziness, and nausea, but these have generally been mild and may improve after several weeks of treatment. High-fat meals can reduce absorption, and thus patients should be informed not to take ramelteon shortly after a rich meal. Ramelteon is metabolized via cytochrome P450 3A4, and serum levels may be increased by fluvoxamine and decreased by carbamazepine. It is not an unreasonable question to ask what the benefits of ramelteon are over less-expensive melatonin supplements. Certainly, the consistency of the manufacturing of ramelteon over the much more variable manufacturing of over-the-counter food supplements such as melatonin is an advantage. The potency of ramelteon might be expected to also be greater than that of over-the-counter melatonin, but this has not been established, and no direct comparisons of ramelteon and over-the-counter melatonin have been reported. Nonetheless, ramelteon has a unique niche among currently available hypnotics as a well-tolerated agent with no abuse potential. In patients with a history of substance abuse, geriatric patients, and patients with initial insomnia, ramelteon might be worth trying before other agents. Our general sense is that ramelteon may not be as consistently effective as more traditional hypnotics but is far less likely to cause mischief as well.

Sedative Antihistamines and Other Nonbenzodiazepine Psychoactive Drugs With Hypnotic Properties

Hydroxyzine compounds are the only antihistamines with some documented efficacy in the treatment of anxiety disorders. They also have an indication for preoperative and postanesthesia sedation. These drugs are available in capsules or tablets ranging from 10 to 100 mg each. However, our clinical experience with psychiatric patients suggests that the drugs are neither much appreciated by patients nor particularly effective on the few occasions when we have tried them. They are reasonably free of side effects, although hydroxyzine and the other antihistamines exert anticholinergic effects. When taken with other anticholinergic agents, hydroxyzine and related compounds can pose problems, particularly at high doses. Their main value may be as a delaying action for patients who are inclined to abuse sedative-hypnotic or benzodiazepine drugs, because they do not produce either physical or psychological dependence.

Diphenhydramine (Benadryl) is another antihistamine sometimes used for its sedative or alleged hypnotic effects. It has not been well studied in either capacity but has some sedative properties and is occasionally judged by patients to be acceptable. There is a well-controlled study showing some efficacy for diphenhydramine in treating insomnia (Rickels et al. 1983). The dose for sleep is 50–100 mg. Diphenhydramine is now available over the counter in 25-mg formulations. The drug is anticholinergic and can be used for acute dystonic reactions to antipsychotics (see Chapter 4: "Antipsychotic Drugs"). Promethazine (Phenergan) is a phenothiazine without antipsychotic properties that is marketed as an antihistamine with sedative properties. Again, it is occasionally found useful as a mild sedative at doses of 25–100 mg, but it is not a major psychiatric drug. Doxylamine, another antihistamine, is the ingredient used in most over-the-counter preparations (e.g., Unisom) that are used for either tranquilization or hypnosis.

Several TCAs exert marked antihistaminergic effects and are excellent hypnotics. So is trazodone, a heterocyclic antidepressant. Doxepin, amitriptyline, and trimipramine can be used in doses of 25–75 mg at bedtime. Trazodone is best begun, as a hypnotic, at a dose of 50 mg hs, with 50-mg increments up to 200 mg hs. At some dose in that range improved sleep should occur, perhaps with undesirable sedation on the following morning. Some patients lose this side effect if the dose is held steady for 3–5 days; others require a lower dose that, it is hoped, will be effective without inducing a hangover. Sometimes adult patients taking trazodone on an empty stomach will faint from postural hypotension if they do not go to bed soon after taking it as a hypnotic. Occasionally, elderly patients develop orthostatic hypotension the next day after taking this agent at bedtime. Some studies of trazodone's effects on sleep and of its utility in other unexpected areas (agitation in the elderly, if given in 25-mg doses; PTSD [Hertzberg et al. 1996]) have emerged. It retains, so far, its record with us of mixing innocuously with all other psychiatric drugs, including SSRIs and monoamine oxidase inhibitors (MAOIs). There is even a study showing that vis-à-vis triazolam or zolpidem, trazodone has no euphoriant effects in individuals with a history of substance abuse (Rush et al. 1999). Mirtazapine can also be an effective hypnotic at dosages of 7.5–15 mg/day. The drug is a potent serotonin$_2$ (5-HT$_2$) receptor antagonist and has antihistaminic properties as well.

Gabapentin and pregabalin are probably also as safe and useful as trazodone in treating insomnia. They have the added potential benefit of having both analgesic and hypnotic effects, as shown in large placebo-controlled studies involving patients with postherpetic or diabetic neuralgia, and are reported to be potentially useful in the treatment of other painful conditions that interfere with sleep. The dose to be used is more of a problem, with the dosage ranging between 300 mg and 1,200 mg taken at bedtime for gabapentin and between 150 and 600 mg/day for pregabalin. γ-Aminobutyric acid (GABA) analogs such as gabapentin and pregabalin appear to be more useful for insomnia or anxiety symptoms in psychiatric patients than as a primary mood stabilizer, although occasional patients with bipolar disorder appear to do uniquely well while taking gabapentin (see Chapter 5: "Mood Stabilizers") (Ketter et al. 1999). There is one disturbing report describing withdrawal symptoms (anxiety, agitation, and dysphoria) that were worse than those occurring at baseline (Cora-Locatelli et al. 1998), but no one we know of locally has observed or heard of such a phenomenon. Again, gabapentin has been mixed with a wide variety of other psychoactive drugs, mainly in treating bipolar patients, without evidence of adverse interactions (Chouinard et al. 1998).

TCAs may also be effective as hypnotics (Gursky and Krahn 2000) and, like gabapentin and pregabalin, may have analgesic properties as well if given a prolonged trial in patients with chronic pain and insomnia. Most TCAs, as well as most other antidepressants, suppress or delay REM sleep. Nefazodone and mirtazapine do not appear to do so, and the importance of suppressing (or encouraging) various sleep phases in depressed patients is still unclear despite many studies. Trimipramine, among the TCAs, may be the least likely to affect sleep architecture, but it may cause dry mouth, constipation, and weight gain. It seems less likely to cause orthostatic hypotension or to affect penile tumescence than other TCAs in doses of 25–100 mg hs. Independent evidence that TCAs (at least amitriptyline and imipramine) can improve sleep without relieving depression comes from the NIMH Collaborative Depression Study (Katz et al. 1991). Doxepin (Silenor) is currently under FDA review as a treatment for insomnia. Small dosages (3–6 mg/day) appear effective as a hypnotic. However, doxepin is a very antihistaminic/anticholinergic drug and thus is probably a less-than-ideal hypnotic in the elderly.

It is hard to make clear recommendations about the use of benzodiazepine or related hypnotics versus trazodone, mirtazapine, gabapentin, or pregabalin. Clearly, patients with an abuse potential may be at greater risk for dependence while taking benzodiazepines and related agents. Those patients with significant anxiety or depression might do better when an agent such as pregabalin or mirtazapine is used to also help sleep. The TCAs are less safe in overdose than other potential hypnotics and should generally be avoided for hypnotic use.

Barbiturates

A number of barbiturates have or had an FDA-approved indication for use as sedative-hypnotics (Table 7–2). Their use as oral hypnotics now is rarely justified. However, the barbiturates continue to be used as intravenous agents of choice in anesthesia and occasionally in critical care settings. The structures of these compounds are shown in Figure 6–3 (see Chapter 6: "Antianxiety Agents"). Pentobarbital, secobarbital, amobarbital, and a combination of secobarbital and amobarbital are most commonly used for nighttime sedation. In addition, several of these have indications for both daytime and nighttime sedation. (The use of amobarbital, butabarbital, and other barbiturates for daytime sedation is discussed in Chapter 6: "Antianxiety Agents.") Dosage ranges of these compounds and routes of administration are listed in Table 7–2.

For many years barbiturates were widely used for their hypnotic effects, but their use has dwindled with the introduction of the safer benzodiazepines. The half-lives of barbiturates determine their clinical applications. The extremely short-acting barbiturates (e.g., hexobarbital) are used for preanesthesia or anesthesia. Intermediate-duration barbiturates (e.g., pentobarbital) are used for induction and maintenance of sleep. Longer-acting compounds may be used for agitation or anxiety (see Chapter 6: "Antianxiety Agents"). Barbiturate preparations are variations of a barbituric acid structure with substitutions at one or more key positions (see Figure 6–3), resulting in differences in lipophilia and half-lives.

The barbiturates have become less widely used because of their limited safety margin in overdose, their potential for dependence, and the degree of central nervous system (CNS) depression they induce. These drugs are extremely potent hypnotics, particularly for patients who have not previously taken barbiturates. Indeed, some patients may demonstrate considerable somnolence 24 hours after ingestion. Moreover, these agents pose potential problems when mixed with alcohol or other CNS depressants and are contraindicated in patients with acute intermittent porphyria or attention-deficit/hyperactivity disorder.

Table 7–2. Barbiturates for insomnia

Generic name	Brand name	Formulations and strengths	Nighttime dose (mg)[a]
butabarbital sodium	Butisol Sodium	Tablets: 30, 50 mg Elixir: 30 mg/5 mL (480-mL bottle)	50–100
pentobarbital	Nembutal	Injection: 50 mg/mL (20-mL, 50-mL vials) Capsule: 100 mg	150–200
phenobarbital	Various generics	Tablets: 15, 30, 60, 100 mg Tablets: 16.2, 32.4, 64.8, 97.2 mg[b] Concentrate: 20 mg/5 mL (480-mL) Injection: 65 mg/mL (1-mL prefilled syringe[c] and single-dose vial), 130 mg/mL (1-mL prefilled syringe)	
secobarbital	Seconal	Capsule: 100 mg	100
secobarbital and amobarbital	Tuinal	Capsule: 50, 50 mg each	50–200

[a]Adult dosages. For child dosages, consult the latest edition of *Physicians' Desk Reference* (PDR) or a similar reference.
[b]16.2 mg equivalent to ¼ grain, 32.4 to ½ grain, and so forth.
[c]Tubex, Carpuject.

In depressed patients, the administration of barbiturates often resulted in a marked reduction in TCA plasma levels and diminution of antidepressant effects because of their induction of liver microsomal enzymes and accelerated degradation of the TCA. Clinicians should keep this in mind when considering adjunctive use of hypnotics in depressed patients. Indeed, we saw depressed patients who were chronically treated with barbiturates for sleep and failed to respond to amitriptyline and other TCAs but who did respond after discontinuing their barbiturates (see Chapter 9: "Augmentation Strategies for Treatment-Resistant Disorders").

Currently, the main remaining use in outpatient psychiatry for intermediate-acting sedative-hypnotic barbiturates, such as pentobarbital, is probably limited to the older patient who occasionally needs a hypnotic for insomnia and, because of prolonged past experience with barbiturates, finds a barbiturate sleeping pill preferable to any of the newer benzodiazepines. Such prescribing is, of course, a matter of giving in to a patient's experience and preference rather than a mandatory or necessary clinical maneuver. (For discussion of various uses of amobarbital, including its use in treating catatonia and in analytically oriented interviews, see Chapter 6: "Antianxiety Agents.")

For patients who have become dependent on barbiturates, detoxification is necessary. Abrupt withdrawal should be avoided because it can result in seizures, delirium, and even death. When the daily dose of barbiturate is not known, physicians can give test doses of a barbiturate (watching for the emergence of nystagmus, slurred speech, ataxia, and sedation) to determine the currently needed dosage. The test dose can then act as a barometer of the dose at which to begin a detoxification program (see Chapter 11: "Pharmacotherapy for Substance Use Disorders").

Nonbarbiturate Hypnotics

In the late 1940s and the 1950s, several nonbarbiturate hypnotic drugs were developed in the hope that they would be safer and better than the barbiturates. Unfortunately, this hope was not realized. They proved, generally, to have as many limitations as the barbiturates.

Only one of these drugs currently available for use—chloral hydrate (see Figure 7–3)—is generally viewed as effective. The rest are no longer available. Chloral hydrate is a somewhat effective and reasonably safe sleeping medica-

Figure 7–3.   Chemical structures of nonbarbiturate hypnotics.

tion in doses between 500 and 1,500 mg at bedtime (Table 7–3). Early prescription levels of 500 mg at bedtime often proved inadequate to produce sedation, and most prescribers have come to favor 1,000 mg, particularly in younger adult patients. The drug is often used in double-blind trials of other psychiatric medications as an adjunct medication because of its presumed safety and "cleanliness." It is unlikely that this reputation is fully deserved, particularly because chloral hydrate itself was once widely abused in England in the early 1900s. It also has a very low margin of safety, the lethal dose being about 10 times the hypnotic dose. Chloral hydrate is irritating to the stomach. It was also used with alcohol as a "Mickey Finn" to knock out victims who were being shanghaied. Alcohol and trichlorethanol, the metabolite and active principal of chloral hydrate, are presumed to interact to increase the combination potency. Trichlorethanol slows the metabolism of ethanol, while ethanol speeds the conversion of chloral hydrate to trichlorethanol (Rall 1993).

Another hypnotic, paraldehyde, is a colorless liquid with a very pungent odor and a burning, disagreeable taste. The oral hypnotic dose is 5 or 10 mL. However, the medication has no advantages and may be quite toxic if the material is old and deteriorated. It is too irritating to be given parenterally, although intramuscular and rectal administration were once common. Paraldehyde's former use in the detoxification of patients with chronic alcoholism has been supplanted by use of the longer-acting and safer benzodiazepines.

Other nonbarbiturate hypnotics, including glutethimide, ethinamate, methyprylon, and ethchlorvynol, were developed because of the known dangers of addiction and lethality on suicidal ingestion of barbiturates. Unfortunately, none of these drugs proved to be either safer or less capable of producing physical or psychological dependence than the drugs that they were supposed to replace. There are currently no logical reasons for using them in preference to the safer benzodiazepines.

Methaqualone

Methaqualone (Quaalude), a drug that still deserves passing mention (Figure 7–3), was a nonbarbiturate hypnotic marketed as a safe and effective replacement for the more dangerous older sleeping pills. It became widely abused in the illicit street market and achieved a good deal of publicity as the "love" drug in the 1960s. Methaqualone was alleged to have aphrodisiac properties, a proposition that has never been specifically tested in any scientific way. The drug, however, can cause paresthesias, which may somehow increase sexual feelings.

Methaqualone has acquired a remarkably tainted reputation and is now no longer available for prescription use in the United States. Whether the drug was really more likely to be abused or was more euphoriant than the barbiturates is quite unclear. The one available study relevant to the point suggested that it was really no different from pentobarbital in its subjective effects. In

Table 7–3.   Other nighttime hypnotic agents

Generic name	Brand name	Formulations and strengths	Dosage (mg/day)[a]
zolpidem	Ambien[b]	Tablets: 5, 10 mg	5–10
	Ambien-CR	Tablets (extended release): 6.25, 12.5 mg	
	Edular	Sublingual: 5, 10 mg	
	Zolpimist	Oral spray solution: 5 mg/spray (60 mL)	
zaleplon	Sonata[b]	Capsules: 5, 10 mg	5–10
eszopiclone	Lunesta[b]	Tablets: 1, 2, 3 mg	1–3
ramelteon	Rozerem	Tablet: 8 mg	8
chloral hydrate	Noctec	Capsule: 500 mg	500–1,500
		Syrup: 500 mg/5 mL (480 mL)	

[a]Adult dosages. Patients may require slightly higher dosages of chloral hydrate or ethchlorvynol. For child dosages, consult the latest edition of *Goodman & Gilman's*.

[b]Lower doses may be indicated when combined with potent cytochrome P450 3A4 inhibitors (e.g., fluoxetine).

our local clinical experience, we found occasional patients with severe insomnia who claimed that methaqualone was far superior as a hypnotic—in terms of both speed of onset and lack of hangover—than other available hypnotics, even comparable barbiturates. In any event, methaqualone, for good or for bad, is no longer available.

Over-the-Counter Sleeping Agents

L-Tryptophan

A hypnotic drug that seems to be free of dependence or abuse liability is the amino acid L-tryptophan. It has not been formally approved for medical use as a hypnotic drug in the United States, but it was available in both drugstores and health food stores as a dietary supplement, either in the pure form or combined with other nutriments. There was reasonable evidence that, at doses of 1–6 g at bedtime, L-tryptophan had some efficacy as a sleeping pill in some patients with insomnia. It was neither as powerful as the major hypnotics nor, presumably, as dangerous. It would be, however, a rather expensive way to get a night's sleep, because the drug used to cost (in the 1980s) almost $1 per gram.

In 1989, a small series of seriously ill patients with fever, myalgia, and massive eosinophilia were identified. All had had exposure to L-tryptophan, and most had persistent illness requiring steroids for relief. There were at least 37 deaths and 1,500 cases of eosinophilia-myalgia syndrome reported. The cause was thought to be a foreign manufacturer's producing a toxic variant of the compound. On this basis, the FDA withdrew all L-tryptophan from the market. It is currently available only as an investigational new drug or by order from Canadian pharmacies.

The risk of this serious disease is unknown, but L-tryptophan was used for years without evidence of massive eosinophilia. If it were to be considered safe to use again, the starting dose should be 1–2 g at bedtime, with an increase to 3–4 g after two to three nights. The amount of available L-tryptophan in milk—particularly when warmed—rivals a 2-g dose, and some clinicians have advocated this time-honored approach for insomnia. Some workers have further noted that carbohydrates facilitate the absorption of L-tryptophan, suggesting that milk and cookies may be better than milk alone. We know of no double-blind studies of this approach, however.

The ill-considered use of L-tryptophan to treat insomnia in patients who are being treated with fluoxetine or MAOIs should be avoided. The serotonin syndrome, manifested by myoclonic jerks, hyperpyrexia, confusion, and coma, can be precipitated if doses of 1–4 g are given initially to patients taking fluoxetine or MAOIs. The manufacturer of fluoxetine notes that the addition of L-tryptophan to the regimen of patients already being treated with fluoxetine is contraindicated. It is unclear whether beginning with 500 mg of L-tryptophan at bedtime and titrating upward is clinically useful or safe in patients taking MAOIs. We have tried L-tryptophan for MAOI-related insomnia in doses of 1–2 g at bedtime with little success but without adverse effects.

In recent years, a substitute for tryptophan, 5-hydroxytryptophan (or 5-HTP), has been marketed in the United States for the treatment of depression and anxiety. Over the years, there have been a number of small open and controlled trials supporting the use of 5-HTP. Most of these trials involved fewer than 20 patients, and definitive studies are lacking.

Melatonin

Melatonin, a naturally occurring hormone, is often used over the counter to treat insomnia and jet lag. The prescription drug ramelteon is a melatonin agonist that became available in 2006 as a hypnotic with no abuse potential. In humans, at least, melatonin appears to be excreted by the pineal gland early during the sleep cycle and may well contribute to our "natural" circadian rhythms. Blind subjects do not have a regular 24-hour rhythm as sighted people do. The melatonin excretion patterns of blind subjects are also irregular. Elderly subjects with insomnia have low levels of melatonin.

Melatonin has been shown to act as a hypnotic in small, brief studies of insomnia due to factors such as jet lag or bad diurnal rhythm, but the correct dose and the effects of chronic (i.e., over 7 days) administration are unknown. Doses between 0.2 mg and 5 mg seem to be effective; higher doses may be less effective (Zhdanova et al. 1997).

The substance is available over the counter in drugstores in at least (locally) 0.2-mg and 3-mg dose units. It is sold as a dietary supplement. It is said that oral ingestion of melatonin has no effect on the pineal gland's daily production of the material—an odd state of affairs for a hormone. The *Medical Letter on Drugs and Therapeutics* ("Melatonin" 1995) says that the commercial melatonin can be synthetic or can be extracted from hog pineal glands. Some preparations contain unidentified impurities. Experts on melatonin claim that it is a remarkably efficient antioxidant, more potent than any other currently available. There is considerable variation in melatonin levels produced by specific preparations.

Informal reports from friends and patients who have tried over-the-counter melatonin for mild insomnia or jet lag have been favorable; it does feel subjectively as if it were a mild sedative. It also appears to help overcome insomnia in elderly persons. However, so far, no single reliable producer's melatonin has been adequately tested for either efficacy or safety. This lack of adequate study points to the discouraging object lesson of the disastrous effects of badly made L-tryptophan on a few health food store patrons. Melatonin can be tried as a hypnotic, but unanticipated adverse effects might occur ("Melatonin" 1995).

Valerian Extract

Valerian has come to be popularly assumed to be a useful herbal preparation for improving sleep or decreasing anxiety. It binds to GABA receptors, perhaps because the extract actually contains GABA. Valerian's innate GABA cannot cross the blood-brain barrier and should not, therefore, help with insomnia or anxiety. Valerian extract is also believed to bind to serotonin and adenosine receptors (Houghton 1999; Wong et al. 1998). The adenosine receptor may be responsible for meprobamate's sedative-hypnotic actions.

Several small studies suggest that valerian extract may affect sleep positively, but the studies were small and the findings were inconsistent (Buysse and Dorsey 2002). One can only repeat the warning from L-tryptophan: "dietary supplements," under which category valerian falls, are not evaluated for safety and efficacy, and the user runs the risk of unpredictable adverse effects. On the other hand, if one were to see a patient who had used valerian extract for months or years for periodic insomnia with satisfaction, such a patient may be better off continuing to use valerian than shifting to a benzodiazepine-like hypnotic.

If valerian proves to be effective for insomnia, it will be a very delayed lesson for Dr. Harry Gold, an early clinical pharmacologist who pioneered double-blind studies in angina and pain at Cornell Medical College in the 1940s. He used to assert that valerian extract was the ideal placebo—it had an interesting color and taste, it had multiple uses (the pharmacopoeia of the time listed about 50 uses for it), it could be given either in drops or in cupfuls, and it was perfectly benign and without pharmacological effects. Maybe he was wrong.

General Conclusions

For the physician seeing a patient with recent-onset insomnia without evident primary medical, psychiatric, or sleep diagnoses (e.g., restless legs, sleep apnea) that would account for it, prescribing a small amount of a shorter-acting hypnotic (zolpidem, temazepam, lorazepam) in the lowest dose size taken every 3 days for up to 4 weeks seems reasonable, assuming the patient has no history of substance abuse.

For short-term relief of insomnia, zolpidem 5–10 mg hs has been generally satisfactory, although it would be hard to prove that it is the best of the available benzodiazepine-like drugs. Zaleplon probably produces a briefer hypnotic effect than zolpidem, and it has not been as well adopted as has zolpidem. Eszopiclone may turn out to be a major addition—effective acutely as well as over extended periods. Patients who awaken too early after taking zolpidem may do better taking temazepam as a longer-acting sedative. However, any of the benzodiazepines may be effective when the right dose for the patient is determined, though flurazepam, quazepam, and possibly clonazepam may have long enough half-lives to cause morning sedation and, perhaps, psychomotor impairment.

For patients with long-standing insomnia who are already accustomed to a nightly hypnotic of the benzodiazepine class, physical dependence probably exists and a slow but purposeful taper of dosage over months, not days or weeks, may be needed. If shifting to a nonbenzodiazepine hypnotic (e.g., trazodone), it would seem sensible to first add the new hypnotic and make sure it improves sleep for at least 2 weeks before beginning to taper the benzodiazepine.

Trazodone 25–50 mg hs, mirtazapine 7.5–15 mg hs, amitriptyline 10–50 mg hs, or gabapentin 100–500 mg hs may do as well as a benzodiazepine and can be taken nightly with little concern about physical dependence; but because these are "off-label" (non–FDA-approved) uses, written justification for their use should be made in the medical record. Likewise, sedating second-generation antipsychotics such as quetiapine at doses of 25–100 mg may benefit some patients with insomnia, including those with depression or anxiety. However, the side effects and dangers of medications like amitriptyline or quetiapine may outweigh the advantages for many patients. Over-the-counter Benadryl (diphenhydramine), at two 25-mg capsules, may be almost as effective. The rare occurrence of priapism with trazodone deserves mention to male patients, with a warning to seek emergency room help if an erection persists beyond 4 hours (Thompson et al. 1999).

All the above except the benzodiazepine-like drugs could be used in patients with a history of substance abuse problems, although such patients can sometimes escalate the dose of any drug rapidly and unwisely. In very unstable, impulsive individuals, gabapentin or trazodone are probably safest. On the other hand, if an alcoholic individual in prolonged remission comes to a physician's office with either a credible history of intractable, severe, untreated insomnia or a history of safe, cautious, appropriate use of a hypnotic like clonazepam for months or years, continuing or starting a benzodiazepine-like hypnotic with careful monitoring is probably safe.

For patients with long-term insomnia being treated with hypnotics and without diagnosable sleep problems that require treatment with nonhypnotics, having the patient continue to take the hypnotic while evaluating and treating any concurrent Axis I psychiatric disorders is sensible. Once the patient's condition and the patient-physician relationship are stable, alternatives can be considered. These include shifting to nonbenzodiazepine sleep-inducing drugs, tapering the original hypnotic very slowly, referring the patient to a sleep program for more specialized diagnosis and possible behavioral or other nonsedative treatments, or making and documenting a conscious, responsible treatment plan in which the patient continues to take a stable benzodiazepine dose for a defined period, say a year, for sensible reasons (e.g., waiting for a divorce to become final, finishing a major job, recovering fully from a manic episode).

At the other extreme, one sees patients with a desperate, frantic need for a full night's sleep who have been taking large doses of several drugs (e.g., temazepam 90 mg plus trazodone 200 mg plus gabapentin 600 mg per night) with little benefit. In our experience such patients need to be referred to a sleep program. If the program fails or a program is unavailable, they need to be told that hypnotic medications are not the answer, that even 90 mg of temazepam either will not work or will harm them, and that they need to have their bedtime medications gradually but firmly tapered while they engage in psychotherapy and a search is made for other, more treatable conditions.

Bibliography

Backonja M, Beydoun A, Edwards KR, et al: Gabapentin for the symptomatic treatment of painful neuropathy in patients with diabetes mellitus: a randomized controlled trial. JAMA 280:1831–1836, 1998

Bunney WE, Azarnoff DL, Brown BW, et al: Report of the Institute of Medicine Committee on the Efficacy and Safety of Halcion. Arch Gen Psychiatry 56:349–352, 1999

Buysse DJ, Dorsey CM: Current and experimental therapeutics of insomnia, in American College of Neuro-Psychopharmacology: A Fifth Generation of Progress. Edited by Davis JM, Charney D, Coyle J, et al. Philadelphia, PA, Lippincott Williams & Wilkins, 2002, pp 1931–1943

Chouinard G, Beauclair L, Belanger M: Gabapentin: long-term antianxiety and hypnotic effects in psychiatric patients with comorbid anxiety-related disorders (letter). Can J Psychiatry 43:305, 1998

Cora-Locatelli G, Greenberg BD, Martin JD, et al: Rebound psychiatric and physical symptoms after gabapentin discontinuation (letter). J Clin Psychiatry 59:131, 1998

Dement W, Seidel W, Carskadon M, et al: Changes in daytime sleepiness/alertness with nighttime benzodiazepines, in Pharmacology of Benzodiazepines. Edited by Usdin E, Skolnick P, Tallman JF, et al. New York, Macmillan, 1982, pp 219–228

Earley CJ, Allen RP: Pergolide and carbidopa/levodopa treatment of restless legs syndrome and periodic leg movements in sleep in a consecutive series of patients. Sleep 19:801–810, 1996

Edinger JD, Means MK: Cognitive-behavioral therapy for primary insomnia. Clin Psychol Rev 25:539–558, 2005

Ehrenberg BL, Eisensher I, Corbett KE, et al: Valproate for sleep consolidation in periodic limb movement disorder. J Clin Psychopharmacol 20:574–578, 2000

Elie R, Ruther E, Farr I, et al: Sleep latency is shortened during 4 weeks of treatment with zaleplon, a novel nonbenzodiazepine hypnotic. J Clin Psychiatry 60:536–544, 1999

Erman M, Seiden D, Zammit G, et al: An efficacy, safety, and dose-response study of ramelteon in patients with chronic primary insomnia. Sleep Med 7:17–24, 2006

Falco M: Methaqualone misuse: foreign experience and US drug control policy. Int J Addict 11:597–610, 1976

Garfinkel D, Laudon M, Nof D, et al: Improvement in sleep quality in elderly people by controlled-release melatonin. Lancet 346:541–544, 1995

Gelenberg A (ed): Zaleplon: a new nonbenzodiazepine hypnotic. Biological Therapies in Psychiatry 23:5–6, 2000

Gillin JC, Byerley WF: Drug therapy: the diagnosis and management of insomnia. N Engl J Med 322:239–248, 1990

Gillin JC, Reynolds CF, Shipley JE: Sleep studies in selected adult neuropsychiatric disorders, in Psychiatry Update: American Psychiatric Association Annual Review, Vol 4. Edited by Hales RE, Frances AJ. Washington, DC, American Psychiatric Press, 1985, pp 352–360

Greenblatt DJ, Shader RI, Abernethy DR: Current status of benzodiazepines, I. N Engl J Med 309:354–359, 1983a

Greenblatt DJ, Shader RI, Abernethy DR: Current status of benzodiazepines, II. N Engl J Med 309:410–415, 1983b

Gursky JT, Krahn LE: The effects of antidepressants on sleep: a review. Harv Rev Psychiatry 8:298–306, 2000

Hajak G, Muller WE, Wittchen H-U, et al: Abuse and dependence potential for the nonbenzodiazepine hypnotics zolpidem and zopiclone: a review of case reports and epidemiological data. Addiction 98:1371–1378, 2003

Hauri PJ, Sateia MJ: Nonpharmacological treatment of sleep disorders, in Psychiatry Update: American Psychiatric Association Annual Review, Vol 4. Edited by Hales RE, Frances AJ. Washington, DC, American Psychiatric Press, 1985, pp 361–378

Hertzberg MA, Feldman ME, Beckham JC, et al: Trial of trazodone for posttraumatic stress disorder using a multiple baseline group design. J Clin Psychopharmacol 16:294–298, 1996

Hertzman PA, Blevins WL, Mayer J, et al: Association of the eosinophilia-myalgia syndrome with the ingestion of tryptophan. N Engl J Med 322:869–873, 1990

Houghton PJ: The scientific basis for the reputed activity of valerian. J Pharm Pharmacol 51:505–512, 1999

Hughes RJ, Sack RL, Lewy AJ: The role of melatonin and circadian phase in age-related sleep-maintenance insomnia: assessment in a clinical trial of melatonin replacement. Sleep 21:52–68, 1998

Johnson MW, Suess PE, Griffiths RR: Ramelteon: a novel hypnotic lacking abuse liability and sedative adverse effects. Arch Gen Psychiatry 63:1149–1157, 2006

Kales A: Benzodiazepines in the treatment of insomnia, in Pharmacology of Benzodiazepines. Edited by Usdin E, Skolnick P, Tallman JF, et al. New York, Macmillan, 1982, pp 199–217

Kales A: Quazepam: hypnotic efficacy and side effects. Pharmacotherapy 10:1–12, 1990

Karam-Hage M, Brower KJ: Open pilot study of gabapentin versus trazodone to treat insomnia in alcoholic outpatients. Psychiatry Clin Neurosci 57(5):542–544, 2003

Katz MM, Koslow SH, Maas JW, et al: The timing, specificity and clinical prediction of tricyclic drug effects in depression. Psychol Med 17:297–309, 1987

Katz MM, Koslow SH, Maas JW, et al: Identifying the specific clinical actions of amitriptyline: interrelationships of behavior, affect and plasma level in depression. Psychol Med 21:599–611, 1991

Ketter TA, Post RM, Theodore WH: Positive and negative psychiatric effects of antiepileptic drugs in patients with seizure disorders. Neurology 53 (5, suppl 2):S53–S67, 1999

Lasagna L: Over-the-counter hypnotics and chronic insomnia in the elderly. J Clin Psychopharmacol 15:383–386, 1996

McGechan A, Wellington K: Ramelteon. CNS Drugs 19(12):1057–1065 [discussion: 1066–1067], 2005

Melatonin. Med Lett Drugs Ther 37:111–112, 1995

Mendelson WB (ed): Current strategies in the treatment of insomnia. J Clin Psychiatry 53 (12, suppl):1–45, 1992

National Center on Sleep Disorders Research: Insomnia: Assessment and Management in Primary Care (NIH Publ No 98-4088). Washington, DC, National Center on Sleep Disorders Research, 1998

NIH State of the Science Conference Statement on Manifestations and Management of Chronic Insomnia in Adults Statement. J Clin Sleep Med 1:412–421, 2005

Nishino S, Okuro M: Armodafinil for excessive daytime sleepiness. Drugs Today (Barc) 44:395–414, 2008

Rall TW: Hypnotics and sedatives, ethanol, in Goodman and Gilman's The Pharmacologic Basis of Therapeutics, 8th Edition. Edited by Gilman AG, Rall TW, Nies AS, et al. New York, McGraw-Hill, 1993, pp 345–382

Regenstein Q: Specific effects of sedative/hypnotic drugs in the treatment of incapacitating insomnia. Am J Med 83:909–916, 1987

Reiter RJ, Melchiorri D, Sewerynek E, et al: A review of the evidence supporting melatonin's role as an antioxidant. J Pineal Res 18:1–11, 1995

Reynolds CF, Buysse DJ, Kupfer DJ: Disordered sleep: developmental and biopsychosocial perspectives on the diagnosis and treatment of persistent insomnia, in Psychopharmacology: The Fourth Generation of Progress. Edited by Bloom FE, Kupfer DJ. New York, Raven, 1995, pp 1617–1629

Rickels K, Morris RJ, Newman H, et al: Diphenhydramine in insomnia. J Clin Psychiatry 23:235–242, 1983

Rickels K, Ginsberg J, Morris RJ, et al: Doxylamine succinate in insomniac family practice patients: a double-blind study. Current Therapeutic Research 35:532–540, 1984

Roffwarg H, Erman M: Evaluation and diagnosis of the sleep disorders: implications for psychiatry and other clinical specialties, in Psychiatry Update: American Psychiatric Association Annual Review, Vol 4. Edited by Hales RE, Frances AJ. Washington, DC, American Psychiatric Press, 1985, pp 294–328

Roth T, Seiden D, Sainati S, et al: Effects of ramelteon on patient-reported sleep latency in older adults with chronic insomnia. Sleep Med 7(4):312–318, 2006

Rowbotham M, Harden N, Stacey B, et al: Gabapentin for the treatment of postherpetic neuralgia: A randomized controlled trial. JAMA 280:1837–1842, 1998

Rush C, Griffiths R: Zolpidem, triazolam, and temazepam: behavioral and subject-rated effects in normal volunteers. J Clin Psychopharmacol 16:146–157, 1996

Rush CR, Baker RW, Wright K: Acute behavioral effects and abuse potential of trazodone, zolpidem and triazolam in humans. Psychopharmacology (Berl) 144:220–233, 1999

Scharf MB, Mayleben DW, Kaffeman M, et al: Dose response effects of zolpidem in normal geriatric subjects. J Clin Psychiatry 52:77–83, 1991

Schneider-Helmert D: Why low-dose benzodiazepine dependent insomniacs can't escape their sleeping pills. Acta Psychiatr Scand 78:706–711, 1988

Seidel WF, Roth T, Roehrs T, et al: Treatment of a 12-hour shift of sleep schedule with benzodiazepines. Science 224:1262–1264, 1985

Shamir E, Landon M, Barak Y, et al: Melatonin improves sleep quality in patients with chronic schizophrenia. J Clin Psychiatry 61:373–377, 2000

Thompson JW, Ware M, Blashfield R: Psychotropic medications and priapism: a comprehensive review. J Clin Psychiatry 51:430–433, 1999

Victorri-Vigneau C, Dailly E, Veyrac G, et al: Evidence of zolpidem abuse and dependence: results of the French Centre for Evaluation and Information on Pharmacodependence (CEIP) network survey. Br J Clin Pharmacol 64:198–209, 2007

Wang MY, Wang SY, Tsai PS: Cognitive behavioural therapy for primary insomnia: a systematic review. J Adv Nurs 50:553–564, 2005

Wong AH, Smith M, Boon HS: Herbal remedies in psychiatric practice. Arch Gen Psychiatry 55:1033–1044, 1998

Zhdanova IV, Lynch JH, Wurtman RJ: Melatonin: a sleep-promoting hormone. Sleep 20:899–907, 1997

8

Stimulants and Other Fast-Acting Drugs

Like all other drug classifications in clinical psychopharmacology, the term *stimulants* covers a range of drugs, with some overlapping actions, that may be useful in treating some disorders, syndromes, or symptoms (Table 8–1). Here, as elsewhere, we lack a tidy one-to-one correlation of drug efficacy and syndrome.

The concept of stimulants began early with caffeine and then, in 1887, with synthesis of amphetamine in Germany. However, amphetamine was a drug without an indication and largely forgotten until the 1930s. Another stimulant, phedrine, was extracted from a Chinese herbal remedy in the 1930s. Ephedrine was known to cause euphoria, sympathetic activation, and alertness. Ephedrine was used in treating asthma and has never been tested for efficacy in attention-deficit/hyperactivity disorder (ADHD), obesity, or, to our knowledge, narcolepsy. From ephedrine, K. K. Chen synthesized a variant, amphetamine (Benzedrine), which was, within 10 years, separated into its two stereoisomers, D-amphetamine (Dexedrine) and L-amphetamine. The dextro isomer was much more potent and is almost the only one used clinically today.

Table 8–1.   Stimulants: names, formulations, and strengths

Generic name	Brand name	Formulations and strengths
D-amphetamine[a]	Dexedrine	Tablets: 5, 10 mg
	Dexedrine Spansule	Spansules: 5, 10, 15 mg
amphetamine/ dextroamphetamine[b]	Adderall Adderall XR	Tablets: 5, 7.5, 10, 12.5, 15, 20, 30 mg Capsules: 5, 10, 15, 20, 25, 30 mg
D-methamphetamine	Desoxyn	Tablet: 5 mg
methylphenidate[a]	Ritalin	Tablets: 5, 10, 20 mg
	Methylin	Tablets, chewable: 2.5, 5, 10 mg Oral solution: 5 mg/5 mL, 10 mg/5 mL (500 mL)
	Methylin ER	Tablets: 10, 20 mg
	Ritalin SR	Tablet: 20 mg
	Ritalin LA	Capsules: 10, 20, 30, 40 mg
	Metadate ER	Tablets: 10, 20 mg
	Metadate CD	Capsules: 10, 20, 30, 40, 50, 60 mg
	Concerta	Tablets: 18, 27, 36, 54 mg
	Daytrana	Transdermal patch: 10, 15, 20, 30 mg/ 9 hours[c]
dexmethylphenidate[b]	Focalin	Tablets: 2.5, 5, 10 mg
	Focalin XR	Capsules: 5, 10, 15, 20 mg
lisdexamfetamine	Vyvanse	Capsules: 30, 40, 50, 60, 70 mg
modafinil	Provigil	Tablets: 100, 200 mg
armodafinil	Nuvigil	Tablets: 50, 150, 250 mg
guanfacine	Intuniv	Tablets: 1, 2, 3, 4 mg

[a]Available in generic form.
[b]Available in generic except the extended-release form.
[c]Delivery rate of 1.1, 1.6, 2.2, and 3.3 mg/hour for the 10-, 15-, 20-, and 30-mg patches, respectively. In vivo delivery rate is based on a wear period of 9 hours of pediatric patients ages 6–12 years.

It turned out to be effective in focusing attention and/or decreasing maladaptive behaviors in children who would now be diagnosed as having ADHD; in reducing sleepiness (i.e., in narcolepsy); and in reducing fatigue-induced decrements in behavior. It decreases appetite and has been widely used as an antiobesity medication. For some years, D-amphetamine was sold as a cold remedy, in an inhaler, to shrink swollen nasal membranes when inhaled. It was also used in treating depression and related fatigue states, until the widespread abuse of its analog D-methamphetamine (speed) by self-injection in the 1960s led to legislation scheduling most stimulants into Drug Enforcement Agency (DEA) Schedule II along with morphine and the potent opiates. This decision was made despite the fact that almost all illicit methamphetamine was made illegally and not diverted from drug companies, pharmacies, or doctors.

As a result of the legislative scheduling, the use of stimulants in medicine decreased sharply, and their use was sanctioned only for ADHD, narcolepsy, and obesity. Methylphenidate (Ritalin) was marketed just before the law changed and has become much more widely used than D-amphetamine for ADHD. In the last few years, Adderall, an "old" drug because it was effective in treating obesity when all old drugs were assessed in the early 1960s, was more recently resurrected as a treatment for ADHD (Horrigan and Barnhill 2000). Adderall contains three different salts of D-amphetamine and one of L-amphetamine. So far, no studies are available comparing Adderall with either D-amphetamine or methylphenidate in treating ADHD, but it seems likely to be about as active as the total of its D-amphetamine salts in any of the situations in which D-amphetamine is useful. Adderall is available in tablets of various strengths (see Table 8–1); its potency is probably slightly less than the same dose of D-amphetamine, but its duration of action may be longer. It had taken over a 33% market share by 2001 (Rosack 2001). A long-acting form of Adderall, Adderall XR, lasts as long as 10 hours and is given at a dosage of 10–30 mg/day, with the dose taken in the morning.

D-Methamphetamine is still available in immediate-release form by prescription as Desoxyn. Its sustained-release form was believed by Wender to be superior in duration of action to either the current Ritalin SR (available in a 20-mg dose) or the current Dexedrine Spansule. The last two have a reputation for discharging their main dose of stimulant in the first hour or two and may not have the prolonged effect their makers intended. Unfortunately, Abbott Laboratories stopped distributing long-acting Desoxyn, so its possible benefits are irrelevant. (As of this writing, an immediate-release form is still manufactured by Lundbeck, Inc.) Alternatively, it is possible that the brain responds only to rising stimulant levels and that a prolonged, even elevation of blood level over hours might lead to rapid loss of all behavioral effect. Newer and better long-acting forms of methylphenidate and amphetamine are now available. One of these, Concerta, a long-acting methylphenidate formulation that lasts 12 hours, was released in July 2000 and is available in strengths of 18, 27, 36, and 54 mg. It appears to be truly long-acting.

A number of new stimulant dosing options have become available in the past few years, and relevant studies of these agents were discussed by Dr. Lawrence Greenhill at the 2001 American Academy of Child and Adolescent Psychiatry meeting as reported in *Psychiatric News* (Rosack 2001). Methylphenidate is available in its old, familiar immediate-release form, racemic *dl*-methylphenidate, with its effectiveness for ADHD symptoms lasting 3–4 hours, and *l*-methylphenidate–sustained release (Ritalin SR), which has been available for several years and is believed to be weaker, both in onset of action and possibly in duration of action, than immediate-release Ritalin. Novartis, manufacturer of Ritalin and Ritalin SR, has developed Ritalin LA (long acting), designed to release half of each dosage unit quickly and the other half slowly. However, Novartis also has obtained pure *d*-methylphenidate (Focalin), which is twice as potent as racemic Ritalin—2.5 mg of Focalin equals 5 mg of *d,l*-methylphenidate. The *d* isomer even appears to be slightly—but statistically—more effective than twice the dose of *d,l*-methylphenidate.

To add options and perhaps confusion to the field, Celltech Pharmaceuticals brought out a long-acting methylphenidate (Metadate CD), which produces about 8 hours of effect, compared with Concerta's 12 hours of action. Both seem "better" in duration of action than Ritalin SR and, presumably, Focalin. Further, another company has developed a transdermal methylphenidate patch (Daytrana), which has recently become available.

Adderall XR also releases half its dosage of mixed amphetamine metabolites rapidly and the other half slowly, both from little coated beads like those in a Dexedrine Spansule. These beads can be taken out of the capsule and sprinkled on applesauce and swallowed (but *not* chewed).

Lisdexamfetamine (Vyvanse) represents another approach: once-a-day dosing. Lisdexamfetamine is essentially a pro-drug that is metabolized to dextroamphetamine. It has been studied primarily in 6- to 12-year-olds with ADHD, and doses of 30–70 mg taken in the morning appear to be effective throughout the day.

All these long-acting preparations cannot be smashed up without losing their prolonged action. Concerta tablets, or their residua, can sometimes be seen in the taker's feces.

The original idea behind all this ingenuity was to avoid the midday pill that may embarass schoolchildren or complicate the lives of school nurses or that could be diverted to others. Also, some youngsters with ADHD need continued medication effect to be able to do homework or other evening activities well. These various forms allow the prescribing physician to adjust the drug formulation to the needs and side effects of individual patients. If a patient has loss of appetite for supper and insomnia, he or she may not need a 12-hour stimulant like Concerta.

One approach to all this is to determine the bid or tid dose of *dl*-methylphenidate or D-amphetamine and then replace these multiple doses with the appropriate longer-acting formulation.

Adderall was already believed to have a 5-hour duration of action in ADHD, and Adderall XR should stretch this to possibly 10 hours.

Not all stimulants work in an identical way. Methylphenidate, D-amphetamine, and cocaine all increase release of dopamine into the postsynaptic cleft. D-Amphetamine affects presynaptic receptors as well, whereas methylphenidate does not. Pemoline (Cylert), which resembles methylphenidate in its mechanism of action, was longer acting than D-amphetamine or methylphenidate and was only in Schedule IV. However, it caused rare but lethal liver toxicity (see below), which made it undesirable as a first-line drug, and has since been taken off the market.

Clinicians have had experience with D-amphetamine, methylphenidate, pemoline, and several anorexiant drugs like phentermine for many years. It is clear that occasional patients will do very well while taking one of these drugs but fail to respond to any of the others for no apparent reason. The use of stimulants in psychiatric practice has been reviewed extensively elsewhere (Chiarello and Cole 1987; Klein and Wender 1995; Satel and Nelson 1989; Wilens et al. 1995). It should also be noted that in hospital pharmacies, stimulants have been made into suppositories for rectal administration to patients unable to swallow pills.

Fenfluramine (Pondimin), which in 1997 was available for use in decreasing appetite, was presumed to exert its effects through a serotonergic mechanism, but it was not a stimulant. In 1987 *d*-fenfluramine, one of its isomers, was introduced in the United States after having been available in Europe for some time and was widely used alone or in combination with phentermine (Ionamin) as "fen-phen" in obesity programs. *d*-Fenfluramine was associated with heart valve damage and occasionally with fatal pulmonary hypertension and was withdrawn from the U.S. market.

At about the same time, sibutramine (Meridia) was introduced for the treatment of mild to moderate obesity. It was free of any evidence of abuse liability in premarketing studies but was placed in Schedule IV anyway by the Food and Drug Administration (FDA) because other drugs approved for the treatment of obesity were of abuse potential. Sibutramine started life as a potential antidepressant; it blocks reuptake of norepinephrine, serotonin, and dopamine. However, in its first two clinical trials in depression, the weight loss of the patients seemed even more impressive than the effects on depression. Hence, we have an appetite-suppressing drug that is not particularly stimulant-like in other respects.

Late in 1998 modafinil (Provigil) was marketed for the treatment of daytime sleepiness related to narcolepsy. This drug had been in use in France for several years and had not been noted to be abused. It was reported to "feel" like a stimulant in some human abuse liability trials but has slower onset of action and longer duration of action than D-amphetamine. Further, it appears to have no observable effect on any receptor or any biogenic amine in the brain. Radioactive modafinil concentrates in the hypothalamus, whereas conventional stimulants do not. So we have yet another "stimulant" that is not conventional. A number of studies have suggested that modafinil may help lessen the fatigue and sleepiness associated with a variety of conditions, such as shift work and obstructive sleep apnea. In addition, preliminary work also suggests that modafinil may be effective in the treatment of ADHD. Studies by our group and others suggest that a dosage of 100–200 mg/day of modafinil added to a selective serotonin reuptake inhibitor (SSRI) helps with fatigue and hypersomnia associated with depression.

The R enantiomer of modafinil, armodafinil, was approved in 2008 for the same indications as modafinil. Armodafinil has a somewhat longer half-life than does modafinil and may have a slightly different side-effect profile. Armodafinil is being explored in the treatment of a number of conditions beyond sleep disorders, including fatigue associated with cancer and bipolar depression.

The current dilemma is that ADHD and narcolepsy (and depression when it responds) may require amphetamines as maintenance therapy for years or at least months, so that the DEA Schedule II restriction that each prescription must be rewritten each month becomes a burden on both the doctor and the patient.

As can be seen, this chapter on stimulant drugs covers drugs used for the core indications of the older stimulants—ADHD, narcolepsy, and obesity—whether or not they have obvious stimulant effects in man or animals. Monoamine oxidase inhibitors (MAOIs) could be included here, but drugs whose major use is in treating depression are considered in Chapter 3 ("Antidepressants") instead.

Amphetamine Abuse

D-Amphetamine and methylphenidate, but not magnesium pemoline or modafinil, are spontaneously self-administered intravenously by laboratory animals and are well known to have abuse liability in humans. An unpublished study by the second author showed pemoline, in single doses of 75 mg and 150 mg, to have no euphoriant effects in casual recreational users. Sibutramine is also without euphoriant effects (Cole et al. 1998).

One of the most abused stimulants to date is methamphetamine. This drug was used intravenously in very high doses during the flower-child period of the 1960s, resulting in some individuals, known as "speed freaks," becoming heavily dependent. Such individuals usually took the medication in relatively large doses in runs of a few days and then withdrew from the drug for a day or two, experiencing a crash, before starting again. Patterns of oral abuse were less intense and dramatic (Grinspoon and Hedblom 1975).

Methamphetamine abuse has reemerged in recent years. The original formulation, known as "speed," was the hydrochloride. Crystalline methamphetamine base, known as "ice," has been widely abused in Hawaii and California. It is chiefly smoked but is also used intravenously, the preferred route during the 1960s. When smoked, it appears to give a rush (immediate pleasurable feeling) similar to that of cocaine but with a longer duration of the euphoric state. This effect fits with the known relative pharmacokinetics: methamphetamine is metabolized more slowly than cocaine. In monkeys, cocaine is more abusable intravenously than is methamphetamine; monkeys will work harder and longer to get cocaine and will continue self-administration for days without stopping, until death occurs. In contrast, amphetamines are less reinforcing. It is too early to tell whether smoked ice will be more or less of a problem than cocaine. Cho (1990) reviewed the pharmacology of ice, but no studies and almost no other published reports on ice are available.

There is reasonable evidence that very high doses of D-amphetamine, generally higher than 80 mg/day and sometimes as high as 1,000–2,000 mg/day, can produce an acute psychosis that generally resembles paranoid schizophrenia but can occasionally present with delirium and other conventional signs of toxic drug psychosis. This condition is sometimes considered a model for schizophrenia, or at least for acute paranoid psychosis. In addition, parenteral administration of methylphenidate has been used as a test to predict risk of psychotic relapse in patients with schizophrenia. These studies stirred ethical concerns and have largely been discontinued.

Magnesium pemoline was a little different from the other two drugs, having had a somewhat slower onset and offset of action, and for a while was preferred in treating occasional patients who get symptom relief for 3–4 hours from a single dose of methylphenidate or D-amphetamine but who experienced an abrupt change in status as the drug wore off. For such patients, magnesium pemoline may have been smoother and better tolerated. Unfortunately, the risk of serious liver damage with magnesium pemoline use in both children and adults was increasingly judged to be more serious (Young and Findling 1998), and the drug was eventually taken off the market.

Although modafinil is a Schedule IV drug, no evidence of an abuse potential has occurred in postmarketing surveys since 1998. Since modafinil, unlike amphetamine, does not affect the dopaminergic systems that mediate reward in the cortex, there is no physiological basis for abuse or dependence. Rapid discontinuation of the drug has not been associated with withdrawal symptoms.

Uses of Stimulants

Attention-Deficit/Hyperactivity Disorder

ADHD is the only condition other than narcolepsy and weight reduction for which stimulants are currently approved by the FDA. In children, the syndrome is manifested by very short attention span, overactivity, irritability, poor social relations, impulsivity, occasional angry or assaultive behavior, poor school performance, and apparent inability to benefit from instruction or limit setting. Some children with the syndrome have a parent with a history or current symptoms of a similar condition. Occasional children with the syndrome have clear evidence of central nervous system (CNS) damage at birth or subsequently; the majority of such patients, however, do not have "hard" neurological signs of clearly diagnosable brain injury or abnormality.

In children with ADHD, any of the three drugs is likely to be clinically better than placebo in about 70%–80% of those treated; about 30% show a clear and highly impressive degree of clinical improvement, and another 40% show some modulation of behavior that may be of some clinical importance. Occasionally, children are made more active by these drugs. In the first weeks of treatment, children often look drawn and even somewhat depressed and rarely show any euphoriant effect from the medication. It is not clear that the drugs dramatically reduce activity level. They probably act by improving attention span and organizing behavior more effectively. Some degree of growth inhibition or weight loss has been reported occasionally in children, but these are generally not major problems. (See Chapter 12: "Pharmacotherapy in Special Situations" for further discussion of the use of stimulants in children.)

Huessey (1979), at the University of Vermont; Ratey et al. (1994) and Spencer et al. (1995) in Boston; and Wender et al. (1985) at the University of Utah identified adults with symptoms resembling those seen in children with ADHD and showed that such adults respond to stimulant therapy. These drug responders are very likely to be remembered as hyperkinetic children by their parents. Some individuals who have had clear clinical benefit from stimulants in childhood continue to require and to benefit from stimulant medication well into adult life. Many children with ADHD, however, seem to grow out of the major manifestations of the illness at some time in adolescence, although they are often left with residual symptoms of impaired concentration or coping ability, which may or may not be benefited by further stimulant administration. This issue is well discussed by Klein and Wender (1995). Further, Ward et al. (1993) developed a useful self-report form for use by adult patients suspected of having had ADHD behaviors in childhood.

The interesting and clinically useful aspect of stimulant therapy in treating either children or adults with ADHD is that clinical effects are often clear and dramatic within a day or two of reaching the appropriate dosage. Stimulant therapy, with this rapid clinical response, stands in dramatic contrast to the more conventional antidepressants and antipsychotics, which often take days or even weeks to achieve a satisfactory clinical result.

In clinical practice, adults with personality disorder, short attention span, restlessness, hyperactivity, irritability, impulsivity, and related symptoms sometimes present with a history of illicit drug abuse. In treating such individuals, a trial of a stimulant raises an ethical problem: when it is clear that any stimulant will be abused, the drug cannot be used. Stimulants might be used in patients with a history of drug abuse under the following circumstances:

1. The stimulant drug has clearly been used to improve functioning rather than to get high (produce euphoria).
2. A good therapeutic alliance is available.
3. The medication can be closely monitored, perhaps in an inpatient setting.
4. Other approaches have failed.
5. The patient's problems are seriously interfering with his or her life functioning.

Some children and adults with ADHD respond to bupropion, a serotonin-norepinephrine reuptake inhibitor, atomoxetine, or desipramine, which can be used with patients who might abuse a stimulant. Clonidine may also be an alternative for patients who cannot use stimulants. Emerging data suggest that the nonstimulant modafinil also may be useful in the treatment of ADHD.

The utility of stimulant therapy in treating substance abusers with a clear history of ADHD, including individuals addicted to cocaine (Schubiner et al. 1995), has been documented in open trials, as has the lack of utility of stimulant therapy in treating cocaine users without ADHD during the early post–cocaine withdrawal period; methylphenidate facilitates return to cocaine use in such patients. There is now a smattering of studies of the use of various antidepressants (desipramine, phenelzine, bupropion, SSRIs, selegiline, and venlafaxine) in treating patients with ADHD, both childhood and adult varieties. Desipramine and bupropion are the best-documented drugs for this purpose. Most controlled studies have been positive. Some clinicians believe that, in children at least, desipramine tends to lose its effectiveness over time. With all these drugs, it is best to start with low dosages (e.g., 10 mg/day of desipramine, 75 mg/day of bupropion sustained-release [SR] formulation) on the presumption that some ADHD patients will be likely to respond to low doses and show undesirable side effects at higher dosages.

The issue of the existence of ADHD (or attention-deficit disorder without hyperactivity) in adults has received more attention in the last few years.

Ratey et al. (1994), in a clinical report, described patients with these conditions and their responses to various medications, and Spencer et al. (1995) reported positive results in a placebo-controlled trial of methylphenidate in treating adult ADHD patients at Massachusetts General Hospital. The superior effectiveness of stimulants, compared with psychosocial treatment, for childhood ADHD received strong support from a federally sponsored multicenter study (Jensen et al. 2001). Further, the breadth of stimulant effect in conduct disorder in children was strongly supported by the results of a study by Klein et al. (1997).

Depression

In the early literature on the use of amphetamines in psychiatry, there were a number of case reports of individuals presenting with the full syndrome of endogenous depression who responded dramatically to racemic amphetamine. A few double-blind trials completed since the early 1970s showed some evidence of clinical efficacy of stimulants in depressed outpatients. Findings from some studies were only weakly positive, and most others were clearly negative (Satel and Nelson 1987). The use of stimulants as adjunctive agents in depression is suggested by a number of uncontrolled studies.

Given the lack of data, it is probably not reasonable to use stimulant monotherapy in the early treatment of MDD. However, in patients with a chronic treatment-resistant depression who have failed to respond to a range of standard antidepressants, stimulants occasionally provide excellent symptomatic relief and often enable patients to function adequately for prolonged periods without side effects or any indication that the drug is being abused or misused. Some of these patients have clear-cut vegetative symptoms, others appear to have atypical depressions, and still others have major symptoms of fatigue or executive dysfunction. As it has become increasingly clear that antidepressants often do an unsatisfactory job of treating cognitive symptoms and fatigue, stimulants are being reevaluated to target those symptoms specifically.

It is not possible to tell in advance which depressed patients will benefit from stimulant therapy. Rickels et al. (1970) suggested some time ago that relatively heavy intake of coffee (four cups a day or more) was a predictor of good clinical response, at least to magnesium pemoline. In contrast, patients who are intolerant of caffeine sometimes cannot tolerate stimulants.

However, experience at McLean Hospital, in an informal study involving 30 patients who had done well while taking prescribed stimulants for more than 2 years, suggests that some depressed patients with excellent response to stimulants dislike or avoid caffeine-containing beverages. Only three of the patients in the study had histories suggestive of childhood ADHD, but many had a significant "thought disorder" (i.e., difficulty in organizing their thoughts and in functioning effectively at work or school). Almost all had significant depression, and several had bulimia. All but three had had persistent benefit from stimulants for a period ranging from 2 to 30 years.

The cases of the three patients with poor outcomes can be summarized as follows: one took stimulants at very high doses for 20 years, initially to lose weight, but instead he gained weight massively, finally requiring a gut bypass operation. His career was probably adversely affected, and a family disaster, with resulting major depression, led to his referral to McLean from another state. One professional with clear ADHD symptoms from childhood who succeeded academically without stimulant therapy ended up taking methylphenidate 80–120 mg/day, which, paradoxically, caused fatigue and inability to function professionally. The third, after having had a favorable response for a decade, began to experience marital stress and developed paranoid hypomania alternating with depression. Each retrial of a stimulant to relieve her chronic depression led to hospitalization, with the patient in a paranoid excitement.

The poor outcomes in these three cases must be balanced against the substantial symptom relief and improved role functioning in all the other patients seen in consultation. Many were followed for up to 15 years with continuing benefit (Cole et al. 1993).

Stimulants also have a place in the crisis management of individuals whose functioning is impaired by depression and whose life situation would deteriorate rapidly if they were not able to resume functioning within a few days. In such situations, a trial of modafinil, methylphenidate, D-amphetamine, or Adderall is worth initiating to attempt to get a patient through a crisis when failure to function might result in getting fired from a job or flunking out of college. In such situations, weaker semistimulants such as bupropion are unlikely to work rapidly enough to be useful. Modafinil, with a favorable side-effect profile, would seem like a good choice for many patients. However, it is not approved for any psychiatric indication as of this writing, and insurance companies are hesitant to pay for it. For now, D-amphetamine in its generic form costs less and is a bit more likely to be effective than methylphenidate. One might begin with D-amphetamine 5 mg in the morning and increase the dosage by 5 mg every morning until the patient either feels better or feels unpleasantly stimulated. The patient should check in daily during this process. If the morning dose helps, a second, equal dose 4–6 hours later should be added. If the D-amphetamine has an unpleasant effect, it should be stopped and methylphenidate 10 mg (5 mg in elderly or hypertensive patients) should be tried instead. Adderall, the mixture of amphetamine salts, at an initial dose of 10 mg can also be tried. Dosages up to 20 or 30 mg/day of D-amphetamine or twice that amount of methylphenidate also can be used to see whether a response occurs.

The major problem in recommending stimulant therapy to other psychiatrists for a specific patient is the likelihood that the patient will be left taking an ineffective dosage (e.g., initial dose 5–10 mg once or twice a day) for a couple of weeks, until the drug is stopped for lack of efficacy. Using a stimulant in adult psychiatric patients requires close—almost daily—monitoring, at least by telephone, so that the treating psychiatrist can determine whether the drug at the dosage given had any effect. In the absence of any effect, positive or negative, the dosage should be steadily increased until something happens—up to 40 mg/day of D-amphetamine or 80 mg/day of methylphenidate. This dosing method is infrequently used, perhaps because of fear of the abuse potential of the drug (uncommon in psychiatric patients) or because psychiatrists are so accustomed to using drugs that take 7–30 days to act that they do not change their prescribing behavior when using unfamiliar but rapid-acting drugs like D-amphetamine.

Some patients show an initial excellent response to a stimulant medication and then develop rapid tolerance and all effect is lost, whereas others continue to benefit from the same low dose of the stimulant for months or even years. Still other patients feel anxious, agitated, and unpleasantly "wired" while taking some or all stimulants. If the drug is to be stopped, it can be either tapered or stopped abruptly. Some rebound depression may occur (see Chapter 11: "Pharmacotherapy for Substance Use Disorders"). Patients with a history of pronounced mood disturbances may require hospitalization.

D-Amphetamine is available in 5-mg, 10-mg, and 15-mg Spansule (slow-release) formulations. Methamphetamine (Desoxyn) is available in a 5-mg tablet. Adderall is available in 5-mg, 7.5-mg, 10-mg, 12.5-mg, 15-mg, 20-mg, and 30-mg tablets, about equivalent in efficacy to that dose of dextroamphet-amine. Methylphenidate is available in a 20-mg SR formulation. Better, really longer-acting preparations of several stimulants have recently been marketed or are now under development (see discussion earlier in chapter). One of these, Concerta, is available in 18-mg, 27-mg, 36-mg, and 54-mg 12-hour SR tablets. Several years ago, the increasingly common use of methylphenidate was a concern to many in the community, and there has been considerable debate as to whether it is being overused. The debate has subsided in the past few years.

Some depressed patients prefer taking ordinary tablets of D-amphetamine or methylphenidate and may take the entire daily dose at once on arising, even if 30–60 mg/day is being given. Such patients feel no rush or high but are relieved of depression for at least 24 hours. Others take single fast-release tablets several times a day, taking another as the effect of the first dose wears off. Some dislike this on-off effect and prefer to use SR preparations.

After decades in which only single-dosage forms of D-amphetamine and methylphenidate were available, there are now several forms of methylpheni-date with different lengths and forms of sustained release. Several appear de-signed to avoid the necessity for the child with ADHD to take a second dose of stimulant around noon, which entails involving the school and making the child's "problem" obvious to teachers or classmates. The most recent variant, the "patch," bypasses the oral route and uses a "bandaid"-like approach. It is too early to tell if this or other available formulations are better or worse than other established formulations. We suggest that ordinary immediate-release pills be used initially and that the dose and the formulation be adjusted to im-prove drug response (e.g., ability to study after school) or avoid side effects (i.e., anorexia or initial insomnia).

Phenylpropanolamine was marketed as an over-the-counter antiobesity pill in 37.5-mg and 75-mg strengths, usually in a SR preparation. We have seen occasional patients with either depression or ADHD who had found phenylpropanolamine helpful in the way a standard stimulant sometimes is. However, most patients and most recreational users of drugs find the subjec-tive effects of pseudoephedrine or phenylpropanolamine mildly unpleasant. When phenylpropanolamine was abused in "triple-threat" illicit pills containing ephedrine and caffeine as well, it is likely that the ephedrine or the combination accounted for the pills' amphetamine-like properties. Phenylpropanolamine alone may reduce appetite and increase pulse and blood pressure a little, but it is not a useful stimulant. It should be noted that the drug marketed in Europe as phenylpropanolamine is a different stereoisomer and probably has amphetamine-like stimulant effects.

In November 2000, the FDA issued a public health advisory concerning phenylpropanolamine in over-the-counter and prescription drug products. There was growing evidence that phenylpropanolamine increases the risk of hemorrhagic stroke in women and, perhaps, in men (though the risk appears to be lower in men). The advisory committee recommended that drug companies discontinue marketing drug products containing phenylpropanolamine. Then in December 2005, the FDA stated their position in a bulletin: "The Food and Drug Administration (FDA) is taking steps to remove phenylpropanolamine . . . from all drug products and request that all drug companies discontinue drug products containing phenylpropanolamine." Currently, drug products (OTC or prescription) do not contain phenylpropanolamine (see the FDA's information page on phenylpropanolamine (www.fda.gov/cder/drug/infopage/ppa).

Acquired Immunodeficiency Syndrome

Patients with AIDS often have a mixture of depression, fatigue, and difficulty initiating activities, perhaps a form of akinesia (see Chapter 12: "Pharmacotherapy in Special Situations"). Such patients may have CNS complications of AIDS, including shrinking of the basal ganglia. Standard tricyclic antidepressants (TCAs) may or may not be poorly tolerated, but one fears that they may cause increased memory problems or delirium. Methylphenidate appears to be widely used in treating such patients, with excellent results, though little has been written about this use. Patients can begin taking low dosages (e.g., 5 mg bid), titrated to a level relieving symptoms without causing side effects. The dose may need to be increased gradually as the disease progresses. Local experts in Boston give us the impression that methylphenidate in treating AIDS-related depression, inertia, and confusion resembles L-dopa in treating parkinsonism— a replacement therapy needed because of changes in the brain. This idea is, of course, purely speculative.

Other stimulants have not, to our knowledge, been tried in AIDS patients, but there is no obvious reason why D-amphetamine, D-methamphetamine, or Adderall should not be tried. Some children with ADHD do better on one than on another, and stimulant-responsive depressed patients often have clearly better responses to one of these drugs than to the others, for no known reason. Appetite suppressants, such as phenmetrazine, phentermine, and Biphetamine, sometimes work as antidepressants in individual patients. Sibutramine, an appetite suppressant at dosages of 5–15 mg/day, was originally developed to be an antidepressant; it would not be surprising if it also was useful in treating "ordinary" depression as well as anhedonia in patients with AIDS. There is, however, some evidence that standard antidepressants, both TCAs and SSRIs, are useful in treating depressive disorders in patients testing positive for HIV, with or without overt AIDS, and are well tolerated (Markowitz et al. 1994).

Stimulants may have unique abilities to improve energy or cognitive functioning of AIDS patients, but all studies in this important area are uncontrolled and the findings are relatively impressionistic (Angrist et al. 1992).

Other Medical Conditions

A growing series of case reports has documented the usefulness of stimulants in treating patients on the medical wards of general hospitals. These patients have various combinations of debilitating depression and fatigue that make them unable to cooperate in necessary treatments, and they lose weight rapidly. In this situation, standard antidepressants simply do not have a fast enough onset of action. Stimulants do, probably about 50% of the time, have a fast enough onset of effects. For this indication, therefore, they are being used more commonly and appear to be safe (Wallace et al. 1995).

Drug Combinations

Methylphenidate and D-amphetamine both interact with imipramine in laboratory animals to potentiate response to electrical stimulation of pleasure centers. Part of this potentiation is pharmacokinetic, in the sense that the stimulant and the TCA interfere with each other's metabolism, causing higher blood levels of each. This property was sometimes used clinically, when methylphenidate was prescribed early in TCA therapy to hasten response. If a patient improved with methylphenidate plus imipramine, it was impossible to know whether the clinical response was due to 1) the methylphenidate alone, 2) a longer period taking imipramine, 3) the elevation of imipramine blood level caused by methylphenidate, or 4) a true combined effect of the two drugs. Generally, we do not recommend this combination approach (see Chapter 9: "Augmentation Strategies in Treatment-Resistant Disorders"). Stimulants have been used to counteract anergia secondary to SSRI therapy in depression. Here, the plasma levels of the SSRI may be increased.

Intuitively, it should be considered clinically dangerous to combine a stimulant with an MAOI, because the addition of a stimulant might precipitate a hypertensive crisis. However, we know of a few patients who have, on their own responsibility, added magnesium pemoline, methylphenidate, or D-amphetamine to reverse MAOI-induced sedation or lack of clinical response, with alleged good subjective effects and no apparent effect on blood pressure. Other such patients have been described in the literature. We have seen hypertensive crises when phenylpropanolamine or pseudoephedrine was added to an MAOI, but so far we have not encountered any such crises with stimulant-MAOI combinations. Stimulant-MAOI combinations are not recommended in general practice; however, the combination has been used cautiously to counteract MAOI-induced hypotension (see Chapter 3: "Antidepressants") and, by us, to reverse MAOI-induced daytime sedation, so far without adverse effects.

Psychosis

The older literature, from the 1930s and 1940s, on the use of racemic amphetamine, D-amphetamine, and methylphenidate in treating patients with what was then called chronic schizophrenia reported mixed results: some patients improved on a stimulant given alone, some showed no change, and some worsened. However, more recent studies of single doses of intravenous methylphenidate showed that this drug increases psychosis in drug-free acutely ill patients with mania or schizophrenia but has only a mild stimulant effect when such patients are in remission. Studies by Angrist et al. (1980) and Robinson et al. (1991) demonstrated that chronically ill schizophrenic outpatients who showed increased psychosis after a single dose of a stimulant were much more likely to relapse into a psychotic exacerbation than were patients who showed no worsening on stimulant administration. Other work by Lieberman et al. (1994) also supports the finding that an exacerbation of psychosis to a single dose of methylphenidate may predict higher relapse risk in stable patients whose antipsychotic dose is reduced or discontinued. This type of research has become extremely controversial in recent years because of ethical concerns about worsening patients' conditions.

Another "stimulant," fenfluramine in its racemic form, was used in the past to raise TCA blood levels and to lower blood serotonin in autism. It has been shown to have weak antimanic effects. Unfortunately, the release of its *d*-isomer in the United States for obesity was followed by intensive use in combination with phentermine (so-called fen-phen). A number of patients developed pulmonary hypertension with serious consequences, and both forms of the drug, the earlier *dl* form and *d*-fenfluramine, were withdrawn from clinical use in the United States.

Stimulant Use Versus Abuse

We have occasionally seen patients who had taken prescribed stimulants for years, with claimed excellent relief from depression, fatigue, or disorganized behavior, and had had the drug withdrawn by a physician concerned about drug abuse. Such patients then often failed to respond to a variety of more conventional TCAs and were dysphoric and unable to function adequately for years. When the stimulant was represcribed, these patients often did quite well again for prolonged periods. It may be very hard to tell whether such individuals (who rarely have histories suggestive of ADHD) really have a uniquely stimulant-responsive disorder or whether they have somehow become dependent on stimulants. In either case, if they cope well and feel well only when taking stimulants, take low to moderate dosages as prescribed, and do not develop tolerance, the stimulant should be continued. If the physician feels uncomfortable about prescribing stimulants for such patients, consultation with a clinical psychopharmacologist may provide helpful clinical and ethical support.

More difficult permutations of the problem exist, of course. What about a patient who recalls D-amphetamine as making him feel "better," but not better enough to actually complete graduate courses or even to motivate him to pay the bill of the psychiatrist who was prescribing the pills? What about a patient for whom a host of antidepressants have failed but who refuses to try an MAOI because of the restricted diet and risks? Should she be forced to fail on an MAOI before a stimulant is tried or retried? What about a marginally employed, distant, mildly paranoid young man with severe ear pain of an undiagnosable nature who buys illicit stimulants to relieve the pain? The stimulants do not help him function, and they do not make him more paranoid—they only make him feel better. What about the chronically very depressed woman who feels better only when taking 200 mg of methylphenidate a day? We feel more comfortable prescribing stimulants when they either obviously improve functioning or, at least, relieve incapacitating distress. We would not force a patient to try an MAOI if he or she has already improved while taking a stimulant in the past, but these are personal judgments.

In summary, we suspect that the useful, rapidly acting stimulant drugs are underused in American adult psychiatric practice. They do not always work or even help, but when they do, they can be very effective. It is still unclear whether bupropion, which resembles the stimulants in some respects, or other new drugs, which do not (see Chapter 3: "Antidepressants"), will provide safer, less abusable drugs that will help those psychiatric patients who now respond only to standard stimulants.

Atomoxetine

Atomoxetine is a pure norepinephrine reuptake blocker that is FDA approved for the treatment of ADHD in children and adults. It appears to have no abuse liability potential and has been shown to be significantly more effective than placebo in children and adolescents as well as in adults with the disorder. It carries the same black-box warning around suicidality as do the antidepressants. In a small study in adults, Spencer et al. (1998) reported that the drug was significantly more effective than placebo. The average dosage was 76 mg/day. Subsequently, several positive trials in adults have been reported (Michelson et al. 2003). Similarly, the drug has been reported to be effective in a large study in children and adolescents (Michelson et al. 2002) (see Chapter 12: "Pharmacotherapy in Special Situations"). Atomoxetine appears to be more effective in improving attention than in controlling hyperactivity. Relative to the effects of stimulants, the effects of atomoxetine on ADHD are also more gradual. Stimulants tend to show more rapid benefits.

The adult daily dose is 40–100 mg; in children, the daily dose is approximately 1.2 mg/kg and should not exceed 1.4 mg/kg, or 100 mg, whichever is less. Primary side effects appear to be, in children, loss of appetite and gastrointestinal upset and, in adults, gastrointestinal upset, orthostatic blood pressure effects, and insomnia. In contrast to the older stimulants, the dosage of atomoxetine has to be increased slowly to avoid somatic side effects.

Guanfacine

In 2009, guanfacine, in its extended-release formulation, became the second nonstimulant, after atomoxetine, to be approved for the treatment of ADHD. Guanfacine is an old medication, used historically as an antihypertensive but rarely used for this indication currently. The drug is a selective α_{2A} antagonist whose efficacy in the treatment of ADHD in children and adolescents has been established in two randomized, controlled, fixed-dose trials. Both trials included children ages 6–17. One of the trials evaluated guanfacine at dosages of 2–4 mg/day over 8 weeks (Biederman et al. 2008a, 2008b), and the other used dosages of 1–4 mg/day over 9 weeks (Sallee et al. 2009). Both studies used the ADHD Rating Scale IV (ADHD R4) to assess changes from baseline to the end of the study. Guanfacine at all dosages was reported to be superior to placebo at improving overall scores on the ADHD R4. Interestingly, there did appear to be a dose-response relationship, with higher dosages being more effective but also having more side effects than lower dosages. No comparison studies with stimulants or atomoxetine have yet been completed, so it is unclear if there are any efficacy advantages of guanfacine over other agents.

The side effects of guanfacine can be anticipated from its α-adrenergic effects: somnolence, sedation, hypotension/dizziness, bradycardia, dry mouth, abdominal pain, and constipation. About 33% of children treated with guanfacine experienced sedation/somnolence compared with about 12% of placebo-treated children. Sedation was the most common reason for discontinuing the drug. About 6% of children had some evidence of hypotension, and 1% had syncopal episodes. GI adverse events were not common reasons for discontinuing guanfacine in the acute ADHD trials.

Guanfacine is metabolized via CYP3A4, and concurrent administration of inhibitors such as ketoconazole can increase plasma concentrations of the drug, whereas inducers such as carbamazepine or rifampin may lower serum levels.

Guanfacine extended-release is usually dosed at 1 mg/day given in the morning. Daytime sedation may benefit from evening dosing of guanfacine. The dosage is increased by no more than 1 mg/week to a maximum of 4 mg/day. Measuring blood pressure at the start of treatment and with dosage changes is recommended.

Guanfacine, then, represents another nonstimulant that appears to be effective for the treatment of ADHD. We would anticipate that as a nonscheduled agent that does not have a black-box warning around suicidality, guanfacine should have an important niche in the treatment of ADHD. It remains to be seen how much of an issue the cardiovascular and sedating effects of the drug will be in clinical practice.

Other Fast-Acting Drugs

Psychopharmacology mainly concerns itself with complex drugs shown to be relatively useful in depression, mania, psychosis, and, more recently, dementia—drugs with complicated mechanisms of action taking days to weeks to get full clinical effect.

Two hundred years ago the pharmacopoeia used in asylums was much more limited and quite different. Opiates have been a mainstay of treatment for violent or agitated patients for centuries. By the late 1800s sedatives—barbiturates, chloral hydrate, and paraldehyde—came into use to manage excitement. Marijuana was reported (in a letter to the editor of the *British Medical Journal* in the late nineteenth century) to be useful in reducing nighttime agitated wandering. Apomorphine and hyoscine were used in combination to "snow" patients being transported from Bellevue's psychiatric facility in Manhattan to the several surrounding state hospitals.

Then several biological therapies (electroconvulsive and pentylenetetrazol convulsive treatment, continuous sleep therapy, insulin coma therapy, and psychosurgery) were introduced, each on the basis of initially striking rapid clinical improvement in a few of patients. These therapies were dramatically more effective but had problems.

To our knowledge stimulants—caffeine, theophylline, cocaine—did not become part of asylum therapies, though one suspects that Freud was not the only psychiatrist to explore the subjective effects of cocaine.

By the 1930s the stage was set for LSD-25 which rapidly "invaded" the mind of a Swiss pharmacologist who had unknowingly absorbed the miniscule amount of lysergic acid diethylamide needed to get a striking psychedelic experience. At the same time ephedrine was found in China where it was known as a *ma huang* and permuted into *d*-amphetamine. The later was tried in children being treated at the Bradley Home in Rhode Island, allegedly to reduce headache caused by radiological brain studies. Anyway *dl*-amphetamine had a striking immediate good behavioral effect—one that was easily replicated in smaller, blinded studies (Cole 1969).

Most recently, tetrahydrocannabinol (Marinol, 5-mg tablets) has been available for use in the nausea and vomiting associated with cancer treatments. We know of a handful of noncancer patients with severe anxiety, nausea, and weight loss who have responded well to Marinol when standard methods have failed. Moreover, a patient with painful, incapacitating dystonia has had significant relief of spasms for 3 months on 5-mg delta-tetrahydrocannabinol three times a day.

The stimulants are widely used examples of this broadening group of drugs. They do a particularly good job of illustrating shifts in attitudes to drug classes over time from anathema to, more recently, quite wide acceptance of the diagnoses of ADHD in both children and adults and even the rebirth of older drugs like Adderall and Ritalin into a variety of formulations.

Finally, the study of hallucinogens as treatment approaches appears to have been finally made possible by changes in procedures and attitudes at the U.S. Food and Drug Administration (FDA) and by the gradual increase in evidence that regular users of peyote in the Southwest United States and of another hallucinogen in Brazil are not appreciably harmed by this use. Furthermore, perusual of the World Wide Web shows that a number of Web users claim that a single dose of psilocybin is enough to stop a highly painful run of cluster headaches in its tracks.

All these treatments share, to some degree, rapid action and in some ways are related to other drugs taken socially such as opiates, cocaine, and alcohol. Even alcohol has been prescribed in psychiatry. In the 1970s there was an elderly agitated professional man with a 6-month stay at McLean who was regularly prescribed two martinis two nights a week to reduce his anxiety over going off grounds to have dinner with his wife. We have heard of alcohol by stomach tube having been used to handle hysterical paralyses (or catatonia)

successfully before the newer barbiturates or benzodiazepines became readily
available.

Bibliography

Angrist B, Rotrosen J, Gershon S: Responses to apomorphine, amphetamine, and
neuroleptics in schizophrenic subjects. Psychopharmacology (Berl) 67:31–38,
1980

Angrist B, Peselow E, Rubinstein M, et al: Amphetamine response and relapse risk
after depot neuroleptic discontinuation. Psychopharmacology (Berl) 85:277–283,
1985

Angrist B, D'Hollosy M, Sanfillipo M, et al: Central nervous system stimulants as symptomatic treatments for AIDS-related neuropsychiatric impairment. J Clin Psychopharmacol 12:268–272, 1992

August GJ, Naftali R, Papanicolaou AC, et al: Fenfluramine treatment in infantile
autism: neurochemical, electrophysiological and behavioral effects. J Nerv Ment
Dis 172:604–612, 1984

Biederman G: Fenfluramine (Pondimin) in autism. Biological Therapies in Psychiatry
Newsletter 8:25–28, 1985

Biederman J, Faraone SV: Attention-deficit hyperactivity disorder. Lancet 366:237–
248, 2005

Biederman J, Melmed RD, Patel A, et al: Long-term, open-label extension study of
guanfacine extended release in children and adolescents with ADHD. CNS Spectr
13:1047-1055, 2008a

Biederman J, Melmed RD, Patel A, et al, and SPD503 Study Group: A randomized,
double-blind, placebo-controlled study of guanfacine extended release in children
and adolescents with attention-deficit/hyperactivity disorder. Pediatrics 121:e73-
e84, 2008b (Epub)

Bodkin JA, Zornberg GL, Lukas SE, et al: Buprenorphine treatment of refractory
depression. J Clin Psychopharmacol 15:49–57, 1995

Chiarello RJ, Cole JO: The use of psychostimulants in general psychiatry: a reconsid-
eration. Arch Gen Psychiatry 44:286–295, 1987

Cho AK: Ice: a new dosage form of an old drug. Science 249:631–634, 1990

Cole JO (ed): The amphetamines in psychiatry. Semin Psychiatry 1:128–137, 1969

Cole JO: Drug therapy of adult minimal brain dysfunction, in Psychopharmacology Update. Edited by Cole JO. Lexington, MA, Collamore Press, 1981, pp 69–
80

Cole JO, Boling LA, Beake BJ: Stimulant drugs: medical needs, alternative indications and related problems, in Impact of Prescription Drug Diversion Control Systems on Medical Practice and Patient Care (NIDA Monogr No 131). Edited by Cooper JR, Czechowicz DJ, Molinari SP. Rockville, MD, National Institute on Drug Abuse, 1993, pp 89–108

Cole JO, Levin A, Beake B, et al: Sibutramine: a new weight loss agent without evidence of the abuse potential associated with amphetamines. J Clin Psychopharmacol 18:231–236, 1998

Davidoff E, Reifenstein E: Treatment of schizophrenia with sympathomimetic drugs: Benzedrine sulfate. Psychiatr Q 13:127–144, 1939

Elizur A, Wintner I, Davidson S: The clinical and psychological effects of pemoline in depressed patients: a controlled study. Int Pharmacopsychiatry 14:127–134, 1979

Ellinwood EH: Amphetamine psychosis: individuals, settings, and sequences, in Current Concepts on Amphetamine Abuse (DHEW Publ No HSM-729085). Edited by Ellinwood EH, Cohen S. Washington, DC, U.S. Government Printing Office, 1972, pp 143–158

Expert Roundtable Highlights: Stimulants and atomoxetine in the treatment of attention-deficit/hyperactivity disorder. J Clin Psychiatry Monograph 19(1):1–23, 2004

Faraone SV, Glatt SJ: Effects of extended-release guanfacine on ADHD symptoms and sedation-related adverse events in children with ADHD. J Atten Disord 13:532–538, 2009

Feighner JP, Herbstein J, Damlouji N: Combined MAOI, TCA, and direct stimulant therapy of treatment-resistant depression. J Clin Psychiatry 46:206–209, 1985

Feldman PE: Ancient psychopharmacotherapy. Bull Menninger Clin 29:256–263, 1965

Fernandez F, Levy JK, Galizzi H: Response of HIV-related depression to psychostimulants: case reports. Hosp Community Psychiatry 39:628–631, 1988

Greenhill LL, Osman BB (eds): Ritalin: Theory and Practice, 2nd Edition. Larchmont, NY, Mary Ann Liebert, 2000

Grinspoon L, Hedblom P: The Speed Culture: Amphetamine Use and Abuse in America. Cambridge, MA, Harvard University Press, 1975

Horrigan JP, Barnhill LJ: Low-dose amphetamine salts and adult attention/hyperactivity disorder. J Clin Psychiatry 61:414–417, 2000

Huessey H: Clinical explorations in adult minimal brain dysfunction, in Psychiatric Aspects of Minimal Brain Dysfunction in Adults. Edited by Bellak L. New York, Grune & Stratton, 1979

Hughes CH: Tranquilizer for maniacs. Alienist and Neurologist 32:163–166, 1911

Jackson JG: Hazards of smokable methamphetamine (letter). N Engl J Med 321:907, 1989

Jensen PS, Hinshaw SP, Swanson JM, et al: Findings of the NIMH Multimodal Treatment Study of ADHD: implications and applications for primary care providers. J Dev Behav Pediatrics 22:60–73, 2001

Kaufmann M, Murray G, Cassem N: Use of psychostimulants in medically ill depressed patients. Psychosomatics 23:817–819, 1982

Klein R, Mannuzza S: Hyperactive boys almost grown up, III: methylphenidate effects on ultimate height. Arch Gen Psychiatry 45:1131–1134, 1988

Klein RG, Wender P: The role of methylphenidate in psychiatry (commentary). Arch Gen Psychiatry 52:429–433, 1995

Klein RG, Abikoff H, Klass E: Clinical efficacy of methylphenidate in conduct disorder with and without attention deficit hyperactivity disorder. Arch Gen Psychiatry 54:1073–1080, 1997

Kroft C, Cole JO: Adverse behavioral effects of psychostimulants, in Adverse Effects of Psychotropic Drugs. Edited by Kane JM, Lieberman JA. New York, Guilford, 1992, pp 153–162

Lieberman JA, Alvir J, Geisler S, et al: Methylphenidate response, psychopathology and tardive dyskinesia as predictors of relapse in schizophrenia. Neuropsychopharmacology 11:107–118, 1994

Markowitz JC, Rabkin JG, Perry SW: Treating depression in HIV-positive patients. AIDS 8:403–412, 1994

Masand P, Olin J: Psychostimulants for depression in hospitalized cancer patients. Psychosomatics 37:57–62, 1996

Mattes JA, Boswell L, Oliver H: Methylphenidate effects on symptoms of attention-deficit disorder in adults. Arch Gen Psychiatry 41:59–63, 1984

Michelson D, Allen AJ, Busner J, et al: Once-daily atomoxetine treatment for children and adolescents with attention-deficit/hyperactivity disorder: a randomized, placebo-controlled study. Am J Psychiatry 159:1896–1901, 2002

Michelson D, Allen AJ, Spencer T, et al: Atomoxetine in adults with ADHD: two randomized, placebo-controlled studies. Biol Psychiatry 53:112–120, 2003

The MTA Group: A 14-month randomized clinical trial of treatment strategies for AD/HD. Arch Gen Psychiatry 56:1073–1088, 1999

Myerson A: The effect of benzedrine sulfate on mood and fatigue in normal and neurotic persons. AMA Arch Neurol Psychiatry 36: 816–822, 1936

Ratey J, Greenberg MS, Bemporad JR, et al: Unrecognized ADHD in adults. Journal of Child and Adolescent Psychiatry 2:267–275, 1994

Rickels K, Gordon P, Gansman D, et al: Pemoline and methylphenidate in mildly depressed outpatients. Clin Pharmacol Ther 11:698–710, 1970

Ritvo ER, Freeman BJ, Yuwiler A: Study of fenfluramine in outpatients with the syndrome of autism. J Pediatr 105:823–828, 1984

Robinson D, Jody D, Lieberman JA: Provocative tests with methylphenidate in schizophrenia and schizophrenia spectrum disorders, in Ritalin: Theory and Patient Management. Edited by Greenhill LL, Osman BB. New York, Mary Ann Liebert, 1991, pp 309–320

Rosack J: ADHD treatment arsenal increasing rapidly. Psychiatr News 36(24):17, 28, 2001

Sallee FR, Lyne A, Wigal T, et al: Long-term safety and efficacy of guanfacine extended release in children and adolescents with attention-deficit/hyperactivity disorder. J Child Adolesc Psychopharmacol 19:215–226, 2009

Satel S, Nelson JC: Stimulants in the treatment of depression: a critical overview. J Clin Psychiatry 50:241–249, 1989

Savage GH: Hyoscyamine, and its uses. Journal of Mental Science 25:177–184, 1879

Schubiner H, Tzelepis A, Isaacson H, et al: The dual diagnosis of attention deficit/hyperactivity disorder and substance abuse: case reports and literature review. J Clin Psychiatry 56:146–150, 1995

Shekim WO, Asarnow RF, Hess E, et al: A clinical and demographic profile of a sample of adults with attention-deficit hyperactivity disorder. Compt Psychiatry 31:416–425, 1990

Spencer T, Wilens T, Biederman J, et al: A double-blind, crossover comparison of methylphenidate and placebo in adults with childhood-onset attention deficit/hyperactivity disorder. Arch Gen Psychiatry 52:434–443, 1995

Spencer T, Biederman J, Wilens T, et al: Effectiveness and tolerability of tomoxetine in adults with attention-deficit/hyperactivity disorder. Am J Psychiatry 155:693–695, 1998

Spencer T, Biederman J, Wilens T, et al: A large, double-blind randomized clinical trial of methylphenidate in the treatment of adults with attention-deficit/hyperactivity disorder. Biol Psychiatry 57:456–463, 2005

Stoll A, Pillay S, Diamond L, et al: Methylphenidate augmentation of SSRIs: a case series. J Clin Psychopharmacol 57:72–76, 1996

U.S. Modafinil in Narcolepsy Multicenter Study Group: Randomized trial of modafinil for the treatment of pathological somnolence in narcolepsy. Ann Neurol 43:88–97, 1998

Wallace AE, Kofoed LL, West AN: Double-blind placebo-controlled trial of methylphenidate in older depressed, medically ill patients. Am J Psychiatry 152:929–931, 1995

Ward M, Wender PH, Reimherr FW: The Wender Utah Rating Scale: an aid in the retrospective diagnosis of childhood attention-deficit hyperactivity disorder. Am J Psychiatry 150:885–890, 1993

Wender PH, Reimherr FW, Wood D, et al: A controlled study of methylphenidate in the treatment of attention deficit disorder, residual type in adults. Am J Psychiatry 142:547–552, 1985

Wilens TE, Biederman J, Spencer T, et al: Pharmacotherapy of adult attention-deficit/hyperactivity disorder: a review. J Clin Psychopharmacol 15:270–279, 1995

Wood DR, Reimherr FW, Wender PH, et al: Diagnosis and treatment of minimal brain dysfunction in adults: a preliminary report. Arch Gen Psychiatry 33:1453–1460, 1976

Young CM, Findling RL: Pemoline and hepatotoxicity. Int Drug Ther Newsl 33(9):46–47, 1998

9

Augmentation Strategies for Treatment-Resistant Disorders

It is the general hope of all clinicians that patients will respond to a single therapeutic agent. However, such a response may be the exception rather than the rule. Although for a long time there was much warranted consternation regarding polypharmacy (patients receiving too many different types of medications), many patients do require simultaneous treatment with different classes of drugs to achieve an adequate response. There are a number of reasons for combining medications. Among the most common is to augment the effect of one agent—for example, lithium is combined with an antidepressant to enhance or bring about an antidepressant effect, or two mood stabilizers are combined to reduce breakthrough mania. A second common reason for adding one medication to another is to treat one aspect of the illness—for example, a hypnotic added to an antidepressant to help with sleep, or a stimulant is added to combat residual fatigue. Medications are also commonly combined to reduce side effects of particular agents—for example, antiparkinsonian drugs are added to standard antipsychotics.

495

Unfortunately, research on combination treatments has lagged behind research on monotherapy. For many years, neither the pharmaceutical industry nor the National Institute of Mental Health (NIMH) had been particularly motivated to study the effects of medication combinations, except for adverse effects. However, recently, pharmaceutical companies have pursued approval for combination strategies. The NIMH has funded several large effectiveness trials, such as Sequenced Treatment Alternatives for Resistant Depression (STAR*D) in major depression and the Systematic Treatment Enhancement Program for Bipolar Disorder (STEP-BD), that have provided some important information regarding optimal combination strategies. However, the conclusions that can be drawn from these studies are limited by the lack of placebo arms and the tendency of open-label (often nonrandomized) comparison studies to yield similar results across treatment groups. In addition, these studies tend to not employ much clinical judgment; rather, they randomly assign patients to different augmenting strategies regardless of symptom profile or other historical diagnoses. Until more is learned about the biochemistry of various disorders and the range of pharmacological effects of available and future medications, clinicians will constantly be faced with using more than one agent to effect a positive response in individual patients.

Obviously, the number of potential combinations is vast, and consideration of all of them is beyond the scope of our discussion in this chapter. Instead, we focus on combinations of agents used in augmentation (Table 9–1) (medications used to counteract side effects have been discussed in the previous chapters). We recommend that clinicians become familiar with a number of commonly used combination drugs or combination regimens that have been reported in recent years to be particularly effective in specific clinical situations. In addition, clinicians should become familiar with combinations that can pose difficulties because of drug-drug interactions or additive side effects.

Augmentation Strategies for Depression
Lithium-Antidepressant Combinations

Lithium is perhaps the *best-studied* augmenter to antidepressants in patients with treatment-resistant depression (TRD). There are more lithium augmentation trials than there are augmentation studies using any other agent in TRD. However, the total number of subjects in all of these trials probably does not

Table 9–1. Potential augmenting agents for antidepressants

Antidepressant	Augmenting agent
Tricyclics/tetracyclics	lithium thyroid supplements amphetamines SSRIs monoamine precursors MAOIs
SSRIs	lithium thyroid supplements TCAs trazodone buspirone pindolol modafinil stimulants atomoxetine/reboxetine SGAs folate pramipexole/ropinirole mirtazapine bupropion
MAOIs	lithium SGAs thyroid supplements TCAs

Note. SGA = second-generation antipsychotic; SSRI = selective serotonin reuptake inhibitor; MAOI = monoamine oxidase inhibitor; TCA = tricyclic antidepressant.

equal the number of subjects in the registration trials of one SGA in the treatment of TRD. In addition, saying lithium is the best studied augmenter is different from saying lithium is the best augmenter or the strategy that should be used before others are attempted. Lithium can be cumbersome to use, requiring careful titration and serum level monitoring, and can be lethal in overdose. An ever-growing number of augmentation strategies have been proposed, but lithium remains an important option for TRD.

Lithium has been well studied in its own right as an antidepressant. Overall, the drug is effective in some 50% of patients, with suggestions that it is best used in treating males with bipolar depression (see Chapter 3: "Antidepressants," and Chapter 5: "Mood Stabilizers"). de Montigny et al. (1981) reported that the addition of lithium to a tricyclic antidepressant (TCA) trial resulted in clinical improvement within 72 hours in patients who did not have a response to a TCA alone. Before 1986, studies of lithium augmentation, which were typically open-label studies, suggested that the response rate to lithium augmentation of TCAs was as high as 75%. More recent, placebo-controlled studies have not typically confirmed this rapid clinical improvement or the more robust response rate. They have, however, demonstrated that the addition of lithium is more effective than is placebo. Although approximately one in four patients responds to lithium augmentation within 1 week, the most robust responses have typically required 3 weeks or more. Response often occurs at low dosages (600–1,200 mg/day) and at relatively low serum levels. Current data suggest that serum levels in the range of 0.5 to 0.8 mEq/L are effective in lithium augmentation of antidepressant effects (Bauer and Dopfmer 1999). The mechanism of action has been hypothesized as a potentiation of serotonergic activity, via either increased biosynthesis or receptor adaptation. Our experience with the combination has generally been favorable, and we have been particularly impressed with results obtained in depressed patients with pronounced obsessionality and agitation. However, there are no controlled trial data to support the clinical impression. Price et al. (1983) reported that lithium also elicited a response in patients with delusional depression who had not responded to the combination of amitriptyline and perphenazine.

Lithium also appears to augment responses to other antidepressants. For example, patients with bipolar depression with hypersomnia and hyperphagia (formerly termed "atypical") may respond dramatically to the combination of lithium and the monoamine oxidase inhibitor (MAOI) tranylcypromine. In an open-label study, Price et al. (1985) found that 11 of 12 patients with TRD responded to the combination of lithium and tranylcypromine. Many of these patients had not had a response to lithium-TCA combinations. In a New Haven follow-up study, patients with unipolar depression who were treated with desipramine plus lithium remained euthymic in the community for much longer periods when not taking medication than did patients who improved while taking desipramine plus placebo (Nierenberg et al. 1990).

A number of studies have confirmed the efficacy of lithium augmentation of selective serotonin reuptake inhibitors (SSRIs). In an early report, Pope et al.

(1988) found that lithium appeared to augment the antidepressant effects of fluoxetine. More recent, double-blind studies have confirmed this finding (Fava et al. 1994; Katona et al. 1995). Some evidence suggests that lithium may do a better job augmenting SSRIs than augmenting TCAs. In a double-blind study, lithium more effectively boosted the antidepressant actions of paroxetine than it did amitriptyline, and these effects were seen as early as 2 weeks and continued for the 6 weeks of the study (Bauer et al. 1999). In the STAR*D trial, lithium augmentation was compared with addition of L-triiodothyronine (T_3) in patients who did not respond to two previous medication trials (Nierenberg et al. 2006a). At this level (3) of the STAR*D protocol, patients received augmentation with a variety of antidepressants that could include citalopram, venlafaxine, bupropion, and sertraline. Both augmenting strategies had modest, statistically equal efficacy, but lithium was much more poorly tolerated than was T_3. About 16% of the group receiving lithium augmentation achieved a remission versus about 25% of the group receiving T_3 augmentation. As with lithium augmentation of TCA response, the maximum potentiation of SSRI response appears to require adequate lithium serum levels and may require trials of 4 weeks or longer. (For further discussion of maintenance treatment, see Chapter 3.) Overall, we would expect about 50% of patients who did not have a response to a TCA or an SSRI to have a response after the addition of lithium.

There are probably certain characteristics in depressed patients that predict response to the addition of lithium to their antidepressant regimen. Depressed patients may be more likely to improve with lithium augmentation if they exhibit significant psychomotor retardation, have significant anorexia and weight loss, and have low serum cortisol levels (Alvarez et al. 1997).

If lithium is to be added, it should be initiated at 300 mg bid for 2 days, and the dosage should be increased to 900 mg/day for 3–4 days, with a further increase to 1,200 mg/day for 10–14 days. A serum level of at least 0.5 mEq/L should be achieved. If there is no response, then the dose should be gradually increased as tolerated to a serum level of 1.2 mEq/L. Given that there is probably a bimodal distribution to response, with some patients responding within the first 2 weeks and others requiring a month or more to achieve response (Thase et al. 1998), we tend to not regard a lithium augmentation trial as failed until serum levels greater than 0.5 mEq/L are obtained for at least 6 weeks, and we would prefer a level of 0.6 mEq/L or more.

Thyroid Supplement–Antidepressant Combinations

A number of years ago a debate emerged in the literature regarding whether thyroid preparations (e.g., thyroxine [T_4] and T_3) prescribed with a TCA hastened the onset of the antidepressant effect. Early studies in women suggested that it did, although subsequent studies in men, which also employed higher dosages of TCAs, failed to substantiate the earlier finding. Then a fallow period followed for this combination until 1982, when Goodwin et al. reported that the addition of 25–50 µg/day of T_3 (Cytomel) elicited within 7 days a clinical response in patients who had previously not had a response to a seemingly adequate TCA trial. A number of subsequent clinical reports have confirmed this observation, although some clinicians have reported responses requiring 14 days or more of combined therapy. In a trial by R. T. Joffe et al. (1993), T_3 augmentation of TCAs appeared to be as effective as lithium, and both were significantly more effective than placebo. A subsequent head-to-head crossover trial also suggested that patients receiving T_3 augmentation were more likely to respond than were lithium-treated patients (Spoov and Lahdelma 1998). Statistical equivalence of T_3 augmentation to lithium augmentation was found in the STAR*D study reviewed in the previous section (Nierenberg et al. 2006a). If thyroid and lithium augmentation are both helpful in resistant depression, perhaps combining both lithium and thyroid with an antidepressant would have additive effects. Unfortunately, a study by Joffe and colleagues (2006) did not find that combining lithium with thyroid hormone had any advantages over either one alone.

Thyroid augmentation of MAOIs has been less well studied than that of TCAs. The response to thyroid supplementation of MAOIs also appears to be somewhat less consistent than for other antidepressants. Nonetheless, the combination of T_3 and an MAOI appears to be well tolerated and may be considered if lithium augmentation is not successful.

Several case reports have suggested that thyroid augmentation of the SSRIs may also be effective. For example, R. T. Joffe (1992) found that Cytomel (T_3) at 25–50 µg/mL/day when added to fluoxetine enhanced the antidepressant effects of the drug and was well tolerated. A number of other case reports suggested that thyroid supplements may potentiate SSRI antidepressant effects (Crowe et al. 1990; Gupta et al. 1991). Whether the T_3 is added at the initiation of SSRI therapy or after a patient fails a trial of an SSRI may be important in the efficacy of this intervention. For example a meta-analysis of randomized controlled trials in which the T_3 was combined with SSRIs at the beginning of treatment did not find a benefit of thyroid augmentation (Papakostas et al. 2009). However, a review of studies that examined the utility of T_3 added to an SSRI after an unsuccessful trial of SSRI monotherapy indicated that this strategy might be beneficial (Cooper-Kazaz et al. 2009).

The data suggest that thyroid supplementation may be effective in combination with a wide spectrum of antidepressants. However, good studies are still lacking, and the available studies have shown mixed results.

The mechanism of action of T_3 potentiation of antidepressants is undetermined. Generally, theories have revolved around the role of T_3 in facilitating adrenergic receptor adaptation. However, Targum et al. (1984) reported that patients who had a response to T_3 demonstrated relatively enhanced thyroid-stimulating hormone (TSH) responses to thyrotropin-releasing hormone (TRH) infusions, suggesting that a subtle form of thyroid dysfunction might play a role in these patients' condition. Targum et al. suggested that patients with refractory depression who have a normal TSH but a blunted response to the TRH stimulation test may be good candidates for thyroid augmentation.

Clinicians frequently ask whether T_4 (Synthroid) is as effective as T_3 in augmenting response to TCAs. T_4 is metabolized to T_3 in humans. One double-blind study comparing 2-week treatments of T_4 and T_3 indicated that T_3 was significantly more effective. However, because T_4 has a much longer half-life, the patients may not have achieved steady state on T_4, leaving the conclusions of the study open to question (R. T. Joffe and Singer 1987). Possible explanations of the greater effectiveness of T_3 in some patients include difficulty in converting T_4 to T_3 or in transporting thyroid into the brain. Data suggest that depressed patients may demonstrate decreased cerebrospinal fluid levels of thyroid transport protein, which would limit the effect of T_4 on the brain. Clinically, we have seen a number of patients who did not respond to an antidepressant in combination with T_4 who did have a response when T_3 was substituted. In addition, an occasional patient benefits from high-dose T_4 added to his or her antidepressant regimen. A number of years ago Arthur Prange's group (Bunevicius et al. 1999) reported that in patients with thyroid disease who were treated with T_4, the addition of T_3 significantly improved both mood and cognition in comparison with placebo, suggesting that individuals could have relative T_3 deficiencies in brain. An open-label trial using T_4 at an average of 482 μg/day for 8 weeks found that more than 50% of the patients in a treatment-resistant population had a robust response (Bauer et al. 1998). Although side effects were not common in this trial, the use of supraphysiological doses of T_4 for an extended time might be problematic for some patients.

Can one predict those patients who are the best candidates for thyroid augmentation? Clearly, those who have any evidence of thyroid abnormalities, including subclinical hypothyroidism, appear to be good candidates. There is evidence that patients with mild thyroid abnormalities (slightly elevated TSH, normal T_3 and T_4) are less likely to respond to antidepressants alone but do respond to the addition of a thyroid supplement (Sokolov et al. 1997). Women over the age of 50, perhaps because they are most susceptible to hypothyroidism, also appear to have high responses to thyroid augmentation. Overall, it is our impression that Cytomel (T_3) is useful in patients with pronounced psychomotor retardation. Cytomel may be experienced as energizing and may actually help with weight loss in patients with atypical features. We have on occasion found that Cytomel can also bring about a response in patients who have experienced a relapse while taking a TCA to which they had previously responded.

Cytomel (T_3) is typically started at 12.5–25 μg/day, with dosage increases in 1-week increments to 50 μg/day. Levothroid or Synthroid (T_4) is typically initiated at 50 μg/day and increased every week or two, up to 200 μg/day. Whereas an adequate trial of T_3 may be 1–4 weeks, preparations of T_4 will probably require duration of 4–8 weeks because of its longer half-life. Thyroid preparations tend to be well tolerated, but they should be used with caution in patients who have a history of coronary artery disease, hypertension, or arrhythmia. If thyroid supplementation results in significant suppression of TSH, it is thought that bone demineralization may occur during extended treatment. However, Whybrow's group (Whybrow 1994) did not observe demineralization in bipolar patients with rapid cycling treated with high doses of T_4. Overdoses occasionally result in cardiac decompensation. If a patient responds positively, we recommend continuing the T_3 for an additional 60 days and then tapering by 12.5 μg every 3 days. Some patients will demonstrate a resumption of symptoms and will require resumption of the T_3. One of our patients required resumption of dose and maintenance for more than 1 year before T$_3$ could finally be tapered off. Results of thyroid function tests while the patient was taking T$_3$ were essentially normal. After the T$_3$ was tapered, the patient's T$_3$ uptake, TSH, and T$_4$ levels were all lower than normal but normalized within 2–3 weeks. This patient demonstrated none of the stigmata of decreased thyroid status immediately after discontinuation.

Estrogen, DHEA, and Testosterone Combinations With Antidepressants

For many years, estrogens have sometimes been used alone or in combination with antidepressants to treat depression in women who are postmenopausal or postpartum whose conditions are refractory to standard treatments. The results of using estrogens for depression have been uneven. Some studies found estrogens to be useful in the treatment of depression in some women, and others did not. The findings of an increased risk of breast cancer, heart attacks, and strokes in the Women's Health Initiative study in 2002 resulted in many women abandoning hormone replacement therapy. However, estrogen does have some effects on mood, and some women clearly have benefited from these effects. Coope (1981) found that estrogen had no significant antidepressant effect when used alone for perimenopausal depression. On the other hand, studies using higher doses of conjugated estrogens (5–25 mg/day) found some partial antidepressant benefit in postmenopausal women. One published study in this area (Soares et al. 2001) found that a transdermal patch of 17-β-estradiol was significantly more effective than placebo in reducing depressive symptoms in perimenopausal women. This was a reasonably sized study (50 subjects) with a sufficient duration of treatment. On the other hand, a study by Rasgon and colleagues (2007) failed to show much benefit of adding transdermal estrogen to sertraline in depressed postmenopausal women.

The utility of estrogens in postpartum depression is also uneven. Some studies have failed to show benefit. However, another study found estrogen to be an effective prophylaxis against recurrent affective illness in the postpartum period (Sichel et al. 1995). In a Cochrane Review, the administration of progesterone in the postpartum period was associated with an enhanced risk of developing depression, while the administration of estrogen was concluded to have modest benefit for postpartum depression (Dennis et al. 2008). Our experience with using estrogens alone in women with refractory depression has not been particularly encouraging.

The combination of estrogens with antidepressants has yielded more consistent results. Several studies before 1985 failed to show any additional benefit of combining estrogens with TCAs in depressed women. However, there have been case reports of oral contraceptives augmenting the effects of antidepressants in patients with refractory depression (Sherwin 1991). In addition, postmenopausal women may respond better to fluoxetine if they are on hormone replacement therapy than if they are not (Schneider et al. 1997, 2001).

Some cautions are worth considering when administering estrogens to women with mood disorders. Estrogens appear to be capable of inducing rapid cycling in some women with bipolar disorder, and progesterone may suppress rapid cycling. In addition, estrogen use carries the risk of thrombophlebitis and an increased risk of breast, cervical, and uterine cancer. Unfortunately, progesterone may induce depression in some women. Estrogens also appear to increase the bioavailability and serum levels of TCAs. Thus, lower doses of TCAs are sometimes indicated when an estrogen is added to the regimen.

At this time, the routine combination of estrogen with antidepressants is unwarranted. However, some women with refractory depression in the postpartum or perimenopausal periods might benefit from such a combination. Typical dosages of estrogens in successful studies ranged from 5 to 25 mg/day of conjugated estrogens. The risks of long-term use of high-dose, unopposed estrogen, however, are probably too great to justify use of that approach for mild depression.

Dehydroepiandrosterone (DHEA), a steroid precursor of both androgens and estrogens, has become a very popular over-the-counter remedy for dysphoria ("Dehydroepiandrosterone" 1996). Some controlled reports suggested that dosages of 50–100 mg/day result in increases in physical and psychological well-being in women ages 40–70. An early study found that DHEA is more effective in augmenting a standard antidepressant at dosages up to 90 mg/day than is placebo (Wolkowitz et al. 1997). Likewise, there is some evidence that DHEA is significantly more effective than placebo as a monotherapy for the treatment of dysthymia (Bloch et al. 1999). A number of studies have also found DHEA to be effective in the treatment of depressive symptoms in midlife (Schmidt et al. 2005) and in patients with HIV-related illness (Rabkin et al. 2006).

The problem with DHEA, however, is that it is not a simple food supplement; it is a prohormone of adrenal origin. Androgenic effects, including irreversible hair loss, hirsutism, and deepening of voice, have occasionally been reported. In addition, there is some concern that DHEA could accelerate tumor growth, because many malignancies, including those of the breast, endometrium, and prostate, are hormone sensitive. It will be important to collect safety data concerning long-term use of DHEA. Thus, we encourage prudence in using DHEA until further study is completed.

Testosterone gel has been reported to be effective in a small double-blind, placebo-controlled trial in men with refractory depression (Pope et al. 2003). This 8-week study was undertaken in men with low or borderline low testosterone levels. In a previous trial, intramuscular testosterone had failed to separate from placebo (Seidman et al. 2001). Likewise, a later study by Seidman and colleagues (2005) in patients with SSRI-resistant depression did not show benefit to intramuscular testosterone supplementation versus the injection of a placebo. Overall, it appears that testosterone's antidepressant benefits are most consistently seen in men with hypogonadism, and perhaps elderly men and those with HIV-related depressive symptoms (Zarrouf et al. 2009). Among the more significant risks of testosterone supplementation is an increased risk of prostate cancer, although increased levels of other androgens and estrogens may play more of a role than testosterone in enhancing the risk of prostate cancer (Raynaud 2006). Regardless of the prostate risks, there may also be cardiovascular risks and altered insulin resistance with testosterone supplements. Given the unknown risks, testosterone therapy in depressed men with normal testosterone levels does not appear warranted.

Dopamine Agonist–Antidepressant Combinations

In the early 1970s, Wharton and colleagues (1971) reported that the addition of methylphenidate increased plasma levels of TCAs through inhibition of microsomal degradation of the TCA in the liver (similar to the competitive inhibition observed with antipsychotic agents). This approach offers a possible way of increasing TCA plasma levels without increasing TCA dose. In addition to this effect, methylphenidate is a stimulant and may be useful in treating the anergia and psychomotor retardation of endogenous depression. However, as described in Chapter 8, we do not recommend adding methylphenidate to increase plasma levels, because higher TCA plasma levels can be obtained by increasing the TCA doses. Rather, clinicians might want to use methylphenidate for its energizing properties, but they should keep in mind that it may increase TCA plasma levels and side effects. Fawcett et al. (1991) found that pemoline or dextroamphetamine was effective in inducing improvement when added to an MAOI in patients with severe, treatment-refractory depression. Although this combination was safe and no hypertensive crises were reported, approximately one in five patients treated developed either hypomania or mania.

The traditional stimulants do appear to still have a role in patients with TRD, those with concurrent attention-deficit disorders, and medically ill patients. Stimulants can improve energy and concentration in medically ill patients and appear to be useful adjuvants to most classes of antidepressants. Although less well studied in combination with newer antidepressants, amphetamine-type drugs have been reported in case series to augment venlafaxine and the SSRIs.

A number of new kinds of dopamine agonists have potential as augmenting agents in TRD. For example, the D_2, D_3 agonist pramipexole (Mirapex), which has an FDA-approved indication for the treatment of Parkinson's disease, has also been evaluated as a treatment for major depression. In one study, pramipexole separated from placebo to a comparable degree as fluoxetine (Corrigan et al. 2000). We have found it useful as an adjunctive agent to SSRIs in some patients with TRD at dosages up to 1 mg/day (DeBattista 1997). In addition, pramipexole appears to help with restless legs, including restless legs exacerbated by the use of SSRIs (DeBattista et al. 2000). More recently, pramipexole was found to improve depression in two small double-blind, placebo-controlled studies of bipolar depressed patients (Goldberg et al. 2004; Zarate et al. 2004). In an open-label study, we found that adjunctive ropinirole at dosages of 3–12 mg/day helped about half the 72 patients who had not had an adequate response to a standard antidepressant (DeBattista et al. 2008). These results were similar to those reported by Cassano and colleagues (2005), who used ropinirole at an average dosage of just 1 mg/day to augment standard antidepressants. Side effects of ropinirole commonly include nausea, dizziness, and headache. More rare side effects have included compulsive behaviors such as gambling and visual hallucinations. In general, ropinirole appears to better tolerated at lower dosages than at higher dosages, and just 1 mg/day may prove a reasonable augmentation dose if its effectiveness is confirmed by subsequent studies.

Monoamine Precursor–Antidepressant Combinations

The addition of amino acids to antidepressants is based on the rationale that supplementing the diet with precursors of monoamines may help correct a deficiency of the monoaminergic system. Phenylalanine is a precursor of dopamine and norepinephrine; tryptophan is ultimately converted into serotonin (5-HT). These amino acids have been combined with MAOIs, TCAs, and SSRIs in the treatment of refractory depression, with varying degrees of success. The "Newcastle cocktail," which has been used for treatment-refractory depression, employed a combination of clomipramine or phenelzine, lithium, and tryptophan (Montgomery 1991). This was said to be an effective combination, but one that carried some risk of serotonin syndrome. Dosages of tryptophan used for augmentation have ranged from 2 to 6 g/day. Phenylalanine has been used in dosages of 500 mg/day to 5 g/day as a supplement. We have not been particularly impressed with phenylalanine augmentation. A related strategy is the use of inositol, a precursor of an important intracellular second-messenger system: the phosphatidylinositol (PI) system. The PI system may be important in mediating the effects of lithium and various antidepressants. Levine et al. (1995) reported a small double-blind study suggesting that inositol 6 g bid was useful and was more effective than placebo in treating patients with major depression. However, in a follow-up study, no difference could be found between placebo and inositol in the augmentation of SSRIs (Levine et al. 1999). In bipolar depression, the addition of inositol 10–15 g was found to be as effective (or ineffective) as adding lamotrigine or risperidone to lithium, valproate, or carbamazepine (Nierenberg et al. 2006b). However, a small placebo-controlled trial did not demonstrate clear efficacy over placebo in the adjunctive treatment of bipolar depression (Eden Evins et al. 2006b). In fact, a few subjects, especially those with high baseline irritability, appeared to get substantially worse while taking the inositol. The small size of the study ($N=17$) precludes definitive conclusions.

SSRI Combinations

Since the SSRIs are now the most common agents used to treat depression, a number of potential augmenting agents have been combined with the SSRIs in patients with TRD. Lithium and thyroid augmentation are often used to enhance SSRI response, but a number of other agents may also be useful (see Table 9–1).

Among the most common augmenting agents currently used in clinical practice is bupropion. A number of studies have suggested that bupropion, as a noradrenergic-dopaminergic agent, can enhance the antidepressant effects of SSRIs and venlafaxine (Bodkin et al. 1997; Fatemi et al. 1999; Kirsch and Louie 1999). We have studied the addition of sustained-release bupropion (Wellbutrin SR) to SSRIs and believe it is a convenient and well-tolerated method of improving antidepressant response (DeBattista et al. 2003). Since all formulations of bupropion are now generic, we tend to use the XL because of the added convenience of once-a-day dosing. We start bupropion at 150 mg and then go to 300 mg by the end of the second week of treatment. Still, no good double-blind studies are yet available to confirm the efficacy of this approach, and the termination of the patent life makes it less likely that such a study will ever be completed. The largest trial of bupropion augmentation, the open-label but randomized STAR*D trial, found that augmenting citalopram with bupropion was about as effective as augmenting with buspirone in producing a remission-level response (Trivedi et al. 2006; see also Chapter 3, this volume). However, there was an advantage of bupropion over buspirone when focusing on absolute change on one of the standard depression scales used in the study (QID-SR-16). Improvement in the scale score was 25% with bupropion and only 17% with buspirone. The target dosage for bupropion was 300–400 mg/day and 45–60 mg/day for buspirone.

We recently reported on a placebo-controlled study in which atomoxetine was added to sertraline in patients who had not responded to monotherapy. Atomoxetine was not found to be superior to placebo (Michelson et al. 2006).

Modafinil is a wake-promoting agent used in the treatment of narcolepsy (Ferraro et al. 1997). It lacks the addictive potential and the hemodynamic side effects of stimulants. We have found that 100–200 mg of modafinil taken in the morning with an SSRI is well tolerated and helps with fatigue and hypersomnia in depressed patients (DeBattista et al. 2003, 2004; Fava et al. 2007). The drug appears to work quickly, within the first 2 weeks, if it is going to help. Modafinil is generally well tolerated in combination with SSRIs. Side effects of modafinil such as headache, nausea, and anxiety are usually mild and easy to manage.

In animal models, the combination of fluoxetine with desipramine produced marked and rapid downregulation of postsynaptic β-adrenergic receptors (Baron et al. 1988), suggesting that the combination should be effective.

Several reports have suggested this is the case (Nelson and Price 1995; Weilburg et al. 1989). In a randomized controlled trial, Nelson and colleagues (2004) reported that depressed inpatients treated with the combination of desipramine and fluoxetine were far more likely to achieve remission than those patients treated with either agent alone. However, the TCA dosing must be done conservatively, because the SSRIs slow the hepatic degradation of TCAs via competitive inhibition of cytochrome P450 (CYP) 2D6 and other CYP enzymes (see Chapter 3), resulting in potential elevation of TCA levels and increased side effects (Aranow et al. 1989; Bell and Cole 1988). If a TCA is added in patients already being treated with an SSRI, initiation of the TCA should be at low dosages: 25 mg/day of nortriptyline or 50 mg/day of imipramine, with a further increase of 25 mg every 3 days as tolerated to a target dosage of 75 mg/day of nortriptyline or 150–300 mg/day of imipramine. Plasma levels of the TCA should be monitored closely, and electrocardiograms should be taken and also monitored closely. When an SSRI is added to the TCA, we recommend first gradually reducing the dosage of the TCA to 100 mg/day of nortriptyline or 150 mg/day of imipramine and monitoring plasma levels. TCA levels should be obtained before and after dosage reduction as well as after starting an SSRI.

Trazodone is often safe and useful as a hypnotic in patients who have insomnia as a result of taking fluoxetine. In the course of such use, we found patients whose depressions cleared nicely after trazodone was added to the fluoxetine. One study (Nierenberg et al. 1994) found that trazodone 100 mg at night counteracted fluoxetine- or bupropion-induced insomnia in 10 of 15 patients treated. Doses of trazodone ranging from 25 to 300 mg are used for drug-induced insomnia. The literature on trazodone augmentation of fluoxetine is sparse; in one study (Nierenberg et al. 1992), trazodone seemed to potentiate the effects of fluoxetine in 3 of 8 patients treated. The combination of trazodone and the SSRIs appears to be generally well tolerated and useful but needs further study. The SSRIs have been combined with agents that act on the serotonin$_{1A}$ (5-HT$_{1A}$) receptor to augment response and reduce side effects. Also, Nierenberg and Keck (1989) have reported on the use of trazodone to overcome insomnia associated with MAOI therapy.

Buspirone, which is a 5-HT$_{1A}$ partial agonist, has been shown to potentiate the antidepressant effects of fluoxetine in open-label studies, including the study by R. T. Joffe and Schuller (1993). Dosages of buspirone as low as 5 mg/day and as high as 50 mg/day in these studies were enough to effect a full response in the majority of patients who had not had a response or had only a partial response. On the other hand, double-blind studies have failed to show any advantage to adding buspirone to fluoxetine in the treatment of obsessive-compulsive disorder. Double-blind trials for buspirone augmentation of SSRIs for TRD have yielded mixed results; one study showed a benefit of buspirone over placebo (Bouwer and Stein 1997), and a more recent study showed negative results (Landen et al. 1998). As reported earlier in this section, buspirone was similar in efficacy to bupropion in augmenting SSRI response in the STAR*D trial (Trivedi et al. 2006). Because buspirone is such a relatively benign agent compared with other potential augmenting agents, it is worth considering in treatment-resistant cases. A 4- to 6-week trial of dosages of buspirone from 30 to 60 mg/day is probably adequate to determine whether combination with an SSRI will be useful. In addition, buspirone may help attenuate SSRI-induced sexual dysfunction, as reported in Chapter 3. However, we have not been impressed with buspirone as an augmenting agent or in the treatment of SSRI-induced sexual dysfunction.

Another SSRI augmentation strategy is the use of pindolol, a β-blocker that also has 5-HT$_{1A}$ antagonist properties. In two open-label studies (Artigas et al. 1994; Blier and Bergeson 1995), it was found to potentiate antidepressant response. In both studies, pindolol 2.5 mg tid seemed to speed the onset of action and lead to a response in the vast majority of patients who had not had a response. A few patients did drop out of both studies because they became more irritable. Subsequent studies of pindolol augmentation of SSRIs suggest that in addition to possibly speeding response, pindolol also resulted in more sustained response in acute treatment than monotherapy with an SSRI. In one study, 70% of patients treated with pindolol were able to sustain a response to the end of the acute trial, while only 40% of patients treated with fluoxetine alone had similar sustained benefits (Portella et al. 2009). Similar benefits of sustaining initial response with pindolol augmentation have also been seen in studies that have included bipolar depressed patients (Geretsegger et al. 2008). However, it is not clear whether a more rapid and sustained acute response with pindolol augmentation would have any benefits in preventing later recurrence and relapse. Such studies have not been done. Pindolol may enhance serotonergic tone by acting on somatodendritic autoreceptors.

We have attempted to use pindolol to augment SSRI response, with mixed results. A controlled trial from Yale University apparently found an increase in speed of onset. In a total of six controlled trials of pindolol augmentation that had been completed to date, three had had positive results and three had had negative results (McAskill et al. 1998). Still, pindolol may represent another fairly benign augmentation strategy that could be considered when a patient fails to continue responding to an SSRI after months of good response. There is a general impression that pindolol may hasten antidepressant response but is relatively weak as an augmenter. The most common side effects of pindolol include hypotension, dizziness, and fatigue, particularly at higher dosages. Some patients report CNS activation—for example, insomnia, anxiety, and irritability. We recommend starting at 2.5 mg bid and increasing to 5 mg bid in the second week. Blood pressure should be monitored, and if no response is seen in 3 weeks, the trial can be discontinued.

The use of mirtazapine to augment SSRIs in treating depression has proved very useful for some patients. Some evidence suggests that the combination of venlafaxine or an SSRI plus mirtazapine, although poorly studied, is efficacious and well tolerated in some patients with TRD (Carpenter et al. 1999, 2002). In the STAR*D trial, the addition of mirtazapine to venlafaxine in patients in whom three consecutive trials for depression had failed was at least as effective as switching to an MAOI and was far better tolerated (McGrath et al. 2006). Unfortunately, both treatments were only modestly beneficial in these patients with TRD. Only 6.9% achieved remission when a switch was made to tranylcypromine versus 13.7% when mirtazapine was added to venlafaxine. We have found that mirtazapine 15–45 mg qhs is probably more effective than is the addition of trazodone in helping with sleep, anxiety, and depression. Clearly, more study is needed on the utility and tolerability of mirtazapine augmentation.

L-Methylfolate is a cofactor in the synthesis of monoamines. Depression has been associated with low serum and CNS folate levels. It thus follows that supplementation with methylfolate or folic acid may have a role to play in the treatment of depression. Research to date on methylfolate in the treatment of depression has been limited and mostly open label. However, a few controlled studies exist. For example, Godfrey and colleagues (1990) found that the addition of 15 mg of methylfolate to a TCA in depressed patients with low RBC folate levels showed greater improvement over a 6-month period than did those who were treated with a TCA alone. Likewise, Alpert and colleagues (2002) found that the open-label addition of folinic acid in 22 patients who had failed at least 4 weeks of SSRI therapy resulted in a modest but significant benefit. L-Methylfolate has been generally well tolerated, with side effects that do not differ in clinical trials from those seen with placebo. Methylfolate may lower the serum levels of concomitant anticonvulsants, including valproate and carbamazepine, and thus dosage adjustments may be required.

Several reports indicate that adding clonazepam to an SSRI provides more rapid responses in patients with panic disorder or major depression. In a study by Smith et al. (1998), clonazepam at a dosage of 0.5–1.0 mg hs for the first 3 weeks of fluoxetine therapy appeared to have calming effects and to accelerate overall antidepressant response. In another study (Goddard et al. 2001), clonazepam at doses of up to 1.5 mg hs accelerated response to sertraline in panic disorder patients.

Antipsychotic-Antidepressant Combinations

The combination of antidepressants and antipsychotics has been used in the treatment of both psychotic and nonpsychotic depression. Psychotic depression occurs in up to 25% of inpatients with major depression and tends to be less responsive to antidepressant therapy alone than are nondelusional depressions. The data indicate that with the exception of amoxapine, which is chemically related to the antipsychotic loxapine, an antipsychotic-antidepressant combination or electroconvulsive therapy is probably required for effective treatment of this disorder. However, some studies have suggested that monotherapy with SSRIs and newer agents may be effective in the treatment of psychotic depression (Wijkstra et al. 2006; Zanardi et al. 2000). In addition, patients with schizophrenia or schizoaffective disorder frequently develop depressive episodes that may require the addition of an antidepressant to their antipsychotic regimen.

Most studies on psychotic depression have involved combining a TCA with a standard antipsychotic. A prepackaged amitriptyline-perphenazine combination drug is available for use in psychotic and anxious depression. This combination had appeared under two trade names (Triavil and Etrafon), since discontinued. Various combinations of strengths are available, coded according to the dose of each drug contained in the capsule (Table 9–2); the dose of perphenazine is given first. For example, 2-25 contains 2 mg of perphenazine

Table 9–2.   Prepackaged combination antidepressants: names, formulations and strengths, and dosages

Generic name	Brand name	Formulation and strengths[a]	Dosage[b]
chlordiazepoxide–amitriptyline	Limbitrol	Tablets: 5-12.5, 10-25	3 tablets 10-25 to 6 tablets 10-25
perphenazine–amitriptyline	—[c]	Tablets: 2-10, 2-25, 4-10, 4-25, 4-50	2-25 tid to 4-50 qid
olanzapine–fluoxetine	Symbyax	Capsules: 3-25, 6-25, 6-50, 12-25, 12-50	

[a]Formulation strengths list amount (in milligrams) of first and second ingredients, respectively.
[b]Adult dosages; some patients may require lower dosages.
[c]Available in generic form only.

and 25 mg of amitriptyline. This neuroleptic-TCA combination was widely used in the United States and was generally prescribed by primary care practitioners. However, experienced psychopharmacologists advocate prescribing each drug individually to allow for optional flexibility in dosing.

A newer antipsychotic-antidepressant combination pill is the combination of olanzapine and fluoxetine (OFC, or Symbyax). Symbyax was the first drug approved for the treatment of bipolar depression (in 2003) (see Chapter 5: "Mood Stabilizers") and also the first drug treatment approved for TRD (in 2009). In a controlled trial in 853 bipolar patients treated with olanzapine alone, placebo, or OFC (6 mg/25 mg to 12 mg/50 mg), both OFC and olanzapine were better than placebo. OFC was faster and more effective than olanzapine alone (Keck 2002).

A second-generation antipsychotic (SGA), with its serotonin$_{2C}$ receptor (5-HT$_{2C}$) antagonism, would appear to be a useful adjunctive agent with an SSRI. Research in the rat suggests that olanzapine in combination with an SSRI may increase release of prefrontal dopamine. Since 2003, the evidence has steadily mounted that the SGAs are effective augmenters and currently are the only FDA-approved drugs for the adjunctive treatment of depression. (For a more complete review of this topic, see Chapter 4, "Antipsychotic Drugs"). Aripiprazole was approved as an adjunctive treatment for unipolar depression in 2007, and the combination OFC was approved in 2009 for patients who had failed trials with at least two standard antidepressants. Quetiapine's approval for the adjunctive treatment of TRD is pending as of this writing but is expected to be approved. Although the wording of the FDA indications vary a little, in general the studied SGAs appear to be helpful in TRD. However, questions remain about how to best use these agents, including how long they should be used. Because of concerns about metabolic issues, extrapyramidal symptoms (EPS), and cost, it seems reasonable to try to taper the SGA in a patient who has responded to the combination for at least 3-6 months. Our experience is that many patients successfully treated with the combination of an antidepressant plus an SGA may be able to have the SGA discontinued after a period of stabilization. However, no studies exist to guide on whether the combination substantially diminishes the risk of relapse and whether this risk is outweighed by the risk of adverse effects. Some patients clearly do relapse readily after the SGA is discontinued. Thus, the decision to continue a successful trial of an SGA should be discussed with patients on an individual basis.

Anecdotally, we have used all of the atypical agents as augmenters in nonpsychotic depression with variable success. Anxious, agitated depressed patients often seem to benefit from the addition of 5–15 mg/day of olanzapine or 100–200 mg/day of quetiapine. More lethargic patients or those in whom there is a greater concern about weight gain might benefit from augmentation with aripiprazole 10–15 mg/day.

Other TCA Combinations

One of the most controversial TCA combinations is that with MAOIs. Although proscribed in the *Physicians' Desk Reference*, the combination can be relatively safe and is occasionally effective in patients who have failed to respond to treatment with an MAOI or a TCA alone. As indicated in Chapter 3, combining MAOIs with sympathomimetic agents can result in acute hypertensive crises. Because TCAs exert an effect on sympathetic systems, prudence is warranted. Early fears of the combination came largely from a number of deaths that resulted from overdoses of the combination. However, overdoses of either TCAs or MAOIs alone can be lethal.

In contrast to earlier reports, some clinicians have argued that the combination can be of unique benefit. However, double-blind studies comparing a TCA, an MAOI, and their combination in patients with non-TRD have failed to show that the combination is of added benefit. The lack of superior efficacy for the MAOI-TCA combination could reflect the limited doses of both drugs used (e.g., 45 mg of phenelzine and 150 mg of amitriptyline). Some investigators have reported to us that combining higher doses of both is effective, and we have noted positive results from this treatment with some patients. However, generally speaking, a number of important caveats about the combination of an MAOI and a TCA should be noted:

1. It appears safest to start the two drugs together. Adding the TCA to the MAOI is far more dangerous than adding the MAOI to the TCA.
2. Clomipramine combined with an MAOI (particularly tranylcypromine) is far more likely to produce serotonin syndromes than are other TCAs. This combination is to be avoided. Lader, in the United Kingdom (personal communication, 1988), recommended that when switching between an MAOI and clomipramine in either direction, a 4-week interval be observed.
3. Amitriptyline and trimipramine are believed to be the TCAs that best mix with an MAOI—that is, that produce fewer hypertensive crises and, probably, serotonin syndromes. This is largely unproven, although suggestive data do exist.
4. Phenelzine and isocarboxazid appear to be less problematic than does tranylcypromine, which may have an amphetamine-like action.

An early TCA combination drug, Limbitrol (Table 9–2), available in the United States since 1980, contains chlordiazepoxide. It carries an FDA-approved indication for the treatment of mixed anxiety and depression. The numerical designation parallels that of Triavil. Limbitrol 10-25 contains 10 mg of chlordiazepoxide and 25 mg of amitriptyline. It is also available in a 5-12.5 form (Table 9–2). The recommended starting dosage in adults is three or four tablets a day of the 10-25 strength, with a recommended maximum daily dosage of six tablets. In elderly patients, the recommended starting dosage is one 5-12.5 tablet three or four times a day. Although data from previous studies indicated that chlordiazepoxide alone was not an effective antidepressant, the combination was shown to decrease anxiety, to aid sleep early in treatment (within the first 2 weeks), and to be associated with better patient compliance. However, published studies have not indicated that continued additional benefit can be obtained after the initial 4–6 weeks. Whenever possible, clinicians who have used the combination for this initial period should consider switching to prescribing these agents individually and eventually tapering the benzodiazepine. Limbitrol is used quite rarely now, because the sedating effects of chlordiazepoxide are additive to those of amitriptyline. Many patients taking amitriptyline do not require the addition of a benzodiazepine. Thus, the advantages of Limbitrol in ease of use may be outweighed by the disadvantages of the drug. Other benzodiazepines, such as lorazepam and alprazolam, are commonly added to TCAs to treat concurrent agitation or panic in the weeks before the TCA begins working.

Augmentation/Combination Strategies for Bipolar Disorder

Combinations of Two or More Mood Stabilizers

While monotherapy with lithium was the standard treatment for bipolar disorder in 1970, the availability of many newer agents and the limited efficacy of lithium in a large percentage of patients have resulted in polypharmacy as the new standard of care in many, if not most, bipolar patients. Lithium may be combined with anticonvulsants in the treatment of patients with refractory mania. There are few prospective data using such combinations; however, a number of reports indicated that lithium-carbamazepine combinations are effective with patients who have failed to respond to these two agents given separately (see Chapter 5: "Mood Stabilizers"). Retrospective reviews have generally found the combination of lithium and carbamazepine to be useful and synergistic (Lipinski and Pope 1982; Peselow et al. 1994). However, at least one retrospective study (Fritze et al. 1994) failed to find any benefit from combining lithium and carbamazepine in bipolar patients. There is also evidence that the combination of lithium and carbamazepine may be particularly useful in rapid-cycling bipolar disorder. The combination of lithium and carbamazepine appears to be well tolerated. There is one report of increased risk of sinus node dysfunction with this combination (Steckler 1994), but this effect appears to be rare. In addition, the combination of lithium and carbamazepine may have a cumulative antithyroid effect (Kramlinger and Post 1990). There is no evidence of increased neurotoxicity or blood dyscrasias with this combination. Dosing schedules of the lithium and carbamazepine should parallel regimens used for prescribing each drug alone. The therapeutic serum levels of both drugs should be monitored and maintained.

Lithium has also been combined with valproate with good results in patients with treatment-refractory bipolar disorder. One study reported that patients who were older, whose illness lasted longer, who were hospitalized more frequently, and who maintained higher valproate levels might have a better response to the combination of valproate and lithium (McCoy et al. 1993). Few prospective studies are available to evaluate the combination of valproate and lithium in the treatment of refractory bipolar disorder. One of the few prospective studies to date is an open-label study by Sharma et al. (1993), who reported that eight of nine rapid-cycling patients with bipolar disorder, most of whom failed to respond to the combination of lithium and carbamazepine, responded when lithium was combined with valproate. In addition, combining the two drugs also appeared to help the depressive phase of the illness in three of eight subjects. A similar study found that the augmentation of lithium with valproate was successful in stabilizing rapid cycling in four geriatric patients (A. L. Schneider and Wilcox 1998). On the other hand, there did not appear to be a clear advantage of the combination of lithium and valproate in a small randomized controlled trial in patients with rapid cycling and concurrent substance abuse issues (Kemp et al. 2009). A number of small prospective studies suggested that the combination of lithium and valproate may be more effective in the prophylaxis of bipolar episodes than either one alone (Denicoff et al. 1997; Solomon et al. 1997, 1998). The combination of lithium and valproate seems to be well tolerated, and the dosing should achieve adequate serum levels for both drugs. Occasionally, valproate has been combined with carbamazepine when lithium is poorly tolerated or ineffective. There are anecdotal reports that this combination is sometimes useful. However, valproate and carbamazepine compete for hepatic metabolism, an effect that increases the risk of carbamazepine toxicity. For this reason, some investigators have suggested that the combination of valproate and carbamazepine is contraindicated. Our experience suggests that the combination may be used safely if serum levels of both drugs are closely monitored and the doses are adjusted as necessary.

As reported in Chapter 5, other anticonvulsants such as gabapentin, topiramate, and lamotrigine have sometimes been combined with lithium and divalproex sodium in patients with treatment-resistant bipolar disorder. As with most other combination treatments for bipolar disorder, combining lithium or valproate with newer anticonvulsants is poorly studied. Gabapentin has probably been best studied as an adjuvant to lithium in the treatment of bipolar disorder, and the results have been mixed. Some evidence from open-label trials and case reports suggests that gabapentin can help with both manic and depressive symptoms when added to an existing regimen (Ghaemi et al. 1998; Perugi et al. 1999; Young et al. 1999). However, an unpublished double-blind augmentation study found that gabapentin was not significantly more effective than placebo as an add-on. Clearly, the combination of gabapentin with standard mood stabilizers is quite benign and may help with anxiety and agitation even if it proves to be less robust as a mood stabilizer. We typically use 900–2,700 mg/day as an adjuvant and do not recommend gabapentin as a monotherapy for bipolar disorder.

Lamotrigine may prove to be a better mood stabilizer than gabapentin, and we have a number of patients with treatment-resistant illnesses who have done well with the addition of lamotrigine. There are very few data, other than case reports, on the utility of lamotrigine combinations. The combination of lamotrigine with valproate or carbamazepine is more difficult to manage than the combination with lithium. Valproate doubles the serum level of lamotrigine, increasing the risk of rash, whereas carbamazepine cuts the lamotrigine serum levels in half. We have found lamotrigine at dosages in the range of 50–200 mg/day particularly helpful in treating bipolar depression in combination with lithium.

Topiramate may be more useful as an adjuvant than as an augmenting agent. The addition of 50–200 mg of topiramate to a standard mood-stabilizing regimen can help mitigate weight gain. Whether topiramate also helps augment mood-stabilizing effects is less clear at this time. Controlled monotherapy trials have been disappointing.

Mood Stabilizer–Antipsychotic Combinations

The combinations of an SGA and lithium or valproate are perhaps the most common combinations used in all phases of bipolar disorder. Most of the SGAs are FDA approved as an adjunctive treatment to lithium or valproate in the treatment of acute mania or mixed states. The American Psychiatric Association Treatment Guidelines have, since 2002, recommended that SGAs be combined with mood stabilizers for severe acute manic or mixed states. In addition, the combination of olanzapine and fluoxetine, and the SGA quetiapine, are approved for bipolar depression. In the maintenance phase, the only approved adjunctive treatment as of this writing is quetiapine combined with a mood stabilizer. Lithium does have some antidopaminergic properties, and some patients may have a greater proclivity for developing EPS when lithium is combined with antipsychotics. This appears to be particularly true at higher or toxic lithium serum levels. Likewise, it has been suggested that lithium increases the risk of tardive dyskinesia in patients also treated with first-generation antipsychotics. However, whether lithium really adds to the risk of antipsychotic-induced tardive dyskinesia is still unanswered. As reported earlier, there does not appear to be evidence of an increased risk of neurotoxicity when lithium is combined with a high-potency first-generation antipsychotic.

In a pooled analysis of five of the larger controlled trials of SGAs combined with lithium or valproate in acute mania versus a mood stabilizer alone, Ketter and colleagues (2006) concluded that there was about a 20% advantage of combination treatment versus monotherapy. This is roughly equivalent to the advantage of monotherapy with a mood stabilizer or SGA over placebo in the treatment of acute mania. Thus, the authors concluded that there appeared to be a distinct advantage of combining an SGA with lithium or valproate in acute mania. On the other hand, the combination of an SGA with carbamazepine has been less successful. For example, there appeared to be no advantage to combining olanzapine with carbamazepine in the treatment of acute mania relative to carbamazepine monotherapy (Tohen et al. 2008). In addition, the combination was more poorly tolerated than was carbamazepine monotherapy.

Quetiapine was approved in 2008 in combination with valproate or lithium in the maintenance treatment of bipolar I disorder. In patients who had been stabilized on lithium or valproate, the addition of quetiapine was significantly better than the addition of placebo in preventing both depressive and manic episodes over the next 24 weeks (Suppes et al. 2009). Far fewer patients had a relapse of a mood episode while taking the combination treatment (20%) versus monotherapy with lithium or valproate (52%). As expected, the combination of quetiapine with lithium or valproate was also less well tolerated than was adjunctive placebo, with higher rates of weight gain, sedation, and discontinuation due to adverse events.

Clozapine tends to be at the bottom of the treatment algorithm for treatment-resistant bipolar disorder because of its toxicity and complexity of use. As reported in Chapter 5, patients with treatment-resistant bipolar disorder often respond to clozapine therapy. The combination of lithium and clozapine may be synergistic—an effect that is a double-edged sword. On the one hand, some patients with refractory illness have a response after addition of clozapine to their regimens. In addition, lithium may mitigate the leukopenia associated with clozapine (Adityanjee 1995). On the other hand, most of the known cases of neuroleptic malignant syndrome (NMS) associated with clozapine have been associated with concurrent lithium use. Still, for the patient with treatment-resistant bipolar disorder, the addition or substitution of clozapine in the regimen remains an important option if other mood stabilizers and antipsychotics have failed.

Mood Stabilizer–Antidepressant Combinations

It is still common practice to use an antidepressant with a mood stabilizer to treat the depressed phase of bipolar illness. However, the utility of this combination remains questionable. As reported in Chapter 4, most studies evaluating the addition of an antidepressant to a mood stabilizer for the treatment of bipolar depression have not found clear advantages over adding placebo. For example, STEP-BD found that 23% of patients with bipolar depression treated with an antidepressant in combination with a mood stabilizer achieved euthymia for at least 8 consecutive weeks, compared with 27% of patients who had placebo added to a mood stabilizer (Sachs et al. 2007). Likewise, Nemeroff and colleagues (2001) did not find an advantage for adding imipramine or paroxetine to lithium versus adding placebo in bipolar depressed patients. However, patients with lower lithium serum levels (<0.8 mEq/L) did better with the addition of an antidepressant than they did with the addition of placebo. Thus, depressed bipolar patients who cannot tolerate a higher lithium level might benefit from the addition of an antidepressant.

Since antidepressants have not fared well in combination studies, a related question is whether the addition of a second mood stabilizer is superior to the combination of an antidepressant and a mood stabilizer in the treatment of bipolar depression. A study by Young et al. (2000) attempted to answer this question. Twenty-seven depressed bipolar patients were randomly assigned to either paroxetine or an additional mood stabilizer (either lithium or valproate).

Over the 6-week trial, both strategies improved the depression, but patients were more likely to benefit from the paroxetine than they were from the mood stabilizer. Since this was a short trial, it is still conceivable that the addition of an antidepressant may be more problematic in the long run than is the addition of another mood stabilizer. While many depressed bipolar patients do not appear to benefit from the addition of an antidepressant to a mood stabilizer, some patients clearly do. We have observed some bipolar patients who clearly do more poorly when an antidepressant is discontinued. In patients who are tolerating the combination and appear to be benefiting, it makes sense to continue that combination.

Among the potential drawbacks of using antidepressants in bipolar patients is the induction of rapid cycling and switching into mania (Wehr and Goodwin 1979; Wehr et al. 1988). The induction of rapid cycling has mostly been observed with TCAs, but it may occur with MAOIs, SSRIs, and other classes of drugs.

Bupropion was initially thought to be less likely to induce rapid cycling or mixed states, but a few cases of bupropion-induced mixed states and manic episodes have been reported. On the basis of the limited data, we suggest trying bupropion or SSRIs before treating a depressed cycle of bipolar illness with a noradrenergic antidepressant, including a TCA, duloxetine, or venlafaxine. If rapid cycling is induced, the antidepressant should be discontinued if possible, and a combination of mood stabilizers, with or without thyroid supplement, should be considered.

Mood Stabilizers and Omega-3 Fatty Acids

Omega-3 and omega-6 fatty acids are the building blocks of fats in the same way that amino acids are the building blocks of proteins. A number of reports since the early 1990s suggested that affective illness may be associated with deficiencies of some omega-3 fatty acids. For example, there appears to be a higher ratio of arachidonic acid to eicosapentaenoic acid in more severely depressed patients compared with less severely depressed patients. Other studies have suggested that there may be lower omega-3 fatty acids in the red blood cell membranes of depressed patients compared with healthy control subjects. Furthermore, some limited evidence suggests that omega-3 fatty acids may impact signal transduction in a manner analogous to lithium.

A preliminary double-blind study reported that adding supplemental omega-3 fatty acids to the drug regimens of bipolar patients improved their outcomes (Stoll et al. 1999). In this study, 30 bipolar patients were randomly assigned to either 9.6 g/day of omega-3 supplements or olive oil (as a control) for 4 months. They continued taking standard mood stabilizers. The patients treated with omega-3 experienced longer remission and more complete resolution of symptoms than the placebo-treated patients. More recent studies of the adjunctive use of omega-3 fatty acids in both bipolar disorder and unipolar depression have been inconclusive (see Chapters 5 and 13, this volume). A Cochrane review of the five controlled trials completed to date of omega-3 fatty acids in the treatment of bipolar disorder concluded that there was little evidence that these supplements help manic symptoms but might help depressive symptoms in bipolar patients (Montgomery and Richardson 2008).

The American Psychiatric Association has taken the position that patients with a mood disorder might benefit from the addition of omega-3 fatty acids to their diet. The APA has suggested at least two servings of fatty fish, such as salmon, per week or 1 g of EPA/DHA per day. Since these fatty acids are fairly benign and may have other health benefits, we think it is not unreasonable to supplement the mood-stabilizing regimens of bipolar patients with omega-3 fatty acids. Although dramatic benefits are uncommon in our experience, the downsides are minimal. Children and pregnant women should avoid eating those fish with the highest levels of mercury (and other heavy metal) concentration (i.e., shark, mackerel, swordfish). In addition, the FDA recommends eating no more than 12 oz. a week of fish with lower mercury levels, such as canned light tuna, salmon, pollock, and catfish.

Augmentation Strategies for Schizophrenia

Combinations of Two Antipsychotics

Combining two or more antipsychotics is generally frowned upon, since the utility of this approach is not clear. However, an atypical antipsychotic can sometimes be augmented by a standard antipsychotic drug. The most common example is the combination of clozapine, which has limited D_2 antagonism, and haloperidol or perphenazine. Although few data are available on the efficacy of this approach, some patients appear to benefit. Risperidone combined with a standard antipsychotic resulted in a modest but significant improvement in some patients with chronic schizophrenia studied prospectively (Takahashi et al. 1999). The combination of other atypical antipsychotics and standard antipsychotics may also be warranted if the maximum dosage of the atypical agent has been achieved with less than satisfactory benefit. We tend to prefer the addition of high-potency agents, because the weight gain, hypotensive, and sedation problems associated with the atypical antipsychotics complicate the addition of low-potency agents. Since risperidone is such a potent D_2 antagonist by itself, we push the dosage of risperidone as tolerated by the patient up to 12 mg/day rather than add a standard antipsychotic to it.

Does it make any sense to combine two atypical agents? Perhaps. A few case reports have suggested that the addition of risperidone to clozapine might be helpful for some patients with refractory schizophrenia (see Morera et al. 1999). However, the α-adrenergic receptor–blocking properties of risperidone might be problematic in some patients being treated with clozapine, and the addition of haloperidol might work just as well and with fewer complications. Likewise, the combination of clozapine with aripiprazole (Ziegenbein et al. 2006) or ziprasidone (Ziegenbein and Calliess 2006) has been anecdotally suggested to be beneficial and well tolerated in patients with resistant schizophrenia. On the other hand, combining aripiprazole with other antipsychotics has sometimes been associated with a worsening of symptoms (Chan and Sweeting 2007; Chan et al. 2006). In general, the evidence that the combination of two antipsychotics is better than one is not compelling. In a review of studies involving clozapine and various antipsychotics, Cipriani and colleagues (2009) concluded that the benefits of these combinations could not clearly be demonstrated in the studies completed to date.

Combining two standard antipsychotics is sometimes done, but with unclear benefits. The most common combination is a high-potency agent such a haloperidol and a low-potency agent such as chlorpromazine. The rationale for using the low-potency agent is usually to help with sleep. However, the clinician could obtain the same effect from adding higher doses of diphenhydramine (50–100 mg qhs) to the antipsychotic, or better yet, a benzodiazepine. There is the rare patient who clinically does better with two different standard antipsychotics, but there is rarely a time that another class of agents (an atypical antipsychotic, a benzodiazepine, or a mood stabilizer) might not work even better.

Combinations of Antidepressants and Antipsychotics

The SSRIs and other antidepressants have been combined with antipsychotics in the treatment of negative symptoms and depression in schizophrenia, schizoaffective disorder, and psychotic depression. Open-label studies have suggested that fluoxetine and fluvoxamine may help with negative symptoms and mood problems in patients with schizophrenia (Goldman and Janecek 1990; Silver and Nassar 1992). One potential problem is that the SSRIs may raise the serum levels of standard and atypical antipsychotics. In a double-blind trial of fluoxetine added to a depot neuroleptic, negative symptoms were clearly improved with the fluoxetine treatment, but serum levels of the antipsychotic were increased an average of 65% with fluphenazine and 20% with haloperidol decanoate (Goff et al. 1995). Although EPS did not worsen in this study, some patients clearly had a worsening of akathisia and other symptoms with the addition of fluoxetine or other SSRIs to their antipsychotic regimen. Therefore, lower antipsychotic doses may be required when antipsychotics are combined with the SSRIs. As indicated previously, SSRIs, particularly fluvoxamine, can markedly elevate serum clozapine levels.

Other antidepressants may also benefit negative symptoms. Trazodone has shown modest benefits in the treatment of negative symptoms, as has moclobemide. Trazodone produces significant but modest improvements in negative symptoms compared with placebo when added to a standard antipsychotic (Decina et al. 1994). Bodkin et al. (1996) found that selegiline 5 mg bid over 6 weeks significantly improved negative symptoms and EPS in a group of 21 patients with schizophrenia or schizoaffective disorder but had no effect on positive symptoms. At these low dosages, one would not anticipate significant interactions with atypical, serotonergic antipsychotics, but caution should be exercised. Transdermal selegiline at a dosage of 6 mg/day would be expected to be at least as safe as low-dose oral selegiline. However, transdermal selegiline has not been evaluated in schizophrenia as of this writing.

Finally, low doses of standard antipsychotics may actually increase the availability of dopamine synaptically by stimulating presynaptic dopamine autoreceptors to release more dopamine. There have been some anecdotal reports of both worsening of positive symptoms and improvement of negative symptoms with low-dose antipsychotics. In a placebo-controlled study, amisulpride, a dopamine-blocking benzamide antipsychotic not yet available in the United States, was found to significantly improve negative symptoms of schizophrenia at low doses (Boyer et al. 1995). At high doses, amisulpride and standard antipsychotics may worsen negative symptoms by dampening dopaminergic tone throughout the prefrontal cortex.

Combinations of Mood Stabilizers and Antipsychotics

As many as a third of schizophrenic patients do not respond adequately to an antipsychotic. One of the earliest augmentation strategies for treatment-resistant schizophrenia was the addition of lithium. Lithium augmentation of neuroleptics at relatively low dosages (300–900 mg/day) has been said to be helpful in the treatment of schizophrenia (Johns and Thompson 1995). However, most of the reports suggesting that lithium is a useful augmenting agent in treating schizophrenia have been anecdotal. Several randomized, controlled studies have investigated the efficacy of lithium when added to an antipsychotic. None has shown any benefit of adding lithium over adding placebo in patients with well-characterized schizophrenia (Collins et al. 1991; Schulz et al. 1999; Wilson 1993). It may be that earlier reports included patients with schizoaffective disorder or psychotic mania, who may clearly benefit from lithium. Since lithium appears to increase the risk of EPS and perhaps NMS with antipsychotics, we suggest using lithium augmentation primarily in treating patients with suspected schizoaffective disorder. The dosage of the antipsychotic may need to be lowered in some patients treated concurrently with lithium.

Valproate has been shown to be helpful as an adjunctive treatment in combination with antipsychotics in the treatment of acute exacerbations of schizophrenia. Casey and colleagues (2003) reported that adding 15–30 mg/kg/day of valproate resulted in earlier improvement in psychotic symptoms in acutely ill schizophrenic patients. However, the effects of valproate as an augmenter tend not to be evident at the endpoint of most trials (Basan et al. 2004). Thus, valproate's primary utility might be in speeding response, or perhaps as an adjunct in treating agitation in some patients.

It has also been suggested that carbamazepine may boost antipsychotic effects. As with lithium, many anecdotal and open-label studies have suggested a role for carbamazepine in treatment-resistant schizophrenia. However, as with lithium, controlled trials have failed to show much benefit of adding carbamazepine to an antipsychotic (Llorca et al. 1993; Martin Munoz et al. 1992). Since carbamazepine can substantially lower the serum levels of most concurrent antipsychotics, we find it difficult to use carbamazepine as an augmenting agent in treating schizophrenia.

An alternative to carbamazepine or valproate as an adjunctive agent in schizophrenia may be topiramate. The addition of topiramate to antipsychotics has been reported to be beneficial in resistant schizophrenia in a controlled trial (Tiihonen et al. 2005). Topiramate may also have the advantage of mitigating antipsychotic-induced weight gain.

There has been some evidence that adding lamotrigine to clozapine may be helpful in patients with treatment-resistant schizophrenia. At least five small open or controlled trials have been completed to date of adding lamotrigine to clozapine. In general, the addition of lamotrigine appears to modestly help both positive and negative symptoms in patients who have not responded to clozapine monotherapy (Citrome 2009). On the other hand, the addition of lamotrigine 100–400 mg/day to various other SGAs did not show much benefit (Goff et al. 2007). Lamotrigine is currently being investigated as an adjunctive agent in schizophrenia to specifically target cognitive deficits, as this potential benefit has been seen in at least one of the controlled trials.

In general, mood stabilizers have been thought to have a limited role as augmenting agents in the treatment of the core symptoms of schizophrenia. We have believed, on the other hand, that mood stabilizers have a role as adjuvant agents in treating aggressive outbursts and agitation in patients with schizophrenia. We have found gabapentin, at dosages up to 3,600 mg/day, and valproate, at dosages of 750–2,000 mg/day, helpful in treating agitation and aggression in some patients with schizophrenia. In addition, gabapentin may have the added benefit of helping with EPS in patients treated with standard antipsychotics (see Chapter 5: "Mood Stabilizers").

Other Augmentation Strategies

Since cognitive and executive deficits in schizophrenia appear to be one of the major factors that limit functioning in patients with schizophrenia, the NIMH has been interested in fostering research that leads to better treatment of cognitive deficits in this population. The Measurement and Treatment Research to Improve Cognition in Schizophrenia (MATRICS) program has begun to evaluate possible treatments. Among the adjunctive medications that might have a role to play in improving cognition in schizophrenia patients are stimulants, modafinil, atomoxetine, and acetylcholinesterase inhibitors, among other agents. Small studies have suggested that amphetamine can help working memory and executive dysfunction in patients with schizophrenia (Barch et al. 2005). While stimulants can worsen positive symptoms, they often help negative symptoms (see Chapter 4). In contrast, modafinil has not been particularly helpful for treating executive deficits in schizophrenia patients to date (Savedra-Valez et al. 2009), although it may help on some global measures of negative symptoms. Likewise, atomoxetine and acetylcholinesterase inhibitors have also not been particularly efficacious (Kelly et al. 2009). The search continues for viable treatments for cognitive deficits in schizophrenia. A promising experimental strategy is the potential use of $\alpha7$ nicotinic agonists (Barak et al. 2009).

Abnormalities in glutamate transmission, particularly hypofunctioning of the N-methyl-D-aspartate (NMDA) glutamate receptor, have been proposed in the etiology of deficit symptoms in schizophrenia. To this end, a number of studies have examined the role of glycine and D-cycloserine in augmenting the effects of antipsychotics. D-Cycloserine is an agonist of the NMDA receptor, and a number of controlled trials have suggested that D-cycloserine improves negative symptoms and neuropsychological functioning in patients taking standard antipsychotics (Goff et al. 1999b; Rosse et al. 1996; Tsai et al. 1998) but not in those taking clozapine (Goff et al. 1996, 1999a; Tsai et al. 1999). The dosage of D-cycloserine that was most effective was around 50 mg/day and tended to be well tolerated. The effects of D-cycloserine on negative symptoms and cognitive functioning, though significant, have not been particularly robust.

Glycine is an amino acid that is a co-agonist of the NMDA receptor. Early open trials suggested that glycine helps some patients with schizophrenia and worsens symptoms in others (Rosse et al. 1989). A more recent crossover trial of high-dose glycine (0.8 g/kg) added to an antipsychotic found that negative symptoms were significantly improved relative to placebo (Heresco-Levy et al. 1999). Glycine augmentation is a fairly benign strategy for improving negative symptoms. However, it is unlikely that adding glycine to a standard antipsychotic is better in improving negative symptoms than simply switching to an atypical agent. For patients who do not respond as well to an atypical antipsychotic, the addition of glycine or D-cycloserine may be an option.

Cyproheptadine (Periactin) is a general serotonin antagonist used primarily to treat migraines and allergies. Its serotonin receptor antagonist properties have made it of interest to clinicians treating negative symptoms in schizophrenia, since all atypical antipsychotics are also 5-HT$_2$ antagonists. In a controlled trial, cyproheptadine at a dosage of 24 mg/day significantly improved negative symptoms and was well tolerated (Akhondzadeh et al. 1999). Cyproheptadine also has the advantage of being anticholingergic and can help with EPS. The problem with cyproheptadine is that most patients find it quite sedating, and 24 mg/day is a large dosage for many patients. It is unclear whether smaller dosages might work just as well.

Finally, the serotonin$_3$ (5-HT$_3$) antagonist ondansetron has also been reported to be a useful adjunctive or augmenting agent in resistant schizophrenia. Over the past 15 years, a number of anecdotal reports have suggested that ondansetron, which is used primarily as an antinausea medication, might help the cognitive and negative symptoms of schizophrenia. The first double-blind study of ondansetron in resistant schizophrenia also seems to support the benefits of this agent (Zhang et al. 2006). Patients with schizophrenia that is unresponsive to haloperidol were more likely to see a 30% improvement in psychotic symptoms than were patients who had placebo added to the haloperidol. Ondansetron is well tolerated but currently quite expensive. The dosage of ondansetron used in Zhang et al.'s (2006) study was 8 mg/day administered for 12 weeks.

Bibliography

Adityanjee: Modification of clozapine-induced leukopenia and neutropenia with lithium carbonate (letter). Am J Psychiatry 152:648–649, 1995

Akhondzadeh S, Mohammadi MR, Amini-Nooshabadi H, et al: Cyproheptadine in treatment of chronic schizophrenia: a double-blind, placebo-controlled study. J Clin Pharm Ther 24:49–52, 1999

Alpert JE, Mischoulon D, Rubenstein GE, et al: Folinic acid (Leucovorin) as an adjunctive treatment for SSRI-refractory depression. Ann Clin Psychiatry 14:33–38, 2002

Alvarez E, Perez-Sola V, Perez-Blanco J, et al: Predicting outcome of lithium added to antidepressants in resistant depression. J Affect Disord 42:179–186, 1997

Aranow RB, Hudson JL, Pope HG Jr, et al: Elevated antidepressant plasma levels after addition of fluoxetine. Am J Psychiatry 146:911–913, 1989

Artigas F, Perez V, Alvarez E: Pindolol induces a rapid improvement of depressed patients treated with serotonin reuptake inhibitors. Arch Gen Psychiatry 51:248–251, 1994

Austin LS, Arana GW, Melvin JA: Toxicity resulting from lithium augmentation of antidepressant treatment in elderly patients. J Clin Psychiatry 51:344–345, 1990

Bakish D, Hooper CL, Thornton MD, et al: Fast onset: an open study of the treatment of major depressive disorder with nefazodone and pindolol combination therapy. Int Clin Psychopharmacol 12:91–97, 1997

Barak S, Arad M, De Levie A, et al: Pro-cognitive and antipsychotic efficacy of the alpha7 nicotinic partial agonist SSR180711 in pharmacological and neurodevelopmental latent inhibition models of schizophrenia. Neuropsychopharmacology 34:1753–1763, 2009

Barch DM, Carter CS: Amphetamine improves cognitive function in medicated individuals with schizophrenia and in healthy volunteers. Schizophr Res 77:43–58, 2005

Baron BM, Ogden AM, Seigel BW, et al: Rapid down-regulation of beta-adrenoreceptors by co-administration of desipramine and fluoxetine. Eur J Pharmacol 154:125–134, 1988

Basan A, Kissling W, Leucht S: Valproate as an adjunct to antipsychotics for schizophrenia: a systematic review of randomized trials. Schizophr Res 70:33–37, 2004

Bauer M, Dopfmer S: Lithium augmentation in treatment-resistant depression: meta-analysis of placebo-controlled studies. J Clin Psychopharmacol 19:427–434, 1999

Bauer M, Hellweg R, Graf KJ, et al: Treatment of refractory depression with high-dose thyroxine. Neuropsychopharmacology 18:444–455, 1998

Bauer M, Zaninelli R, Muller-Oerlinghausen B, et al: Paroxetine and amitriptyline augmentation of lithium in the treatment of major depression: a double-blind study. J Clin Psychopharmacol 19:164–171, 1999

Bell IR, Cole JO: Fluoxetine induces elevation of desipramine levels and exacerbation of geriatric nonpsychotic depression (letter). J Clin Psychopharmacol 8:447–448, 1988

Blier P, Bergeson R: Effectiveness of pindolol with selected antidepressant drugs in the treatment of major depression. J Clin Psychopharmacol 15:217–222, 1995

Bloch M, Schmidt PJ, Danaceau MA, et al: Dehydroepiandrosterone treatment of midlife dysthymia. Biol Psychiatry 45:1533–1544, 1999

Bodkin JA, Cohen BM, Salomon MS, et al: Treatment of negative symptoms in schizophrenia and schizoaffective disorder by selegiline augmentation of antipsychotic medication: a pilot study examining the role of dopamine. J Nerv Ment Dis 184:295–301, 1996

Bodkin JA, Lasser RA, Wines JD Jr, et al: Combining serotonin reuptake inhibitors and bupropion in partial responders to antidepressant monotherapy. J Clin Psychiatry 58:137–145, 1997

Bommer M, Naber D: Subclinical hypothyroidism in recurrent mania. Biol Psychiatry 31:729–734, 1992 [also see comments]

Bouwer C, Stein DJ: Buspirone is an effective augmenting agent of serotonin selective reuptake inhibitors in severe treatment-refractory depression. S Afr Med J 87 (4, suppl):534–537, 540, 1997

Bowden CL, Myers JE, Grossman F, et al: Risperidone in combination with mood stabilizers: a 10-week continuation phase study in bipolar I disorder. J Clin Psychiatry 65:707–714, 2004

Boyer P, Lecrubier Y, Puech AJ, et al: Treatment of negative symptoms in schizophrenia with amisulpride. Br J Psychiatry 166:68–72, 1995

Buchanan RW, Freedman R, Javitt DC, et al: Recent advances in the development of novel pharmacological agents for the treatment of cognitive impairments in schizophrenia. Schizophr Bull 33:1120–1130, 2007

Bunevicius R, Kazanavicius G, Zalinkevicius R, et al: Effects of thyroxine as compared with thyroxine plus triiodothyronine in patients with hypothyroidism. N Engl J Med 340:424–429, 1999

Carpenter LL, Jocic Z, Hall JM, et al: Mirtazapine augmentation in the treatment of refractory depression. J Clin Psychiatry 60:45–49, 1999

Carpenter LL, Yasmin S, Price LH: A double-blind, placebo-controlled study of antidepressant augmentation with mirtazapine. Biol Psychiatry 51:183–188, 2002

Casey DE, Daniel DG, Wassef AA, et al: Effect of divalproex combined with olanzapine or risperidone in patients with an acute exacerbation of schizophrenia. Neuropsychopharmacology 28:182–192, 2003

Cassano P, Lattanzi L, Fava M, et al: Ropinirole in treatment-resistant depression: a 16-week pilot study. Can J Psychiatry 50:357–360, 2005

Cattell DL, King EA: Estrogen for postnatal depression. J Fam Pract 43:22–23, 1996

Chambers CD, Johnson KA, Dick LM, et al: Birth outcomes in pregnant women taking fluoxetine. N Engl J Med 335:1010–1015, 1996 [also see comments]

Chan J, Sweeting M: Combination therapy with non-clozapine atypical antipsychotic medication: a review of current evidence. J Psychopharmacol 21:657–664, 2007

Chang JS, Ha KS, Young Lee K, et al: The effects of long-term clozapine add-on therapy on the rehospitalization rate and the mood polarity patterns in bipolar disorders. J Clin Psychiatry 67:461–467, 2006

Cipriani A, Boso M, Barbui C: Clozapine combined with different antipsychotic drugs for treatment resistant schizophrenia. Cochrane Database Syst Rev July 8(3):CD006324, 2009

Citrome L: Adjunctive lithium and anticonvulsants for the treatment of schizophrenia: what is the evidence? Expert Rev Neurother 9:55–71, 2009

Collins PJ, Larkin EP, Shubsachs AP: Lithium carbonate in chronic schizophrenia—a brief trial of lithium carbonate added to neuroleptics for treatment of resistant schizophrenic patients. Acta Psychiatr Scand 84:150–154, 1991

Cooke RG, Joffe RT, Levitt AJ: T3 augmentation of antidepressant treatment in T4-replaced thyroid patients. J Clin Psychiatry 53:16–18, 1992 [also see comments]

Coope J: Is estrogen effective in the treatment of menopausal depression? J R Coll Gen Pract 31:134–180, 1981

Cooper-Kazaz R, van der Deure WM, Medici M, et al: Preliminary evidence that a functional polymorphism in type 1 deiodinase is associated with enhanced potentiation of the antidepressant effect of sertraline by triiodothyronine. J Affect Disord 116:113–116, 2009

Corrigan MH, Denahan AQ, Wright CE, et al: Comparison of pramipexole, fluoxetine, and placebo in patients with major depression. Depress Anxiety 11:58–65, 2000

Crowe D, Collins JP, Rosse RB: Thyroid hormone supplementation of fluoxetine treatment (letter). J Clin Psychopharmacol 10:150–151, 1990

DeBattista C: Pramipexole in the treatment of resistant depression. Presentation at the annual meeting of the New Clinical Drug Evaluation Unit (NCDEU), Boca Raton, FL, 1997

DeBattista C, Schatzberg AF: Estrogen modulation of monoamines, in Estrogen in Mental Health: From the Bench to the Bedside. Edited by Liebenluft E. Washington, DC, American Psychiatric Publishing, 1999

DeBattista C, Solvason HB, Breen JA, et al: Pramipexole augmentation of a selective serotonin reuptake inhibitor in the treatment of depression. J Clin Psychopharmacol 20:274–275, 2000

DeBattista C, Solvason HB, Poirer J, et al: A prospective trial of bupropion SR augmentation of partial and nonresponders to serotonergic antidepressants. J Clin Psychopharmacol 23:27–30, 2003

DeBattista C, Lembke A, Solvason HB, et al: A prospective trial of modafinil as an adjunctive treatment of major depression. J Clin Psychopharmacol 24:87–90, 2004

DeBattista C, Patkar P, Hawkins J: Ropinirole augmentation of standard antidepressants in the treatment of resistant depression. Presented at the 48th Annual Meeting of the New Clinical Drug Evaluation Unit (NCDEU), Session 1, Phoenix, AZ, 2008

Decina P, Mukherjee S, Bocola V, et al: Adjunctive trazodone in the treatment of negative symptoms of schizophrenia. Hosp Community Psychiatry 45:1220–1223, 1994

Dehydroepiandrosterone (DHEA). Med Lett Drugs Ther 8 (985; October 11):91–92, 1996

de Montigny C, Grunberg F, Mayer A, et al: Lithium induces rapid relief of depression in tricyclic antidepressant drug non-responders. Br J Psychiatry 138:252–255, 1981

de Montigny C, Cournoyer G, Morissette R, et al: Lithium carbonate addition in tricyclic antidepressant–resistant unipolar depression. Arch Gen Psychiatry 40:1327–1334, 1983

Denicoff KD, Smith-Jackson EE, Bryan AL, et al: Valproate prophylaxis in a prospective clinical trial of refractory bipolar disorder. Am J Psychiatry 154:1456–1458, 1997 [also see comments]

Dennis CL, Ross LE, Herxheimer A: Oestrogens and progestins for preventing and treating postpartum depression. Cochrane Database Syst Rev October 8;(4):CD001690, 2008

Eden Evins A, Demopulos C, Nierenberg A, et al: A double-blind, placebo-controlled trial of adjunctive donepezil in treatment-resistant mania. Bipolar Disord 8:75–80, 2006a

Eden Evins A, Demopulos C, Yovel I, et al: Inositol augmentation of lithium or valproate for bipolar depression. Bipolar Disord 8:168–174, 2006b

Everett HC: The use of bethanechol chloride with tricyclic antidepressants. Am J Psychiatry 132:1202–1206, 1976

Fatemi SH, Emamian ES, Kist DA: Venlafaxine and bupropion combination therapy in a case of treatment-resistant depression. Ann Pharmacother 33:701–703, 1999

Fava M, Rosenbaum JF, McGrath PJ, et al: Lithium and tricyclic augmentation of fluoxetine treatment for resistant major depression: a double-blind, controlled study. Am J Psychiatry 151:1372–1374, 1994

Fava M, Thase ME, DeBattista C, et al: Modafinil augmentation of selective serotonin reuptake inhibitor therapy in MDD partial responders with persistent fatigue and sleepiness. Ann Clin Psychiatry 19:153–159, 2007

Fawcett J, Kravitz HM, Zajeda JM, et al: CNS stimulant potentiation of monoamine oxidase inhibitors in treatment refractory depression. J Clin Psychopharmacol 11:127–132, 1991

Feighner JP, Brauzer B, Gelenberg AJ, et al: A placebo-controlled multicenter trial of Limbitrol versus its components (amitriptyline and chlordiazepoxide) in the symptomatic treatment of depressive illness. Psychopharmacology (Berl) 61:217–225, 1979

Ferraro L, Antonelli T, O'Connor WT, et al: Modafinil: an antinarcoleptic drug with a different neurochemical profile to d-amphetamine and dopamine uptake blockers. Biol Psychiatry 42:1181–1183, 1997

Flint AJ, Rifat SL: A prospective study of lithium augmentation in antidepressant-resistant geriatric depression. J Clin Psychopharmacol 14:353–356, 1994

Fontaine R, Ontiveros A, Elie R, et al: Lithium carbonate augmentation of desipramine and fluoxetine in refractory depression. Biol Psychiatry 29:946–948, 1991 [erratum: Biol Psychiatry 31:322, 1992; also see comments]

Freedman R, Olincy A, Buchanan RW, et al: Initial phase 2 trial of a nicotinic agonist in schizophrenia. Am J Psychiatry 165:1040–1047, 2008

Fritze J, Beneke M, Lanczik M, et al: Carbamazepine as adjunct or alternative to lithium in the prophylaxis of recurrent affective disorders. Pharmacopsychiatry 27:181–185, 1994

Geretsegger C, Bitterlich W, Stelzig R, et al: Paroxetine with pindolol augmentation: a double-blind, randomized, placebo-controlled study in depressed in-patients. Eur Neuropsychopharmacol 18:141–146, 2008

Gerner RH, Stanton A: Algorithm for patient management of acute manic states: lithium, valproate, or carbamazepine? J Clin Psychopharmacol 12 (1, suppl):57S–63S, 1992

Ghaemi SN, Goodwin FK: Use of atypical antipsychotic agents in bipolar and schizoaffective disorders: review of the empirical literature. J Clin Psychopharmacol 19:354–361, 1999

Ghaemi SN, Sachs GS, Baldassano CF, et al: Acute treatment of bipolar disorder with adjunctive risperidone in outpatients. Can J Psychiatry 42:196–199, 1997

Ghaemi SN, Katzow JJ, Desai SP, et al: Gabapentin treatment of mood disorders: a preliminary study. J Clin Psychiatry 59:426–429, 1998

Ghaemi SN, Schrauwen E, Klugman J, et al: Long-term lamotrigine plus lithium for bipolar disorder: one year outcome. J Psychiatr Pract 12:300–305, 2006

Gitlin MJ, Weiner H, Fairbanks L, et al: Failure of T3 to potentiate tricyclic antidepressant response. J Affect Disord 13:267–272, 1987

Goddard AW, Brouette T, Almai A, et al: Early coadministration of clonazepam with sertraline for panic disorder. Arch Gen Psychiatry 58:681–686, 2001

Godfrey PS, Toone BK, Carney MW, et al: Enhancement of recovery from psychiatric illness by methylfolate. Lancet 336(8712):392–395, 1990

Goff DC, Midha KK, Sarid-Segal O, et al: A placebo-controlled trial of fluoxetine added to neuroleptic in patients with schizophrenia. Psychopharmacology (Berl) 117:417–423, 1995

Goff DC, Tsai G, Manoach DS, et al: D-Cycloserine added to clozapine for patients with schizophrenia. Am J Psychiatry 153:1628–1630, 1996

Goff DC, Henderson DC, Evins AE, et al: A placebo-controlled crossover trial of D-cycloserine added to clozapine in patients with schizophrenia. Biol Psychiatry 45:512–514, 1999a

Goff DC, Tsai G, Levitt J, et al: A placebo-controlled trial of D-cycloserine added to conventional neuroleptics in patients with schizophrenia. Arch Gen Psychiatry 56:21–27, 1999b [also see comments]

Goff DC, Keefe R, Citrome L, et al: Lamotrigine as add-on therapy in schizophrenia: results of 2 placebo-controlled trials. J Clin Psychopharmacol 27:582–589, 2007

Goldberg JF, Burdick KE, Endick CJ: Preliminary randomized, double-blind, placebo-controlled trial of pramipexole added to mood stabilizers for treatment-resistant bipolar depression. Am J Psychiatry 161:564–566, 2004

Goldman MB, Janecek HM: Adjunctive fluoxetine improves global functioning in chronic schizophrenia. J Neuropsychiatry Clin Neurosci 2:429–431, 1990

Goodwin FK, Prange A, Post RM, et al: Potentiation of antidepressant effects by L-triiodothyronine in tricyclic nonresponders. Am J Psychiatry 139:34–38, 1982

Granacher RP, Baldessarini RJ: Physostigmine: its use in acute anticholinergic syndrome with antidepressant and antiparkinson drugs. Arch Gen Psychiatry 23:375–380, 1978

Gupta S, Masand P, Tanquary JF: Thyroid hormone supplementation of fluoxetine in the treatment of major depression. Br J Psychiatry 159:866–867, 1991

Hayes SG: Barbiturate anticonvulsants in refractory affective disorders. Ann Clin Psychiatry 5:35–44, 1993

Heninger GR, Charney DS, Sternberg DE: Lithium carbonate augmentation of antidepressant treatment. Arch Gen Psychiatry 40:1335–1342, 1983

Heresco-Levy U, Javitt DC, Ermilov M, et al: Efficacy of high-dose glycine in the treatment of enduring negative symptoms of schizophrenia. Arch Gen Psychiatry 56:29–36, 1999 [also see comments]

Hollander E, DeCaria CM, Schneier FR, et al: Fenfluramine augmentation of serotonin reuptake blockade antiobsessional treatment. J Clin Psychiatry 51:119–123, 1990

Holsboer F, Grasser A, Friess E, et al: Steroid effects on central neurons and implications for psychiatric and neurological disorders. Ann N Y Acad Sci 746:345–359 [discussion 359–361], 1994

Hopwood SE, Bogle S, Wildgust HJ: The combination of fluoxetine and lithium in clinical practice. Int Clin Psychopharmacol 8:325–327, 1993

Howland RH: Lithium augmentation of fluoxetine in the treatment of OCD and major depression: a case report (letter). Can J Psychiatry 36:154–155, 1991

Howland RH: Thyroid dysfunction in refractory depression: implications for pathophysiology and treatment. J Clin Psychiatry 54:47–54, 1993

Hunter MD, Ganesan V, Wilkinson ID, et al: Impact of modafinil on prefrontal executive function in schizophrenia. Am J Psychiatry 163:2184–2186, 2006

Joffe G, Appelberg B, Rimon R: Adjunctive nefazodone in neuroleptic-treated schizophrenic patients with predominantly negative symptoms: an open prospective pilot study. Int Clin Psychopharmacol 14:233–238, 1999

Joffe RT: Triiodothyronine potentiation of fluoxetine in depressed patients. Can J Psychiatry 37:48–50, 1992

Joffe RT, Schuller DR: An open study of buspirone augmentation of serotonin reuptake inhibitors. J Clin Psychiatry 54:269–271, 1993

Joffe RT, Singer W: Thyroid hormone potentiation of antidepressants. Neuroendocrinology Letters (St. Michael's Hospital) 9:172, 1987

Joffe RT, Levitt AJ, Bagby RM, et al: Predictors of response to lithium and triiodothyronine: augmentation of antidepressants in tricyclic nonresponders. Br J Psychiatry 163:574–578, 1993

Joffe RT, Sokolov ST, Levitt AJ: Lithium and triiodothyronine augmentation of antidepressants. Can J Psychiatry 51:791–793, 2006

Johns CA, Thompson JW: Adjunctive treatments in schizophrenia: pharmacotherapies and electroconvulsive therapy. Schizophr Bull 21:607–619, 1995

Karunakaran K, Tungaraza TE, Harborne G: Is clozapine-aripiprazole combination a useful regime in the management of treatment-resistant schizophrenia? J Psychopharmacol 21:453–456, 2007

Katona CL, Robertson MM, Abou-Saleh MT, et al: Placebo-controlled trial of lithium augmentation of fluoxetine and lofepramine. Int Clin Psychopharmacol 8:238, 1993

Katona CL, Abou-Saleh MT, Harrison DA, et al: Placebo-controlled trial of lithium augmentation of fluoxetine and lofepramine. Br J Psychiatry 166: 80–86, 1995

Keck PE: A randomized, placebo-controlled trial of olanzapine and olanzapine-fluoxetine combination in the treatment of bipolar depression. Presentation at the 155th annual meeting of the American Psychiatric Association, Philadelphia, PA, May 2002

Keck PE Jr, McElroy SL, Vuckovic A, et al: Combined valproate and carbamazepine treatment of bipolar disorder. J Neuropsychiatry Clin Neurosci 4:319–322, 1992

Kelly DL, Buchanan RW, Boggs DL, et al: A randomized double-blind trial of atomoxetine for cognitive impairments in 32 people with schizophrenia. J Clin Psychiatry 70:518–525, 2009

Kemp DE, Gao K, Ganocy SJ, et al: A 6-month, double-blind, maintenance trial of lithium monotherapy versus the combination of lithium and divalproex for rapid-cycling bipolar disorder and co-occurring substance abuse or dependence. J Clin Psychiatry 70:113–121, 2009

Ketter TA, Winsberg ME, DeGolia SG, et al: Rapid efficacy of olanzapine augmentation in nonpsychotic bipolar mixed states (letter). J Clin Psychiatry 59:83–85, 1998 [also see comments]

Ketter T, Wang P, Nowakowski C: Treatment of acute mania in bipolar disorder, in Advances in Treatment of Bipolar Disorder. Edited by Ketter TA. Washington, DC, American Psychiatric Publishing, 2005, pp 11–55

Ketter TA, Wang PW, Chandler RA, et al: Adjunctive aripiprazole in treatment-resistant bipolar depression. Ann Clin Psychiatry 18:169–172, 2006

Kirsch MA, Louie AK: Combination treatment with venlafaxine and bupropion (letter). Am J Psychiatry 156:494, 1999

Kishimoto A: The treatment of affective disorder with carbamazepine: prophylactic synergism of lithium and carbamazepine combination. Prog Neuropsychopharmacol Biol Psychiatry 16:483–493, 1992

Kline NS, Pare M, Hallstrom C, et al: Amitriptyline protects patients on MAOIs from tyramine reactions. J Clin Psychopharmacol 2:434–435, 1982

Kramlinger KG, Post RM: Addition of lithium carbonate to carbamazepine: hematological and thyroid effects. Am J Psychiatry 147:615–620, 1990 [also see comments]

Kusalic M: Grade II and grade III hypothyroidism in rapid-cycling bipolar patients. Neuropsychobiology 25:177–181, 1992

Landen M, Bjorling G, Agren H, et al: A randomized, double-blind, placebo-controlled trial of buspirone in combination with an SSRI in patients with treatment-refractory depression. J Clin Psychiatry 59:664–668, 1998

Lemberger L, Rowe H, Bosomworth J, et al: The effect of fluoxetine on the pharmacokinetics and psychomotor responses of diazepam. Clin Pharmacol Ther 43: 412–419, 1988

Levine J, Brak Y, Gonzalves M, et al: Double-blind controlled trial of inositol treatment of major depression. Am J Psychiatry 152:792–794, 1995

Levine J, Mishori A, Susnosky M, et al: Combination of inositol and serotonin reuptake inhibitors in the treatment of depression. Biol Psychiatry 45:270–273, 1999

Lipinski JF, Pope HG Jr: Possible synergistic action between carbamazepine and lithium carbonate in the treatment of three acutely manic patients. Am J Psychiatry 139:948–949, 1982

Llorca PM, Wolf MA, Lancon C, et al: Comparative efficacy of bromocriptine, carbamazepine and cyproheptadine with neuroleptics in 24 refractory chronic schizophrenic patients [in French]. Encephale 19:565–571, 1993

Martin Munoz JC, Morinigo Dominguez AV, Mateo Martin I, et al: Carbamazepine: an efficient adjuvant treatment in schizophrenian [in Spanish]. Actas Luso-Esp Neurol Psiquiatr y Cienc Afines 20:11–16, 1992

McAskill R, Mir S, Taylor D: Pindolol augmentation of antidepressant therapy. Br J Psychiatry 173:203–208, 1998 [also see comments] [erratum: Br J Psychiatry 173:443, 1998]

McCoy L, Votolato NA, Schwarzkopf SB, et al: Clinical correlates of valproate augmentation in refractory bipolar disorder. Ann Clin Psychiatry 5:29–33, 1993

McElroy SL, Pope HG Jr (eds): Use of Anticonvulsants in Psychiatry: Recent Advances. Clifton, NJ, Oxford Health Care, 1988

McGinness J, Kishimoto A, Hollister LE: Avoiding neurotoxicity with lithium-carbamazepine combinations. Psychopharmacol Bull 26:181–184, 1990

McGrath PJ, Stewart JW, Fava M, et al: Tranylcypromine versus venlafaxine plus mirtazapine following three failed antidepressant medication trials for depression: a STAR*D report. Am J Psychiatry 163:1531–1541 [quiz 1666], 2006

McIntyre A, Gendron A, McIntyre A: Quetiapine adjunct to selective serotonin reuptake inhibitors or venlafaxine in patients with major depression, comorbid anxiety, and residual depressive symptoms: a randomized, placebo-controlled pilot study. Depress Anxiety 24:487–494, 2007

Michelson D, Aller AA, Amsterdam JD, et al: Addition of atomoxetine for depression incompletely responsive to sertraline: a randomized, double-blind, placebo-controlled study, in Syllabus and Proceedings Summary, American Psychiatric Association Annual Meeting, Toronto, ON, Canada, May 20–25, 2006, p 74

Mitchell P, Withers K, Jacobs G, et al: Combining lithium and sodium valproate for bipolar disorder. Aust N Z J Psychiatry 28:141–143, 1994

Montgomery P, Richardson AJ: Omega-3 fatty acids for bipolar disorder. Cochrane Database Syst Rev April 16;(2):CD005169, 2008

Montgomery SA: Selectivity of antidepressants and resistant depression, in Advances in Neuropsychiatry and Psychopharmacology, Vol 2: Refractory Depression. Edited by Amsterdam JD. New York, Raven, 1991, pp 93–104

Morera AL, Barreiro P, Cano-Munoz JL: Risperidone and clozapine combination for the treatment of refractory schizophrenia. Acta Psychiatr Scand 99:305–306 [discussion: 306–307], 1999

Mouaffak F, Tranulis C, Gourevitch R, et al: Augmentation strategies of clozapine with antipsychotics in the treatment of ultraresistant schizophrenia. Clin Neuropharmacol 29:28–33, 2006

Muly EC, McDonald W, Steffens D, et al: Serotonin syndrome produced by a combination of fluoxetine and lithium (letter). Am J Psychiatry 150:1565, 1993

Nelson JC, Price LH: Lithium or desipramine augmentation of fluoxetine treatment (letter). Am J Psychiatry 152:1538–1539, 1995

Nelson JC, Mazure CM, Jatlow PI, et al: Combining norepinephrine and serotonin reuptake inhibition mechanisms for treatment of depression: a double-blind, randomized study. Biol Psychiatry 55:296–300, 2004

Nemeroff CB, Evans DL, Gyulai L, et al: Double-blind, placebo-controlled comparison of imipramine and paroxetine in the treatment of bipolar depression. Am J Psychiatry 158:906–912, 2001

Nierenberg AA, Keck PE: Management of monoamine oxidase inhibitor–associated insomnia with trazodone. J Clin Psychopharmacol 9:45–54, 1989

Nierenberg AA, Price CH, Charney DS, et al: After lithium augmentation: a retrospective follow-up of patients with antidepressant-refractory depression. J Affect Disord 18:67–75, 1990

Nierenberg AA, Cole JO, Glass L: Possible trazodone potentiation of fluoxetine: a case series. J Clin Psychiatry 53:83–85, 1992

Nierenberg AA, Adler LA, Pelow E, et al: Trazodone for antidepressant associated insomnia. Am J Psychiatry 151:1069–1072, 1994

Nierenberg AA, Fava M, Trivedi MH, et al: A comparison of lithium and T$_3$ augmentation following two failed medication treatments for depression: a STAR*D report. Am J Psychiatry 163:1519–1530 [quiz 1665], 2006a

Nierenberg AA, Ostacher MJ, Calabrese JR, et al: Treatment-resistant bipolar depression: a STEP-BD equipoise randomized effectiveness trial of antidepressant augmentation with lamotrigine, inositol, or risperidone. Am J Psychiatry 163:210–216, 2006b

Okuma T: Effects of carbamazepine and lithium on affective disorders. Neuropsychobiology 27:138–145, 1993

Ontiveros A, Fontaine R, Elie R: Refractory depression: the addition of lithium to fluoxetine or desipramine. Acta Psychiatr Scand 83:188–192, 1991

Palinkas LA, Barrett-Connor E: Estrogen use and depressive symptoms in postmenopausal women. Obstet Gynecol 80:30–36, 1992

Papakostas GI, Cooper-Kazaz R, Appelhof BC, et al: Simultaneous initiation (co-initiation) of pharmacotherapy with triiodothyronine and a selective serotonin reuptake inhibitor for major depressive disorder: a quantitative synthesis of double-blind studies. Int Clin Psychopharmacol 24:19–25, 2009

Pare CMB, Kline N, Hallstrom C, et al: Will amitriptyline prevent the "cheese" reaction of monoamine oxidase inhibitors? Lancet 2:183–186, 1982

Perugi G, Toni C, Ruffolo G, et al: Clinical experience using adjunctive gabapentin in treatment-resistant bipolar mixed states. Pharmacopsychiatry 32:136–141, 1999

Peselow ED, Fieve RR, Difiglia C, et al: Lithium prophylaxis of bipolar illness: the value of combination treatment. Br J Psychiatry 164:208–214, 1994

Pope HG Jr, McElroy SL, Nixon RA: Possible synergism between fluoxetine and lithium in refractory depression. Am J Psychiatry 145:1292–1294, 1988

Pope HG Jr, Cohane GH, Kanayama G, et al: Testosterone gel supplementation for men with refractory depression: a randomized, placebo-controlled trial. Am J Psychiatry 160:105–111, 2003

Portella MJ, de Diego-Adeliño J, Puigdemont D, et al: Pindolol augmentation enhances response outcomes in first depressive episodes. Eur Neuropsychopharmacol 19:516–519, 2009

Price LH, Conwell Y, Nelson JC: Lithium augmentation of combined neuroleptic-tricyclic treatment in delusional depression. Am J Psychiatry 140:318–322, 1983

Price LH, Charry DS, Heninger GR: Efficacy of lithium-tranylcypromine treatment in refractory depression. Am J Psychiatry 142:619–623, 1985

Rabkin JG, McElhiney MC, Rabkin R, et al: Placebo-controlled trial of dehydroepiandrosterone (DHEA) for treatment of nonmajor depression in patients with HIV/AIDS. Am J Psychiatry 163:59–66, 2006

Rapaport MH, Gharabawi GM, Canuso CM, et al: Effects of risperidone augmentation in patients with treatment-resistant depression: results of open-label treatment followed by double-blind continuation. Neuropsychopharmacology 31:2505–2513, 2006 [erratum: Neuropsychopharmacology 31:2514, 2006)]

Rasgon NL, Dunkin J, Fairbanks L, et al: Estrogen and response to sertraline in post-menopausal women with major depressive disorder: a pilot study. J Psychiatr Res 41:338–343, 2007

Raynaud JP: Prostate cancer risk in testosterone-treated men. J Steroid Biochem Mol Biol 102:261–266, 2006

Remington G, Saha A, Chong SA, et al: Augmentation strategies in clozapine-resistant schizophrenia. CNS Drugs 19:843–872, 2005

Rosse RB, Theut SK, Banay-Schwartz M, et al: Glycine adjuvant therapy to conventional neuroleptic treatment in schizophrenia: an open-label, pilot study. Clin Neuropharmacol 12:416–424, 1989

Rosse RB, Fay-McCarthy M, Kendrick K, et al: D-Cycloserine adjuvant therapy to molindone in the treatment of schizophrenia. Clin Neuropharmacol 19: 444–450, 1996

Rothschild AJ, Samson JA, Besset MP, et al: Efficacy of the combination of fluoxetine and perphenazine in the treatment of psychotic depression. J Clin Psychiatry 54:338–342, 1993

Rothschild AJ, Williamson DJ, Tohen MF, et al: A double-blind, randomized study of olanzapine and olanzapine/fluoxetine combination for major depression with psychotic features. J Clin Psychopharmacol 24:365–373, 2004

Saavedra-Velez C, Yusim A, Anbarasan D, et al: Modafinil as an adjunctive treatment of sedation, negative symptoms, and cognition in schizophrenia: a critical review. J Clin Psychiatry 70:104–112, 2009

Sachs GS, Weilburg JB, Rosenbaum JF: Clonazepam vs. neuroleptics as adjuncts to lithium maintenance. Psychopharmacol Bull 26:137–143, 1990

Sachs GS, Grossman F, Ghaemi SN, et al: Combination of a mood stabilizer with risperidone or haloperidol for treatment of acute mania: a double-blind, placebo-controlled comparison of efficacy and safety. Am J Psychiatry 159:1146–1154, 2002

Sachs GS, Nierenberg AA, Calabrese JR, et al: Effectiveness of adjunctive antidepressant treatment for bipolar depression. N Engl J Med 356:1711–1722, 2007

Schatzberg AF, DeBattista CB, DeGolia S: Valproate in the treatment of agitation associated with depression. Psychiatr Ann 26:1–4, 1996

Schmidt PJ, Daly RC, Bloch M, et al: Dehydroepiandrosterone monotherapy in midlife-onset major and minor depression. Arch Gen Psychiatry 62:154–162, 2005

Schneider AL, Wilcox CS: Divalproate augmentation in lithium-resistant rapid cycling mania in four geriatric patients. J Affect Disord 47:201–205, 1998

Schneider LS, Small GW, Hamilton SH, et al: Estrogen replacement and response to fluoxetine in a multicenter geriatric depression trial. Fluoxetine Collaborative Study Group. Am J Geriatr Psychiatry 5:97–106, 1997

Schneider LS, Small GW, Clary CM: Estrogen replacement therapy and antidepressant response to sertraline in older depressed women. Am J Geriatr Psychiatry 9:393–399, 2001

Schulz SC, Thompson PA, Jacobs M, et al: Lithium augmentation fails to reduce symptoms in poorly responsive schizophrenic outpatients. J Clin Psychiatry 60:366–372, 1999

Seidman SN, Spatz E, Rizzo C, et al: Testosterone replacement therapy for hypogonadal men with major depressive disorder: a randomized, placebo-controlled clinical trial. J Clin Psychiatry 62:406–412, 2001

Seidman SN, Miyazaki M, Roose SP: Intramuscular testosterone supplementation to selective serotonin reuptake inhibitor in treatment-resistant depressed men: randomized placebo-controlled clinical trial. J Clin Psychopharmacol 25:584–588, 2005

Sharma V, Persad E: Augmentation of valproate with lithium in a case of rapid cycling affective disorder. Can J Psychiatry 37:584–585, 1992

Sharma V, Persad E, Mazmanian D, et al: Treatment of rapid cycling bipolar disorder with combination therapy of valproate and lithium. Can J Psychiatry 38:137–139, 1993

Shelton RC: The combination of olanzapine and fluoxetine in mood disorders. Expert Opin Pharmacother 4:1175–1183, 2003

Shelton RC, Tollefson GD, Tohen M, et al: A novel augmentation strategy for treating resistant major depression. Am J Psychiatry 158:131–134, 2001

Shelton RC, Williamson DJ, Corya SA, et al: Olanzapine/fluoxetine combination for treatment-resistant depression: a controlled study of SSRI and nortriptyline resistance. J Clin Psychiatry 66:1289–1297, 2005

Sherwin BB: Estrogen in refractory depression, in Advances in Neuropsychiatry and Psychopharmacology, Vol 2: Refractory Depression. Edited by Amsterdam JD. New York, Raven, 1991, pp 209–218

Sichel DA, Cohen LS, Robertson LM, et al: Prophylactic estrogen in recurrent postpartum affective disorder. Biol Psychiatry 38:814–818, 1995

Silver H, Nassar A: Fluvoxamine improves negative symptoms in treated chronic schizophrenia. Biol Psychiatry 31:698–704, 1992

Simhandl C, Denk E, Thau K: The comparative efficacy of carbamazepine low and high serum level and lithium carbonate in the prophylaxis of affective disorders. J Affect Disord 28:221–231, 1993

Smith WT, Londborg PD, Glaudin V, et al: Short-term augmentation of fluoxetine with clonazepam in the treatment of depression: a double-blind study. Am J Psychiatry 155:1339–1345, 1998

Soares CN, Almeida OP, Joffe H, et al: Efficacy of estradiol for the treatment of depressive disorders in perimenopausal women. Arch Gen Psychiatry 58:529–534, 2001

Sokolov ST, Levitt AJ, Joffe RT: Thyroid hormone levels before unsuccessful antidepressant therapy are associated with later response to T3 augmentation. Psychiatry Res 69:203–206, 1997

Solomon DA, Ryan CE, Keitner GI, et al: A pilot study of lithium carbonate plus divalproex sodium for the continuation and maintenance treatment of patients with bipolar I disorder. J Clin Psychiatry 58:95–99, 1997

Solomon DA, Keitner GI, Ryan CE, et al: Lithium plus valproate as maintenance polypharmacy for patients with bipolar I disorder: a review. J Clin Psychopharmacol 18:38–49, 1998

Spiker DG, Weiss JC, Dealy RS: The pharmacological treatment of delusional depression. Am J Psychiatry 142:430–436, 1985

Spoov J, Lahdelma L: Should thyroid augmentation precede lithium augmentation? A pilot study. J Affect Disord 49:235–239, 1998

Steckler TL: Lithium- and carbamazepine-associated sinus node dysfunction: nine-year experience in a psychiatric hospital. J Clin Psychopharmacol 14:336–339, 1994

Stein G, Bernadt M: Lithium augmentation therapy in tricyclic resistant depression: a controlled trial using lithium in low and normal doses. Br J Psychiatry 162:639–640, 1993

Stoll AL, Locke CA, Marangell LB, et al: Omega-3 fatty acids and bipolar disorder: a review. Prostaglandins Leukot Essent Fatty Acids 60:329–337, 1999

Stromgren LS: The combination of lithium and carbamazepine in treatment and prevention of manic-depressive disorder: a review and a case report. Compr Psychiatry 31:261–265, 1990

Suppes T, Vieta E, Liu S, et al, and Trial 127 Investigators: Maintenance treatment for patients with bipolar I disorder: results from a North American study of quetiapine in combination with lithium or divalproex (Trial 127). Am J Psychiatry 166:476–488, 2009

Takahashi N, Terao T, Oga T, et al: Comparison of risperidone and mosapramine addition to neuroleptic treatment in chronic schizophrenia. Neuropsychobiology 39:81–85, 1999

Targum SD, Grengberg RD, Harmon RL, et al: Thyroid hormone and the TRH stimulation test in refractory depression. J Clin Psychiatry 45:345–346, 1984

Thase ME, Kupfer DJ, Frank E, et al: Treatment of imipramine-resistant recurrent depression: an open clinical trial of lithium augmentation. J Clin Psychiatry 50:385–388, 1989

Thase ME, Howland RH, Friedman ES: Treating antidepressant nonresponders with augmentation strategies: an overview. J Clin Psychiatry 59 (5, suppl):5-12 [discussion:13–15], 1998

Tiihonen J, Halonen P, Wahlbeck K, et al: Topiramate add-on in treatment-resistant schizophrenia: a randomized, double-blind, placebo-controlled, crossover trial. J Clin Psychiatry 66:1012–1015, 2005

Tiihonen J, Wahlbeck K, Kiviniemi V: The efficacy of lamotrigine in clozapine-resistant schizophrenia: a systematic review and meta-analysis. Schizophr Res 109:10–14, 2009

Tohen M, Chengappa KN, Suppes T, et al: Efficacy of olanzapine in combination with valproate or lithium in the treatment of mania in patients partially nonresponsive to valproate or lithium monotherapy. Arch Gen Psychiatry 59:62–69, 2002

Tohen M, Bowden CL, Smulevich AB, et al: Olanzapine plus carbamazepine v carbamazepine alone in treating manic episodes. Br J Psychiatry 192:135–143, 2008

Tollefson GD, Sanger TM, Anderson SW: The use of an olanzapine:fluoxetine combination in the treatment of major depression with psychotic features: results from a large, prospective double-blind trial, in Abstracts of the 40th Annual Meeting of the American College of Neuropsychopharmacology, Waikoloa, HI, 2001, p 58

Trivedi MH, Fava M, Wisniewski SR, et al, and STAR*D Study Team: Medication augmentation after the failure of SSRIs for depression. N Engl J Med 354:1243–1252, 2006

Tsai G, Yang P, Chung LC, et al: D-Serine added to antipsychotics for the treatment of schizophrenia. Biol Psychiatry 44:1081–1089, 1998 [also see comments]

Tsai GE, Yang P, Chung LC, et al: D-Serine added to clozapine for the treatment of schizophrenia. Am J Psychiatry 156:1822–1825, 1999

The Upjohn Company: Technical Report Synopsis: A Multicenter Study to Evaluate the Pharmacokinetic and Clinical Interactions Between Alprazolam and Imipramine. Kalamazoo, MI, The Upjohn Company, 1986

The Upjohn Company: Technical Report Synopsis: A Pharmacokinetic/Pharmacodynamic Evaluation of the Combined Administration of Alprazolam and Fluoxetine. Kalamazoo, MI, The Upjohn Company, 1990

Vieta E, Sanchez-Moreno J, Martinez-Aran A, et al: Effects on weight and outcome of long-term olanzapine-topiramate combination treatment in bipolar disorder. J Clin Psychopharmacol 24:374–378, 2004

Vieweg V, Shutty M, Hundley P, et al: Combined treatment with lithium and carbamazepine (letter). Am J Psychiatry 148:398–399, 1991 [also see comments]

Wehr TA, Goodwin FK: Rapid cycling in manic-depressives induced by tricyclic antidepressants. Arch Gen Psychiatry 36:555–559, 1979

Wehr TA, Sack DA, Rosenthal NE, et al: Rapid cycling affective disorder: contributing factors and treatment responses in 51 patients. Am J Psychiatry 145:179–184, 1988

Weilburg JB, Rosenbaum JF, Biederman J, et al: Fluoxetine added to non-MAOI antidepressants converts nonresponders to responders: a preliminary report. J Clin Psychiatry 50:447–449, 1989

Wharton RN, Perel JM, Dayton PG, et al: A potential clinical use for methylphenidate with tricyclic antidepressants. Am J Psychiatry 127:1619–1625, 1971

Wheatley D: Potentiation of amitriptyline by thyroid hormone. Arch Gen Psychiatry 26:229–233, 1972

White K, Simpson G: Combined MAOI–tricyclic antidepressant treatment: a reevaluation. J Clin Psychopharmacol 1:264–282, 1981

Whybrow PC: The therapeutic use of triiodothyronine and high dose thyroxine in psychiatric disorders. Acta Med Austriaca 21:47–52, 1994

Whybrow PC, Bauer MS, Gyulai L: Thyroid axis considerations in patients with rapid cycling affective disorder. Clin Neuropharmacol 15:391A–392A, 1992

Wijkstra J, Lijmer J, Balk FJ, et al: Pharmacological treatment for unipolar psychotic depression: systematic review and meta analysis. Br J Psychiatry 188:410–415, 2006

Wilson WH: Addition of lithium to haloperidol in non-affective, antipsychotic non-responsive schizophrenia: a double blind, placebo controlled, parallel design clinical trial. Psychopharmacology (Berl) 111:359–366, 1993

Wolkowitz OM, Reus VI, Roberts E, et al: Antidepressant and cognition-enhancing effects of DHEA in major depression. Ann N Y Acad Sci 774:337–339, 1993

Wolkowitz OM, Reus VI, Roberts E, et al: Dehydroepiandrosterone (DHEA) treatment of depression. Biol Psychiatry 41:311–318, 1997

Young LT, Robb JC, Hasey GM, et al: Gabapentin as an adjunctive treatment in bipolar disorder. J Affect Disord 55:73–77, 1999

Young LT, Joffe RT, Robb JC, et al: Double-blind comparison of addition of a second mood stabilizer versus an antidepressant to an initial mood stabilizer for treatment of patients with bipolar depression. Am J Psychiatry 157:124–126, 2000

Zanardi R, Franchini L, Serretti A, et al: Venlafaxine versus fluvoxamine in the treatment of delusional depression: a pilot double-blind controlled study. J Clin Psychiatry 61:26–29, 2000

Zarate CA, Payne JL, Singh J, et al: Pramipexole for bipolar II depression: a placebo-controlled proof of concept study. Biol Psychiatry 56:54–60, 2004

Zarrouf FA, Artz S, Griffith J, et al: Testosterone and depression: systematic review and meta-analysis. J Psychiatr Pract Jul;15:289–305, 2009

Zhang ZJ, Kang WH, Li Q, et al: Beneficial effects of ondansetron as an adjunct to haloperidol for chronic, treatment-resistant schizophrenia: A double-blind, randomized, placebo-controlled study. Schizophr Res 88:102–110, 2006

Ziegenbein M, Calliess IT: Clozapine and ziprasidone: a useful combination in patients with treatment-resistant schizophrenia. J Neuropsychiatry Clin Neurosci 18:246–247, 2006

Ziegenbein M, Wittmann G, Kropp S: Aripiprazole augmentation of clozapine in treatment-resistant schizophrenia: a clinical observation. Clin Drug Investig 26:117–124, 2006

10

Emergency Department Treatment

Psychiatrists see patients in crisis not only in emergency departments but also (occasionally) in their offices, during home visits, or in medical or nursing home settings. In this chapter, we address some of the more common emergencies facing the clinical psychiatrist.

In emergency situations, psychiatrists are often faced with the diagnosis and treatment of patients presenting with psychiatric symptoms of sudden or presumed recent onset. Phenomenologically, these symptoms can be crudely subdivided into the following types:

1. Agitation and violent behavior, with or without signs of alcohol or other intoxication
2. Depression with suicidal ideation, with or without a recent suicide attempt
3. Acute psychotic episodes, usually with overt thought disorder, paranoid ideation, and/or hallucinations and marked fear or anger
4. Delirium presenting with disorientation and confusion, with or without psychotic symptoms

5. Severe anxiety without psychotic symptoms but often with physical symptoms

6. Psychogenic stupor/catatonia

In some of these situations a history can be obtained either from the patient or from friends or relatives. Sometimes the patient may be carrying enough identification that friends or relatives can be rapidly contacted. In the worst situation, the psychiatrist will have little to go on besides the patient's behavior and a brief physical examination. When the patient is severely disturbed, obtunded, or confused, can give no history, and has no diagnostic stigmata (e.g., needle tracks, obvious atropine-like toxic signs), hospitalization without specific drug treatment, or at least medical evaluation with toxic screens, electrocardiogram, and so forth in a competent medical emergency facility, is indicated.

We stress the importance of trying to ascertain which drugs the patient has been taking or may have been taking before pharmacotherapy is begun. Deaths have occurred when a tricyclic antidepressant (TCA) or meperidine was given to patients who were already taking monoamine oxidase inhibitors (MAOIs). Adding sedative drugs in a patient already intoxicated on alcohol or other sedative drugs is unwise. Adding a neuroleptic in a patient with possible neuroleptic malignant syndrome (NMS) is obviously contraindicated. Similarly, drugs must be carefully chosen if a TCA overdose may have affected cardiac function. In short, when the patient may have been taking preexisting medication or may have overdosed on an unknown drug, it is better to avoid medication until the situation can be clarified.

Agitation and Violence

Few emergency department encounters are more difficult than having to contend with an agitated, violent patient. Individuals representing many diagnostic groups may present to the emergency department in an agitated, violent state. In one survey, 80% of teaching hospital emergency departments reported patient assaults of staff members, and at least 25% of these emergency departments had to restrain patients daily (Lavoie et al. 1988). It is difficult to ascertain how frequently assaults occur against medical personnel by patients, as the vast majority of these assaults are not reported (Barlow et al. 1997). Violence often represents an attempt by the patient to assert control in the context of feeling frightened and helpless.

In nonpsychotic patients presenting to emergency rooms with angry tantrums, as well as in similar patients with severe anxiety that seems to be based on family fights or other interpersonal crises, supportive listening, reassurance, and the elixir of time often enable the patient to gradually become calm and reasonable without specific medication. Sedative- or alcohol-related angry intoxication also often passes gradually with time, talk, and external limit setting.

From the legal perspective, the use of external restraints is sometimes considered a less invasive intervention than the involuntary administration of psychotropic medications. No intervention is more effective for potentially violent patients than a sufficient show of force to restrain the patient, if necessary, along with calm reassurance. The use of restraints generally should be a last resort, when all less-restrictive options have been exhausted or are impractical. Thus, this option should be employed if the patient represents an imminent danger to himself or herself or others. However, some patients are quite capable of exhausting or injuring themselves while in restraints. In these cases the addition of medications is frequently required.

A number of open-label studies have investigated the use of various psychotropic agents in the "rapid tranquilization" of agitated patients. Dr. William Dubin of Temple University has used that term to describe the use of antipsychotics and benzodiazepines given every half hour or hour to treat the target symptoms of agitation, motor excitement, tension, and hostility. Although the strategy of rapid tranquilization as described by Dubin is over 20 years old, emergency psychiatrists still tend to employ some variation of this strategy (Allen et al. 2005). There has been some movement to using second-generation antipsychotics (SGAs) as first-line agents and a greater reliance on benzodiazepines in nonpsychotic conditions. Rapid tranquilization is sometimes confused with rapid neuroleptization, which uses large loading doses of first-generation antipsychotics, sometimes as much as 100 mg/day of haloperidol, in an attempt to accelerate remission of psychotic symptoms. Unfortunately, studies have revealed that this strategy is not successful, and side effects are burdensome. Rapid tranquilization strategies have been studied with both psychotic and nonpsychotic patients.

Table 10–1. Medication options for rapid tranquilization of agitated patients (administered every 30–60 minutes)

| Medication | Dose | | Average total dose for tranquilization |
	Intramuscular	Oral	
haloperidol	2.5–5 mg	5–10 mg	10–20 mg
thiothixene[a]	10–20 mg	5–10 mg	15–30 mg
droperidol	2.5–5 mg	Not available	5–20 mg
loxapine[a]	10–15 mg	25 mg	30–60 mg
chlorpromazine	50 mg	100 mg	300–600 mg
lorazepam	0.5–1 mg	1–2 mg	4–8 mg
diazepam	Not applicable	5–10 mg	20–60 mg
olanzapine	2.5–10 mg	2.5–5 mg	10–20 mg
ziprasidone	10–20 mg	40–160 mg	10–20 mg
aripiprazole	9.75 mg	10–30 mg	9.75–19.5 mg

[a]No longer available in the United States.

The typical rapid tranquilization approach employs an intramuscular route of administration for rapid absorption and increased bioavailability (Table 10–1). However, Dubin et al. (1985) suggested that oral concentrate forms of antipsychotics also provide rapid response and may decrease feelings of helplessness in an already vulnerable patient, relative to being approached with a needle. In a study of 159 agitated psychiatric patients randomized to either intramuscular or oral concentrate forms of thiothixene, haloperidol, or thioridazine, there was a minimal time advantage to using the intramuscular route of administration, but fewer intramuscular doses were required to achieve a satisfactory response (Dubin et al. 1985). The SGAs also tend to be available in oral solution form, which may have similar advantages over intramuscular forms. In medical-surgical patients, the intravenous route of administration is also a common option. Moller et al. (1982) found that patients given intravenous haloperidol improved more rapidly than patients taking oral haloperidol in the first 3 hours. However, after 3 hours there was no significant difference between the oral and the intravenous haloperidol–treated groups. Several other open-label studies have confirmed the utility of intravenous haloperidol and benzodiazepines (lorazepam) in the management of agitated medical-surgical patients.

Intramuscular SGAs such as intramuscular olanzapine, aripiprazole, and ziprasidone are being employed with increasing frequency relative to intramuscular first-generation antipsychotics such as haloperidol. However, there is little evidence that they are more effective than first-generation antipsychotics. Rather, the advantage of intramuscular SGAs is a reduced rate of acute extrapyramidal symptoms (EPS), especially akathisia and dystonic reactions. On the other hand, a significant disadvantage of the atypical intramuscular formulations is that they are substantially more costly than generic agents such as haloperidol. Intramuscular olanzapine has now been approved for use in treating agitation associated with psychosis. It has been studied in the acute management of schizophrenia, dementia, and bipolar disorder. In acutely agitated patients with dementia, olanzapine at 2.5 or 5 mg im was significantly more effective than placebo in reducing agitation 2 and 24 hours postinjection (lorazepam at 1 mg was not) (Meehan et al. 2002). In patients with schizophrenia, olanzapine at 5–10 mg im was significantly more effective than placebo at 2 and 24 hours postinjection (Breier et al. 2001); similar data at 10–25 mg were observed in acutely manic patients (Meehan et al. 2001). The primary advantages of intramuscular olanzapine over intramuscular haloperidol are a faster onset of action and less EPS (Wright et al. 2003). The onset of action of intramuscular olanzapine is within 30 minutes, and minimal EPS have been reported. The most common side effects were somnolence and dizziness. Occasional mild hypotension and bradycardia have been reported.

An injectable form of ziprasidone has been available since 2002. Ziprasidone has been evaluated in several double-blind trials in the treatment of acute agitation. Both 10 mg and 20 mg im appear to be effective, but 2 mg im was not effective. Like olanzapine, intramuscular ziprasidone has a low incidence of EPS. In studies of acute agitation in psychotic patients, dosages of 10–20 mg/day were as effective as haloperidol in treating agitation and more effective in treating psychosis. The most common side effects with intramuscular ziprasidone were headache, nausea, and somnolence.

Aripiprazole became the latest atypical antipsychotic to be indicated in the treatment of acute agitation associated with bipolar disorder, schizoaffective disorder, and schizophrenia. Several studies of the acute effects of aripiprazole in the reduction of agitation have demonstrated the superiority of this agent to placebo and its equivalence to intramuscular haloperidol (see Andrezina et al. 2006a, 2006b). Intramuscular aripiprazole appears to produce EPS much less commonly than does intramuscular haloperidol, with about 2% of aripiprazole-treated patients experiencing akathisia and 1% experiencing dystonic reactions. It is likely, but untested, that repeated doses may increase the risk of EPS. Other side effects more commonly seen with intramuscular aripiprazole than with placebo include headache, somnolence, nausea, and dizziness.

For severely agitated or imminently violent patients, rapid tranquilization strategies employ antipsychotics every 30–60 minutes until the target symptoms of hostility, agitation, and assaultiveness are reduced. Most studies suggest that the typical dose of antipsychotics required is in the range of 300–600 mg of chlorpromazine, 10–20 mg of haloperidol, or 10–20 mg of olanzapine over a 2- to 4-hour period (see Table 10–1). The high-potency typical antipsychotics have the advantage of not producing significant adrenergic blockade in the acute setting. However, akathisia and dystonic reactions may be problematic, particularly in young males. We have found that alternating the antipsychotic with a benzodiazepine is also a sound strategy. In a common regimen, haloperidol 5 mg im is alternated with lorazepam 1–2 mg im every 30 minutes until tranquilization is achieved. Droperidol was sometimes used for rapid tranquilization but has now received a black box warning secondary to QTc prolongation. Droperidol is also associated with hypotension and respiratory depression. Thus, its use in psychiatric settings is rarely warranted, and the availability of droperidol is more limited than it was previously.

Lorazepam is the only benzodiazepine reliably absorbed from all routes of administration. However, for oral dosing, diazepam may offer the most rapid onset of action. The combination of benzodiazepines and antipsychotics offers several advantages. Frequently, lower doses of both classes of medications are sufficient when they are combined. The lower doses decrease the risks of side effects from either the benzodiazepines or the antipsychotics. Further, benzodiazepines may counter some antipsychotic side effects, including akathisia. Likewise, the combination with high-potency first-generation antipsychotics may reduce the excessive sedation associated with use of benzodiazepines alone. However, some data support the idea that benzodiazepines alone may be as effective as antipsychotics within the first 24 hours, even with floridly psychotic patients (Saklad et al. 1985).

For less severe acute agitation, especially in a nonpsychotic patient or when there is limited information available, the use of benzodiazepines alone appears to be adequate. Lorazepam 1–2 mg po every hour to a maximum of 10 mg or diazepam 5–10 mg every hour to a maximum of 60 mg is usually enough to calm the more moderately agitated patient.

A number of long-term strategies for the management of aggression in patients have been used. Mood-stabilizing agents such as lithium, carbamazepine, and valproate have proved useful in controlling aggressive, violent impulses in some patients. The selective serotonin reuptake inhibitors (SSRIs) have been used with some success in studies of treating patients with aggressive personality disorders. Likewise, buspirone, propranolol, trazodone, and clozapine, with long-term use, may all have a role in reducing aggression in some patients.

Depression and Suicidality

Depressed, suicidal patients, along with agitated patients, represent one of the most common and serious challenges confronted by the emergency department clinician. In many emergency departments, complaints of depression and suicidal ideation, with or without attempts, represent the most frequent reason for psychiatric hospital admission. Predicting imminent suicide is sometimes not an easy matter, even for skilled psychiatrists. Many factors have been known to increase the risk of suicide, including advanced age, a diagnosis of major depression, male gender, concurrent alcohol use, a viable suicide plan, and a history of serious suicide attempts. The significant majority of the successful 30,000 or so suicides that occur in the United States annually involve white males older than 45. In addition, depression or alcohol is implicated in approximately 75% of all suicides (Bongar 1992). Fawcett et al. (1990) attempted to further elucidate factors that may increase the immediate risk of suicide; among these were global insomnia and severe anxiety (Table 10–2).

Suicidal depressed patients brought to an emergency room after suicide threats or nonharmful attempts present a real challenge to clinical judgment. The conservative course is to admit such patients to a secure inpatient unit. Occasionally, this may seem unwise or impractical. If the clinician can develop an alliance with and personally follow the patient, and/or if friends or relatives can reliably supervise the patient until the next appointment, the patient may be followed as an outpatient. In general, any patient with suicidal ideation or

Table 10–2.   Short-term (6- to 12-month) risk factors for suicide in depressed patients

Obsessive-compulsive features
Severe hopelessness
Panic, severe anxiety, and agitation
Global insomnia
Severe cognitive difficulties and psychotic thinking
Lack of friends in adolescence
Acute overuse of alcohol
Recurrent depression

Source.   Adapted from Fawcett et al. 1990.

attempt and depression who is psychotic, who cannot attend to daily needs, who is acutely intoxicated, or about whose well-being the clinician has any significant doubt should be admitted and observed.

Very few somatic interventions work rapidly enough to be useful in the emergency setting. For example, it is generally unwise to start an antidepressant in the emergency department: the older antidepressants may be lethal in overdose, the physician following the patient after the emergency department visit may not agree with the emergency department's choice of agents, and, in any case, it may take several weeks or longer for the antidepressant to work. Thus, not much is lost in waiting to initiate antidepressant treatment until the patient is on the ward or makes the first outpatient visit.

Given the type of imminent risk factors described by Fawcett et al. (1990), benzodiazepines are probably underused in the emergency and acute setting for the treatment of suicidal patients. Benzodiazepines may have an immediate effect on risk factors such as severe insomnia and anxiety. Patients' hopelessness is also attributed, in part, to the belief that they will never feel any better. When they feel better quickly with a benzodiazepine, their belief system may be altered enough to mitigate the risk of imminent suicide. We have found that lorazepam 0.5–1.0 mg qid, with the last dose given at bedtime, can make a dramatic difference even in less agitated suicidal patients. That being said, there is little empirical evidence that benzodiazepines help patients who are acutely suicidal (Youssef et al. 2008). One also has to consider that some suicidal patients may become more depressed or disinhibited while taking benzodiazepines. Therefore, it is important that the suicidal patient be observed when starting a benzodiazepine.

A number of other somatic interventions are worth considering in the acute management of imminently suicidal patients. Among these is electroconvulsive therapy (ECT). ECT may work very rapidly in the profoundly depressed suicidal patient and may therefore be lifesaving. The average number of ECT treatments for depression in the United States is eight to nine; therefore it is not unusual to see significant benefit in the first 2 weeks of treatment. In addition, there is some evidence that the rapid titration of some antidepressants may be associated with an earlier onset of action. For example, premarketing studies (among them Montgomery 1993) suggested that venlafaxine may have a more rapid onset of action when the dose is titrated up to 300 mg or more in the first 7 days of treatment (Montgomery 1993). Unfortunately, we have found that many patients are unable to tolerate this rapid dose titration. Other strategies that may be associated with a more rapid onset of response for depressed suicidal patients include stimulant or lithium augmentation of various antidepressants. There is perhaps more evidence of an anti-suicidal property of lithium than for any other medication. Lithium appears to reduce both completed suicides and suicide attempts in patients with recurrent mood disorders (Cipriani et al. 2005; Kovacsics et al. 2009; Prien et al. 1984). However, a low therapeutic index makes it an inappropriate drug to start in the emergency department. On the other hand, it may be a reasonable drug to consider during the acute hospitalization of the suicidal patient.

Many depressed patients have used their antidepressants in suicide attempts. TCAs are the most commonly used antidepressants in completed overdoses (Table 10–3). The usual cause of death in these cases is malignant arrhythmias. Management of TCA overdoses includes charcoal lavage (50 g slurry followed by repeat doses of 25 g via nasogastric tube), admitting the patient to a unit for cardiac monitoring, fluids to combat the adrenergic blockade, physostigmine 1 mg im for severe anticholinergic symptoms, and correction of acidosis with sodium bicarbonate if necessary.

MAOI overdoses of as little as 2 mg/kg may be lethal. The cause of death in MAOI overdoses ranges from arrhythmia and cardiovascular collapse to rhabdomyolysis and renal failure. Acute management of overdose includes gastric lavage, maintenance of MAOI diet, cardiac monitoring for at least 24 hours, the use of benzodiazepines to treat central nervous system activation,

Table 10–3. Antidepressant overdoses and their management

Drug	Toxic dose	Toxicity manifestations	Management
TCAs	>1,500 mg (imipramine and most TCAs)	Anticholinergic symptoms, arrhythmia, hypotension, delirium, seizures	Gastric lavage, fluid support, cardiac monitoring
MAOIs	≥2 mg/kg	CNS excitation, hypo- or hypertension, delirium, fever, arrhythmia, seizures, rhabdomyolysis	Gastric lavage, fluids, cardiac monitoring, antihypertensives, body cooling, benzodiazepines for CNS symptoms, maintenance of MAOI diet
Bupropion	>2 g	CNS excitation, seizures	Gastric lavage, benzodiazepines, anticonvulsants
SSRIs	Unknown	CNS excitation, somnolence, GI irritation	Gastric lavage, supportive care
SNRIs (venlafaxine, duloxetine)	Unknown	Cardiotoxicity, hypertension, seizures, serotonin effects	Gastric lavage, supportive care

Note. CNS = central nervous system; GI = gastrointestinal; MAOI = monoamine oxidase inhibitor; SNRI = serotonin-norepinephrine reuptake inhibitor; SSRI = selective serotonin reuptake inhibitor; TCA = tricyclic antidepressant.

and the use of sodium nitroprusside or phentolamine 5 mg iv to treat the hypertension.

MAOIs are also associated with another medical emergency: the development of a serotonin syndrome. The combination of MAOIs with serotonergic drugs such as SSRIs and clomipramine (see Chapter 3: "Antidepressants") is among the more common causes of the serotonin syndrome. Symptoms of the serotonin syndrome are tremor, diaphoresis, rigidity, myoclonus, and autonomic dysregulation, potentially progressing to hyperthermia, rhabdomyolysis, coma, and death. The treatment of serotonin syndrome involves discontinuing the offending drugs, monitoring vital signs, and supporting vital functions. Cooling blankets are often helpful. Cyproheptadine, a general serotonin (5-hydroxytryptamine; 5-HT) antagonist, has been used occasionally in oral doses up to 16 mg/day to counteract the serotonin syndrome. Dantrolene in doses up to 1 mg/kg iv in divided doses has been used in severe cases to treat rigidity and prevent rhabdomyolysis. The key to treatment of the serotonin syndrome, however, is discontinuing the offending agents and providing supportive care.

Fortunately, many of the newer antidepressants present much less of a problem in overdose than do the TCAs and MAOIs. Overdoses of SSRIs and 5-HT antagonists are often asymptomatic or may present with gastrointestinal distress, agitation, and somnolence. The treatment of choice is gastric lavage and supportive care. The British drug authorities warned that venlafaxine overdoses are more likely to be lethal than are SSRI overdoses. Their data suggest that risk of lethality from overdose with venlafaxine is comparable to that with TCAs. A review by the U.S. Food and Drug Administration resulted in a change in the package insert for venlafaxine in 2006 that indicates that venlafaxine may carry a higher risk for a fatal outcome in overdose than SSRIs but less risk than the TCAs. The risk of fatality in overdose is not just from cardiac events but is also associated with seizures, rhabdomyolysis, and other causes. Patients taking venlafaxine tend to be more ill than those taking SSRIs, and this may be associated with a greater risk of overdoses in general (Rubino et al. 2007). One possible mechanism for the increased risk is an effect on sodium channels. Bupropion overdoses also tend to be less dangerous than overdoses of TCAs. There has, however, been at least one death related to neurotoxicity and seizures (see Chapter 3: "Antidepressants").

Acute Psychotic Episodes

Psychotic symptoms can be manifestations of drug intoxication, mania, depression, schizophrenia, dementia, delirium, or a variety of other disorders. An organic basis for the psychosis should be ruled out, whenever possible, by history, physical examination, and urine and/or blood tests for drugs of abuse.

Mixed Psychotic Features

With any psychotic episode presumptively due to toxicity from illicit or licit drugs, a variety of complicated clinical pictures can occur. Illicit drug users often take several kinds of drugs and alcohol simultaneously. Patients with schizophrenia abuse drugs and/or become intoxicated on alcohol, and acute drug-induced psychosis can sometimes persist and blend into a picture indistinguishable from schizophrenia that can continue for days or weeks. The pharmacotherapeutic problem is to choose between acute doses of an antipsychotic, a benzodiazepine, and watchful waiting, while checking for illicit drugs in urine or blood, evaluating possible medical causes, and obtaining a recent history from friends or relatives. Benzodiazepines should not be used with patients who appear to be already intoxicated from alcohol or sedative drugs but are commonly used to manage withdrawal from CNS depressants.

Schizophrenic, Schizophreniform, and Manic Psychoses

When the likelihood of a drug-induced psychosis is low and the patient is manifestly acutely psychotic—paranoid, disorganized, hallucinated, agitated, belligerent, and so forth—the rapid tranquilization strategies described earlier are quite useful. Often oral haloperidol is taken without objection by the patient; in that case, liquid medication is preferred, since ingestion can be ensured.

Parenteral antipsychotics (e.g., chlorpromazine 50 mg, aripiprazole 9.75 mg, olanzapine 10–30 mg, ziprasidone 10–20 mg, haloperidol 5–10 mg) are all effective. An antiparkinsonian drug should usually be given at the same time as the typical antipsychotics to help avert dystonia.

Acute mania is managed with a combination of antipsychotics, benzodiazepines, and mood stabilizers. Although loading doses of lithium have not proved useful, loading doses of valproate may speed the onset of response. Valproate at an oral loading dosage of 20 mg/kg/day has been associated with moderate antimanic effects occurring in as little as a few days. Standard doses of mood stabilizers may take a week or longer to achieve adequate control of mania. Benzodiazepines may be as useful as antipsychotics in the acute management of nonpsychotic manic patients. However, both psychotic and nonpsychotic patients benefit equally well from an atypical agent, and these drugs are more rapidly acting than mood stabilizers in the management of acute mania. Thus, we will typically prescribe an SGA for a manic patient and add a benzodiazepine or mood stabilizer as necessary.

When a psychotic patient can give some history and has a preference among available antipsychotic drugs, or when relatives or past medical records provide relevant information, the drug reported as best for the particular patient should be used.

Patients may present to the emergency room with antipsychotic complications in many forms (Table 10–4). One still fairly common form may be the development of acute EPS. The most worrisome of the acute EPS is *dystonia*. As discussed in Chapter 4 ("Antipsychotic Drugs"), young males are most vulnerable to acute dystonic reactions, which may include oculogyric crisis, opisthotonos, torticollis, trismus, or laryngospasm. Although all dystonic reactions are very frightening to patients, laryngospasm compromises the airway and is potentially fatal. Severe dystonic reactions may occur at any time of treatment, but they usually occur in the first few days of neuroleptic use. Furthermore, high-potency typical antipsychotics may have a greater association with dystonia. The most reliable and rapid treatment for dystonia is intravenous diphenhydramine 50 mg or benztropine 2 mg every 30 minutes until the dystonia resolves. Laryngospasm may require intubation and the use of intravenous lorazepam to treat the spasm. If intravenous access cannot be secured, intramuscular injections of the drugs will be necessary. Although atypical agents are less commonly associated with dystonic reactions, such reactions still sometimes occur.

An overdose of antipsychotics is rarely fatal. However, overdoses may result in hypothermia, hyperthermia, severe EPS, and occasional arrhythmias. Low-potency agents may additionally produce anticholinergic toxicity and hypotension. Hypotension is a complication of risperidone overdose as well. All antipsychotics reduce the seizure threshold, but clozapine may be particularly problematic in overdose. Psychotically depressed patients and young, educated male schizophrenic patients may be at greatest risk for antipsychotic overdoses. Antipsychotic overdoses usually respond to gastric lavage and supportive measures, including hydration, antiparkinsonian drugs for EPS, and cardiac monitoring.

NMS is a relatively rare complication of antipsychotic use that was discussed in Chapter 4. It represents a medical emergency and is characterized by severe EPS, delirium, hyperthermia, and autonomic abnormalities. Both typical and atypical antipsychotics, including clozapine, are sometimes associated with NMS. The major risk factors for EPS appear to be dehydration, concurrent use of lithium, and rapid titration to higher doses of all standard neuroleptics. Treatment involves immediate cessation of antipsychotics, sup-

Table 10–4. Emergency complications of antipsychotic use

Complication	Risk factors	Clinical findings	Management
Dystonia	Age < 40, male, high-potency agents	Torticollis, opisthotonos, oculogyric crisis, trismus, laryngospasm	Diphenhydramine (iv) or benztropine (iv); lorazepam and maintain airway for laryngospasm
Overdose	Age < 40, male, educated; schizophrenic, psychotic depression	Hypothermia/ hyperthermia, EPS, hypotension, anticholinergic toxicity, seizures, arrhythmia	Gastric lavage, hydration, antiparkinsonian agents for EPS, cardiac monitoring
Neuroleptic malignant syndrome	Dehydration; lithium use; high doses	Delirium, hyperthermia, severe EPS, autonomic instability, elevated CK and LFTs	Stop antipsychotics; dantrolene (iv), bromocriptine, lorazepam (iv)

Note. CK = creatine kinase; EPS = extrapyramidal symptoms; iv = intravenous; LFT = liver function tests.

port of vital functions, and prescription of dantrolene sodium as a muscle relaxant in doses of 0.8–1 mg/kg iv every 6 hours for up to 2 weeks. Longer use may be associated with extreme respiratory suppression and muscle atrophy. Bromocriptine at a dosage of up to 5 mg tid may help relieve some of the EPS, and lorazepam 1 mg iv tid may also provide relief. In refractory cases, ECT is also reported to be of utility.

Delirium

DSM-IV-TR (American Psychiatric Association 2000) criteria for delirium include a disturbance of consciousness, a change in cognition, a fluctuating course, and an organic basis for the disorder. Common causes of delirium include withdrawal syndromes, medication overdoses, endocrinopathies, metabolic abnormalities, and infections. Very old persons appear to be at greatest risk for the development of delirium, but it may occur at any age. The presence of delirium is a medical emergency and is associated with significant morbidity and mortality.

Clinical management of delirium centers on assessment of the underlying cause and supportive care. Physical restraints are often necessary and tend to be preferable to the administration of psychoactive agents, which may further cloud the clinical picture. When medications are required for control of an agitated, delirious patient, small doses of high-potency antipsychotics may be the treatment of choice. Drugs such as haloperidol do not cause significant anticholinergic or α-adrenergic symptoms and tend not to present problems of cardiac or respiratory depression. A typical dosage of haloperidol in the management of elderly delirious patients is 0.5 mg bid. Another pharmacological option is the use of small doses of 3-hydroxy-benzodiazepines, such as lorazepam and oxazepam, that have no active metabolites, have short half-lives, and are well metabolized even in elderly patients. Lorazepam can be administered in doses of 0.5–1 mg iv every 30 minutes, if administered slowly to avoid very high peak serum levels and subsequent respiratory depression. Oxazepam is not available in a parenteral form and has the second disadvantage of slow absorption and thus slower onset of action. If the patient is able to take medication orally, oxazepam 15 mg tid as needed for agitation is worth considering but is generally less desirable than lorazepam. Another strategy with which clinicians have had some success in the treatment of postoperative delirium include gabapentin (Leung et al. 2006). Gabapentin has also been associated with reducing perioperative pain and reducing the need for analgesics.

Severe Anxiety

Patients can present with panic, severe fear and anxiety, or multiple somatic symptoms. The symptoms of severe anxiety may be associated with a variety of medical conditions, including hypothyroidism, hypoglycemia, coronary artery disease, carcinoid syndrome, and pheochromocytoma. In addition, severe anxiety may be a feature of other psychiatric disorders, including schizophrenia, acute drug intoxication, alcohol withdrawal, and depression.

The anxiety disorders with which patients are most likely to present to the emergency room are panic disorder and posttraumatic stress disorder (PTSD). If medical illness can be rapidly ruled out or the patient has a known history of panic attacks, oral diazepam offers significant advantages because of its rapid onset of action after administration. Either 5- or 10-mg doses prn can be tried, depending on the severity of the anxiety and the patient's past responses to sedatives. If intramuscular administration is required, however, diazepam is not an ideal choice because of its erratic absorption. Lorazepam 1 mg im repeated hourly is effective in the acute management of severe anxiety. Antidepressant drugs are indicated in the longer-term treatment of panic disorders, but they are slow in onset and of no immediate value in patients experiencing acute, severe anxiety. Thus, it may be appropriate to use a benzodiazepine with an antidepressant in the initial weeks of antipanic therapy. A month later, the benzodiazepine may be tapered off after the antidepressant has begun to work. Clonazepam is also an effective antipanic agent and can be initiated at a dosage of 0.5 mg bid. Although anticonvulsants such as gabapentin and tiagabine are occasionally useful, they do not appear to be as rapidly acting as the benzodiazepines.

PTSD patients may present to the emergency room with significant symptoms of autonomic arousal from flashback experiences, intrusive thoughts, and insomnia. It is important to evaluate patients for comorbid disorders such as depression and substance abuse. Violent or agitated PTSD patients should be managed by the rapid tranquilization methods described earlier. β-Blockers may also be helpful in the initial management of autonomic hyperarousal. However, long-term treatments, including the use of antidepressants and mood-stabilizing agents, are best initiated after the acute distress is reduced and long-term follow-up is secured.

Some experts prefer low-dose antipsychotic drugs in patients with borderline or other personality disorders who present in an acute crisis. If the patient has a past history of sedative abuse, olanzapine 5–10 mg or chlorpromazine could be used. Chlorpromazine's sedation is likely to persist for many hours—at times, longer than is desired. If the patient is currently dependent on sedative drugs, consideration must be given to the problem of withdrawal reactions if the drugs are stopped abruptly. Buspirone is available for use in anxiety, but single doses are not helpful in reducing acute symptoms.

Stupor and Catatonia

Catatonia is a syndrome that may be induced by a variety of medical and psychiatric disorders. It is characterized by cataplexy and waxy flexibility, mutism, resistance to instructions or attempts to be moved (negativism), and intermittent agitation. The causes of catatonia range from metabolic disorders such as hepatic encephalopathy and ketoacidosis to postictal states and basal ganglia lesions. Affective disorders represent the most common psychiatric cause of catatonia, although the syndrome often occurs in schizophrenia. Nonpsychiatric etiologies account for a large percentage of catatonia cases. Therefore, a thorough history, a physical examination, and laboratory assessment are required. If medical or neurological causes for stupor can be ruled out, hospital admission to a psychiatric ward is generally indicated. If no information on the patient is available, intravenous benzodiazepines (e.g., lorazepam 1–2 mg) can sometimes facilitate obtaining a history by letting the patient talk relatively freely. (Historically, intravenous amobarbital sodium was used. However, this approach required the clinician to be experienced in the technique, and, again, it was best done in an inpatient setting (see Chapter 6: "Antianxiety Agents"). Intravenous amobarbital sodium is given at a rate up to 50 mg/minute to a maximum of 700 mg. The dose is titrated to the size and age of the patient; smaller and older patients require smaller amounts. There is a significant risk of respiratory depression with larger doses, which necessitates having a crash cart available and perhaps having a second IV line in case of difficulties.

There are lethal forms of catatonia in which patients present with hyperthermia, extreme rigidity, mental status changes, muscle breakdown, rhabdomyolysis, and renal failure. This so-called lethal or malignant catatonia may be quite difficult to distinguish from NMS. The distinction may be important, because lethal catatonia sometimes responds to antipsychotics, whereas antipsychotics are contraindicated in treating NMS. Fortunately, both NMS and lethal catatonia may respond to ECT.

Emergency Department Referrals

Psychiatric patients are occasionally referred to a general hospital emergency department by their psychiatrist after telephone calls or office visits. Definite or possible overdose attempts, unexplained confusional states, or serious drug side effects (such as MAOI-related hypertensive crises or acute dystonia) are reasonable examples of appropriate referrals.

It is important for psychiatrists to remember that emergency department physicians may know less about the pharmacological effects of psychiatric drugs than they do, despite the natural hope that the emergency department doctor will be all-knowing and highly resourceful. Therefore, to ensure that no major gaps in knowledge exist, it is worthwhile to call the emergency department before the patient gets there and/or after the patient has been initially evaluated. Many physicians have never heard that meperidine can be fatal when added to an MAOI. Some who do not know that TCAs have quinidine-like effects on cardiac conduction might give quinidine to treat an arrhythmia resulting from TCA overdose. Not uncommonly in emergency departments, a patient with a severe headache due to a hypertensive crisis may be ignored (i.e., made to wait) until the headache has passed on its own.

If a patient is sick enough to be admitted to a hospital and the psychiatrist knows of a history of benzodiazepine use, the psychiatrist should encourage the hospital staff to be concerned about withdrawal symptoms such as seizures or delirium. Also, the emergency physician may be reassured to know that overdoses of SSRIs, serotonin$_2$ (5-HT$_2$) antagonists, venlafaxine, and bupropion are likely to be relatively benign. In our experience, emergency department staff seem interested and appreciative when the responsible psychiatrist calls and provides both clinical and psychopharmacological input.

Bibliography

Allen MH, Currier GW, Carpenter D, et al; Expert Consensus Panel for Behavioral Emergencies 2005: The Expert Consensus Guideline Series. Treatment of behavioral emergencies 2005. J Psychiatr Pract 11 (suppl 1):5–108, 2005

American Psychiatric Association: Diagnostic and Statistical Manual of Mental Disorders, 4th Edition, Text Revision. Washington, DC, American Psychiatric Association, 2000

Andrezina R, Josiassen RC, Marcus RN, et al: Intramuscular aripiprazole for the treatment of acute agitation in patients with schizophrenia or schizoaffective disorder: a double-blind, placebo-controlled comparison with intramuscular haloperidol. Psychopharmacology (Berl) 188:281–292, 2006a

Andrezina R, Marcus RN, Oren DA, et al: Intramuscular aripiprazole or haloperidol and transition to oral therapy in patients with agitation associated with schizophrenia: subanalysis of a double-blind study. Curr Med Res Opin 22:2209–2219, 2006b

Barlow CB, Rizzo AG: Violence against surgical residents. West J Med 167:74–78, 1997

Bazire S: MAOIs and narcotic analgesics (letter). Br J Psychiatry 151:701–710, 1987

Bongar B: Suicide Guidelines for Assessment, Management and Treatment. New York, Oxford University Press, 1992

Breier A, Wright P, Birkett M, et al: Intramuscular olanzapine: dose-related improvement in acutely agitated patients with schizophrenia. Presentation at the 154th annual meeting of the American Psychiatric Association, New Orleans, May 5–10, 2001

Browne B, Lintner S: Monoamine oxidase inhibitors and narcotic analgesics: a critical review of the implications for treatment. Br J Psychiatry 151:210–212, 1987

Cipriani A, Pretty H, Hawton K, et al: Lithium in the prevention of suicidal behavior and all-cause mortality in patients with mood disorders: a systematic review of randomized trials. Am J Psychiatry 162:1805–1819, 2005

Cole J: Drugs and seclusion and restraint. McLean Hospital Journal 10:37–53, 1985

Crome P: Antidepressant overdosage. Drugs 23:431–461, 1982

Dubin WR, Field JA: Rapid tranquilization of the violent patient. Am J Emerg Med 7:313–319, 1989

Dubin W, Stolberg R: Emergency Psychiatry for the House Officer. New York, SP Medical & Scientific Books, 1981

Dubin WR, Waxman MH, Weiss KJ, et al: Rapid tranquilization: the efficacy of oral concentrate. J Clin Psychiatry 46:475–478, 1985

Fawcett J, Scheftner WA, Clark DC: Time related predictors of suicide. Am J Psychiatry 147:1189–1194, 1990

Goldberg RJ, Dubin WR, Fogel BS: Behavioral emergencies: assessment and psychopharmacologic management. Clin Neuropharmacol 12:233–248, 1989

Hillard JR (ed): Manual of Clinical Emergency Psychiatry. Washington, DC, American Psychiatric Press, 1990

Hughes DH: Trends and treatment models in emergency psychiatry. Hosp Community Psychiatry 44:927–928, 1993

Hyman SE, Tesar GE: Manual of Psychiatric Emergencies, 3rd Edition. Boston, MA, Little, Brown, 1994

Kovacsics CE, Gottesman II, Gould TD: Lithium's antisuicidal efficacy: elucidation of neurobiological targets using endophenotype strategies. Annu Rev Pharmacol Toxicol 49:175–198, 2009

Lavoie FIV, Carter GL, Danzl DF, et al: Emergency department violence in United States teaching hospitals. Ann Emerg Med 17:1227–1232, 1988

Leung JM, Sands LP, Rico M, et al: Pilot clinical trial of gabapentin to decrease post-operative delirium in older patients. Neurology 67:1251–1253, 2006

Meehan KM, Zhang F, David SR, et al: A double-blind, randomized comparison of the efficacy and safety of intramuscular injections of olanzapine, lorazepam, or placebo in treating acutely agitated patients diagnosed with bipolar mania. J Clin Psychopharmacol 21:389–397, 2001

Meehan KM, Wang H, David SR, et al: Comparison of rapidly acting intramuscular olanzapine, lorazepam, and placebo: a double-blind, randomized study in acutely agitated patients with dementia. Neuropsychopharmacology 26:494–504, 2002

Moller HJ, Kissling W, Lang C, et al: Efficacy and side effects of haloperidol in psychotic patients: oral vs. intravenous administration. Am J Psychiatry 139:1571–1575, 1982

Montgomery SA: Venlafaxine: a new dimension in antidepressant pharmacotherapy. J Clin Psychiatry 54:119–124, 1993

Müller-Oerlinghausen B, Berghöfer A, Ahrens B: The antisuicidal and mortality-reducing effect of lithium prophylaxis: consequences for guidelines in clinical psychiatry. Can J Psychiatry 48:433–439, 2003

Munizza C, Furlan PM, d'Elia A, et al: Emergency psychiatry: a review of the literature. Acta Psychiatr Scand Suppl 374:1–51, 1993

Prien RF, Kupfer DJ, Mansky PA, et al: Drug therapy in the prevention of recurrences in unipolar and bipolar affective disorders: report of the NIMH Collaborative Study Group comparing lithium carbonate, imipramine, and a lithium carbonate–imipramine combination. Arch Gen Psychiatry 41:1096–1104, 1984

Puryear DA: Proposed standards in emergency psychiatry. Hosp Community Psychiatry 43:14–15, 1992

Rubino A, Roskell N, Tennis P, et al: Risk of suicide during treatment with venlafaxine, citalopram, fluoxetine, and dothiepin: retrospective cohort study. BMJ 334(7587):242, 2007

Saklad SR, Ereshefsky L, Jann MW, et al: Usefulness of injectable and oral lorazepam in psychotic and developmentally disabled patients. Paper presented at the 138th annual meeting of the American Psychiatric Association, Dallas, TX, May 20–23, 1985

Szuster RR, Schanbacher BL, McCann SC, et al: Underdiagnosis of psychoactive-substance-induced organic mental disorders in emergency psychiatry. Am J Drug Alcohol Abuse 16:319–327, 1990

Weissberg MP: Emergency psychiatry: a critical educational omission (editorial). Ann Intern Med 114:246–247, 1991

Wright P, Lindberg SR, Birkett M, et al: Intramuscular olanzapine and intramuscular haloperidol in acute schizophrenia: antipsychotic efficacy and extrapyramidal safety during the first 24 hours of treatment. Can J Psychiatry 48:716–721, 2003

Youssef NA, Rich CL: Does acute treatment with sedatives/hypnotics for anxiety in depressed patients affect suicide risk? A literature review. Ann Clin Psychiatry 20:157–169, 2008

11

Pharmacotherapy for Substance Use Disorders

Drug therapies for patients with substance use disorders are sometimes necessary or useful, but they are rarely sufficient to cure the disorder. If illicit drugs are overused by a patient with major depression to reduce psychic pain, by a patient with mania manifested as overactivity and uncontrolled hedonism, or by a patient with some other comorbid major Axis I disorder, appropriate drug therapy for the underlying major psychiatric condition can be very helpful. Unfortunately, some patients with clear syndromes (e.g., depression, bipolar disorder, schizophrenia) continue to abuse illicit drugs even when the syndromes are in full or partial remission, though others show improvement in both conditions with appropriate drug therapy.

Specific drug therapies are, however, available for some aspects of chemical dependence. Medications are useful for ameliorating withdrawal symptoms caused by physical dependence on sedative or opiate drugs. Either methadone or buprenorphine, as maintenance therapy, is a longer-acting, more manageable, less dangerous drug than heroin and can be given indefinitely in an attempt to replace heroin. Naltrexone, an opiate antagonist, can also be given in-

565

definitely to prevent the patient from obtaining euphoria from heroin and has been found to be useful in the maintenance therapy of alcoholism. Disulfiram (Antabuse) is sometimes used in treating chronic alcoholism to ensure that patients will become unpleasantly sick if they were to consume alcohol. Alternatively, a medication such as naltrexone or acamprosate can reduce the risk of relapse in an alchohol-dependent patient.

Some classes of illicit drugs, of course, do not cause any serious degree of physical dependence. These include cannabis, inhalants, and the hallucinogens (e.g., lysergic acid diethylamide [LSD] and mescaline). Withdrawal symptoms are also seldom seen with phencyclidine (PCP) use. Such drugs can sometimes be abruptly discontinued, even in heavy and frequent users. Nevertheless, a drug therapy that would decrease or stop the use of these agents might well be clinically useful. Drug dependence syndromes for which drug therapies are sometimes or regularly useful involve stimulants, opiates, sedative-hypnotics, and alcohol.

A large variety of interesting, even promising, drug therapies for various substance use disorders have been proposed and studied, but the basic, approved, and available drug therapies have changed very little. The situation is exciting, frustrating, and, even sometimes, irritating. However, there is general agreement that a variety of psychosocial approaches to substance use disorders, especially opiate, cocaine, and alcohol dependence, are effective, probably more so than most available or even potential drug therapies. There is also agreement that drug therapies must be used in the context of psychosocial treatments, including 12-step and compulsory aspects of treatment.

The only new drug to be approved for the treatment of alcoholism in more than a decade is acamprosate (Campral). Acamprosate was approved by the U.S. Food and Drug Administration (FDA) in 2004 but has been used in Europe since the early 1990s.

On the basis of published evidence, buprenorphine, a mixed opiate agonist-antagonist, appears to be effective both in opiate detoxification and as a maintenance treatment potentially superior to methadone, particularly if it is allowed to be used without all the legalistic complications surrounding the use of methadone and L-α-acetylmethadol (LAAM). Buprenorphine was approved for the maintenance treatment of opiate dependence in 2002. It is currently available in 2-mg and 8-mg sublingual tablets (Subutex) and in an injection form (Buprenex). Buprenorphine is also available in combination with naloxone (Suboxone) in sublingual tablets (2 mg buprenorphine/0.5 mg naloxone and 8 mg buprenorphine/2 mg naloxone).

A number of drug therapies (e.g., tricyclic antidepressants [TCAs]) were found to be better than placebo in the treatment of cocaine users in early controlled studies but not effective in many other similar controlled studies. Old drugs in new bottles (e.g., disulfiram for cocaine abuse) and totally new approaches (e.g., antibodies against cocaine) wait in the wings.

The only other relatively solid advance in the pharmacotherapy of substance use disorders is the handful of well-controlled studies showing that patients with substance use disorders and major depression can benefit from standard antidepressants without being forced to become drug free first.

Drug Testing

A variety of sensitive assays are available to monitor and test for illicit drug use. The most common of these are urine drug screens that evaluate the "NIDA 5," which are the five classes of drugs typically evaluated in federal drug testing programs: cannabinoids, opiates, cocaine, amphetamine, and PCP. Many labs are also equipped to evaluate benzodiazepines, barbiturates, hallucinogens, and inhalants.

Urine drug screens are the least intrusive tests, and they are inexpensive and, typically, quite reliable. The cost for in-office tests range from about $5 to $50 dollars. Urine drug screens can be influenced by abstaining before the drug screen and primarily detect drugs taken within 7 days of the test. However, chronic cannabis use up to 12 weeks before a urine drug screen can be detected by the screen, while a single use a few days before the test might be picked up. Saliva tests are usually processed in a laboratory and tend to be more expensive ($20–$100) than urine drug screens. Salivary tests are capable of detecting very recent use (the past hour or so) that may be missed in a urine test. Like urine tests, they primarily pick up drugs that have been used in the previous 3 days. Serum blood screens are the most sensitive assays and the most expensive. For most drugs, a serum assay is best at detecting drug use in the previous 3–7 days. Other types of tests include hair assays, which can detect most drugs that have been used in the previous 90 days, and patch or sweat tests, which are neither very accurate nor convenient. In most offices, a urine drug screen offers the best combination of convenience, cost, and reliability.

Stimulants

Stimulants, including cocaine, amphetamine, and their various forms, are among the most common drugs of abuse in the United States. The U.S. National Institute on Drug Abuse (NIDA) estimates that at least 1%–2% of the population currently abuses cocaine but that rates of amphetamine abuse are lower. Stimulant overdose or abuse represents a fairly common reason for emergency room (ER) visits and hospitalization in urban settings. When a patient who is dependent on stimulants is hospitalized, stimulant administration should be stopped abruptly. No tapered withdrawal is necessary. Patients who have been taking stimulants in large amounts (e.g., more than 50 mg of D-amphetamine or several doses of cocaine a day) often have a withdrawal syndrome consisting of depression, fatigue, hyperphagia, and hypersomnia. In unstable individuals, this rebound depression can reach serious clinical proportions for a few days and may persist for weeks, usually in less severe form.

A variety of drugs, mainly dopaminergic or noradrenergic drugs (desipramine, amantadine, bromocriptine, bupropion), but even fluoxetine, have been tried in cocaine withdrawal or as possible longer-term treatments, but with no consistent effect. Imipramine, desipramine, and venlafaxine have shown "promising results" in treating depressed cocaine-dependent patients, reducing both depressive symptoms and cocaine use, but the full value of these controlled but preliminary studies does not yet constitute a clear, valid guide for the use of such drugs in patients with major depression who use cocaine.

Carbamazepine has been used, without success, in an attempt to reduce brain stimulation caused by cocaine. Topiramate has shown preliminary success in cocaine dependence (Reis et al. 2008) and may have a role to play in alcohol and nicotine dependence. Calcium channel blockers have been tried as a way to improve brain blood flow in cocaine users, but this work is only in the preliminary stages.

Disulfiram (Antabuse) has been resurrected from its declining use in treating chronic alcoholism, because it inhibits dopamine-β-hydroxylase, thereby raising brain cocaine and dopamine levels. One might imagine that this effect would only make the cocaine "high" better and longer, but disulfiram seems to increase anxiety, paranoia, and dysphoria when cocaine is taken. Several small studies have shown reduction in cocaine use, perhaps secondary to subjects' fear of using alcohol to modulate cocaine-induced agitation. In one study the reduction in cocaine use in the disulfiram group occurred even in patients who disclaimed prior use of alcohol (Petrakis et al. 2000). The dosage of disulfiram used appears to be 250 mg/day. It is unclear how safe this therapy will be in the long run if patients drink alcohol despite warnings and get severe reactions.

Other investigational approaches include ecopipam, a dopamine$_1$ receptor blocker, and citicoline, previously used in treating neurological disorders to repair damaged cell membranes. Even aspirin has been used to prevent platelet aggregation and improve brain blood flow and, in one study, to improve neuropsychological function (O'Leary and Weiss 2000).

As noted earlier, a cocaine "vaccine"—a large antibody that binds cocaine in body fluids—is being developed. Animal experiments suggest this approach might have promise. A very recent study suggested some potential efficacy in a trial in humans; however, the authors concluded that the vaccine did not produce sufficient effect and that better vaccines were required (Martell et al. 2009).

Any or all of the forementioned potential therapies should be combined with appropriate addiction-focused psychotherapies (Najavits and Weiss 1994).

Amphetamine abuse, even the relatively recent advent of "crack"-style D-methamphetamine ("ice") inhalation, has not stimulated any new pharmacotherapy—either conceptually or empirically—though treatments useful for cocaine use would likely be effective for "speed" use.

The issue of abuse can be a problem with medically prescribable stimulants. If the patient has a clinical depression that responds uniquely to stimulants or clearly has adult attention-deficit/hyperactivity disorder and takes moderate doses in a stable manner to produce socially responsible functioning, stimulant use can be therapeutically helpful (see Chapter 8: "Stimulants"). If the patient takes stimulants in large doses for euphoriant purposes or pushes the dosage to the point that paranoia or other serious symptoms develop, prescribing stimulants is obviously contraindicated.

Opiates

Detoxification

Opiates include heroin, the most common street narcotic, and its variants. In addition, this large class includes commonly used therapeutic agents such as morphine, codeine, methadone, and other prescription narcotic analgesics. Abstinence symptoms can begin as early as 6 hours after the last dose of heroin or other short-acting opiate. Withdrawal symptoms include anxiety, insomnia, yawning, sweating, and rhinorrhea, followed by dilated pupils, tremor, goose flesh, chills, anorexia, and muscle cramps. About a day after the last dose, pulse, blood pressure, respiration, and temperature may all increase, and diarrhea, nausea, and vomiting can occur. The syndrome, untreated, peaks at 2–3 days and resolves within about 10 days, although mild variable complaints may persist for weeks.

Because a great deal of street heroin is so weak, some illicit heroin users may not have developed true physical dependence. In addition, both street and medical users of opiates, with or without real physical dependence, often consciously or unconsciously exaggerate their withdrawal distress in an effort to obtain more opiate medication from the physician. For these reasons, the drug treatment of the withdrawal syndrome should be based on objective signs of opiate withdrawal, not on subjective complaints. These signs are listed in Table 11–1.

Methadone, a long-acting opiate, is used to treat withdrawal because of its superior pharmacokinetics (a long half-life). A short-acting drug like morphine would have to be given every few hours to block withdrawal, whereas methadone accomplishes this when given only twice a day. The initial methadone dose should be 10 mg orally, in liquid or crushed tablet form, so as to blind the patient to that dosage and subsequent dosages during detoxification. The patient should be evaluated every 4 hours, and an additional 10 mg of methadone should be administered if at least two of the four criteria in Table 11–1 are met. Unless the patient is being withdrawn from high-dose methadone maintenance therapy, no more than 40 mg of methadone should be required in the first 24 hours.

The total dose of methadone given in the first 24 hours should be considered the stabilization dose. This dose is then given the next day in two divided doses (e.g., 15 mg at 8:00 A.M. and 8:00 P.M.) in crushed or liquid form. It should be consumed under the direct observation of a staff member

Table 11–1.   Objective opiate withdrawal signs

1. Pulse 10 bpm or more over baseline or more than 90 if no history of tachycardia and baseline unknown (baseline: vital-sign values 1 hour after receiving 10 mg of methadone)
2. Systolic blood pressure 10 mm Hg or more above baseline or greater than 160/95 in nonhypertensive patients
3. Dilated pupils
4. Gooseflesh, sweating, rhinorrhea, or lacrimation

to avoid illicit diversion. The stabilization dose should then be reduced by 5 mg/day until the patient is completely withdrawn from the drug. A patient who is physically dependent on sedative drugs and opiates should continue taking the stabilization methadone dose without tapering until he or she is completely withdrawn from the sedative drug.

An alternative pharmacological approach to the management of opiate withdrawal has been used for the last few years at some centers. This approach involves the use of the nonopiate antihypertensive drug clonidine, which is mainly an α_2-adrenergic agonist. It can suppress both objective and subjective symptoms of opiate withdrawal. In beginning clonidine treatment, the method of Kleber et al. (1985) is worth following: an initial dose of 0.1 mg of clonidine should be given to assess the patient's tolerance of this approach. Hypotension, dizziness, sedation, and dry mouth are common adverse effects. If the initial dose is tolerated well by the patient, doses of 0.1–0.2 mg every 8 hours can be given during the early phases of opiate withdrawal, with increases to as high as 0.2–0.4 mg every 8 hours after 2–3 days. Blood pressure should be checked before each dose, and the dose should not be given if blood pressure is less than 85/55. Amelioration of withdrawal symptoms reaches a peak 2 or 3 hours after each dose. Muscle aches, irritability, and insomnia are not well suppressed by clonidine.

In one inpatient study of the use of clonidine in the detoxification of patients withdrawing from maintenance methadone, an average dosage of about 1 mg/day of clonidine was required for the first 8 days the patients were withdrawing from methadone. In a study using clonidine in outpatient detoxification, the medication was begun at 0.1 mg every 4–6 hours as needed, and the dose was increased to 0.2 mg every 4–6 hours, with a maximum dosage of 1.2 mg/day (average maximum total daily dose was 0.8 mg). Some variation of these dosing strategies could be used if a methadone detoxification program is to be avoided.

Physicians interested in using this approach should carefully read the article by Kosten et al. (1989) or consult with a local program where this approach is being actively used.

Outpatient use of clonidine for opiate detoxification has generally met with much less success than has use in inpatient studies. Clonidine (Catapres) is available in 0.1-mg, 0.2-mg, and 0.3-mg tablets, as well as in transdermal patches that may be administered weekly.

Three interlocking developments are taking place in the area of opiate detoxification. One is the use of buprenorphine, the mixed opiate agonist-antagonist, instead of methadone to speed the detoxification process and as a maintenance treatment (Umbricht et al. 1999). Another, more experimental use of buprenorphine is to combine it with the opiate antagonist naltrexone or naloxone to precipitate rapid, severe abstinence of short duration, leaving the patient no longer physically dependent on (or having tolerance for) opiates after a day or two.

Neither buprenorphine-assisted withdrawal nor very rapid antagonist withdrawal is a procedure to be undertaken outside a specialized treatment facility. Buprenorphine certification is generally required for practitioners, and courses are available at the annual meetings organized by the American Psychiatric Association.

Maintenance

For many years, methadone maintenance has been available in major urban areas in specially licensed clinics as a replacement therapy for heroin or other illicit opiates for confirmed addicts who have failed to stay drug free after detoxification. The dose adjustment varies from program to program; dosages as high as 80 mg/day are used in some clinics; it now has been repeatedly shown that a dosage of 60 mg/day provides much better long-term results than lower maintenance dosages.

Patients usually take the drug once a day at the clinic under direct supervision and have their urine samples checked for other illicit drug use. If the patient is drug free and doing generally well, take-home doses are often allowed so that the patient takes the methadone dose at the clinic only every other day. The drug is often dispensed in a fruit drink to avoid intravenous misuse of the alternate-day dose taken at home. Although this regimen would appear to provide a popular and useful alternative for confirmed opiate addicts, patients often drop out of methadone maintenance programs after weeks or months of participation.

Over the years it has become ever clearer that the purpose of methadone maintenance and related programs is not to gradually wean all patients off methadone entirely over weeks or months, but to stabilize the patients so they can improve their psychosocial adjustment or, at least, not have to resort to criminal activity to obtain heroin. Concomitantly, "dirty" urine samples showing that the patient is using other abusable drugs have become issues for counseling, not reasons to throw the patient out of the methadone program.

LAAM is even longer acting than methadone and is effective even if administered only three times a week. This feature eliminates the complications of daily clinic visits and the potential diversion of take-home doses. LAAM was approved by the FDA for the treatment of opiate dependence in 1993. However, LAAM has been associated with ventricular arrythmias and was removed from the European market in 2001. In 2003, the most common formulation of LAAM, Orlaam, was discontinued in the United States.

Either methadone or LAAM was intended to avert withdrawal symptoms and to abolish craving for opiates in heroin-addicted individuals. Either agent was also supposed to provide so high a level of tolerance to opiates that self-administration of street heroin or other illicit morphinelike drugs will no longer cause euphoria.

Maintenance methadone is stabilizing for some opiate addicts, but it does not completely suppress drug-seeking behavior, even for heroin; patients in methadone programs often continue to get in trouble with other drugs of abuse, especially alcohol and cocaine. Maintenance therapy, even coupled with good support programs, cannot solve the multiple problems of many heroin users.

Maintenance methadone is a specialized modality in which psychiatrists cannot get involved in the ordinary course of practice. Consider the plight of the psychiatrist involved in caring for an opiate-dependent patient who is seeking, or claims to be seeking, admission to a detoxification program but has an admission date that is several days off. What can or should the physician do? It is illegal to prescribe opiates to sustain an addiction. The best procedure is to consult with the detoxification program staff as to how to proceed. It is our understanding of U.S. Drug Enforcement Administration (DEA) regulations that a physician is allowed to dispense daily doses of an opiate each day for up to three successive days to avert acute withdrawal while awaiting a planned admission for detoxification. In addition, physicians may provide maintenance treatment to an addict "who is hospitalized for medical conditions other than addiction and who requires temporary maintenance during the critical period of his [or her] hospitalization or whose enrollment in an approved program has been verified" (AHFS Drug Information 2003, p. 2040). Physicians should check with their local DEA office before embarking on such an enterprise. It is legal to prescribe opiates for prolonged periods outside a methadone clinic if the patient has bona fide chronic pain of substantial degree. Before getting into such a situation, the physician should certainly obtain a consultation from a pain specialist or refer the patient to a pain clinic.

Another available maintenance treatment is the opiate antagonist naltrexone (ReVia). This drug is similar to naloxone (Narcan), the opiate antagonist that has long been available for treating opiate overdose. However, naltrexone is much longer acting and is available in oral form. Either drug could, in theory, be given orally in large daily doses to create a chronic blockade of opiate receptors, which would reliably block the euphoriant effects of heroin or other morphinelike drugs. Naloxone is too weak and short acting orally to be usable. Naltrexone is adequate for the purpose, but it has been even less popular with opiate addicts than methadone has. However, now that naltrexone has become available to the clinician, it may perhaps find a useful niche in the long-term maintenance treatment of some opiate-addicted individuals, particularly those who are highly motivated. The problem, of course, is that naltrexone is as easy as disulfiram to circumvent. An opiate addict needs to simply hold the dose of naltrexone for 2 or 3 days and then inject heroin to experience the full effects of the drug. For the moment, however, naltrexone is still a drug to be used mainly in special programs and not by general psychiatrists, unless they are asked to take over the care of a patient who has already been stabilized by being given naltrexone in a specialty program. The usual dosage of naltrexone for maintenance treatment of opiate addiction is 50 mg/day. It can be given three times a week (100 mg, 100 mg, then 150 mg), but gastrointestinal side effects are more common with that regimen. A recent report from Australia indicates an implantable form of naltrexone was more effective than oral naltrexone in promoting abstinence in a long-term trial (Hulse et al. 2009).

Buprenorphine (Subutex; Suboxone [buprenorphine and naloxone]), a mixed agonist-antagonist, was approved by the FDA in 2002 as an alternative to methadone for maintenance treatment of opiate addiction. The approval of buprenorphine allowed the possibility of an office-based treatment outside the highly regulated methadone clinics. Buprenorphine is available as a schedule III drug, whereas methadone is a schedule II drug and requires stricter regulations for usage. Studies support the contention that outpatient-based buprenorphine therapy is highly effective in reducing relapse and enhancing adherence in 12-step programs and may be safer than methadone treatment (Bell et al. 2009; Parran et al. 2010). The drug is given usually at dosages of 6–20 mg/day, with a target dosage of around 16 mg/day. Buprenorphine is taken sublingually to avoid excessive drug destruction in the liver, which occurs if the drug is taken as an ordinary pill and swallowed. This sublingual form, which is said to be the most widely used analgesic in many European countries, has been placed by the DEA in schedule III.

Buprenorphine is a good analgesic, but so are many other opiates and mixed agonist-antagonists (e.g., pentazocine). However, when buprenorphine was tested for abuse liability in humans by Jasinski et al. (1978) at the NIDA Addiction Research Center, it proved to be well tolerated and to elicit very mild dependence and withdrawal symptoms, even after prolonged high-dose administration.

Buprenorphine can substitute for other opiates and can block opiate-induced euphoria. Testing for periods of several weeks with opiate-addicted individuals has suggested that the drug is much more acceptable to patients than is naltrexone, perhaps because of the former's mild euphoriant effect. It decreases illicit drug use, as measured by urine screens, as effectively as methadone—not completely, but substantially. Studies of buprenorphine in opiate withdrawal suggest that it is equivalent in efficacy to methadone and superior to other drugs, such as clonidine (Janiri et al. 1994).

Withdrawing patients from maintenance buprenorphine is much easier than withdrawing them from methadone. The drug is already in pharmacies, in vials, and, as noted above, has a less restrictive schedule status (III) than does methadone, which is schedule II. Buprenorphine may become the first reasonably good maintenance therapy for chronic opiate users that could be prescribed in ordinary hospitals, clinics, and doctors' offices and dispensed in ordinary pharmacies. Such availability would avoid the bad side of methadone clinics: the massing of a lot of street users all in one clinic to "re-infect" each other. Another change, in process, is in our attitude toward the treatment of depression in methadone patients and other substance users. In a study by Nunes and colleagues (1998), imipramine was superior to placebo in decreasing depression in methadone-maintained patients with coexisting primary major depression. There was also some concomitant decrease in illicit drug use.

Anyone contemplating using psychiatric drugs to treat Axis I disorders in methadone clinic patients should be aware of potential drug-drug interactions. Carbamazepine, but not valproic acid or lithium, enhances hepatic metabolism and lowers methadone blood levels, perhaps justifying an increase in the daily methadone dose. Fluvoxamine, however, blocks methadone metabolism and raises the blood level (which will fall again if the fluvoxamine is discontinued).

In general, selective serotonin reuptake inhibitors (SSRIs) or other newer antidepressants that can be taken once a day and do not need much dose adjustment are easier for patients with depression and substance use disorders. With other agents, these patients are likely to be undercompliant and not experience improvement or to raise their dosages unilaterally and induce toxicity. One of us has seen such an outpatient become delirious after 5 days of taking amitriptyline; because the prescribed dosage (50 mg) did not give rapid relief, the patient took 500 mg/day.

Sedatives and Hypnotics

Detoxification

Over the past 50 years, the problem of sedative addiction (physical and psychological dependence) shifted from being almost completely an abuse of short- or intermediate-acting barbiturates (e.g., amobarbital, pentobarbital, secobarbital) to being an abuse of newer hypnotics (glutethimide, methaqualone) and, most recently, benzodiazepines (e.g., diazepam, alprazolam). All these agents (and alcohol) produce cross-tolerance—that is, physical withdrawal symptoms in a patient who is dependent on any one of these drugs can be relieved by an adequate dose of another. The time course of withdrawal symptoms differs with the half-lives of the drugs involved, beginning within 12–16 hours after the last dose of a short-acting agent (e.g., amobarbital, alprazolam) and perhaps 2–5 days after the last dose of diazepam.

Early withdrawal symptoms include anxiety, restlessness, agitation, nausea, vomiting, and fatigue. Later, weakness develops, often with abdominal cramps, plus tachycardia, postural hypotension, hyperreflexia, and gross resting tremor. Insomnia and nightmares may occur. Peak symptoms, including grand mal seizures in some instances, occur at about 1–3 days after the last dose of short-acting drugs (amobarbital, lorazepam, alprazolam) and 5–10 days after the last dose of long-acting drugs (diazepam, clorazepate). Of patients who have seizures, about half develop delirium with disorientation, anxiety, and visual hallucinations. Even without seizures, patients in benzodiazepine withdrawal may be mildly confused, perceive lights as being too bright and sounds as too loud, become mildly paranoid, and feel depersonalized.

Sedative withdrawal, particularly from barbiturates, can be fatal once it has progressed to delirium and is not readily reversible then. For this reason, withdrawal from sedative dependence should be considered a medical emergency, and patients presenting in withdrawal should be treated as emergency patients. Withdrawal syndromes from benzodiazepines may be less severe. In contrast, opiate withdrawal symptoms are rarely life-threatening and always reversible if an opiate is given.

There are current regimens that use a long-acting sedative, such as phenobarbital, chlordiazepoxide, or diazepam, to ameliorate withdrawal from sedatives. In previous years, the most commonly recommended regimen involved using the short-acting barbiturate pentobarbital (Nembutal) to establish the degree of dependence and then converting the patient to the longer-acting phenobarbital for the real detoxification phase. This regimen, the *pentobarbital tolerance test,* is very rarely used now; the favored regimen is treatment of sedative dependence with a taper of a long-acting benzodiazepine.

Benzodiazepines

For the more common psychiatric patient who has probably become physically dependent on a prescribed benzodiazepine at moderate doses taken for more than a year, the benzodiazepine dose can be gradually decreased while the patient is followed as an outpatient, if the patient can tolerate such a program. There are reports that in panic patients who have responded to relatively higher dosages (e.g., 6 mg/day) of alprazolam, reduction in dosage at a rate of 0.5 mg every week to 2 mg/day is generally well tolerated. Further reduction below 2 mg/day at this rate of discontinuation will cause patients considerable discomfort. At or below 2 mg/day, a more gradual reduction—0.25 mg/day every week—is recommended.

A shift from short-acting benzodiazepines, such as lorazepam or alprazolam, to longer-acting ones like clonazepam can be tried if tapering of the shorter-acting drug leads to uncomfortable symptoms. For patients with such discomfort, it is not clear whether rapid inpatient withdrawal is required, but that approach seems legitimate if outpatient withdrawal is poorly tolerated. It may be that slow withdrawal over weeks produces more discomfort than would a rapid, systematic inpatient regimen. Even with systematic inpatient withdrawal, however, there is a significant risk of relapse. A study by Joughin et al. (1991) found that most patients with long-term benzodiazepine dependence did not fare well even after successful inpatient detoxification. Only 38% of patients studied had had a "good" outcome in 6-month follow-up, and many had relapsed or encountered other difficulties, including suicide. Elderly patients and those with concurrent depressive symptoms fared particularly poorly. The authors concluded that for some patients, maintenance benzodiazepine therapy might be preferable to withdrawal.

Herman et al. (1987) reported good results in shifting patients from alprazolam to clonazepam. They substituted 1 mg of clonazepam abruptly for every 2 mg of alprazolam and allowed patients to take extra doses of alprazolam as needed during the first week they were receiving clonazepam. Patients stabilized on clonazepam could then be withdrawn more easily from the longer-acting drug.

Animal studies (Galpern et al. 1991) suggested that clonazepam probably has a risk for dependence and tolerance problems similar to that of other benzodiazepines but that its long half-life may make for a smoother withdrawal. Still, we have seen patients who had difficulty in withdrawing from clonazepam.

Carbamazepine has also been used, with mixed results, to facilitate withdrawal from alprazolam and other short-acting benzodiazepines. Patients given carbamazepine at dosages of 200–800 mg/day, initiated before a benzodiazepine taper, showed longer benzodiazepine abstinence after the taper than did patients treated concurrently with placebo (Schweizer et al. 1991). Likewise, geriatric patients who failed to respond to previous tapers of alprazolam were able to achieve success when the taper was initiated with concurrent carbamazepine use (Swantek et al. 1991). However, it has been difficult to demonstrate that the withdrawal is any less severe in patients using carbamazepine as an adjunct in benzodiazepine withdrawal, and not all studies have found a robust effect for this regimen. It is important to keep in mind that carbamazepine may induce cytochrome P450 3A3/4 and other P450 enzymes in the liver, thus lowering alprazolam plasma levels and intensifying withdrawal symptoms. Some clinicians use valproate instead.

Another issue that warrants attention is that mild benzodiazepine withdrawal symptoms should be looked for more carefully in patients who have been admitted to psychiatric hospitals and whose prior sedative benzodiazepine medication was abruptly stopped. A few patients appear to become quite uncomfortable and to have typical withdrawal symptoms after discontinuation of dosages as low as 5 mg/day of diazepam or 30 mg/day of flurazepam if the dosages were taken regularly for many years. Withdrawal symptoms in such patients can last for weeks. Physicians may forget that sedative withdrawal may be occurring when a depressed or schizophrenic patient begins to get more agitated, and they may be painfully surprised and discomfited when the patient suddenly has a grand mal seizure.

There is a real question as to whether outpatients receiving long-term regular benzodiazepine therapy for anxiety—say clonazepam 0.5 mg tid and 1 mg hs—need to be firmly tapered off the drug over their objections. If they have a history of a substance use disorder and have been stable while taking such a dose for months or even years, does the chronic use of prescribed drug put them at significant risk of relapse into serious substance abuse? Physicians who see "ordinary" psychiatric outpatients outside of specialized drug abuse programs are sometimes not aware of their patients' history of past substance abuse. Physicians actively treating patients with serious substance use disorders are often horrified if patients are given maintenance benzodiazepines for chronic anxiety disorder.

The published literature is mixed. Expert opinion is generally against using benzodiazepines in patients with substance use disorders, but clinical reports on the adverse effects of such prescribing are lacking. On the basis of guesswork and of experience supervising residents treating such patients, we surmise that soon after alcohol, sedative, or other detoxification, patients may be at much increased risk of returning to substance abuse if they are prescribed benzodiazepines, but a bit later they may use such sedative drugs sensibly and with benefit.

Some patients with substance use disorders probably have anxiety disorders of such severity that they will relapse rapidly into taking whatever is available to relieve their discomfort; some of these patients may do better on prescribed, well-monitored sedatives than on illicit drugs (Mueller et al. 1996). Any physician regularly prescribing maintenance benzodiazepines to a large number of patients with substance use disorders needs to document the reasons for his or her prescribing in detail in each case and to get outside consultations to forestall accusations of substandard practice.

Alcohol

Ethyl alcohol is a short-acting sedative drug that produces withdrawal syndromes similar to those caused by barbiturates. The symptoms and signs of withdrawal are the same as those described in the "Detoxification" subsection of "Sedatives and Hypnotics" in this chapter, with the caveat that alcoholic patients may be either very slightly dependent physically but in trouble with alcohol for other reasons or malnourished and/or medically quite ill. Because alcoholism programs tend to treat large numbers of patients, they usually choose a "standard" detoxification program—a program that is standard for a given institution but that may differ substantially from one facility to another. McLean Hospital has used chlordiazepoxide in alcohol detoxification for at least 30 years; it may be a good choice because it has a long half-life and may be less euphoriant than diazepam. The use of benzodiazepines for the management of acute alcohol withdrawal has become the standard of care in patients with complicated withdrawal in acute medical settings (Blondell 2005). Because of the risk of Wernicke's syndrome in alcoholic patients, thiamine 100 mg po or im must be given on admission. Thereafter, for 1 month, 50 mg/day is given. Folate 1 mg/day po is also a common component of the alcohol detoxification regimen. Chlordiazepoxide is initiated at a maximum of 200 mg/day for the first 2 days, and then the dosage is reduced by approximately 25% per day to zero, with extra doses given intramuscularly or orally on a prn basis if the withdrawal symptoms are not adequately controlled.

An alternative and perhaps simpler approach, developed by Sellers et al. (1983) (see Table 11–2), for alcoholic patients in withdrawal is to administer

Table 11–2. Pharmacological strategies for acute detoxification of alcohol alone

	Dosage regimen	
Agent	**Fixed**	**Flexible**
diazepam	10–20 mg q 4–6 hours × 2–3 days, then decrease by 25% per day	5–10 mg q 1–2 hours per DBP, pulse > 100
chlordiazepoxide	25–50 mg q 4–6 hours × 2 days, then decrease by 25% per day	25–50 mg q 1–2 hours per DBP, pulse > 100
clonidine	0.1–0.2 mg q 4–6 hours × 2 days, then decrease by 25%–33% per day	Titrate to BP and pulse

Note. BP = blood pressure; DBP = diastolic blood pressure; q = every.

diazepam in 20-mg doses every 1–2 hours until withdrawal symptoms are relieved. Medication is then stopped. Detoxification was reported to proceed comfortably without further drug treatment once this loading dose of a long-acting benzodiazepine has achieved symptom suppression.

Because only about 5% of alcohol-dependent patients are subject to serious withdrawal, some detoxification centers do not use pharmacological strategies at all. In some hospital settings, patients without a history of complicated withdrawal are observed, and the dosing of benzodiazepines is titrated to physiological parameters. A dose of 5–10 mg of diazepam or 25–50 mg of chlordiazepoxide may be given every hour when the diastolic blood pressure or pulse is greater than 100.

Some clinicians have adopted lorazepam as the drug of choice in detoxifying alcoholic patients because it undergoes glucuronidation, has no active metabolites, and has an intermediate half-life. Therefore, patients with alcoholic liver disease might be at less risk of developing toxicity from detoxification with lorazepam than from detoxification with other benzodiazepines. On the other hand, the shorter half-life of lorazepam may be less than ideal for achieving smooth withdrawal. Unfortunately, no controlled studies have ever compared the advantages and disadvantages of various benzodiazepines in alcohol detoxification (Bird and Makela 1994), and there is no evidence for or against the routine use of lorazepam as a first-line agent in the treatment of alcohol withdrawal.

Clonidine has also become popular in some settings for decreasing the discomfort associated with alcohol withdrawal. In one study, transdermal clonidine was as well tolerated and as effective as chlordiazepoxide in the treatment of acute alcohol withdrawal (Baumgartner and Rowen 1991). Clonidine decreases the hypertension, tachycardia, and tremulousness associated with withdrawal. However, it does not prevent seizures or delirium tremens in the rarer instance of complicated withdrawal. Vital signs need to be monitored regularly with this drug. Typical oral dosages average 0.4–0.6 mg/day in two to four divided doses. Clonidine is also available in a transcutaneous patch. Each clonidine patch lasts approximately 1 week and delivers a fixed dose of 0.1–0.3 mg/day, depending on the strength of the patch. Patches, however, do not allow for the day-to-day adjustments in dose that are often required in detoxification.

Phenytoin (Dilantin) is sometimes added in patients with a history of withdrawal seizures or in patients unable to give an adequate history. The very rare patient who develops delirium tremens despite the above regimens should be transferred to a major medical hospital for treatment.

Outpatient detoxification has been carried out in patients with adequate motivation and an adequate social support system. In the managed care era, outpatient detoxification became more common than inpatient detoxification. For outpatient detoxification, chlordiazepoxide 25 mg taken every 4 hours, or less often if not needed, is probably reasonable for the first day, with tapering thereafter. For very tremulous patients who have to be handled as outpatients, chlordiazepoxide 100 mg im initially may be indicated. In this situation, the drug's slow absorption from the tissues is an asset rather than the liability it is in treating psychiatric conditions in which rapid sedation is desired.

As in opiate withdrawal and maintenance treatment, the general psychiatrist will often be well advised to refer patients to specialized alcoholism programs for at least the management of detoxification and possible medical or neurological complications.

Maintenance Treatment

Most alcoholism programs rely for maintenance treatment mainly on Alcoholics Anonymous plus other educational, psychotherapeutic, and psychosocial modalities. Disulfiram (Antabuse) is sometimes prescribed (or recommended). McLean Hospital has used a daily dose of 125 mg for occasional patients with chronic alcoholism. If the disulfiram is taken daily and alcohol is ingested, the following symptoms appear in this general order: flushing, sweating, palpitations, dyspnea, hyperventilation, tachycardia, hypotension, nausea, and vomiting. These events are usually followed by drowsiness and are usually gone after the patient has slept for a period.

Diphenhydramine 50 mg parenterally may be helpful in cases of severe disulfiram-alcohol reactions. Hypotension, shock, and arrhythmias are treated symptomatically. Oxygen is useful in respiratory distress. Hypokalemia may occur. Severe reactions require emergency treatment in a medical setting.

Obviously, willingness to take disulfiram, and thereby to commit oneself to not ingesting alcohol or suffering unpleasant effects if one drinks, is a test of motivation to remain abstinent. It is still, after all these years, not firmly established that the drug is more than a test of motivation or of compliance with therapy. Long-acting injectable or implantable disulfiram preparations have been tested abroad, but they are not available in this country.

Patients whose motivation to remain abstinent at all costs while taking disulfiram is questionable or weak should not be prescribed disulfiram. In fact, doubts about the utility of disulfiram have probably led to the gradual decrease in its use in alcohol treatment programs over the years. Disulfiram can cause side effects such as fatigue, a metallic taste, impotence (rarely), toxic psychosis (even more rarely), and a severe, occasionally fatal toxic hepatitis (very rarely). The last-named side effect comes early in treatment, usually within 2–8 weeks after disulfiram is begun, and is the basis for a labeling recommendation that liver function tests be carried out before disulfiram is begun and again after about 8 weeks of treatment. Disulfiram is a potent inhibitor of cytochrome P450 enzymes and can substantially raise the levels of phenytoin, oral anticoagulants, and other drugs.

Metronidazole (Flagyl) has mild disulfiram-like properties and can cause adverse effects when alcohol is taken with it. Studies of the use of metronidazole in alcoholism have been generally negative.

Naltrexone joined disulfiram as a strategy for the maintenance treatment of alcoholism in the early 1990s. Volpicelli et al. (1992) found that naltrexone 50 mg/day was twice as effective as placebo in preventing relapse from alcohol in a 12-week period. In a similar study, which also incorporated either supportive therapy or coping skills and relapse-prevention approaches, naltrexone was superior to placebo; it worked best when combined with supportive therapy

(O'Malley et al. 1992). Naltrexone appears to modify the reinforcing effects of alcohol through its effect on endogenous opioids (Swift 1995). Further naltrexone studies have yielded mixed results; still, the drug, at dosages of approximately 50 mg/day, is an option for the maintenance treatment of alcohol dependence. Naltrexone does not stop alcohol consumption entirely, but it appears to significantly decrease the likelihood that one drink will lead to uncontrolled binge drinking. In patients who respond well to the drug and are doing well by 3–6 months, discontinuing the drug and continuing other psychosocial treatments seems reasonable. Patients doing badly by 3 months while taking naltrexone are unlikely to improve significantly with longer treatment. However, experience with opiate users taking naltrexone suggests that prolonged treatment over 1 or more years may well be safe if the patient (or the doctor) feels more secure continuing the drug.

Naltrexone tends to be well tolerated at 50 mg/day. However, a number of side effects are common with this drug (Table 11–3). At least 10% of patients experience gastrointestinal side effects, including nausea, vomiting, anorexia, constipation, and abdominal pain. The gastrointestinal disturbance tends to attenuate with time and may be reduced by the patient's avoiding taking the drug on an empty stomach. Central nervous system (CNS) side effects such as nervousness, headache, somnolence, insomnia, and agitation are also fairly common. Lowering the dose and avoiding the drug at bedtime often help with the CNS symptoms. Joint pain and muscle pain occur in about 10% of patients, and increases in hepatic enzymes, rashes, and chills have also been reported at rates higher than those with placebo.

An alternative maintenance treatment for chronic alcoholism, acamprosate (Campral), has been studied extensively in Europe and was approved in the United States in 2004. Its mechanism of action is unclear. The drug is a taurine analog that reduces alcohol intake in animal models of alcoholism, reduces symptoms of alcohol withdrawal in humans, and, as a chronic treatment, reduces relapse drinking and alcohol craving at a dosage of up to 3,000 mg/day (Sass et al. 1996; Swift 1998). In three of four multicenter U.S. trials, acamprosate was effective in maintaining abstinence in patients who were abstinent at the start of treatment. The failed trial occurred in polysubstance abusers. In contrast, the nearly 20 positive European studies had not required abstinence or detoxification, and this may account for the difference from earlier studies. The combination of acamprosate and naltrexone might be more effective than

Table 11–3.   Common side effects of naltrexone therapy

Gastrointestinal	CNS
Nausea and vomiting	Nervousness
Abdominal pain and cramping	Agitation
Constipation	Headaches
Heartburn	Insomnia
Hepatic enzyme elevation	Somnolence
Anorexia	**Musculoskeletal**
	Joint pain
	Muscle soreness

Note.   CNS = central nervous system.

either drug alone (Carmen et al. 2004). The main side effects seem to be diarrhea and headache. However, the drug is well tolerated overall. The target dose is 666 mg given three times daily. Although the divided dosing presents a compliance challenge, many patients have been able to stick with a long-term maintenance program. There are no significant drug interactions with benzodiazepines, naltrexone, or disulfiram.

There was previously much interest in the potential application of serotonin (5-hydroxytryptamine; 5-HT) agonists and reuptake blockers to the management and treatment of patients with alcohol abuse or alcoholism. The rationale for their use stemmed from a number of observations in animals: in rats that are genetically bred to preferentially drink alcohol rather than water, alcohol consumption is reduced by the administration of L-tryptophan and SSRIs (e.g., fluoxetine), but not by the administration of noradrenergic TCAs (Naranjo and Sellers 1985). Abnormalities in the 5-HT receptors 5-HT_{1B}, 5-HT_2, and 5-HT_3 have been implicated in some cases of alcoholism (Murphy 1990). In early studies of heavy social drinkers, zimelidine, an SSRI that was once available in Europe, significantly increased the interval between bouts of consumption. However, subjects had only about 10 drinks fewer per bout, suggesting that this strategy will be only adjunctive at best. The mechanism of action may involve increasing satiety rather than acting via classical aversive or reinforcement mechanisms. The nausea-producing effects of the SSRIs also do not explain their effects on alcohol consumption. The SSRIs are not currently being pursued by pharmaceutical concerns in the United States as a treatment for alcoholism.

However, there is evidence that major depressive disorder coexisting with alcohol dependence can and probably should be treated with an antidepressant. Mason et al. (1996) and McGrath et al. (1996) showed that TCAs produce significant improvement in depression in active alcoholic patients and decrease alcohol consumption at the same time. Cornelius et al. (1997) showed similar results in a placebo-controlled study of fluoxetine. For many years, most clinicians believed that alcoholic patients should be abstinent for at least 4 weeks (and still be depressed) before receiving a drug therapy for their depression. A study by Greenfield et al. (1998) casts serious doubt on this belief. They found that *all* alcoholic patients hospitalized for detoxification who had a recent major depressive diagnosis relapsed into drinking, two-thirds within a month after discharge from the hospital. None had been prescribed antidepressants, in accordance with the practice of the time. This study was completed prior to the publication of the articles showing a positive effect of antidepressants in nonsober depressed alcoholic patients. These two bodies of data combine to encourage the use of antidepressants in treating depressed alcoholic patients even if patients are or are likely to be drinking.

It has been evident for some time that pharmacotherapy and psychosocial therapies should be coordinated in treating patients with substance use disorders. The old caveat that sobriety must precede antidepressant therapy appears to be dubious. The clinician is better advised to work on the substance abuse and the non-substance-related psychiatric disorder concurrently (Weiss 2003). The SSRIs may not suppress drinking directly, but they, and other newer drugs, may be easier to use and therefore more effective (acceptable) in treating depressed alcoholic patients than the TCAs.

Obviously, if a patient has psychiatric disorder that will respond to pharmacotherapy, such as major depression, in addition to alcoholism, the second disorder should be treated appropriately. The treatment of episodic or chronic residual anxiety symptoms after detoxification is a problem. The use of benzodiazepines is usually frowned upon, probably correctly. (The case could be made, however, that chlordiazepoxide could be considered the sedative equivalent of methadone and might be able to be taken at a stable, controlled rate, whereas alcohol, if used to control anxiety, leads to uncontrolled use.) Nonabusable alternatives to sedative benzodiazepines in the treatment of anxious, abstinent alcoholic patients include propranolol, clonidine, hydroxyzine, TCAs, atypical antipsychotics, buspirone, SSRIs, and serotonin-norepinephrine reuptake inhibitors (SNRIs; e.g., venlafaxine).

Cannabis

Cannabis use continues to be quite prevalent in the United States: 5% of the population are current users of the drug. The resin of the marijuana plant, Δ-9-tetrahydrocannabinol (THC), results in the acute intoxication state. Symptoms of cannabis intoxication include behavioral or psychological changes such as euphoria, anxiety, impaired judgment, increased appetite, dry mouth, and increased heart rate. Motor skills and coordination are frequently affected. Rare instances of cannabis-induced delirium and psychosis have been reported (Luzi et al. 2008; Tunving 1985).

Medications are rarely required for the treatment of cannabis intoxication. The most common symptom requiring intervention is severe anxiety. This anxiety can usually be managed by modest amounts of oral benzodiazepines such as lorazepam, 1 mg every 4 hours. Often, one or two doses is an amount sufficient to control the anxiety. Likewise, if psychotic symptoms are present, one or two doses of haloperidol 2–5 mg po will control these symptoms, which have occasionally been reported in frequent users of high-potency cannabis.

States of withdrawal from long-term cannabis dependence are quite uncommon except in chronic daily users of high-potency or high-dose cannabis. The withdrawal state can include mild insomnia, irritability, tremor, and nausea. These symptoms usually do not require treatment. The treatment of choice for long-term dependence is a combination of education, drug counseling, and support programs.

Hallucinogens

The hallucinogens include LSD, mescaline, psilocybin, and related drugs whose principal effects are increased perceptual sensitivity, derealization, visual illusions, and hallucinations. Occasionally, these perceptual changes are associated with a frank panic reaction (called a "bad trip"), depression, or paranoid ideation. The symptoms of hallucinogen intoxication usually begin 1 hour after the last dose and typically last 8–12 hours. LSD use is still apparently more common in the western United States than in other parts of the country, and it is used by young males more than by other demographic groups.

Time and a calm, supportive environment enable patients who are in the midst of a hallucinogenic hallucinosis associated with panic to be talked down.

Benzodiazepines such as diazepam 10–20 mg po will decrease the anxiety and commonly contribute to the patient's being able to sleep off the effects of the hallucinogen. Antipsychotics have also been used, but they are rarely necessary. Low-potency antipsychotics should probably be avoided, because their anticholinergic effects can exacerbate the hallucinosis. Haloperidol 5–10 mg im or po is preferred over other antipsychotics, but there are no controlled studies to support this common clinical practice. For recurrent hallucinosis (flashbacks), benzodiazepines may be as useful as antipsychotics.

Withdrawal states for chronic hallucinogen use are very rarely reported, and no detoxification is necessary. Chronic hallucinogen use is best managed through psychosocial interventions such as drug counseling and support groups.

Phencyclidine

Phencyclidine (PCP; also called angel dust) has been used on the streets since the mid-1960s and remains relatively popular. The drug is usually smoked and is rapidly absorbed across the blood-brain barrier. PCP appears to enhance dopaminergic transmission and also to modulate N-methyl-D-aspartate (NMDA) and glutamate receptor activity. Acute PCP intoxication produces not only behavior that mimics paranoid schizophrenia or manic states but also even more bizarre, violent behavior than do amphetamines or LSD. There are sometimes muscle tension, tachycardia, hypertension, drooling, and horizontal and vertical nystagmus. Other neurological signs include analgesia, loss of proprioception, and ataxia.

Treatment of the PCP intoxication state may involve seclusion and restraints, because at least one-third to two-thirds of PCP patients who come to ERs present in an agitated or violent state. Trying to talk down such patients is usually unsuccessful and often dangerous; isolation in a quiet area is better. These patients' agitation and violent behavior may be managed with high-potency antipsychotics alternated with benzodiazepines, as described in Chapter 10 ("Emergency Department Treatment"). Low-potency antipsychotics may compound the already significant anticholinergic effects of PCP and are sometimes associated with delirium. Acidifying the patient's urine with ammonium chloride (2.75 mEq/kg in 3 oz saline) may facilitate excretion, as may charcoal lavage.

PCP withdrawal appears very rare in humans but is occasionally reported in animals. No detoxification is necessary other than to control the symptoms of intoxication. Unfortunately, no prospective studies on pharmacological strategies for chronic PCP abuse or dependence have been done.

Maintenance treatment interventions include drug counseling, support groups (including 12-step programs like Narcotics Anonymous), and regular drug testing to monitor progress.

Bibliography

Arndt IO, Dorozynsky L, Woody GE, et al: Desipramine treatment of cocaine dependence in methadone-maintained patients. Arch Gen Psychiatry 49: 888–893, 1992

Arndt IO, McLellan AT, Dorozynsky L, et al: Desipramine treatment for cocaine dependence: role of antisocial personality disorder. J Nerv Ment Dis 182:151–156, 1994

Bagasra O, Forman LJ, Howeedy A, et al: A potential vaccine for cocaine abuse prophylaxis. Immunopharmacology 23:173–179, 1992 [also see comments]

Batki SL, Manfredi LB, Jacob P, et al: Fluoxetine for cocaine dependence in methadone maintenance: quantitative plasma and urine cocaine/benzoylecgonine concentrations. J Clin Psychopharmacol 13:243–250, 1993

Baumgartner F, Rowen RC: Transdermal clonidine versus chlordiazepoxide in the management of acute alcohol withdrawal: a randomized controlled clinical trial. South Med J 84:312–317, 1991

Bell J, Trinh L, Butler B, et al: Comparing retention in treatment and mortality in people after initial entry to methadone and buprenorphine treatment. Addiction 104:1193-1200, 2009

Bird RD, Makela EH: Alcohol withdrawal: what is the benzodiazepine of choice? Ann Pharmacother 28:67–71, 1994

Blondell RD: Ambulatory detoxification of patients with alcohol dependence. Am Fam Physician 71:495–502, 2005

Carmen B, Angeles M, Ana M, et al: Efficacy and safety of naltrexone and acamprosate in the treatment of alcohol dependence: a systematic review. Addiction 99:811–828, 2004

Carroll KM, Rounsaville BJ, Nich C, et al: One-year follow-up of psychotherapy and pharmacotherapy for cocaine dependence: delayed emergence of psychotherapy effects. Arch Gen Psychiatry 51:989–997, 1994

Charney D, Sternberg D, Kleber H, et al: The clinical use of clonidine in abrupt withdrawal from methadone. Arch Gen Psychiatry 38:1273–1277, 1981

Cheskin LJ, Fudala PJ, Johnson RE: A controlled comparison of buprenorphine and clonidine for acute detoxification from opioids. Drug Alcohol Depend 36:115–121, 1994

Cole JO, Ryback RS: Pharmacological therapy, in Alcoholism: Interdisciplinary Approaches to an Enduring Problem. Edited by Tarter R, Sugarman AA. Reading, MA, Addison-Wesley, 1976, pp 687–734

Cornelius JR, Sallonm IM, Ehler JG, et al: Fluoxetine in depressed alcoholics. Arch Gen Psychiatry 54:700–705, 1997

Farrell M, Ward J, Mattick R, et al: Methadone maintenance treatment in opiate dependence: a review. BMJ 309:997–1001, 1994

Franklin JE: Addiction medicine. JAMA 273:1656–1657, 1995

Galanter M: Network therapy for addiction: a model for office practice. Am J Psychiatry 150:28–36, 1993 [also see comments]

Galloway GP, Newmeyer J, Knapp T, et al: Imipramine for the treatment of cocaine and methamphetamine dependence. J Addict Dis 13:201–216, 1994

Galpern WR, Lumpkin M, Greenblatt DJ, et al: Chronic benzodiazepine administration, VII: behavioral tolerance and withdrawal and receptor alterations associated with clonazepam administration. Psychopharmacology (Berl) 104:225–230, 1991

Gawin F, Ellinwood E: Cocaine and other stimulants: action, abuse and treatment. N Engl J Med 318:1173–1182, 1988

Gawin F, Allen D, Humblestone B: Outpatient treatment of "crack" cocaine smoking with flupentixol decanoate: a preliminary report. Arch Gen Psychiatry 46:322–325, 1989a

Gawin F, Kleber H, Buck R, et al: Desipramine facilitation of initial cocaine abstinence. Arch Gen Psychiatry 46:117–121, 1989b

Ginzburg HM: Naltrexone: its clinical utility (DHHS Publ No ADM-84-1358). Washington, DC, U.S. Government Printing Office, 1984

Grabowski J, Rhoades H, Elk R, et al: Fluoxetine is ineffective for treatment of cocaine dependence or concurrent opiate and cocaine dependence: two placebo-controlled double-blind trials. J Clin Psychopharmacol 15:163–174, 1995

Greenfield SF, Weiss RD, Muenz LR, et al: The effect of depression on return to drinking: a prospective study. Arch Gen Psychiatry 55:259–265, 1998

Herman JB, Rosenbaum JF, Brotman AW: The alprazolam to clonazepam switch for the treatment of panic disorder. J Clin Psychopharmacol 7:175–178, 1987

Higgins ST, Budney AJ, Bickel WK, et al: Incentives improve outcome in outpatient behavioral treatment of cocaine dependence. Arch Gen Psychiatry 51:568–576, 1994

Hulse GK, Morris N, Arnold-Reed D, et al: Improving clinical outcomes in treating heroin dependence: randomized, controlled trial of oral or implant naltrexone. Arch Gen Psychiatry 66:1108–1115, 2009

Janiri L, Mannelli P, Persico AM, et al: Opiate detoxification of methadone maintenance patients using lefetamine, clonidine and buprenorphine. Drug Alcohol Depend 36:139–145, 1994

Jasinski DR, Pevnick JS, Griffith JD: Human pharmacology and abuse potential of the analgesic buprenorphine. Arch Gen Psychiatry 35:501–516, 1978

Joughin N, Tata P, Collins M, et al: Inpatient withdrawal from long-term benzodiazepine use. Br J Addict 86:449–455, 1991

Kampman KM, Pettinati H, Lynch KG, et al: A pilot trial of topiramate for the treatment of cocaine dependence. Drug Alcohol Depend 75:233–240, 2004

Kleber HD, Riordan CE, Rounsaville B, et al: Clonidine outpatient detoxification from methadone maintenance. Arch Gen Psychiatry 42:391–394, 1985

Kosten T: Current pharmacotherapies for opioid dependence. Psychopharmacol Bull 26:69–74, 1990

Kosten TA, Kosten TR: Pharmacological blocking agents for treating substance abuse. J Nerv Ment Dis 179:583–592, 1991

Kosten T, Vileber H: Buprenorphine detoxification from opioid dependence: a pilot study. Life Sci 42:635–641, 1988

Kosten TR, Kleber HD, Morgan C: Role of opioid antagonists in treating intravenous cocaine abuse. Life Sci 44:887–892, 1989

Kreek MJ: Rationale for maintenance pharmacotherapy of opiate dependence. Res Publ Assoc Res Nerv Ment Dis 70:205–230, 1992

Landry DW, Zhao K, Yang GX, et al: Antibody-catalyzed degradation of cocaine. Science 259:1899–1901, 1993

Lejoyeux M, Solomon J, Adès J: Benzodiazepine treatment for alcohol-dependent patients. Alcohol Alcohol 33:563–575, 1998

Luzi S, Morrison PD, Powell J, et al: What is the mechanism whereby cannabis use increases risk of psychosis? Neurotox Res 14:105–112, 2008

Mann K: Pharmacotherapy of alcohol dependence: a review of the clinical data. CNS Drugs 18:485–504, 2004

Martell BA, Orson FM, Poling J, et al: Cocaine vaccine for the treatment of cocaine dependence in methadone-maintained patients: a randomized, double-blind, placebo-controlled efficacy trial. Arch Gen Psychiatry 66:1116–1123, 2009

Mason BJ, Kocsis JH, Ritvo EC, et al: A double-blind, placebo-controlled trial of desipramine for primary alcohol dependence stratified on the presence or absence of major depression. JAMA 275:761–767, 1996 [see comments]

Mason NA: Disulfiram-induced hepatitis: case report and review of the literature. DICP 23:872–875, 1989

McGrath PJ, Nunes EV, Stewart JW, et al: Imipramine treatment of alcoholics with primary depression. Arch Gen Psychiatry 53:232–240, 1996

Messinis L, Lyros E, Andrian V, et al: Neuropsychological functioning in buprenorphine maintained patients versus abstinent heroin abusers on naltrexone hydrochloride therapy. Hum Psychopharmacol 24:524–531, 2009

Miller NS: Pharmacotherapy in alcoholism. J Addict Dis 14:23–46, 1995

Miller NS, Sheppart LM: Addiction treatment and continuing care in forensic populations. Psychiatr Ann 30:589–596, 2000

Milne M, Crouch BI, Caravati EM: Buprenorphine for opioid dependence. J Pain Palliat Care Pharmacother 23:153-155, 2009

Moak DH: Assessing the efficacy of medical treatments for alcohol use disorders. Expert Opin Pharmacother 5:2075–2089, 2004

Mueller TI, Goldenberg IM, Gordon AL, et al: Benzodiazepine use in anxiety disordered patient with and without a history of alcoholism. J Clin Psychiatry 57:83–89, 1996

Murphy DL: Neuropsychiatric disorders and 5HT receptors. Neuropsychopharmacology 3:457–471, 1990

Najavits LM, Weiss RD: The role of psychotherapy in the treatment of substance-use disorders. Harv Rev Psychiatry 2:84–96, 1994

Naranjo CA, Sellers EM: Research Advances in New Psychopharmacological Treatments for Alcoholism. New York, Excerpta Medica, 1985

Nunes EV, Quitkin FM, Donovan SJ, et al: Imipramine treatment of opiate-dependent patients with depressive disorders: a placebo-controlled trial. Arch Gen Psychiatry 55:153–160, 1998

O'Connor PG, Kosten TR: Rapid and ultrarapid opioid detoxification techniques. JAMA 279:229–234, 1998

O'Connor PG, Carrol KM, Shi JM, et al: Three methods of opioid detoxification in a primary care setting. Ann Intern Med 127:526–530, 1997

O'Leary G, Weiss RD: Pharmacotherapies for cocaine dependence. Curr Psychiatry Rep 2:508–513, 2000

O'Malley SS: Integration of opioid antagonists and psychosocial therapy in the treatment of narcotic and alcohol dependence. J Clin Psychiatry 7:30–38, 1995

O'Malley SS, Jaffe AJ, Chang G, et al: Naltrexone and coping skills therapy for alcohol dependence: a controlled study. Arch Gen Psychiatry 49:881–887, 1992

O'Mara NB, Wesley LC: Naltrexone in the treatment of alcohol dependence. Ann Pharmacother 28:210–211, 1994

Parran TV, Adelman CA, Merkin B, et al: Long-term outcomes of office-based buprenorphine/naloxone maintenance therapy. Drug Alcohol Depend 106:56–60, 2010

Petrakis IL, Carroll KM, Nich C, et al: Disulfiram treatment for cocaine dependence in methadone maintained opioid addicts. Addiction 95:219–228, 2000

Reis AD, Castro LA, Faria R, et al: Craving decrease with topiramate in outpatient treatment for cocaine dependence: an open label trial. Rev Bras Psiquiatr 30:132–135, 2008

Salvato FR, Mason BJ: Changes in transaminases over the course of a 12-week, double-blind nalmefene trial in a 38-year-old female subject. Alcohol Clin Exp Res 18:1187–1189, 1994

Sass H, Soyka M, Mann K, et al: Relapse prevention by acamprosate: results from a placebo-controlled study on alcohol dependence. Arch Gen Psychiatry 53:673–680, 1996

Schweizer E, Rickels K, Case WG, et al: Carbamazepine treatment in patients discontinuing long-term benzodiazepine therapy: effects on withdrawal severity and outcome. Arch Gen Psychiatry 48:448–452, 1991

Sellers T, Naranjo C, Harrison M, et al: Diazepam loading: simplified treatment of alcohol withdrawal. Clin Pharmacol Ther 34:822–826, 1983

Sinclair JD: Drugs to decrease alcohol drinking. Ann Med 22:357–362, 1990

Smith D, Wesson D: Phenobarbital techniques for treatment of barbiturate dependence. Arch Gen Psychiatry 24:56–60, 1971

Stine SM, Kosten TR: Use of drug combination in treatment of opioid withdrawal. J Clin Psychopharmacol 12:203–209, 1992

Stine SM, Kosten TR: Reduction of opiate withdrawal-like symptoms by cocaine abuse during methadone and buprenorphine maintenance. Am J Drug Alcohol Abuse 20:445–458, 1994

Swantek SS, Grossberg GT, Neppe VM, et al: The use of carbamazepine to treat benzodiazepine withdrawal in a geriatric population. J Geriatr Psychiatry Neurol 4:106–109, 1991

Swift RM: Effect of naltrexone on human alcohol consumption. J Clin Psychiatry 7:24–29, 1995

Swift RM: Pharmacological treatments for drug and alcohol dependence: experimental and standard therapies. Psychiatric Annals 28:697–702, 1998

Teoh SK, Mello NK, Mendelson JH, et al: Buprenorphine effects on morphine and cocaine induced subjective responses by drug dependent men. J Clin Psychopharmacol 14:15–27, 1994

Tunving K: Psychiatric effects of cannabis use. Acta Psychiatr Scand 72:209–214, 1985

Umbricht A, Montoya ID, Hoover DR, et al: Naltrexone shortened opioid detoxification with buprenorphine. Drug Alcohol Depend 56:181–190, 1999

U.S. Department of Justice, Drug Enforcement Administration: Controlled Substances Act as Amended to July 1, 1991. Washington, DC, West Publishing, 1991, pp 977–978

Verheul R, Lehert P, Geerlings PJ, et al: Predictors of acamprosate efficacy: results from a pooled analysis of seven European trials, including 1485 alcohol-dependent patients. Psychopharmacology (Berl) 178:167–173, 2003

Volpicelli JR, Alterman AI, Hayashida M, et al: Naltrexone in the treatment of alcohol dependence. Arch Gen Psychiatry 49:876–880, 1992 [also see comments]

Washton A, Resnick R: Clonidine for opiate detoxification: outpatient clinical trial. Am J Psychiatry 137:1121–1122, 1980

Weiss RD: Pharmacotherapy for co-occurring mood and substance use disorders, in Integrated Treatment for Mood and Substance Disorders. Edited by Westermeyer JJ, Weiss RD, Ziedonis DM. Baltimore, MD, Johns Hopkins University Press, 2003, pp 122–139

12

Pharmacotherapy in Special Situations

One of the difficulties that clinicians face is that a typical clinic patient often does not resemble the sanitized patients selected for in research studies. Most published reports evaluating the efficacy of psychoactive drugs in psychiatric patients carefully select physically healthy adult, but not geriatric, pediatric, or pregnant, patients. Unfortunately, in clinical practice, physicians frequently encounter patients with psychiatric disorders who are also pregnant, juvenile, elderly, brain damaged, or medically ill but who are otherwise appropriate candidates for conventional pharmacotherapy. Since the last edition of this book, much has been learned about treating special populations with psychotropic agents. In this chapter, we address some of these special situations.

Pregnancy

Pregnancy, current or planned, poses a complex problem for the psychiatrist, for the psychiatric patient, and for her fetus. Folk wisdom has suggested that pregnancy is a relatively protected time in which women may be less susceptible to psychiatric difficulties. This, unfortunately, is not the case. Pregnancy does not protect patients against the occurrence, recurrence, or exacerbation of psychiatric conditions. For example, most patients with recurrent depression who stop taking an antidepressant in anticipation of conceiving are back taking an antidepressant before delivery. At least 10% of patients meet criteria for a depressive disorder during pregnancy. Pregnancy appears to increase the risk of obsessive-compulsive disorder (OCD) and other anxiety disorders. Mania and schizophrenia may all occur or worsen during pregnancy.

The risks of drug administration during pregnancy include teratogenesis, particularly during the first trimester, and possibly behavioral teratogenesis (Table 12–1). All psychotropic agents cross the placenta to some degree. Gross physical malformations are easy to detect and document, and the possibility that drugs given during pregnancy may affect brain function and behavior years later exists, but there is no clear evidence that it actually occurs. Direct toxic effects on the fetus can occur later in pregnancy. Drugs can affect labor and delivery, with residual effects on the infant's behavior after delivery. All psychotropic drugs are excreted in the mother's milk during breast-feeding, to different degrees. This puts both doctor and patient in a very unpleasant bind. Ideally, every mother should be totally drug free throughout every pregnancy. However, there are many instances in which the known risks of discontinuing psychiatric medications are greater than the unknown risks of continuing to take them.

Not treating mental illness during pregnancy has significant risks. Severely depressed pregnant women do not take care of themselves optimally, and conflicting reports have suggested a higher risk of low birthweight and preterm delivery in untreated depressed women. When the risk of suicide is added to the equation, the risk can be overwhelming. Similarly, untreated schizophrenia has been associated with an increase in perinatal deaths. Psychosis can jeopardize both mother and fetus. There is at least a theoretical risk that elevated cortisol levels associated with severe stress during pregnancy might impact fetal brain development.

This dilemma is illustrated by the case of a markedly manic drug-free patient believed to be in the sixth week of pregnancy who was admitted a number of years ago to McLean Hospital. She was kept drug free in seclusion, and often in restraint, for a week because the treating psychiatrist was afraid to initiate neuroleptic treatment for fear of harming the fetus. One of us who

Table 12–1.   Teratogenic risks of psychotropic medications

Class	Drug	Risk category[a]	Possible effects
Anxiolytics	benzodiazepines	D	"Floppy baby," withdrawal, increased risk of cleft lip or palate
	hypnotic benzodiazepines	X	Decreased intrauterine growth
	buspirone	C	Unknown
Antidepressants	TCAs	D	Fetal tachycardia, fetal withdrawal, fetal anticholinergic effects, urinary retention, bowel obstruction
	amitriptyline, imipramine, nortriptyline		
	other TCAs	C	
	MAOIs	C	Rare fetal malformations; rarely used in pregnancy due to hypertension
	SSRIs	C	Increased perinatal complications
	paroxetine	D	Cardiovascular malformations, increased perinatal complications
	FGAs	C	Rare anomalies, fetal jaundice, fetal anticholinergic effects at birth
Antipsychotics	SGAs		Gestational diabetes, large birthweight
	clozapine	B	
	aripiprazole, risperidone, olanza-pine, quetiapine, ziprasi-done, iloperidone, asenapine	C	
Mood stabilizers	lithium	D	Associated with increase in birth defects, including cardiac anomalies, especially Ebstein's anomaly; behavioral effects
	valproate	D	Neural tube defects
	carbamazepine	D	Neural tube defects, minor anomalies
	oxcarbazepine	C	Unknown
	lamotrigine	C	Unknown
	gabapentin/pregabalin	C	Unknown

Note.   FGA = first-generation antipsychotic; MAOI = monoamine oxidase inhibitor; SGA = second-generation antipsychotic; SSRI = selective serotonin reuptake inhibitor; TCA = tricyclic antidepressant. [a]U.S. Food and Drug Administration use-in-pregnancy risk categories: A: Controlled studies show no risk to humans. B: No evidence of risk in humans, but adequate human studies may not have been performed. C: Risk cannot be ruled out. D: Positive evidence of risk to humans; risk may be outweighed by potential benefit. X: Contraindicated in pregnancy.

consulted on the case advised proceeding with haloperidol therapy, despite the presumed pregnancy, on the grounds that severe hyperactivity and distress were a risk to both patient and fetus, whereas there was no direct evidence that haloperidol or any other antipsychotic leads to any specific birth defect. The physician in charge disagreed. Finally, an ultrasound examination revealed a false pregnancy, and appropriate drug treatment was begun. This case illustrates one kind of clinical dilemma. Thalidomide, with its gross fetal deformities, still haunts all of pharmacotherapy.

As far as we can determine, the only drugs commonly used in psychiatry with proven relationships to specific birth defects are lithium, most anticonvulsants, paroxetine, and benzodiazepines. Lithium has been associated with cardiac abnormalities, especially Ebstein's anomaly, and anticonvulsants have been associated with a variety of birth defects, including facial deformity and spina bifida. However, studies in the 1990s (Cohen et al. 1994) suggested that first-trimester lithium teratogenic effects had been overestimated in the earlier studies and that the risks of stopping lithium in some patients outweighed the risks of birth defects.

Beyond this, there is no clear evidence that any standard psychiatric drug does not (or does) cause birth defects. Minor congenital abnormalities occur in up to 4% of infants born to drug-free mothers. However, there is a general suspicion that any drug might be bad for the fetus, and no doctor feels totally comfortable recommending drug therapy for a patient who is believed to have recently become pregnant or who intends to become pregnant. Whenever possible, drug therapy should be avoided in such instances.

Unfortunately, some women with severe, even disabling, psychiatric disorders either want to become or actually become pregnant, and a choice must be made between treating the patient and avoiding medicating the fetus. If the situation is not a crisis, as with the patient who is taking maintenance medication but would like to become pregnant, outside consultation can be obtained from a psychiatrist experienced in working collaboratively with obstetricians or from a dysmorphologist (an expert in birth defects), a type of specialist found in major medical centers.

Telephone hotlines providing information about the effects of drugs on the fetus are also available. One of these is the California Teratogen Information Service (CTIS, 1-800-532-3749) based at the University of California, San Diego, and at Stanford. Staff members are willing to accept calls and refer callers to other programs around the country when appropriate. Web sites addressing issues of drugs and pregnancy—such as those of the CTIS (www.ctispregnancy.org), which is a member of the Organization of Teratology Information Services (OTIS) (www.otispregnancy.org), and Illinois Teratogen Information Specialists (www.fetal-exposure.org), are also available. Major reference works in this area are listed in the bibliography of this chapter.

Information from a reproductive psychiatry specialist or a telephone hotline can indicate whether there is any solid evidence that a particular drug is teratogenic, but it does not solve the clinician's whole problem. The final decision must be based on the seriousness of the patient's distress and the reasonableness of the desire to have a child. Documented informed consent from the patient and her family (including her husband or her parents, when appropriate) for the treatment plan is necessary, whether one decides to leave the patient drug free with the risks of that course or to continue with a needed medication despite the pregnancy.

It is likely that stopping most psychotropic medication 2–3 weeks before the pregnancy is early enough to avoid malformations.

If medication can be avoided for the first 3 months of pregnancy, the risk of fetal abnormality is much reduced, but other risks can occur. Babies born to mothers who are physically dependent on sedatives or opiates suffer withdrawal syndromes and need to be treated postnatally. Autonomic withdrawal symptoms presumably can occur in the newborn if the mother has been taking tricyclic antidepressants (TCAs) or short-acting antidepressants such as paroxetine and venlafaxine. One can justify withdrawing medication carefully from pregnant women a few weeks before delivery in some circumstances. However, the risk to the fetus/newborn may be small relative to the risks posed by not treating a vulnerable woman as she begins the postpartum period.

Overall, antidepressants are probably the best-studied class of agents during pregnancy relative to all other medicines. The most recent data and reviews on fluoxetine exposure during pregnancy (Rahimi et al. 2006; Yonkers et al. 2009) suggest that fluoxetine is not associated with a higher rate of birth anomalies. More than 5,000 women in a national database who were taking fluoxetine have been prospectively studied, and there is no clear evidence of teratogenic effects for fluoxetine. However, there has been an association of selective serotonin reuptake inhibitor (SSRI) exposure in pregnancy with higher rates of spontaneous abortions (Rahimi et al. 2006), a self-limiting neonatal behavioral syndrome characterized by motor effects, irritability, and gastrointestinal upset (Moses-Kolko El et al. 2005), and possibly even a small risk of postnatal pulmonary hypertension (Chambers et al. 2006; Källén and Olausson. 2008). In addition, women exposed to high doses of fluoxetine in pregnancy might have a somewhat increased risk of delivering a low-birthweight infant (Hendrick et al. 2003; Simon et al. 2002). The clinical significance of an infant with somewhat lower birthweight is unclear, and depression in pregnancy is also associated with low-birthweight deliveries. Preliminary evidence also suggests that citalopram and sertraline do not appear to be teratogens (Einarson et al. 2009). However, paroxetine may be a potential teratogen associated with an increase in cardiovascular malformations, including atrial and septal defects (Cuzzell 2006). But other studies (e.g., Louik et al. 2007) have not found this association. Nonetheless, on the basis of the available evidence, the FDA changed the classification of paroxetine from a category C to a category D agent, indicating a positive risk of teratogenic effects. Thus, paroxetine generally should be avoided in pregnancy if possible, particularly in the first trimester. Given the known risk of relapse or recurrence when antidepressants are stopped, we have, along with our patients, concluded many times that patients are better off continuing their SSRIs throughout pregnancy.

All the SSRIs except paroxetine are currently considered U.S. Food and Drug Administration (FDA) category C agents, meaning that the risk of teratogenic effects cannot be ruled out because of insufficient evidence. However, the FDA classification of drugs taken during pregnancy is inadequate. Bupropion is a category B drug, suggesting that the known risk with bupropion is less than that of the SSRIs. Although animal data on bupropion may suggest minimal risk of teratogenic effects, there are virtually no clinical data. Thus, we would not suggest using bupropion over an SSRI in pregnancy. Likewise, some TCAs such as nortriptyline are category D agents, suggesting that there is positive evidence of risk. For patients who have clearly responded to nortriptyline, it may be much safer for them to continue the drug than to switch to an SSRI.

There are convincing data that valproate is associated with a variety of neural tube defects in the first trimester, including spina bifida, anencephaly, hydrocephalus, microcephaly, urogenital deficits, and fetal valproate syndrome (see Chapter 5: "Mood Stabilizers"). The rate of major congenital malformations associated with valproate is estimated at 6%–20% (Harden et al. 2009). Hydantoin and carbamazepine may be associated with similar defects. The fetal serum levels of the anticonvulsants are around 50%–80% of the maternal dose. Most of the anticonvulsants are category D agents as a result. We know very little about lamotrigine, topiramate, and gabapentin in pregnancy, although these drugs are currently considered risk category C simply because data do not exist to define a risk. The available data do suggest that lamotrigine does carry some teratogenic risk, although less than lithium, valproate, and carbamazepine. Lamotrigine may be associated with a high rate of cleft lip and palate 4–9/1,000, which appears to be at least 10 times the risk in the general population (Viguera et al. 2007).

In addition to being associated with neural tube defects, valproate use in pregnancy appears, with increasing evidence, to be associated with low IQs in children exposed in utero to the drug. Meador and colleagues (2009) examined the cognitive function of 309 children exposed to various anti-epileptics in utero. At 3 years of age, children who had been exposed to valproate had an IQ 9 points lower than children who had been exposed to lamotrigine and 6 points lower than children who had been exposed to carbamazepine. In addition, Meador et al. found an association between higher doses of maternal valproate and lower IQ in their offspring. This study supports earlier work suggesting an association of valproate with higher rates of mental retardation in exposed offspring (Thomas et al. 2008; Vinten et al. 2005). The growing evidence supporting an association of maternal valproate use with diminished cognitive function in their offspring suggests that valproate should not be used in pregnancy as a first-line agent in bipolar patients.

Second-generation antipsychotics (except clozapine) are currently class C. Thus far, experience with the SGAs has not suggested that these agents are teratogens (Einarson et al. 2009; McKenna et al. 2005). However, SGAs carry other risks in pregnancy, including gestational diabetes and large–for–gestation age infants. We are more confident about the first-generation antipsychotics in pregnancy, since so many women have been exposed to these agents since the 1950s. Many women have been treated with phenothiazine-like agents for nausea during the first trimester, and there is no clear evidence of a teratogenic effect. Since psychosis can be such a hazard during pregnancy, the benefits of the typical agents often outweigh the risks of untreated psychosis. At this time, it is probably preferable to employ high-potency first-generation agents during pregnancy rather than either SGAs with metabolic risks or low-potency typical agents with significant anticholinergic properties.

Benzodiazepines were traditionally considered to be contraindicated in pregnancy. Many benzodiazepines carried an FDA X category risk in pregnancy, indicating that the teratogenic risks of these agents generally outweigh the potential benefits and are therefore contraindicated. The concern was that first-trimester exposure was associated with an increased risk of cleft lip and palate. The association with cleft palate with benzodiazepine exposure has been questioned in studies (Dolovich et al. 1998; Eros et al. 2002). The risk of oral clefts with benzodiazepine exposure in pregnancy appears to be less than we once believed, but there does appear to be some increased risk.

The issue of behavioral teratogenicity of drugs taken during pregnancy is more difficult to assess. Cocaine and alcohol intake during pregnancy are sometimes associated with behavioral problems in child development, even if there are no physical deficits. Although physical anomalies are easy to quantify, behavioral effects may be more subtle. The best study to date could find no difference in language, temperament, activity level, or intelligence in 135 children exposed to fluoxetine or TCAs in utero compared with those who were not (Nulman et al. 1997, 2002). A study done by the Stanford group suggests that there may be mild motoric differences in children exposed to antidepressants in utero but no effects on mental development (Casper et al. 2003). Delayed motor development has also been reported in a rat study of fluoxetine exposure in utero. However, in this same study, prenatal exposure to fluoxetine had an unexpected beneficial effect on subsequent cognitive ability in rat pups (Bairy et al. 2006). Children born to mothers taking first-generation antipsychotics also showed no significant differences in motor development, growth, or intellect up to the age of 4 (Slone et al. 1977). These studies, although important, are insufficient to answer the question of whether in utero exposure to psychotropics has negative behavioral effects. Our clinical experience, however, has not indicated any clear behavioral effects of antidepressant exposure during pregnancy, but further study is certainly warranted.

After the baby is born, nursing mothers taking medication excrete some drug in breast milk, because all known psychoactive drugs are secreted in breast milk. While fetal serum levels of antidepressant may approach 50% of the maternal serum levels, less than 1% of the maternal dose is present in breast milk. In the absence of data on breast milk concentrations of a specific drug, it is hard to estimate the seriousness of this problem; generally, however, breast milk concentrations are much lower than drug levels in the blood, and the total dose ingested by the infant may be quite small (Berle et al. 2004). Studies have suggested that antidepressant serum levels are often undetectable in infants who breast-fed while their mothers were taking antidepressants (Birnbaum et al. 1999; Gentile et al. 2007). Stowe et al. (1995) followed seven nursing women with severe postpartum depression who were taking sertraline and found that the maximum daily dose to which their infants were exposed was 0.026–0.044 mg/kg. In related work (Winn et al. 1995), nursing infants exposed to sertraline in breast milk were monitored by growth charts, number of illnesses, and developmental milestones; no adverse effects were noted, compared with controls. As with many risk-benefit situations in medicine, the suffering of the mother must be weighed against the often unknown risk to the infant, as interpreted by the doctor, the patient, and the patient's family.

Pediatric Psychopharmacology

The decision to use a drug treatment for a psychiatrically ill child or young adolescent must be based on a clear clinical need. There are few data on the long-term consequences of psychiatric drug therapy in childhood for brain function, behavior, or physical health in adult life. The psychiatric disorder should pose significant danger to the child's development and well-being and should be undertaken only after considered medical and psychiatric evaluation.

Prepubescent children have relatively efficient livers. This generally allows them to metabolize drugs rapidly and enables them to tolerate somewhat higher doses of psychiatric drugs per unit of weight than adults tolerate. After puberty, drug metabolism resembles that seen in young adults. The lesson here, of course, is not that 7-year-olds should be given huge doses of drugs, but that they should be started on very small doses and, if there is no response, that the dose can be gradually increased to adult dosages, adjusted for weight, without fear of unusual toxicity.

It should be noted that most standard psychiatric drugs have not received FDA approval for use in children or even in adolescents, mainly because the necessary studies have not been carried out. Recently, the FDA has begun to require that manufacturers of antidepressants do studies in children and adolescents.

Stimulants

The best-studied and best-validated drug therapy for psychiatrically ill children is the use of stimulants (D-amphetamine and methylphenidate; see Chapter 8: "Stimulants") in attention-deficit/hyperactivity disorder (ADHD). More than 170 trials of stimulants in the treatment of ADHD involving 5,000 children attest to the benefits of these drugs. Since the early 1990s, the number of children taking stimulants has risen dramatically. Between 1990 and 1993, the number of outpatient visits devoted to ADHD increased from 1.6 million to 4.2 million per year, with 90% of children diagnosed with ADHD receiving a stimulant at some point in their treatment (Swanson et al. 1995). In 1996 alone, more than 10 million prescriptions for methylphenidate were written. By 2004, the rate of stimulant prescription (4.63/1,000) had doubled from the rate observed just 10 years earlier (Winterstein et al. 2008). It is unclear whether the marked increase in stimulant prescriptions is the result of better ADHD recognition or overprescription, but both factors are likely involved (Greenhill et al. 1999). However, the suggestion in some quarters that ADHD is simply an excuse to medicate annoying behavior in children or to sell more drugs does not appear sound.

Research regarding the effects of stimulants on various kinds of behavior suggests that the drug effects are complex. The dose that controls overactivity best may be too high for optimal improvement in learning. The stimulants may cause a slight decrease in body growth, perhaps 1–3 cm in height over the entire developmental period, although a recent follow-up study showed no effect of stimulant exposure on adult height (Kramer et al. 2000). Children taking stimulants may show side effects such as anorexia, insomnia, dysphoria, and even tics.

Some children with ADHD are markedly benefited—generally more in behavior than in academic performance—whereas others received only some benefit and a few are not benefited or even become more agitated. Distractibility, overt aggression, and daily class performance are improved with stimulant use and worsen when the drug is stopped or a placebo is substituted. Most of the studies have been for 12 weeks or less. However, long-term trials with both stimulants and atomoxetine have confirmed that the benefits of pharmacotherapy in children treated for ADHD are sustained (Arnold et al. 1997; Barbaresi et al. 2006; Kratochvil et al. 2006).

A number of long-acting or once-a-day stimulant preparations are currently available. A long-acting form of methylphenidate (Concerta) is now widely being used in the treatment of ADHD. Concerta circumvents the problem of trying to fit in tid dosing during the school day and appears to be as effective as the short-acting form of methylphenidate. Dosing of Concerta is about 20% higher than the total methylphenidate dose. Thus, the total Concerta dose is 18–54 mg taken once a day. Methylphenidate is also available in a transdermal, once-a-day patch and in several other long-acting oral formulations. Lisdexamfetamine is a prodrug of dextroamphetamine that also is taken once a day.

Some children respond better, unpredictably, to one of the two standard stimulants than to the other. Methylphenidate is usually started at 5 mg bid, and the dosage may be increased over time up to 20 mg tid. Dextroamphetamine is less expensive than branded Ritalin, but most stimulant preparations now have generic equivalents. It is initiated at 2.5 mg bid, and the dosage is gradually increased to a maximum of 40 mg in two to four divided doses. The common clinical practice with the shorter-acting stimulants is to prescribe dosing twice a day, with the last dose around noontime to reduce the risk of insomnia. A report by Kent et al. (1995) suggested that adding a third dose in the late afternoon rarely disrupted sleep. Lunchtime doses are frequently a problem, however, for schoolchildren. Sustained-release preparations of D-amphetamine, methylphenidate, and methamphetamine are available, but their usefulness in children with ADHD is not well documented. These preparations can certainly be tried if once-a-day dosing is desired or needed. In patients with a good stimulant response, drug holidays every few months to discover whether the drug is still needed are worth trying. The practice of giving a child with ADHD his or her medication only on school days may have the disadvantage of impairing the child's family and peer relationships as well as impairing learning outside school. Some children continue to benefit from stimulants into adolescence or even adulthood. The dosage may need to be adjusted, up or down, over time as the child grows and matures.

A number of other agents have proved useful in the treatment of ADHD. TCAs (e.g., desipramine) at low dosages (10–25 mg qid) may be useful but may act more slowly: it may take several weeks for them to work. In addition, their effects have been said to fade after a few months. Another antidepressant that has shown promise in the treatment of ADHD is bupropion. Studies have reported that bupropion may be effective in the behavioral and cognitive problems associated with ADHD (Casat et al. 1989) and in the treatment of adult ADHD (Wilens et al. 2005). In children, the bupropion dosage is 3–6 mg/kg/day in divided doses. One case report suggested that there may be a role for the SSRIs in the treatment of ADHD (Frankenburg and Kando 1994). Guanfacine (Tenex), an antihypertensive agent, was used off-label in the treatment of ADHD over the years. In 2009, only the extended-release formulation of guanfacine (Intuniv) received an official indication for treatment of ADHD. The efficacy of guanfacine may be less than that of an antidepressant in the treatment of ADHD.

Finally, clonidine is often used in combination with stimulants to reduce side effects and enhance effects on hyperactivity and hyperkinesis. Clonidine at dosages of 0.1 mg tid has been reported to reduce stimulant-induced insomnia as well as impulsivity. As a monotherapy of ADHD, however, clonidine appears to be inferior to desipramine (Singer et al. 1995).

Various antidepressants, including venlafaxine, bupropion, and desipramine, have been found to be effective in the treatment of ADHD and are discussed later in this section.

Two newer, "nonstimulant," agents—atomoxetine and modafinil—have been studied in the treatment of ADHD. Atomoxetine is a pure inhibitor of the presynaptic norepinephrine transporter that was approved in 2003 for the treatment of ADHD in both children and adults. Atomoxetine has been reported, at dosages of 1.2 mg/kg/day and 1.8 mg/kg/day, to be significantly more effective than placebo in children and adolescents with ADHD (Buitelaar et al. 2004; Kelsey et al. 2004). Most children are treated once a day, with the dosage in the range of 40–80 mg/day.

Atomoxetine is well absorbed orally and has a half-life that averages about 4 hours. However, slow metabolizers of cytochrome P450 (CYP) 2D6 metabolize the drug more slowly. We would anticipate that the combination of atomoxetine with SSRIs might increase toxicity. Thus, lower doses of atomoxetine may be needed when a patient is already taking fluoxetine or paroxetine.

Atomoxetine has the advantage over standard stimulants of not having a significant abuse potential. Thus, atomoxetine does not require a special prescription for controlled substances as do standard stimulants. On the other hand, atomoxetine shares with the stimulants a tendency to suppress weight and to increase heart rate and blood pressure. Both the anorexic and cardiovascular effects of atomoxetine appear to be dose related. Other reported side effects include rash, anxiety, somnolence, and, most recently, liver function test abnormalities. Atomoxetine also carries the same black-box warning around suicidality that the antidepressants carry.

Several studies have evaluated the efficacy of atomoxetine compared with placebo or standard stimulants. In a randomized comparison of atomoxetine and methylphenidate in 228 children with ADHD, both drugs were equally effective (Kratochvil et al. 2002). In a placebo-controlled study of 297 children with ADHD, atomoxetine consistently beat placebo on measures of attention and hyperactivity (Michelson et al. 2001). In addition, atomoxetine also improved social and family functioning relative to placebo.

Modafinil, which is FDA approved for the treatment of narcolepsy, has also been studied for the treatment of ADHD. Modafinil has the distinct advantage over stimulants of not requiring a triplicate prescription, because its abuse potential appears to be very low. In addition, it is better tolerated than amphetamines and simple to dose.

Like atomoxetine, modafinil does not act on the dopaminergic system and, as noted earlier, does not have a significant abuse potential. Modafinil is therefore in Drug Enforcement Administration (DEA) schedule IV and does not require a triplicate prescription. Modafinil appears to act on excitatory histamine projections in very specific regions of the brain and lacks the generalized effects of stimulants. It may also have effects on the hypocretin/orexin system. As such, it is less likely to produce cardiovascular changes of weight gain than either amphetamine or atomoxetine. The most common side effect of modafinil has been headache, but the drug can also produce some mild gastrointestinal side effects. Central nervous system (CNS) side effects such as anxiety or insomnia occur infrequently. Modafinil is an inducer of the CYP 3A3/4 enzyme, so it can speed up the metabolism of oral contraceptives, steroids, and other 3A3/4-dependent compounds. Thus, women taking birth control pills should be advised that there is a theoretical risk of contraceptive failure when modafinil is taken concurrently.

Modafinil has been studied in many conditions associated with producing fatigue, including shift work, sleep apnea, multiple sclerosis, fibromyalgia, Parkinson's disease, and depression (see Chapter 9: "Augmentation Strategies for Treatment-Resistant Disorders"). Preliminary results suggest that modafinil may have a role in the treatment of fatigue in many disorders without a significant downside.

The efficacy of modafinil in the treatment of ADHD has been evaluated in a number of trials. Studies of modafinil in the treatment of ADHD in children have suggested a benefit over placebo and effectiveness equal to that of dextroamphetamine (Rugino and Copley 2001; Taylor and Russo 2000). In a 4-week study of 248 children with ADHD, modafinil at a dosage of 300–400 mg/day was more effective than placebo in treating the symptoms of ADHD and was well tolerated (Biederman et al. 2006). Likewise, in a 9-week double-blind trial of 194 children and adolescents with ADHD, 52% of patients randomly assigned to modafinil improved versus 18% of children randomly assigned to placebo (Greenhill et al. 2006). These data appeared to be sufficient to prompt an approvable letter in 2005 for the treatment of ADHD in children with modafinil. However, there was a report of possible Stevens-Johnson syndrome in a child participating in one of the trials. The etiology of this rash was unclear but might have been related to the study drug. This report resulted in the FDA requesting additional safety information. The company decided to withdraw its application for modafinil in the treatment of ADHD, apparently because of the extensive safety studies that would be required for final approval. The R-enantiomer of modafinil is currently being investigated in the treatment of ADHD and other indications such as bipolar depression.

Antipsychotics

Very few trials of antipsychotics have ever been done with children who have schizophrenia. There has been a general impression that children benefit less from antipsychotics that do adults. However, with the limited data on drug therapy in childhood schizophrenia, it is difficult to make any generalizations. To date, relatively few controlled trials with antipsychotics have ever been done with children. The first showed a modest benefit of haloperidol and loxapine compared with placebo in 75 adolescents with schizophrenia (Pool et al. 1976). Another study showed that haloperidol was superior to placebo in the treatment of childhood schizophrenia (Spencer et al. 1992).

There are growing data on the efficacy and safety of SGAs in the treatment of childhood schizophrenia and bipolar disorder (Kumra et al. 2008). Aripiprazole was approved in the treatment of schizophrenia and bipolar disorder in adolescents in 2008. In 2009, an FDA advisory panel recommended the approval of both quetiapine and olanzapine in the treatment of childhood psychotic disorders. Clozapine has been investigated in small pediatric studies. Even fewer data exist on the efficacy and safety of atypical agents in the treatment of childhood schizophrenia. In one controlled trial, clozapine was compared with haloperidol in 21 patients over 6 weeks (Kumra et al. 1996). The group that was randomly assigned to clozapine showed superior improvement in both positive and negative symptoms relative to the haloperidol-treated children. However, the clozapine was poorly tolerated. Five of 10 clozapine-treated children had significant drops in their neutrophils. In addition, 2 of the 10 children experienced seizures. The average dosage of clozapine was 237 mg/day. Another small randomized controlled trial found that olanzapine and risperidone were somewhat more effective than haloperidol in the treatment of childhood schizophrenia (Sikich et al. 2004). However, weight gain was significantly more problematic in the children treated with SGAs.

Despite the lack of published reports, SGAs such as risperidone and aripiprazole offer clear advantages in a population that may need to be treated for many years. The risk of extrapyramidal symptoms (EPS) with typical antipsychotics is substantial in children who need to be treated through adulthood. While akathisia and dystonic reactions are seen in children treated with SGAs, the risk of tardive dyskinesia is apparently small (Correll et al. 2004). On the other hand, obesity may be a limiting factor for some SGAs. Low-dose risperidone (at dosages of 1–2 mg/day) and perhaps aripiprazole appear to be effective for many without the weight gain associated with other SGAs. Clozapine is a last resort in children in whom trials of both typical and atypical agents have failed.

Table 12–2 lists common pediatric therapeutic dosages of selected antipsychotics in children. In children with developmental disorders such as autism, antipsychotics have a more clear utility. In fact, risperidone became the first drug approved by the FDA for the treatment of some behavioral aspects of autism in 2006. Developmental disorders in children younger than age 15 rarely show marked improvement with antipsychotic treatment, although some decrease in overactive, disorganized behavior can occur. In fact, among the best studies of the SGAs for any condition in childhood are studies of the use of risperidone in children with pervasive developmental disorders. For example, in a multisite study of 101 autistic children, risperidone was significantly more

Table 12–2.   Antipsychotic dosages in children

Drug	Common pediatric therapeutic dosage
Chlorpromazine	0.25 mg/kg tid
Trifluoperazine	0.5–10 mg bid
Haloperidol	0.15–0.5 mg/kg/day (in divided doses [bid])
Aripiprazole	2–10 mg/day
Olanzapine	2.5–5 mg qhs
Quetiapine	25–300 mg/day
Risperidone	1–2 mg/day

effective than placebo in controlling tantrums, aggression, and self-injurious behavior (McCracken et al. 2002). Additionally, the effects were sustained for at least 6 months.

Psychosis associated with affective disorders in children is also helped by antipsychotics. There is no evidence that children are any less tolerant of these drugs than are adults, except perhaps for an even higher rate of dystonia early in treatment in adolescent males. However, the risk of tardive dyskinesia and the lower likelihood of marked improvement make it necessary that clinicians use these agents cautiously, documenting carefully the clinical effects observed and periodically assessing the patient without the medication to make sure that the treatment is really useful as a maintenance therapy. In older adolescents, acute psychotic syndromes begin to resemble those seen in adults and may be treated in the same manner (see Chapter 4: "Antipsychotic Drugs").

Sedative first-generation antipsychotics (e.g., thioridazine and chlorpromazine) may interfere with learning. Of the nonsedative neuroleptics, haloperidol has been best studied in children with autism (pervasive developmental disorder) and has limited efficacy. Recent reports have discussed the utility of atypical antipsychotics such as risperidone and clozapine in treating psychotic children. Earlier case reports attested to the utility of clozapine in child and adolescent schizophrenic patients (Mozes et al. 1994). Although we know of no controlled studies on risperidone that have been completed at the time of this writing, preliminary experience with the drug in children has been positive (Armenteros et al. 1995).

Antipsychotics used at low dosages (e.g., 0.5–3 mg/day of haloperidol or 2–10 mg/day of pimozide) can also control the tics of Tourette's disorder. Clonidine has also been reported to be helpful in severe cases of this disorder. Clonidine can suppress tics fairly well, but it may be more effective in Tourette's disorder patients with explosive violent behaviors. Clonidine causes dry mouth, sedation, constipation, and hypotension.

Antipsychotics have often been used to control the behavior of angry, impulsive children and adolescents without psychosis. This use is not well validated, but most clinicians use low doses of antipsychotics to control angry, violent behavior in child or adolescent inpatients. Some prefer haloperidol in low doses (e.g., 2 mg every hour until the patient is calm), whereas others use more sedative drugs like chlorpromazine in 10- to 50-mg doses three or four times a day. Risperidone has been studied in the treatment of aggression associated with autism in adults and is clearly more effective than placebo (McDougle et al. 1998). Open studies and reports of risperidone in the treatment of aggression in children have also been positive at dosages of 1–2 mg/day (Horrigan and Barnhill 1997; Schreier 1998).

A well-controlled study (Platt et al. 1984) comparing haloperidol (2–6 mg/day), lithium carbonate, and placebo in hospitalized nonpsychotic aggressive children with conduct disorder showed the two drug regimens to be more effective than placebo on various measures. The nursing staff judged the lithium responders to have done best. Sedation and dystonia were problems in patients taking haloperidol. The risks and benefits of this use are unclear. If antipsychotics are used to reduce aggression in children with conduct disorder and actually are effective, the continued use of these potentially harmful drugs to control deviant behavior must be strongly justified. For each particular patient, the drug must make a major and clinically important difference.

Another growing use of antipsychotics in children is for the treatment of anorexia. There are no known effective pharmacotherapies for anorexia nervosa. However, preliminary studies have reported that atypical antipsychotics may help with the agitation, obsessiveness, and disturbing cognitions associated with anorexia nervosa (Dennis et al. 2006; Mondraty et al. 2005). Olanzapine and quetiapine have been most investigated and, as expected, also may be associated with steady weight gain. Additional trials are clearly called for on the utility of antipsychotics in pediatric anorexia.

The side effects and risks of antipsychotics, including tardive dyskinesia with typical agents and weight gain with atypical agents, are similar in children as in adults. However, the possibility of cognitive blunting with these drugs may be relatively more of a problem in children. An inert child who is not learning or functioning may be less trouble to others, but the child may develop more normally if medication is reduced or stopped. In addition, it appears that adolescent males are at much greater risk for dystonic reactions than are older adults (Rosenberg et al. 1994).

When antipsychotics are prescribed for children or adolescents, documented informed consent from the responsible parent or parents is mandatory. Even if the child or adolescent patient is too young to give informed consent, the risks and benefits of the drug should be explained to the patient, and his or her assent to the treatment should be obtained when possible (see Chapter 1: "General Principles of Psychopharmacological Treatment").

Antidepressants

The 2004 decision of an FDA advisory panel to put a black box warning on antidepressants used in children appeared to have resulted in fewer parents seeking or accepting pharmacotherapy for their children in 2005, but antidepressant use in children rebounded somewhat in 2006 (see Chapter 3: "Antidepressants"). While the FDA's review of 25 studies involving 4,600 children suggested an increased risk of suicidal thoughts or gestures by 3% in antidepressant-treated patients versus 1.5% in patients receiving placebo, the review did not adequately weigh the risks of no treatment at all. Child psychiatrists are also more reluctant to prescribe antidepressants because of the enhanced risk of liability associated with a black box warning. That is not to discount the findings of the FDA. Some children appear to be at increased risk for more suicidal thoughts while taking antidepressants. We suspect that pediatric depression is more likely to be associated with bipolar spectrum disorders, and those patients with treatment-emergent akathisia may be at greatest risk. However, the slightly increased risk associated with antidepressants must be weighed against the clear risk of completed suicide in depressed children who are inadequately treated or not treated at all.

The SSRIs have been considered the pharmacotherapy of choice for depression in childhood and adolescence. Fluoxetine remains the only antidepressant that is FDA approved in the treatment of childhood depression, while sertraline and fluvoxamine are approved for pediatric OCD. Although it has been difficult to demonstrate that the TCAs or other antidepressants are more effective than placebo in the treatment of childhood depression, there is some evidence of at least fluoxetine's superiority to placebo in children. In addition, the safety and side-effect profiles of the SSRIs are superior to those of the TCAs. Emslie and colleagues (1997) randomized 76 children (ages 7–17) to either fluoxetine 20 mg/day or placebo. Whereas 56% of the fluoxetine-treated patients responded in 8 weeks, only 33% of the placebo-treated patients responded. Nonetheless, remission was rare for both groups. A more recent study by Emslie and colleagues (2002) in 219 children also found fluoxetine well tolerated and effective in the treatment of pediatric depression. In addition, fluoxetine maintenance treatment appears to be effective in preventing relapse in children (Emslie et al. 2004).

Fluoxetine's oral elixir is quite useful in children. Experience has shown that children are better off starting at lower dosages of fluoxetine. We tend to start at 5 mg/day and increase the dosage every 1–2 weeks to a maximum dosage of 60 mg/day.

Studies on the efficacy of other SSRIs in pediatric depression have been less convincing. Two published trials of sertraline in the treatment of depression in childhood suggest a modest but statistically significant benefit of sertraline after 10 weeks of treatment (Wagner et al. 2003). One published study indicated a somewhat higher rate of remission in depressed children treated with paroxetine but little difference in mean depression scores at the end of 8 weeks (Keller et al. 2001). In another study, paroxetine (20–40 mg/day) and imipramine (200–300 mg/day) at their maximum did not separate from placebo in adolescent depression (Keller et al. 2001). In addition, two unpublished studies of paroxetine did not find benefit in adolescents. One study indicated that citalopram at an average dosage of about 23 mg/day was significantly more effective than placebo in childhood/adolescent depression (Wagner et al. 2001). However, response rates to both drug (36%) and placebo (24%) were relatively low. The drug was well tolerated.

The sum of published and unpublished studies suggests that the benefits of SSRIs in children appear most solid with fluoxetine. Other SSRIs, including paroxetine, citalopram, escitalopram, and sertraline, do appear to have some benefits, but these benefits are more modest and not established in controlled studies. Some investigators have concluded that when unpublished studies are considered and the risks of SSRIs are weighed against the benefits in children, the benefits are not overwhelming (Whittington et al. 2004). However, the FDA warning about the risk for suicidal behavior with the SSRIs had a chilling effect on prescribing, particularly on the part of pediatricians (Nemeroff et al. 2007). Unfortunately, such decreases in prescribing have been accompanied by spikes in the rates of suicides in adolescents (Gibbons et al. 2007). Given that only a relatively small handful of studies on the use of SSRIs in treating pediatric depression have been completed, we believe that it is too early to draw strong conclusions about the utility of SSRIs in children. There is obviously a need for clinicians to have access to previously unpublished studies. But there are children and adolescents who benefit from antidepressants, and they should be both treated and monitored carefully.

It has been even more difficult to demonstrate clear efficacy of TCAs and other antidepressants in controlled studies of childhood depression. For example, a meta-analysis of 12 randomized studies of TCAs in pediatric depression failed to demonstrate a significant difference relative to placebo (Hazell et al. 1995). However, some children who clearly meet criteria for major depressive disorder do appear to respond to TCAs. FDA guidelines recommend an upper dose limit of 2.5 mg/kg for imipramine; however, some studies report doses up to 5.0 mg/kg as often being necessary for clinical response (Table 12–3).

Monitoring of cardiac function is wise when TCAs are used in children: electrocardiograms (ECGs) should be done prior to starting therapy, again when the dose exceeds 3 mg/kg, and then every 2 weeks if the dose is being increased. Doses greater than 5 mg/kg should not be given without outside consultation. Significant slowing of cardiac conduction (PR interval over 0.20 msec, QRS interval over 0.12 msec) may require lowering the dose. Between 1986 and 1992, at least four cases of sudden death occurred in children taking desipramine. The cardiac long QT syndrome has been proposed as a mechanism of action in these sudden deaths. A more recent review of the topic (Biederman et al. 1995) failed to find a strong association between desipramine use and sudden death in children 5–14 years old.

TCAs are effective in the treatment of enuresis at doses of 0.3–1.0 mg/kg of imipramine or an equivalent drug, but behavioral treatments are generally preferred because they are also effective and may have a lower relapse rate. ADHD tends to respond in the same dosage range. It is interesting to note that TCAs improve enuresis within a few days, whereas response to ADHD or depression takes 1–4 weeks. Monoamine oxidase inhibitors (MAOIs) are also said to be effective in the treatment of both enuresis and ADHD, but their use has not been

Table 12–3. Common antidepressant dosages in children

Drug	Dosage range	Serum level (ng/mL)
imipramine	1–5 mg/kg/day	150–250
desipramine	1–5 mg/kg/day	150–250
nortriptyline	0.5–2 mg/kg/day	75–150
phenelzine	0.25–1 mg/kg/day	NA
fluoxetine	5–30 mg/day	NA
bupropion	1–7 mg/kg/day	NA
citalopram	10–20 mg/day	NA

Note. NA = not applicable.

well studied. Clomipramine is available for the treatment of OCD; it has been shown to be effective in children and adolescents with this condition (see Chapter 6: "Antianxiety Agents" for additional discussion).

Side effects of antidepressants in children resemble those seen in adults. Blood level monitoring is about as useful as it is in adults. That is, it is useful for the TCAs but not for other antidepressants, except, perhaps, to test for compliance. Imipramine is the best-studied TCA, and positive correlations between blood level and improvement are often found in clinical trials. Our experience at McLean Hospital and Stanford University Hospital suggests that depressive symptoms in adolescents rarely include major appetite changes or early-morning awakening. Overly sound and lengthy sleep and dysphoria on awakening are more common. Physical symptoms, fatigue, irritability, anger, and retardation for the first few hours in the day may be present without subjective recognition of depression or sadness. Sex drive is decreased. These adolescents often have a family history of affective disorder. This pattern often responds to TCA therapy, although formal controlled studies have not been done. Panic agoraphobia can occur in adolescents and can be treated with antidepressants.

There is little published data on the use of serotonin$_2$ (5-HT$_2$) antagonists, selective serotonin-norepinephrine reuptake inhibitors (SNRIs), and bupropion in pediatric depression. One small, controlled trial of venlafaxine in pediatric depression showed no benefit (Mandoki et al. 1997). In addition, two unpublished trials did not show benefits for venlafaxine in pediatric depression. However, cautious trials with bupropion may be indicated if the patient has failed to respond to trials of SSRIs or TCAs. Bupropion has been used for ADHD at dosages of 3–7 mg/kg/day in divided doses. In addition, we (Killen et al. 2004) recently reported on a trial of bupropion SR in combination with a nicotine patch in adolescent smoking cessation. The drug was well tolerated. In addition, open-label studies have suggested that there may be a role for bupropion in treating adolescents with depression and comorbid ADHD (Daviss et al. 2001; Solhkhah et al. 2005). Anorexia and the risk of seizures may be problems for some children, and, particularly in those cases, the dose should be titrated upward slowly. The few small studies of MAOIs in the treatment of children with depression and phobias have generally yielded positive findings, but the results are inconclusive.

Mood Stabilizers

Adolescents can show a typical bipolar picture that often responds to lithium therapy or treatment with an SGA. Preadolescent children rarely show mania, but they can show cyclic mood and behavior shifts with periods of impulsivity, hyperactivity, social intrusiveness, tantrums, mood lability, and nonpsychotic euphoria, with parallel shifts in vegetative symptoms, which sometimes respond to lithium. However, there are no controlled studies with adequate sample size that have demonstrated the efficacy of lithium in childhood bipolar illness (Kafantaris 1995; Lopez-Larson and Frazier 2006). One of the better studies was a study in adolescents treated with lithium who had bipolar disorder with comorbid substance abuse (B. Geller et al. 1998). Lithium appeared to help both the bipolar disorder and the substance abuse. A randomized comparison of lithium and divalproex in the maintenance treatment of pediatric bipolar patients (average age = 10.8 years) found that valproate was about as effective as lithium in the time it took to require an additional intervention (Findling et al. 2006). Smaller open-label studies have suggested that lithium is effective and often well tolerated in treating bipolar depression (Patel et al. 2006) and in restabilizing bipolar disorder when combined with valproate in children (Findling et al. 2006).

Explosive, violent behavior in pediatric patients with conduct disorder, mental retardation, and hyperactivity has also responded to lithium treatment in a number of studies (Campbell et al. 1984; Lopez-Larson and Frazier 2006; Vetro et al. 1985).

No one knows the long-term consequences of long-term maintenance lithium treatment begun in childhood or adolescence. Children have increased renal clearance relative to adults and may tolerate larger doses of lithium. For children older than 12, the lithium may often be dosed as it is for adults (Table 12–4). However, younger children under 25 kg are best started at 150–300 mg/day. The dosage may then be increased in 150- to 300-mg increments every 3–7 days in a tid regimen as tolerated. It is not unusual for children to require more than 2,100 mg/day in divided doses to maintain adequate serum levels. The serum levels should be monitored carefully and checked every 3–5 days after each increase in dosage. The side effects of lithium in children are the same as in adults.

Carbamazepine, oxcarbazepine, lamotrigine, and valproate appear to also have a role in pediatric psychiatric disorders. Controlled data demonstrate carbamazepine's efficacy in conduct disorder and intermittent explosive disorder in children and adolescents. There are also data suggesting that anticonvulsants may have utility in the treatment of bipolar disorder and other pediatric conditions. Oxcarbazepine may be somewhat easier to use in children, but the only double-blind study in a pediatric bipolar population failed to show a benefit of oxcarbazepine in this population (Wagner et al. 2006). In Canadian studies, there is a suggestion that adolescents with bipolar disorder prefer valproate to lithium. Valproate has also been reported to help aggressive behavior in adolescents who do and who do not have mood disorders (Saxena et al. 2006; Steiner et al. 2003). While there have been no controlled studies of lamotrigine in pediatric bipolar disorder, open-label studies have reported benefit in the treatment of bipolar depression (Chang et al. 2006). Side effects of anticonvulsants in children parallel those in adults. However, very young children (younger than 2 years) appear at greatest risk for hepatic toxicity with valproate. As with lithium, children often require higher doses of carbamazepine or valproate on a mg/kg basis than adults because of their more efficient hepatic and renal metabolism, as already mentioned. Children may be more at risk for rash while taking lamotrigine than are adults, and slow titration of the drug to therapeutic levels is prudent. The dosage range of carbamazepine in children is 10–50 mg/kg/day in divided doses; the dosage range of valproate is 15–60 mg/kg/day.

Antianxiety Drugs

Benzodiazepines are sometimes of use for short periods in treating pavor nocturnus or sleepwalking in children. Of course, benzodiazepines and nonben-

Table 12–4. Common mood stabilizer dosages in children

Drug	Dosage range	Serum level
lithium	300–2,400 mg/day	0.5–1.2 mEq/L
valproate	15–60 mg/kg/day	50–100 µg/mL
carbamazepine	10–50 mg/kg/day	8–12 µg/mL
oxcarbazepine	5–30 mg/kg/day (150–1,200 mg/day)	NA
lamotrigine	0.15–5.0 mg/kg/day (25–200 mg/day)	NA

zodiazepine hypnotics such as zolpidem also have been associated with somnambulism and amnesia in both children and adults. If used for daytime anxiety, they can increase activity and produce or aggravate behavior disorders, particularly in children with ADHD. Severe school phobia may be better treated with an antidepressant, although a single dose of a benzodiazepine may be used occasionally to allay anticipatory anxiety and help a child return to a feared situation for the first time. Alprazolam has been used successfully to treat panic disorder, generalized anxiety disorder, and avoidant personality disorder in children. Buspirone also appears to have some utility in childhood anxiety disorders (Simeon 1993). Sedative antihistamines are believed to have some antianxiety or hypnotic utility in children for short periods. Prolonged use may lead to anticholinergic side effects and cognitive impairment. Venlafaxine and paroxetine are also being studied in adolescents with social phobia. It is worth remembering that newer drugs are rarely studied in children or adolescents before marketing, and even the older drugs are often only partially studied in children and adolescents. Newer anticonvulsants, such as pregabalin, have not been studied in pediatric anxiety but could prove a useful alternative to benzodiazepines.

The place of drug therapy for children and adolescents is still controversial. Drugs should be reserved for clearly distressed or dysfunctional conditions for which psychosocial treatments either have failed or are likely to be only of short-term benefit. Drug therapy needs to be carefully monitored and requires close collaboration among the physician, the parents, and often school personnel or other caregivers. Prolonged maintenance drug therapy is sometimes justifiable, but there should be strong clinical evidence of benefit, and trials of withdrawal from medication are often indicated to make sure the drug is still making a useful difference.

Geriatric Psychopharmacology

Elderly psychiatric patients present a variety of potential problems for the psychiatrist considering prescribing psychoactive drugs. Elderly persons may have decreased ability to metabolize some drugs, although it has been documented only infrequently. These patients may have low serum protein levels, which could lead them to have relatively higher levels of free drug (not bound to protein) at any given blood level. Free drug is usually presumed to be more active and more likely to cross the blood-brain barrier. Elderly patients may be more sensitive to peripheral side effects (e.g., hypotension, constipation) than younger patients at the same dose or blood level. They may also be more prone to CNS side effects (e.g., delirium, tremor, tardive dyskinesia). None of these presumptions is well documented except for delirium and tardive dyskinesia, chiefly because no adequate studies have been done.

Elderly persons appear to have a reduced reserve of both brain function and cardiovascular competence, which leaves them more vulnerable to drug side effects. Decreased hepatic function and renal function also contribute to side effects in geriatric patients. In addition, the consequences of side effects—such as falls due to orthostatic hypotension, falls due to confusion, or ataxia or decubitus ulcers due to prolonged oversedation—are more likely to be serious in elderly persons. The situation is made worse by the higher likelihood of coexisting medical illness and the use of other drugs for these illnesses in elderly patients. In addition, there is a lack of clear criteria for predicting which elderly patients need very low, cautious dosage regimens of psychoactive drugs and which patients require (and tolerate) rather large dosages to attain adequate treatment response.

Moreover, the definition of geriatrics has changed over the years. The average 60-year-old of today is far more fit than his or her counterpart of 20 years ago and probably does not demonstrate any significant decrease in drug metabolism or tolerability. For the standard psychiatric conditions, such as depression, mania, chronic schizophrenia, and generalized anxiety disorder, the only safe and reasonable approach is to begin with a very low drug dosage and to increase the dosage cautiously after other organic etiologies are ruled out.

As an example, 25 mg of imipramine or trimipramine at bedtime is a reasonable starting dose for healthy patients older than 65, and a 10-mg dose is reasonable for patients older than 70 or for patients older than 60 with concurrent medical problems or with evidence of dementia. In such patients, dosage increments should be scheduled for every 3–7 days, not every day, so that the clinician has a chance to assess side effects before increasing the dose.

Antidepressants

Most antidepressants and electroconvulsive therapy (ECT) have been used effectively in elderly patients with major depression. In the past 20 years, SSRIs, particularly sertraline, citalopram, and escitalopram, have grown more popular in the first-line treatment of geriatric depression. In addition, controlled trials of mirtazapine suggest that the sedating and weight-gain effects of the drug are useful in many elderly depressed patients. Furthermore, mirtazapine may be better tolerated in geriatric patients than some SSRIs with which it has been compared, such as paroxetine. The SSRI side-effect profile is superior to that of the TCAs in most geriatric patients. All TCAs, including the secondary amines, have the disadvantage of producing at least some anticholinergic side effects and orthostasis. However, for more serious depressive episodes in geriatric patients, many clinicians prefer venlafaxine or nortriptyline to SSRIs. Some controversial data suggest that nortriptyline may be superior to fluoxetine in geriatric melancholic depression (see Chapter 3: "Antidepressants"). Our experience, confirmed by discussions with other geriatric psychiatrists and family practitioners, suggests that fluoxetine and other SSRIs are sometimes less useful than TCAs in hospitalized elderly depressed patients.

Five geriatric depression studies are worthy of comment. In one, venlafaxine, fluoxetine, and placebo were all of similar efficacy in depressed patients over 65 years of age. The high response rate with placebo limits the inferences that can be drawn from this study. Both active drugs were well tolerated. ECG and blood pressure effects were minimal with both drugs (Schatzberg and Roose 2006). In contrast, a study involving frail nursing home patients reported higher rates, and perhaps less safety, with venlafaxine than with sertraline (Oslin et al. 2003). In another study, citalopram was not more effective than placebo in so-called old old patients (Roose et al. 2004). Again, a high placebo response was observed. In another presentation, duloxetine was significantly more effective than placebo in depressed geriatric patients (Raskin et al. 2004). A composite cognition score was used as the primary outcome measure. In the last study, mirtazapine was significantly more effective than paroxetine in the first 6 weeks of an 8-week trial. Mirtazapine was associated with significantly fewer dropouts due to adverse events than was paroxetine. The average dosage in this study was approximately 30 mg/day for both (Schatzberg et al. 2002).

Trazodone has been a somewhat effective antidepressant in elderly depressed patients and is an excellent hypnotic. It should not cause orthostatic hypotension except for a couple of hours after a bedtime dose. However, some patients in their 70s and 80s have daytime hypotension when treated with trazodone.

Nefazodone was generally well tolerated in the elderly but was associated with orthostasis and dysphoric activation in some geriatric patients. The risk of hepatotoxicity has limited the use of nefazodone in the elderly, and it is now rarely used. Lower doses of both trazodone and nefazodone are often necessary in older patients, particularly when treatment is being started.

Bupropion appears to be well tolerated in the treatment of geriatric depression but is experienced as too activating by some patients. Dosages in the range of 200–300 mg/day appear to be adequate in many cases of geriatric depression.

ECT remains the major treatment for depressed elderly patients when drug therapy fails. ECT is often very effective. However, some patients with recurring depressions stop responding to ECT after the third to the tenth course of treatment in the same way that some patients may "poop out" with use of some antidepressants.

Although stimulants are occasionally quite helpful in the treatment of recent-onset depressions in elderly patients with medical problems, they often only induce agitation in treatment-resistant elderly depressed patients. We have seen some benefits of adding 100–200 mg in the morning of modafinil (Provigil) to standard antidepressants in geriatric patients. Alexopoulos (2005) has suggested that some late-life depression that is characterized by problems with executive function and white matter changes might respond better to dopamine agonists and perhaps modafinil.

Another presumption in the treatment of elderly patients is that anticholinergic drugs increase the likelihood of delirium. On this basis, desipramine should be safer than amitriptyline, and fluphenazine should be safer than thioridazine. Our review of the literature on TCA use in elderly patients suggests, however, that delirium more often occurs in patients taking a TCA-antipsychotic combination and that this side effect can be transient and relatively easily managed. Again, there are no adequate controlled trials documenting this issue.

Hypnotics and Anxiolytics

If benzodiazepines are to be used as hypnotics or for daytime anxiety, again use the lowest dose first to observe whether this dose is adequate and to determine whether the drug is well tolerated. Elderly patients appear more likely than younger patients to have cognitive side effects, falls, and impaired driving while taking benzodiazepines (Madhusoodanan et al. 2004). These are all very serious issues in a geriatric population. In general, 3-hydroxy-benzodiazepines such as temazepam and lorazepam are the preferred agents for geriatric patients because of their lack of active metabolites and simpler metabolism. There is evidence that benzodiazepine metabolism is slowed in elderly persons, and there is a presumption that higher cumulative blood levels are associated with behavioral toxicity.

Occasionally, elderly (and young adult) patients complain of excessive morning sedation after taking slowly metabolized hypnotics like flurazepam. However, there is a good deal of individual variability in the extent to which this consequence of slowed metabolism causes demonstrable clinical problems. Nonetheless, the long-acting benzodiazepines such as flurazepam, because of their long half-lives and tendency toward residual daytime drowsiness, are not particularly good choices for the treatment of any insomnia. Temazepam is probably the best choice as a benzodiazepine hypnotic because of its shorter half-life and lack of active metabolites.

Currently, zolpidem is among the most widely used hypnotics in geriatric patients. Although a very effective agent, it may be less well tolerated than zaleplon, which is much shorter acting and may be as effective as zolpidem. Zaleplon has been well studied in geriatric patients and has the advantage of being able to be taken in the middle of the night, when some patients are most distressed about not being able to go back to sleep. A dose of 0.5 mg at night or on awakening is often sufficient. Likewise, eszopiclone may be dosed at 1–2 mg per night. The abuse potential appears low, and the chance of significant drug interactions or exacerbation of sleep apnea also appears low.

Trazodone continues to be valuable as a hypnotic in the elderly. At higher doses in geriatric patients, the risk of orthostatic hypotension increases. Thus, we suggest checking orthostatic blood pressures at baseline and as the dose is titrated. The most common dosing is 50–100 mg 1–2 hours before bedtime. Mirtazapine is another fine agent to use as a sleeper. Like trazodone, it carries no risk of dependence and tends to be well tolerated. A dose of 7.5–15 mg at night works at least as well as trazodone without the risk of orthostatic hypotension. Ramelteon may be worth trying before other hypnotics in geriatric patients. Unlike standard hypnotics, ramelteon is not likely to contribute to confusion or amnesia, nor is it associated with orthostatic hypotension as is trazodone. It appears to be somewhat less effective for maintaining sleep.

Mood Stabilizers

Lithium excretion is, on the average, slowed in elderly patients as a consequence of an age-related decrease in kidney function. Therefore, this drug should be started at low dosages in older patients—300 mg/day in patients in their 60s and early 70s and 150 mg/day in patients who are older. Lithium levels and clinical signs of toxicity should be monitored scrupulously. It is our impression that elderly patients can slip from therapeutic to toxic blood levels more rapidly and insidiously than can young adult patients. In addition, elderly patients are often taking concurrent medications that may increase the risk of lithium toxicity, including nonsteroidal anti-inflammatory drugs (NSAIDs), thiazide diuretics, and angiotensin-converting enzyme (ACE) inhibitors. On the other hand, lithium can be as effective in some older bipolar patients as it is in younger ones, although some elderly patients whose condition is of late onset may have an underlying organic disorder that does not respond well to lithium.

Valproate generally appears better tolerated than lithium in elderly patients. It often takes lower doses of valproate to achieve adequate serum levels in geriatric patients. We have seen dosages as low as 250 mg/day appear to result in adequate mood stabilization for some geriatric patients. However, many more patients will not achieve adequate serum levels with dosages below 750 mg/day.

Gabapentin is well tolerated in geriatric patients but of no utility in the treatment of bipolar disorder. It may be more useful in geriatric agitation and anxiety states as pregabalin appears to be.

Other anticonvulsant agents such as oxcarbazepine and lamotrigine have not been adequately studied in geriatric patients with bipolar disorder but are generally well tolerated. Carbamazepine, with its potential for interactions with so many medications, is often a poor choice in geriatric patients.

Antipsychotics

In older patients with chronic schizophrenia, there is a belief that lower antipsychotic dosages are needed than those used with younger adult patients. There is, again, no real evidence to support this belief, but there is some evidence that the same antipsychotic dose yields blood levels 1.5–2 times higher in elderly than in younger patients. Cautious attempts at gradually tapering dosage are indicated in schizophrenic patients older than 60 who are receiving maintenance neuroleptic treatment. When such patients have stopped their medication and become acutely psychotic, cautious low-dosage medication (e.g., 0.5–2.0 mg/day of haloperidol or risperidone, or 1.25–5 mg of olanzapine) should be tried for the first week to see whether a clinical response can be obtained without resorting to high dosages. However, if the patient fails to improve and has a history of requiring and tolerating a higher neuroleptic dosage, the dose can be gradually raised, again with monitoring of side effects. Quetiapine, even at higher doses, has a very low risk of EPS and and is favored by some geriatric psychiatrists.

The use of antiparkinsonian drugs could cause delirium, but leaving the patient exposed to dystonia or pseudoparkinsonism is equally undesirable; clinicians are forced to feel their way, attempting to maximize benefit and to minimize adverse effects. This applies equally to the use of antipsychotics in younger adult patients, but in the elderly, the problems encountered in attempting to achieve the right balance of medications may be more frequent. Aripiprazole, olanzapine, risperidone, and quetiapine offer alternatives to standard antipsychotics. The orthostasis that may be secondary to use of these drugs has occasionally resulted in falls with serious consequences. The anticholinergic properties of clozapine also tend to be poorly tolerated by geriatric patients. Olanzapine also has some anticholinergic properties. However, older patients are often able to tolerate and respond to lower doses of the atypical antipsychotics.

Tardive dyskinesia has been statistically more prevalent in elderly patients, especially women, who are taking maintenance antipsychotics, but in patients with chronic schizophrenia the dyskinesia usually has already been present for years and is not a contraindication to using antipsychotics to achieve relief of psychotic symptoms. Nonetheless, geriatric patients appear to be more vulnerable to developing some EPS, particularly pseudoparkinsonism, than do younger patients. In the rare older chronic patient showing new-onset dyskinesia, a trial of withdrawal from the antipsychotics is usually indicated. The concurrent presence of pseudoparkinsonism and dyskinesia in the same patient is more common in elderly than in other patients.

The use of SGAs in geriatric patients with dementia has been associated with an increased mortality. In fact, all SGAs carry an FDA black box warning indicating a risk of higher mortality when these drugs have been used in treating elderly patients with dementia. No SGA is approved in the treatment of dementia. Overall, it appears that there is a 1.6–1.7 times greater risk of mortality in geriatric patients with dementia who are treated with SGAs versus placebo. The risk of CVAs in controlled trials of olanzapine in the treatment of dementia was 1.3% versus 0.4% with placebo. Likewise, the risk of CVAs in controlled trials of risperidone was 4% versus 2% with placebo. However, a large observational study of 11,400 patients treated with antipsychotics in the Ontario Healthcare Database failed to find an increased risk of CVAs with either olanzapine or risperidone in patients over age 66 (Herrmann et al. 2004). In fact, typical antipsychotics may be associated with the same mortality risks in elderly patients (Trifirò et al. 2007). When the potential for toxicity is considered along with the relative lack of benefit of antipsychotics in some carefully done studies (Schneider et al. 2006), the routine use of antipsychotics in dementia populations should probably be avoided. In cases of behavioral dyscontrol in dementia patients, nonpharmacological interventions should be attempted first. If those interventions fail, a trial with an antipsychotic might be attempted, but the utility of such a trial should be reassessed on a regular basis.

Medications for Dementia

Most elderly patients with mild, moderate, or severe dementia have Alzheimer's disease, although some have multi-infarct dementia, a few have both, and some have neither. The best treatment for dementia is to diagnose a treatable, reversible cause such as vitamin deficiency, hypothyroidism, or congestive heart failure and to treat the underlying medical condition. The other confounding diagnosis is pseudodementia secondary to major depression. Some authors believe that depression can cause dementia in elderly persons, and depression can certainly aggravate mild, preexisting cognitive dysfunction. Depression probably unmasks some dementias. Thus, "pseudodementias" in geriatric patients tend to represent early progressive dementias if followed over time. The evidence is clear that depression should be carefully and thoroughly treated when cognitive impairment and depression coexist. In recent years, greater attention has been paid to vascular depression, which may be associated with marked cognitive impairments. Optimal treatments have yet to be defined, although investigators in this area have suggested that calcium channel blockers and MAOIs might be useful, perhaps in combination. Data are not yet available as of this writing.

Antidepressants might be used in patients with strokes or organic mood lability, even if the depressive syndrome is only partially present. Results from at least 16 controlled trials confirm that antidepressants are effective in the treatment of poststroke depression and that the benefits extend beyond mood (Chen et al. 2006). Improvements in activities of daily living (ADLs), emotional incontinence, and general sense of well-being have been reported benefits of treating poststroke depression with SSRIs and other agents. The odds favor a substantial improvement over any worsening of organic deficit, although the dosage should be started low and raised cautiously. It is clear that patients with behavioral deficits due to strokes who show insomnia, weight loss, agitation, and inability to participate in rehabilitative programs can do well with TCAs and presumably with other antidepressants. There are several favorable reports on the use of nortriptyline for poststroke depression. This strategy was undertaken because nortriptyline is less likely, at therapeutic blood levels, to produce orthostatic blood pressure changes than are other TCAs (see below). In addition, a controlled trial showed fluoxetine to be superior to maprotiline in the treatment of poststroke depression (Dam et al. 1996). In another study (Robinson et al. 2000), nortriptyline was significantly more effective than fluoxetine or placebo in helping with mood and anxiety problems but not with cognitive function. Treatment should not be withheld just because a stroke patient's dysphoria seems appropriate to the disability: depression appears to be associated with a high mortality in stroke patients.

Until the advent of tacrine, dementia alone was not an indication for drug therapy. The only drug previously marketed in the United States for senile symptoms, ergoloid mesylates (Hydergine), was regularly a bit more effective than placebo in a large number of double-blind, placebo-controlled studies; however, the effects were weak, different in different studies, and usually only manifest after 2–3 months, making the marginal utility of this treatment questionable. A variety of other drugs for dementia, including piracetam, vincamine, lecithin, and oral physostigmine, have been studied, but so far only a few have been shown to be somewhat useful.

The first drug FDA approved for the treatment of Alzheimer's disease was tetrahydroaminoacridine (THA; tacrine). Tacrine was an old drug from Australia, used there to reverse drug-induced coma. It is a central cholinesterase inhibitor that is thought to act by raising brain acetylcholine levels and increasing cholinergic brain activity. After an initial very positive study published in the *New England Journal of Medicine* (Summers et al. 1986), a controlled multicenter trial of tacrine in Alzheimer's dementia was initiated by the National Institute on Aging. Several more controlled studies from the Tacrine Study Group (Davis et al. 1992; Farlow et al. 1992; Knapp et al. 1994) confirmed the utility of tacrine in treating Alzheimer's disease patients who have mild to moderate dementia. Tacrine appeared to have a modest effect on the global cognitive deficits that affect most Alzheimer's disease patients. Unfortunately, tacrine was also hepatotoxic and is rarely used now, although it can be obtained through major drug distributors.

Currently, the drug most commonly prescribed for the treatment of Alzheimer's disease is donepezil (Aricept). While donepezil is considerably more benign than tacrine, it is probably no more effective. A number of studies have been completed that demonstrate a clear benefit of donepezil over placebo in such measures as the Alzheimer's Disease Assessment Scale (ADAS) or the Mini-Mental State Exam (Burns et al. 1999; Greenberg et al. 2000). Donepezil may improve cognitive function by 5%–10% and may improve, though modestly, the quality of life of some patients and their care providers. In addition to Alzheimer's disease, donepezil has also been shown to have mild efficacy in the treatment of other dementias, including Lewy body dementia and vascular dementias.

Donepezil tends to be well tolerated, with a dose-related increase in side effects. Dosages of 5 mg/day tend to be well tolerated; the most common side effects of the 10-mg dose are nausea, diarrhea, insomnia, fatigue, muscle cramps, and anorexia. Some adaptation tends to occur over time to most of these side effects.

Some anecdotal reports suggest that donepezil may help ameliorate depression and exacerbate mania (Benazzi and Rossi 1999). Some patients have reported improvement in cognition, even if they did not have dementia, and some reports suggest that donepezil can help with medication-induced memory problems (Jacobsen and Comas-Diaz 1999).

Another cholinesterase inhibitor, rivastigmine (Exelon), was recently approved for the treatment of dementia. Rivastigmine produces a dose-dependent increase in acetylcholine and appears to bypass hepatic metabolism. Thus, it appears safe for hepatic function. Rivastigmine has a half-life of 10 hours and is more centrally active than peripheral in its effects on the cholinergic system, a feature that makes it reasonably tolerated. Gastrointestinal upset is the most common side effect. There have been two large studies demonstrating the superiority of a dosage of 6–12 mg/day over placebo in the treatment of Alzheimer's dementia (Jann 2000). It may be somewhat better tolerated than donepezil in some patients. Rivastigmine is reported to produce fewer and less severe gastrointestinal effects, including diarrhea, than donepezil; however, it does not appear to be any more effective than donepezil. In 2007, a transdermal form of rivastigmine was approved for use in Alzheimer's dementia. The transdermal administration of rivastigmine bypasses the gut and tends to be far better tolerated than the oral form.

Galantamine (Reminyl) was the next cholinesterase inhibitor, after rivastigmine, on the U.S. market. Galantamine's mechanism of action is a variation on the theme of acetylcholinesterase inhibitors. This agent is a competitive inhibitor of acetylcholinesterase and allosterically modulates nicotinic receptors to enhance cholinergic transmission. This mechanism may theoretically give galantamine some advantages over other acetylcholinesterase inhibitors, but none as yet have been demonstrated. What has been proven is that galantamine is more effective than placebo in treating the cognitive deficits of Alzheimer's disease and that these effects are sustained for at least 12 months. The drug seems to be reasonably well tolerated at doses of 24–32 mg/day, with nausea in up to 40% of treated patients and diarrhea in up to 19% of patients. No significant effects were seen on liver function or any other laboratory tests.

In 2003, memantine (Namenda) became the first drug approved for moderate to severe Alzheimer's disease. Memantine is a moderate N-methyl-D-aspartate (NMDA) antagonist that is thought to mitigate the toxic effects of increased calcium flow into neurons by blocking NMDA receptors. This blockade then reduces the neurodegenerative effects caused by lower glutamate levels and increased calcium influx in Alzheimer's disease. Memantine appears to improve cognition and ADLs significantly more than placebo in patients with moderate or more severe dementia (Reisberg et al. 2003). Importantly, memantine also appears to modestly reduce the amount of time caregivers must spend with an Alzheimer's patient. In addition, patients who are already taking a cholinesterase inhibitor, such as donepezil, appear to improve with the addition of memantine to the regimen (Tariot et al. 2004).

Memantine has been quickly adopted in clinical practice not because it is dramatically efficacious but rather because it is impressively benign. In clinical trials, the rate of side effects was not different than the rate with placebo. In fact, no side effect occurred in more than 5% of patients at statistically different rates than with placebo. The most commonly reported side effects were dizziness, confusion, headaches, and hallucinations.

Memantine is not a potent inhibitor or dependent substrate of any CYP enzyme. As a result, it has few drug interactions. The only condition known to substantially affect serum levels of memantine is alkaline urine. A urine pH > 8, such as caused by urinary tract infections or carbonic anhydrase inhibitors, will substantially reduce the clearance of the drug and may be associated with increased side effects.

Memantine is usually started at 5 mg/day, with a target dosage of 20 mg/day. We have generally had no trouble increasing the dosage by 5 mg per week until the patient is taking 10 mg bid. While many patients will tolerate a more rapid titration, it is unclear whether there are any advantages to more rapid titration.

It is nice for the clinician to have options, but it is unlikely that any acetylcholinesterase inhibitor with or without memantine will produce anything more than moderate benefits for the cognitive function and behavioral difficulties of most dementia patients. Donepezil is currently the first choice for most clinicians only because it is the best studied and there is no evidence yet that the newer agents are any more efficacious. Memantine appears to be an important additional option for patients. However, we appear to be a long way from having interventions that substantially affect the course of the disease or the quality of life of Alzheimer's patients.

Medications for Agitation

Patients with chronic dementia often show agitation, irascibility, night wandering, paranoid ideation, or hallucinations and become major management problems at home or in psychiatric hospitals or nursing homes. Behavioral dyscontrol represents one of the most common reasons geriatric patients are placed in nursing homes. Many of these patients were routinely treated with low-dose, typical antipsychotics such as haloperidol, often with dubious benefit. A review of the few controlled studies in this area suggested that only a third of these patients clearly benefit from low-dose (typical) neuroleptics (Cole 1990).

More recent studies have also cast doubt on the utility and safety of atypical antipsychotics in treating behavioral problems in dementia patients (see "Antipsychotics" subsection earlier in chapter). In our own experience, thioridazine is not better tolerated than low doses of more potent antipsychotics; all typical antipsychotics show an unfortunate tendency to cause pseudoparkinsonism and akathisia in the elderly. These problems, plus the increased risk of tardive dyskinesia and the probably increased risk of confusional states when antiparkinsonian drugs are added, often make typical antipsychotics unsatisfactory drugs in treating agitated patients with dementia. We had found low doses of atypical antipsychotics (0.5–1 mg of risperidone or 2.5–5 mg of olanzapine) sometimes helpful in controlling the agitation and psychosis associated with dementia. These tend to produce few, if any, EPS at low doses. However, as described previously, the recent CATIE study (see Schneider et al. 2006) failed to show much benefit for olanzapine, risperidone, or quetiapine over placebo in terms of efficacy, while these agents had much more side effects.

There are a number of other options for treating agitation in patients with dementia. First, treating the underlying dementia with an acetylcholinesterase inhibitor often helps with behavioral problems associated with dementia. Thus, the acetylcholinesterase inhibitors should be tried first. We have had good success with treating some agitated depressed patients with moderate dosages of valproate (500–1,250 mg/day) (Schatzberg and DeBattista 1999). However, many geriatric patients do not tolerate higher doses of Depakote. Tariot's group first reported that the maximum tolerated dosage in this population is about 800 mg/day, or 11.5 mg/kg per day (Profenno et al. 2005). Also, a recent multicenter trial involving 153 patients failed to find valproate at a mean dosage of 800 mg/day to be significantly more effective than placebo in reducing agitation in nursing home patients (Tariot et al. 2005). A number of studies have also demonstrated the utility of carbamazepine in the treatment of agitated dementia patients (Gleason and Schneider 1990). There is one controlled trial in which a modal dose of 300 mg of carbamazepine was significantly more effective than placebo in reducing agitation in dementia patients (Tariot et al. 1998). We still tend to prefer valproate over carbamazepine because carbamazepine tends to be more poorly tolerated, has a lower therapeutic index, and has more drug interactions in these elderly patients, who tend to be on multiple drugs.

Newer anticonvulsants, such as gabapentin, pregabalin, and tiagabine, make intuitive sense for the treatment of agitation but are largely untested. As with benzodiazepines, there has been the suggestion that gabapentin can induce agitation in some brain-injured patients but can help others (Goldenberg et al. 1998; Miller 2001). Probably some patients would respond to a benzodiazepine, preferably oxazepam, because of its simple metabolism and low abuse potential. This drug at least offers hope of an early response when the dose is adjusted properly. Many dementia patients become confused on benzodiazepines, and we now tend to prefer atypical antipsychotics and valproate over benzodiazepines.

Other drugs have been the subject of individual case reports. Propranolol had been the most widely studied, but mainly for agitation and assaultiveness in nonelderly brain-damaged patients (Greendyke and Kanter 1986; Greendyke et al. 1989; Weiler et al. 1988). Some case reports have suggested that agitation decreases as soon as the right dosage of propranolol is reached, but most studies report improvement after a month of taking the right dosage. In the hospitalized, agitated, restless, irascible dementia patient, a month is a very long time, and propranolol carries the risk of orthostatic hypotension, with resulting falls. If it is to be tried in elderly patients, the starting dosage should be 10 mg bid, and dosage should be increased in increments of 10–20 mg every 2 days to 200 mg/day, stopping at lower dosages if hypotension or other side effects occur. Propranolol can cause delirium. Glassman et al. (1979) showed that orthostatic hypotension due to TCAs is far worse in cardiac patients taking multiple cardiac medications than in medically healthy depressed patients. The same is likely with propranolol—it probably should not be tried in patients taking multiple cardiac or other medications.

There are a number of studies on the helpfulness of trazodone and bus-pirone in treating agitated elderly patients with dementia (Colenda 1988; Lebert et al. 1994; Pinner and Rich 1988; Sultzer et al. 2001). The latter is used quite commonly in some nursing home settings at dosages of 10–45 mg/day More recently, controlled trials of SSRIs, such as citalopram at approximately 20 mg/day, have demonstrated benefits for controlling behavioral outbursts in patients with dementia.

Psychosocial measures may be more useful than drugs in treating agitation in elderly patients with dementia. Simple interventions such as keeping the patient oriented with a calendar and clock and keeping the lights on can substantially reduce agitation in dementia patients. Also, looking for and treating concurrent medical problems such as a urinary tract infection will often do more than any pharmacological treatment for agitation. Better studies of more kinds of drug therapy in elderly patients are needed, but in their absence, clinicians have to cautiously try to do their best with available measures.

Mental Retardation (Intellectual Disability)

As with elderly patients with dementia, institutionalized mentally retarded persons have been treated routinely for decades with antipsychotics, such as small doses of haloperidol or risperidone, for a wide range of behavioral disorders. Many patients with even mild intellectual deficits end up taking either antipsychotics or mood stabilizers at some point to control behavioral problems (Haw and Stubbs 2005). Court decisions have mandated evaluating such patients while they are not taking medications, and it now appears that only a fraction of those receiving long-term antipsychotic medication are clinically better with them than without them. Antipsychotic-responsive retarded patients have not been well characterized, but it seems probable that some show psychotic symptoms that would qualify for a diagnosis of schizophrenia. Since the mid-1990s, the atypical antipsychotics have been increasingly employed for the management of behavioral dyscontrol in mentally retarded and brain-injured patients. The evidence has accumulated that agents such as risperidone appear to be useful in both the acute and the long-term management of disruptive behavior, affective symptoms, or self-injurious behavior in patients with subaverage intelligence (Biederman et al. 2006; Reyes et al. 2006b; Shedlack et al. 2005).

A general principle in the treatment of mentally retarded patients may be useful as a guideline. Such patients often show aberrant behaviors (e.g., disrobing, jumping, poking fingers in eyes) that can increase dramatically when they become psychiatrically upset. Counting (monitoring) these target behaviors can be a useful guide to treatment effect in often nonverbal patients. The real diagnosis may have to be inferred from changes in vegetative symptoms such as sleep, appetite, and motor activity or from family history of psychiatric disorders. All this gives a trial-and-error quality to the drug therapy of behaviorally disturbed mentally retarded patients, reinforcing Sovner's (1989) practice of monitoring target behaviors or symptoms before and during trials. It may take a few weeks to be sure any given drug is or is not useful.

Some articles have documented the existence of depressive and bipolar disorders that manifest somewhat atypically in relatively or completely nonverbal patients (Sovner and Hurley 1983). Such patients are appropriate candidates for treatment with standard antidepressants or mood stabilizers.

If one accepts that overactive, turbulent, and episodically violent behaviors toward others or self are usually not a manifestation of psychosis in retarded patients, or if it has been empirically determined that these are not antipsychotic responsive behaviors, what then? Candidate drugs include atypical antipsychotics, SSRIs, valproate, buspirone, propranolol, gabapentin, and carbamazepine. None of these have been the subject of placebo-controlled clinical trials in disturbed retarded patients. However, all have been the subject of small open trials with reported sustained, if often delayed, benefit in the patients described here.

In addition to the antipsychotics, lithium carbonate and valproate have among the best credentials as anti-anger drugs in a variety of psychiatric populations. If the patient has a seizure disorder, shifting to carbamazepine or valproate seems sensible. Nadolol is of theoretical interest because it is a β-blocker that does not cross the blood-brain barrier and because it is hypothesized to decrease episodic violence by peripheral action on muscles. Propranolol requires more titrating (30–480 mg/day) to determine an effective dosage, and it can cause hypotension, bradycardia, and delirium. The desirable monitoring of vital signs before each dosage greater than 120 mg/day may be impossible in some residential facilities.

Buspirone has been useful at dosages of 15–60 mg/day, but onset of clinical action appears to be delayed. Various experts inform us that buspirone is less useful in treating more violent retarded patients. Preliminary data show

634 Manual of Clinical Psychopharmacology

that the SSRIs may be effective in such patients. Further discussion of many of these drugs is found in Chapter 3 ("Antidepressants"), Chapter 4 ("Antipsychotic Drugs"), and Chapter 5 ("Mood Stabilizers").

In patients with a seizure disorder, in the presence or absence of mental retardation, there is a worry that psychiatric drugs, including TCAs and neuroleptics, may lower the seizure threshold and increase the likelihood or frequency of convulsions. There is no firm evidence that this occurs. Maprotiline, imipramine, and amitriptyline have been more often connected with seizure occurrences in nonretarded depressed patients in our experience, but these drugs were also the most commonly used TCAs in the McLean Hospital system at the time seizures were seen. Trazodone is least likely to affect seizure threshold. Bupropion and clomipramine have also been associated with seizures. There is a belief that haloperidol and molindone, among the typical antipsychotics, are least likely to affect seizure occurrence. In our experience, chlorpromazine and loxapine are occasionally associated with seizures, and seizures are more of a problem with clozapine (see Chapter 4). In patients with a known seizure disorder that is adequately treated with anticonvulsants, it is relatively unlikely that any of the standard psychiatric drugs will make a clinically important difference in seizure frequency. In retarded patients taking phenytoin, phenobarbital, or primidone for seizure control, there is a real possibility that the seizure medication may be causing cognitive dysfunction. It may be worth shifting the patient to carbamazepine to determine whether the patient may function better on that relatively different medication.

Stimulants may also be worth a trial in hyperactive retarded patients who are under close clinical observation. Stimulants have the advantage of causing clear clinical effects (improvement or worsening) within a few hours or days of reaching an adequate dose; therefore, the trials of a stimulant may be completed in 1–2 weeks.

Medical Conditions

Some psychiatric syndromes are caused by or strongly associated with medical disorders. Others are commonly associated with medications used to treat medical or neurological conditions. On the other hand, some medical conditions and some drugs used to treat medical conditions complicate the use of standard psychoactive drugs to treat coexisting psychiatric disorders.

Psychiatric Disorders Resulting From Medical Illness

Psychiatric disorders, especially depression, can occur with (and are presumably caused by) thyroid or adrenal cortical dysfunction, uremia, cancer of the pancreas, and any metastatic carcinomatosis sufficiently often to make it worth ascertaining whether these conditions exist in depressed patients. Other, more obvious conditions, such as strokes, multiple sclerosis, lupus erythematosus, and Parkinson's disease, are often associated with depression, as well as with organic brain dysfunction.

Chronic pain syndromes, including headache and low back pain, are so confounded with depressive syndromes that primary antidepressant therapy is often indicated and effective. For some medical conditions such as hypothyroidism, treating the underlying condition is the first order of business. For others, the presence of an untreatable medical or neurological condition is not per se a contraindication to standard antidepressant therapy.

Hyperthyroidism, caffeinism, hypoglycemia, temporal lobe epilepsy, paroxysmal tachycardias, and pheochromocytoma can all mimic panic disorder and should be ruled out. A medical reevaluation is indicated if standard drug therapies fail. A review by Raj and Sheehan (1988) suggested some useful tips for making such key differential diagnoses. For example, attacks of paroxysmal atrial tachycardia generally begin and end more abruptly than do panic attacks and produce heart rates of 140–200 bpm. In contrast, heart rates in panic disorder rarely exceed 140 bpm. In pheochromocytoma, anxiety is only the fourth most common symptom, and many patients with this condition experience tachycardia and increased blood pressure without becoming unduly fearful; in this disorder there is often an increased familial prevalence of neurofibromatosis and café au lait spots.

Hyperthyroidism is associated with sleep disturbance, heat sensitivity, and a more enduring tremor, among other symptoms. Finally, temporal lobe epilepsy may represent a more difficult diagnostic dilemma. In almost 25% of patients with this disorder, anxiety occurs during the aura or interictally. However, such patients frequently also complain of other symptoms—for example, perceptual distortions and lapses of concentration. In assessing patients with possible panic disorder, a routine medical history and physical examination should be obtained. Laboratory tests should be ordered as needed to rule out suspected conditions.

There is now a growing series of very positive case reports on the use of stimulants—mainly methylphenidate at a dosage of 10 mg once or twice a day—in patients with serious medical or surgical illnesses on medical services. These patients were noted on psychiatric consultation to be depressed, retarded, even almost mute, losing weight, not eating, unable to cooperate in treatment, withdrawn, and hopeless. Stimulants can produce relief in a day or two and can often be discontinued in 2–4 weeks, once the patient is generally improving. Of the 17 such case reports, none describe any serious side effects. By inference, elevated pulse or blood pressure is not a problem. Despite the appetite-reducing effect of stimulants in overweight subjects, these medically ill patients rapidly regain weight while taking methylphenidate. Sometimes stimulants are used because TCAs are contraindicated, but the results are positive enough for stimulants to be considered first-choice drugs in treating these patients. Standard antidepressants rarely improve mood or functioning in a few days.

Depression following stroke has received some special study in recent years. It is clear that depression following CVAs occurs in about half the patients affected and can be relieved by antidepressants. In fact, the majority of studies of antidepressants in the treatment of poststroke depression have found significant benefits in mood and behavior and even improvement in activities of daily living (Chen et al. 2006; Gaete and Bogousslavsky 2008). There have been several controlled studies, one of nortriptyline (Lipsey et al. 1984), one of trazodone (Reding et al. 1986), and one of fluoxetine (Dam et al. 1996). Nortriptyline was generally effective, but 3 of the 17 patients studied developed delirium (Lipsey et al. 1984). Patients treated with medication longer and those with plasma levels over 100 ng/mL did better. Trazodone was less effective relative to placebo, but significant positive effects were found in dexamethasone nonsuppressors and patients with higher levels of depressive symptoms (Reding et al. 1986). Slow, cautious dosage increases are best with both drugs to avoid adverse effects. Fluoxetine (20 mg/day) appeared to substantially facilitate recovery in poststroke patients who were undergoing rehabilitation (Dam et al. 1996). In this study of 52 severely disabled hemiplegic patients, fluoxetine-treated patients showed significant improvements in depression, ADLs, and neurological deficits relative to both maprotiline-treated patients and patients receiving placebo. In fact, maprotiline seemed to hinder rehabilitation, whereas fluoxetine generally helped a variety of indices of recovery in these poststroke patients treated for 3 months. Fluoxetine may also help with the emotional incontinence that often occurs after a stroke (Choi-kwon et al. 2006). ECT has also been reported to be effective in poststroke depression. Most patients with cognitive impairment before ECT had improved cognitive functioning after ECT. In contrast, Robinson et al. (2000) reported that nortriptyline was more effective than fluoxetine or placebo in poststroke depression. As indicated earlier, sertraline can prevent poststroke depression.

Many psychiatric disorders may be seen in patients with AIDS, but the prevalence of these disorders is not higher than in carefully matched controls. Studies suggest that subsyndromal depression is the most common disorder seen in this population, and it is thought that the SSRIs may be useful in treating these patients. However, some psychiatric conditions can be a direct consequence of neurological involvement in HIV infection. HIV encephalitis occurs in most AIDS patients at some point in their illness. Mood and personality changes may occur early in the course of the encephalitis, and psychosis, mania, and dementia may occur later. Patients with other neurological consequences of HIV infection, including cerebral lymphoma and toxoplasmosis, often present with cognitive and psychiatric symptoms. These problems generally occur late in the progress of the disease.

Zidovudine (formerly azidothymidine, or AZT) is often helpful in reversing the psychopathology associated with HIV encephalopathy. Antidepressants, lithium, and high-potency antipsychotics may also help treat HIV-associated psychopathology. However, because AIDS patients tend to be quite sensitive to the side effects of psychotropic medications, caution must be exercised.

The recent introduction of the protease inhibitors has made a tremendous impact on the treatment of HIV-positive patients. All the current protease inhibitors are potent inhibitors of the CYP enzyme 3A3/4 and are themselves metabolized by this enzyme. As a result, caution should be exercised when combining these drugs with nefazodone, fluvoxamine, and St. John's wort. In addition, one protease inhibitor, ritonavir (Norvir), also inhibits the CYP enzyme 2D6 and may raise the serum levels of TCAs and other drugs dependent on this enzyme.

Psychiatric Disorders Associated With Nonpsychiatric Drugs

A variety of older antihypertensive drugs (e.g., reserpine, methyldopa) were sometimes associated with depression. These drugs rarely are used in current clinical practice. However, propranolol is commonly used now and has sometimes been associated with major depression. In many instances the β-blockers do not appear to be inducing depression. Rather, high doses of lipophilic β-blockers such as propranolol can induce a lethargy and indifference that is sometimes confused with depression. Shifting to a thiazide diuretic or to a different, non–centrally acting β-blocker (e.g., atenolol) can be helpful, or a TCA alone can sometimes adequately treat both depression and hypertension.

Diazepam has occasionally been associated with increased depression. Both benzodiazepines and barbiturates can aggravate ADHD. Benzodiazepines may produce memory problems, particularly in the elderly.

Stimulants can aggravate schizophrenia or mania. Steroids and L-dopa can mimic almost any known psychiatric syndrome, including delirium, paranoid psychosis, mania, depression, and anxiety.

The whole range of drugs used in treating Parkinson's disease can cause hallucinosis and confusion. Sometimes anticholinergic drugs used in gastrointestinal disorders can also cause anticholinergic confusion and delirium, as can digitalis-like and cimetidine-like agents. It is impossible to list or predict all the drugs or drug combinations that at some dose in some patient can elicit or aggravate symptoms of a psychiatric disorder. In a patient receiving several drugs for medical conditions who presents with depression, anxiety, or psychosis appearing after the drugs were begun, a careful reevaluation of the patient's pharmacotherapies is necessary. Stopping the less obviously crucial medications and shifting to less centrally active alternative drugs, when some medication is necessary, are reasonable steps.

Psychiatric Disorders Complicated by Medical Disorders

Renal Disease

Many medical disorders could have reasonably predictable effects on the pharmacokinetics of standard psychiatric drugs, but the transition from theoretical data to practical application is often not exact. In the case of kidney failure and lithium therapy, the facts are clear. If renal clearance is decreased, lithium excretion will be decreased in a reasonably proportionate manner. In patients with substantially elevated serum creatinine and blood urea nitrogen who are not in acute renal failure, very small doses of lithium (e.g., 150 mg/day) can be cautiously begun and titrated in the same way as in a healthy patient, but more cautiously and with smaller increments. In this situation, lithium citrate given in milliliter doses could give extra flexibility. Some patients on renal dialysis may be stabilized on lithium, with a single 300-mg dose after each episode of dialysis. This dose may maintain an adequate blood level until the next dialysis removes the lithium ions. Likewise, older patients experience a 30%–40% decrease in glomerular filtration and therefore require lower starting and maximum doses than younger patients.

The hydroxylated metabolites of TCAs and other psychotropic agents may also be elevated in elderly patients and in those with advanced renal disease. This suggests that a more gentle titration of these medications is required in these two groups of patients.

Dehydration states are not uncommon, and they can increase the toxicity of lithium therapy. Furthermore, there is some evidence that dehydration is a risk factor in the development of neuroleptic malignant syndrome, although this association is somewhat tenuous. Finally, dehydration can exacerbate the orthostasis caused by risperidone, clozapine, TCAs, and MAOIs.

Urinary retention can be quite problematic in elderly patients, particularly in males with prostate difficulties. The most anticholinergic agents, including tertiary-amine TCAs (amitriptyline, imipramine), low-potency neuroleptics, and antiparkinsonian drugs such as benztropine, should be avoided if possible in elderly patients.

Liver Disease

When there is liver damage or decreased liver efficiency due to normal aging, the effects are more complicated. Most drugs are partially metabolized in the liver after absorption from the small intestine (the first-pass effect). When liver tissue is damaged, many drugs get into the general circulation at much higher levels. Usually, glucuronidation as a method of drug deactivation is well preserved, whereas demethylation and other metabolic processes are more readily impaired. This is why drugs, such as diazepam, that need to be demethylated cause much higher blood levels per unit dose in cirrhosis, whereas drugs like lorazepam, which are only glucuronidated, are handled normally. Unfortunately, it is not always clear to even a skilled clinical pharmacologist exactly what the effect of chronic liver disease on the clinical actions of any particular drug will be.

It is likely that in patients with partial liver failure, standard TCAs such as amitriptyline and imipramine will be less readily converted to their desmethyl metabolites, nortriptyline and desipramine. The consequences of this shift—perhaps more sedation, confusion, or anticholinergic side effects—are less clear. The obvious lesson is to proceed very cautiously; to use blood level determinations, if available; and to assume that liver damage will markedly increase a drug's half-life, making gradual accumulation of higher and higher blood levels quite possible over a couple of weeks at a constant daily dose. Most psychiatrists find fluoxetine a safe drug to use in spite of its long half-life.

Lowered blood protein levels, common in liver disease, may also increase free-drug levels, unbound to protein, making a drug more potent at lower total blood levels measured in the conventional manner. This is less of a problem with venlafaxine, which demonstrates low protein binding.

An overactive liver can also pose problems. Some known drugs, including barbiturates, phenytoin, carbamazepine, and nicotine, induce hepatic enzymes and increase the rate at which some psychiatric drugs are metabolized, making higher dosages necessary in order to achieve clinical results (see Chapter 3: "Antidepressants; Chapter 5: "Mood Stabilizers"; and Chapter 9: "Augmentation Strategies for Treatment-Resistant Disorders"). It is also worth noting that even drug-free patients can show large degrees of biological variability in their natural rates of drug metabolism. As an example, Glassman et al. (1977, discussed in Chapter 3) found imipramine levels to vary from 40 to 1,040 ng/mL in depressed patients receiving 2.5 mg/kg of imipramine. Again, the lesson is that patients taking other drugs for medical reasons may well have an altered response, based on either increased or decreased hepatic metabolism of the psychiatric drug that has just been added (not to mention pharmacological interactions such as additive sedation or additive postural hypotension).

In the likely absence of clear knowledge about the interactions in a particular patient of, for example, cimetidine, phenytoin, chlorothiazide, and isoniazid with imipramine, the clinician adding imipramine in a patient taking all these other drugs must be prepared to proceed cautiously but to use high dosages of imipramine if neither side effects nor clinical response occurs, if blood levels are low, and if ECG changes are not seen. It has also become evident that a number of psychotropic drugs may be associated with causing elevations in liver enzymes. The SSRIs, the TCAs, carbamazepine, and valproate, among other medications, may be associated with increases in aspartate transaminase (AST; formerly serum glutamic-oxaloacetic transaminase [SGOT]) and alanine transaminase (ALT; formerly serum glutamic-pyruvic transaminase [SGPT]). The clinical significance of these elevations remains unclear. However, persisting elevations to greater than twice the normal levels are of particular concern. There are rare reports of children younger than 2 years who are taking valproate and who have developed fulminant hepatic failure; the risk in adults appears to be minimal. There are also a few isolated reports of hepatic failure in children that was believed to be associated with TCA use. In general, it is prudent practice to obtain baseline liver function tests (LFTs) when initiating therapy with carbamazepine and valproate and to check LFTs every 6–12 months thereafter.

A number of drugs pose less of a problem in patients with advanced liver disease because they are less appreciably metabolized by the liver. These include agents such as gabapentin, pregabalin, and lithium. Transdermal and Zydis selegiline also bypass the liver to a large extent and might be used in patients with advanced liver disease.

Cardiac Illness

There is accumulating evidence that depression both is a risk factor for coronary artery disease and significantly increases the risk of mortality in patients who have suffered a myocardial infarction (MI). In fact, depression in the post-MI period is a stronger predictor of subsequent mortality than many more intuitive factors such as systolic ejection fraction, which is one measure of the extent of heart damage. The mechanism by which depression may increase the risk of an MI or subsequent risk of mortality after an MI is unknown. Current speculation is that depression may increase platelet binding and therefore clotting or that depression may decrease heart rate responsiveness. In any case, it would be helpful to know if antidepressant therapy in the post-MI period decreases mortality. It is evident that sertraline in the post-MI period is well tolerated and effective for concurrent depression (McFarlane et al. 2001). However, in this small open-label study, it was not possible to demonstrate significant benefits on coagulation or heart rhythm.

A number of randomized trials have indicated that the SSRIs work at least as well as TCAs and are better tolerated in heart patients. Studies comparing paroxetine with nortriptyline showed that both drugs are highly effective but that paroxetine is safer and better tolerated (Nelson et al. 1999).

In cardiac patients, there has long been a fear that all TCAs are cardiotoxic and likely to cause disastrous arrhythmias. Although they produce mild tachycardia (an increase of 10 bpm) in medically healthy depressed patients, their arrhythmogenic potential appears to occur primarily if the drugs are taken in overdose. The mechanism by which the TCAs and maprotiline affect cardiac function is a quinidine-like slowing of cardiac conduction. TCAs have an ability to decrease cardiac irritability and to suppress premature contractions. They are therefore not contraindicated at ordinary dosages in depressed patients with premature ventricular contractions, and they may well help both cardiac irritability and depression. Nortriptyline has been shown to be effective and generally well tolerated in cardiac patients with melancholic depression (Roose et al. 1994). More recent studies indicate that paroxetine was as effective as nortriptyline in post-MI patients but was better tolerated from a cardiovascular perspective (Roose et al. 1998).

The TCAs should, however, be used with caution in patients with preexisting conduction defects, such as bundle-branch block. Patients with first-degree block have a 9% rate of 2:1 atrioventricular block development when taking TCAs, compared with a 0.7% rate in patients without first-degree block. TCAs should not be given to patients with known intracardiac conduction delays. This is particularly so in patients already taking cardiac antiarrhythmic drugs, which act by slowing cardiac conduction, because additive effects on conduction could be harmful. Not all cardiologists are aware of the cardiac effects of TCAs, and psychiatrists who collaborate with cardiologists or primary care physicians may need to do some educating of their consultants.

The other antidepressants with a possible effect on cardiac irritability are trazodone and venlafaxine. Trazodone does not affect conduction, but it has occasionally (not regularly) been associated with an increase in premature ventricular contractions (PVCs) and should be avoided in patients with runs of PVCs or ventricular bigeminies. There has been concern that venlafaxine overdoses might be associated with a greater risk of mortality, mostly from cardiac events, than are the SSRIs. Venlafaxine overdoses, often in combination with other drugs or alchohol, have been associated with QT prolongation, bradycardia, ventricular tachycardia, and other arrhythmias. Thus, the package insert for venlafaxine was changed at the request of the FDA to reflect this evidence. The risks appear to be substantially less than with TCA overdoses and may be an artifact of more ill patients typically being treated with venlafaxine than with SSRIs. However, more careful monitoring is recommended. Venlafaxine, like the SSRIs, can produce a mild increase in heart rate. It can also increase diastolic blood pressure. Therefore, patients with current and advanced congestive heart failure may not be the best candidates for treatment with venlafaxine. Patients with a history of hypertension may also require increased vigilance when treatment with venlafaxine is being initiated. In one report, venlafaxine was poorly tolerated cardiovascularly in nursing home patients (Oslin et al. 2003). Because of these effects, and given the recent report of British regulators regarding lethality in overdose, the drug should be prescribed cautiously in vulnerable populations (e.g., elderly patients with cardiac disease).

The SSRIs appear to produce a mild (3-bpm) increase in heart rate in medically healthy depressed patients. Although these agents have not yet been widely studied in post-MI patients, their possible use in such patients is suggested by animal studies and by data available in cardiovascularly healthy depressed patients. In addition, these agents produce milder alterations in blood pressure than do other antidepressants. However, the SSRIs may slow the metabolism of a variety of cardiovascular medications, including digoxin, some β-blockers, and class 1C antiarrhythmics. The SSRIs can raise the levels of these other medications by competitive inhibition of the CYP enzyme 2D6 and require close monitoring (Table 12–5). In one study (Roose et al. 1994), fluoxetine was reported to be less effective than nortriptyline in melancholic cardiac patients, although there are other data indicating that it does have efficacy and relative safety in cardiac patients with milder depression. Moreover, paroxetine has been reported to be effective and better tolerated cardiovascularly than nortriptyline in patients with post-MI depression (Roose et al. 1998).

The more significant effect of TCAs and MAOIs is postural hypotension, which can be aggravated (potentiated) in patients already taking drugs, such as propranolol, that are likely to cause hypotension as well. Although patients who have stable cardiac disease but are not in congestive failure probably tolerate antidepressants well, patients taking multiple cardiac drugs are particularly prone to postural hypotension and other cardiac side effects. For seriously ill cardiac patients with severe depression, ECT may be the treatment of choice.

Table 12–5. Interactions of commonly used psychoactive drugs with cardiovascular medications

Drug	TCA	SSRI	Antipsychotic	Lithium	Carbamazepine
calcium channel blockers	Increase hypotension	NA	Increase hypotension	Raise or lower lithium levels, bradycardia	Increase carbamazepine levels
thiazide diuretics	May increase hypotension	NA	Increase hypotension	Increase lithium levels	NA
β-blockers	May increase hypotension	May increase β-blockers	Increase antipsychotic levels	NA	Decrease β-blocker levels
reserpine, guanethidine	Antagonize antihypertensive agents	NA	Increase hypotension	NA	Unknown
clonidine, prazosin	Increase hypotension	NA	Increase hypotension	NA	Unknown
1A antiarrhythmics	Prolong cardiac conduction	NA	Prolong cardiac conduction	Prolong sinus recovery time	May decrease antiarrhythmic levels
1C antiarrhythmics	Prolong cardiac conduction	Increase 1C levels	May prolong cardiac conduction	Prolong sinus recovery time	May decrease antiarrhythmic levels
digitalis	Increases digoxin and TCA levels	May increase digoxin levels	May increase digoxin levels	Prolongs sinus recovery time	Unknown

Note.   NA=applicable; SSRI = selective serotonin reuptake inhibitor; TCA = tricyclic antidepressant.

Bupropion has been assessed in depressed patients with moderate cardiac disease and seems to be better tolerated than the TCAs. Even in overdose, apparently bupropion does not typically have a major effect on cardiac function (Spiller et al. 1994).

Pulmonary Disorders

Patients with pulmonary disorders, including asthma, emphysema, and sleep apnea, are commonly encountered in psychiatric practice, and some psychotropic medications may present problems in this population. Benzodiazepines, for example, may be contraindicated in patients with sleep apnea; the benzodiazepines may relax the airway further and exacerbate already restricted airflow. Zolpidem may be less likely to produce this problem than the benzodiazepines. In addition, benzodiazepines reduce the hypoxic response to ventilation and therefore should be used with caution in patients with chronic obstructive pulmonary disease who retain CO_2. Furthermore, psychotropic medications with significant anticholinergic activity may decrease bronchial secretions and exacerbate pulmonary disorders. Thus caution should be exercised in treating pulmonary patients with drugs such as amitriptyline or benztropine.

Many medications used to treat pulmonary problems are affected by concurrent use of some psychotropic agents. For example, fluvoxamine inhibits the metabolism of theophylline, which can lead to potentially toxic levels. Thus, theophylline levels should be checked frequently if fluvoxamine must be used concurrently. Conversely, theophylline-like drugs increase the excretion and lower the serum levels of lithium.

Seizure Disorders

Many psychotropic medications are known to lower the seizure threshold and, therefore, must be used with caution in patients with a history of a seizure disorder. Most antipsychotics have this potential, although molindone and thioridazine may be less problematic in seizure disorder patients. Clozapine, among the antipsychotics, has perhaps the greatest potential for inducing seizures: up to 5% of patients develop seizures at dosages greater than 600 mg/day. The TCAs and tetracyclic agents all have some potential for lowering the seizure threshold; amitriptyline and maprotiline are among the more problematic offenders. Bupropion is probably contraindicated in patients with a known seizure disorder, because of its dose-related potential for producing seizures. However, the SSRIs and venlafaxine appear relatively safe in this population.

The anticonvulsants are also associated with a variety of interactions. Carbamazepine is an enzyme inducer that will lower the serum levels of a variety of drugs, including TCAs, clonazepam, and most antipsychotics. Oxcarbazepine is a much weaker inducer of the 3A3/4 enzyme. SSRIs, on the other hand, may substantially increase carbamazepine levels.

Other additive or antagonistic interactions certainly occur. Some of the better-documented ones are discussed in earlier chapters focusing on specific drug classes.

Pain Disorders

Antidepressants and other psychotropic drugs have long been used in the treatment of a variety of pain syndromes, including trigeminal neuralgia, peripheral neuropathy, arthritis, myofascial pain, fibromyalgia, migraine prophylaxis, and the pain associated with some forms of cancer. More than 40 placebo-controlled studies have reported that antidepressants are useful in the management of pain, independent of whether depression is a part of the clinical picture.

The TCAs have the longest track record and may be the most consistently efficacious group of psychotropic agents used in the treatment of pain conditions. Tertiary-amine TCAs, particularly amitriptyline, imipramine, and doxepin, have been well studied and found to be effective for a variety of pain conditions. Initially, it was thought that the mechanism of action of these drugs was to increase the peripheral availability of serotonin, which in turn would modulate the pain response. This explanation does not appear to be correct. Some TCAs, which are more noradrenergic than serotonergic, also appear to be useful in the treatment of pain, whereas the SSRIs, which efficiently increase the availability of peripheral serotonin, are sometimes less useful. For example, a study comparing amitriptyline with citalopram (an SSRI) in the prophylaxis of chronic tension headaches found that amitriptyline was efficacious but citalopram was ineffective (Bendtsen et al. 1996). Dosages as low as 25–50 mg/day of amitriptyline or imipramine are frequently useful in the prophylaxis and treatment of pain problems. However, analgesia of the TCAs appears to be dose related, so higher doses may be more effective than lower doses.

The SSRIs have been disappointing in the management of pain disorders, although there is some evidence that they may help with neuropathic pain. Some patients have reported benefit from the SSRIs for migraine prophylaxis, even though many patients experience a worsening of their headaches at the initiation of treatment. The results of open-label studies of paroxetine, at 10–50 mg/day, for chronic daily headaches have been encouraging (Foster and Bafaloukos 1994), whereas findings from double-blind studies have been less promising (Langemark and Olesen 1994).

Venlafaxine and duloxetine, which have a mechanism of action that closely resembles that of the TCAs, have also been extensively studied in the treatment of chronic pain conditions. Low dosages of venlafaxine, on the order of 25–75 mg/day, appear to be useful, but, as with the TCAs, higher dosages may produce more analgesia. In a 6-week double-blind study, venlafaxine XR at dosages of 150–225 mg/day was signficantly more effective than placebo in reducing diabetic neuropathic pain. Venlafaxine XR at a dosage of 75 mg/day did not separate from placebo (Kunz et al. 2000). Preliminary evidence suggests also that the SNRI duloxetine has benefits similar to those of venlafaxine and the TCAs in the management of neuropathic pain at dosages of 60 to 80 mg/day.

Duloxetine became the first drug approved for the treatment of pain associated with diabetic neuropathy in 2004. In 2009, it was also approved for the treatment of fibromyalgia. Both daytime and nighttime pain were substantially reduced by duloxetine as early as the first week of treatment. The dosages proven effective for diabetic neuropathy in clinical trials were 60–120 mg/day. Duloxetine has also been reported to be effective in patients with fibromyalgia, particularly women (Arnold et al. 2004). Duloxetine also appeared to reduce painful symptoms in depressed patients, including their myalgias and back pain. Thus, duloxetine is being used with growing frequency in pain clinics. For the patient with chronic neuropathic pain who is also depressed, duloxetine appears to be a particularly good choice.

Other psychotropic drugs have also been found to be effective in treating pain conditions. The newer SNRIs, including milnacipran and desvenlafaxine, appear useful in the treatment of some pain conditions. Milnacipran was approved for the treatment of fibromyalgia in 2009. Studies in support of pain indications for desvenlafaxine have not been fruitful to date.

As reported in Chapter 5 ("Mood Stabilizers"), gabapentin and pregabalin have been well studied in neuropathic pain. Gabapentin at dosages up to

3,600 mg/day is both effective and well tolerated for many pain patients. As a result, gabapentin has become a standard in most pain specialty clinics. Pregabalin was also approved for the treatment of diabetic neuropathic pain as well as trigeminal neuralgia. It was also the first drug approved for the treatment of fibromyalgia. The typical therapeutic dosage for pregabalin in pain conditions is 150–300 mg/day taken in two divided doses. Dosages up to 600 mg/day have been studied but are probably not much more effective than smaller dosages.

Haloperidol and chlorpromazine, in a number of open-label studies, have been found to be useful in the management of neuropathic pain. Carbamazepine has been efficacious in the treatment of peripheral neuropathies, and lithium is sometimes used in the treatment of cluster headaches.

A number of common agents used in the management of pain disorders might interact with common psychotropic medications. For example, tramadol, which is indicated for moderate to severe pain, is a SNRI, among its analgesic properties. In addition, it is a CYP 2D6 substrate. Thus, there is the potential for both pharmacokinetic and pharmacodynamic interactions with some SSRIs, and serotonin syndrome has been sporadically reported with the combination. Opiates, when combined with CNS depressants (including benzodiazepines), are sometimes associated with respiratory depression, particularly in overdose. Likewise, carisoprodol (Soma) may interact with other CNS depressants, including barbiturates and benzodiazepines, to contribute to sedation, dizziness, and, in overdose, respiratory depression. Meperidine (Demerol) has long been associated with inducing a serotonin syndrome in combination with MAOIs, and the combination is thus contraindicated. While MAOIs have been used safely with other narcotics, the interaction with opiates such as fentanyl is somewhat unpredictable.

Conclusion

It would be helpful if our current knowledge of drug actions could be put to precise clinical use in assessing the effects of adding a new psychiatric drug to a preexisting mixture of medical and psychiatric drugs. Unfortunately, drugs do not work like sums in an algebraic equation. One would think, for example, that the action of D-amphetamine, an indirect dopamine agonist, would be opposed by haloperidol, a reasonably pure dopamine-blocking drug. In practice, however, some patients feel more lively and functional, without becoming more psychotic, when D-amphetamine is added to haloperidol. Drugs usually act on several receptors and on both pre- and postsynaptic receptors of a single type, leading to potentially complex effects and interactions. The clinician is often faced with treating schizophrenia, agoraphobia with panic, or depression in a patient with several medical problems. This kind of situation requires drug therapy for the medical problems that is likely to influence the metabolism or absorption of a psychiatric drug or to have additive, antagonistic, or (more likely) unknown effects in combination with the most appropriate psychiatric drug treatment.

All drug therapy consists of a series of empirical clinical trials; treatment of medically ill patients simply presents more complicated empirical trials. The psychiatrist can try to guess at the more probable ways in which the new drug will act or be affected by the patient's medical disease and ongoing drug therapies, but it is likely to be only guesswork. If there are semipredictable adverse interactions, one can either try to avoid them by choosing the psychiatric drug least likely to cause trouble or proceed cautiously, with close monitoring of the patient for predictable and unpredictable side effects, in collaboration with the physicians managing the patient's nonpsychiatric disorders. One worries that medically ill patients will be very fragile and easily become toxic while taking psychiatric drugs, but it is likely that this is not a general problem; some patients may develop problems, whereas others tolerate psychiatric drugs unusually well.

Bibliography

ACOG Committee on Practice Bulletins—Obstetrics. ACOG Practice Bulletin: Clinical management guidelines for obstetrician-gynecologists number 92, April 2008: Use of psychiatric medications during pregnancy and lactation. Obstet Gynecol 111:1001–1020, 2008 [replaces Practice Bulletin No 87, November 2007]

Alessi N, Naylor MW, Ghaziuddin M, et al: Update on lithium carbonate therapy in children and adolescents. J Am Acad Child Adolesc Psychiatry 33: 291–304, 1994

Alexopoulos GS, Schultz SK, Lebowitz BD: Late-life depression: a model for medical classification. Biol Psychiatry 58:283–289, 2005

Altshuler LL, Szuba MP: Course of psychiatric disorders in pregnancy: dilemmas in pharmacologic management. Neurol Clin 12:613–635, 1994

Aman MG, De Smedt G, Derivan A, et al: Double-blind, placebo-controlled study of risperidone for the treatment of disruptive behaviors in children with subaverage intelligence. Am J Psychiatry 159:1337–1346, 2002

Aman MG, Gharabawi GM, Special Topic Advisory Panel on Transitioning to Risperidone Therapy in Patients With Mental Retardation and Developmental Disabilities: Treatment of behavior disorders in mental retardation: report on transitioning to atypical antipsychotics, with an emphasis on risperidone. J Clin Psychiatry 65:1197–1210, 2004

Armenteros JL, Whitaker AH, Joachim N, et al: Open trial of risperidone in adolescents with schizophrenia. Paper presented at meeting of the International Academy for Biomedical and Drug Research, Florence, Italy, 1995

Arnold LE, Abikoff HB, Cantwell DP, et al: National Institute of Mental Health Collaborative Multimodal Treatment Study of Children With ADHD (the MTA): design challenges and choices. Arch Gen Psychiatry 54:865–870, 1997

Arnold LM, Lu Y, Crofford LJ, et al: A double-blind, multicenter trial comparing duloxetine with placebo in the treatment of fibromyalgia patients with or without major depressive disorder. Arthritis Rheum 50:2974–2984, 2004

Asarnow JR, Tompson MC, Goldstein MJ: Childhood-onset schizophrenia: a followup study. Schizophr Bull 20:599–617, 1994

Bairy KL, Madhyastha S, Ashok KP, et al: Developmental and behavioral consequences of prenatal fluoxetine. Pharmacology 79(1):1–11, 2006

Barbaresi WJ, Katusic SK, Colligan RC, et al: Long-term stimulant medication treatment of attention-deficit/hyperactivity disorder: results from a population-based study. J Dev Behav Pediatr 27(1):1–10, 2006

Barbarich NC, McConaha CW, Gaskill J, et al: An open trial of olanzapine in anorexia nervosa. J Clin Psychiatry 65:1480–1482, 2004

Barkley R, Cunningham L: Do stimulant drugs improve academic performance of hyperkinetic children? A review of outcome studies. Clin Pediatr (Phila) 17:85–92, 1978

Barrickman LL, Perry PJ, Allen AJ, et al: Bupropion versus methylphenidate in the treatment of attention-deficit hyperactivity disorder. J Am Acad Child Adolesc Psychiatry 34:649–657, 1995

Bellantuono C, Migliarese G, Gentile S: Serotonin reuptake inhibitors in pregnancy and the risk of major malformations: a systematic review. Hum Psychopharmacol 22:121–128, 2007 [Erratum in: Hum Psychopharmacol 22:413, 2007]

Benazzi F: Mania associated with donepezil (letter). Int J Geriatr Psychiatry 13:814–815, 1998

Benazzi F, Rossi E: Mania and donepezil (letter). Can J Psychiatry 44:506–507, 1999

Bendtsen L, Jensen R, Olesen J: A non-selective (amitriptyline), but not a selective (citalopram), serotonin reuptake inhibitor is effective in the prophylactic treatment of chronic tension-type headache. J Neurol Neurosurg Psychiatry 61:285–290, 1996

Berle JO, Steen VM, Aamo TO, et al: Breastfeeding during maternal antidepressant treatment with serotonin reuptake inhibitors: infant exposure, clinical symptoms, and cytochrome p450 genotypes. J Clin Psychiatry 65:1228–1234, 2004

Biederman J, Thisted RA, Greenhill LL, et al: Estimation of the association between desipramine and the risk for sudden death in 5- to 14-year-old children. J Clin Psychiatry 56:87–93, 1995

Biederman J, Mick E, Faraone SV, et al: Risperidone for the treatment of affective symptoms in children with disruptive behavior disorder: a post hoc analysis of data from a 6-week, multicenter, randomized, double-blind, parallel-arm study. Clin Ther 28:794–800, 2005

Biederman J, Swanson JM, Wigal SB, et al, Modafinil ADHD Study Group: A comparison of once-daily and divided doses of modafinil in children with attention-deficit/hyperactivity disorder: a randomized, double-blind, and placebo-controlled study. J Clin Psychiatry 67:727–735, 2006

Birnbaum C, Cohen L, Bailey J, et al: Serum concentrations of antidepressants and benzodiazepines in nursing infants: a case series. Pediatrics 104:e11, 1999

Breuning SE, Ferguson DG, Davidson NA, et al: Effects of thioridazine on the intellectual performance of mentally retarded drug responders and non-responders. Arch Gen Psychiatry 40:309–313, 1983

Briggs G, Bodendorfer T, Freeman R, et al: Drugs in Pregnancy and Lactation: A Reference Guide to Fetal and Neonatal Risk. Baltimore, MD, Williams & Wilkins, 1983

Buitelaar JK, Danckaerts M, Gillberg C, et al: A prospective, multicenter, open-label assessment of atomoxetine in non–North American children and adolescents with ADHD. Eur Child Adolesc Psychiatry 13:249–257, 2004

Burns A, Rossor M, Hecker J, et al: The effects of donepezil in Alzheimer's disease: results from a multinational trial. Dement Geriatr Cogn Disord 10:237–244, 1999

Burt T, Sachs GS, Demopulos C: Donepezil in treatment-resistant bipolar disorder. Biol Psychiatry 45:959–964, 1999

Campbell M: Drug treatment of infantile autism: the past decade, in Psychopharmacology: The Third Generation of Progress. Edited by Meltzer HY. New York, Raven, 1987, pp 1225–1232

Campbell M, Spencer EK: Psychopharmacology in child and adolescent psychiatry: review of past 5 years. J Am Acad Child Psychiatry 27:269–279, 1988

Campbell M, Small AM, Green WH, et al: Behavioral efficacy of haloperidol and lithium carbonate: a comparison in hospitalized aggressive children with conduct disorder. Arch Gen Psychiatry 41:650–656, 1984

Campbell M, Adams PB, Small AM, et al: Lithium in hospitalized aggressive children with conduct disorder: a double-blind and placebo-controlled study. J Am Acad Child Adolesc Psychiatry 34:445–453, 1995

Casat CD, Pleasants DZ, Schroeder DH, et al: Bupropion in children with attention deficit disorder. Psychopharmacol Bull 25:198–201, 1989

Casper RC, Fleisher BE, Lee-Ancajas JC, et al: Follow-up of children of depressed mothers exposed or not exposed to antidepressant drugs during pregnancy. J Pediatrics 142:402–408, 2003

Chambers CD, Johnson KA, Dick LM, et al: Birth outcomes in pregnant women taking fluoxetine. N Engl J Med 335:1010–1015, 1996

Chambers CD, Anderson PO, Thomas RG, et al: Weight gain in infants breastfed by mothers who take fluoxetine. Pediatrics 104:e61, 1999

Chambers CD, Hernandez-Diaz S, Van Marter LJ, et al: Selective serotonin-reuptake inhibitors and risk of persistent pulmonary hypertension of the newborn. N Engl J Med 354:579–587, 2006

Chang K, Saxena K, Howe M: An open-label study of lamotrigine adjunct or mono-therapy for the treatment of adolescents with bipolar depression. J Am Acad Child Adolesc Psychiatry 45:298–304, 2006

Chavez B, Chavez-Brown M, Rey JA: Role of risperidone in children with autism spectrum disorder. Ann Pharmacother 40:909–916, 2006

Chavez B, Sopko MA Jr, Ehret MJ, et al: An update on central nervous system stimulant formulations in children and adolescents with attention-deficit/hyperactivity disorder. Ann Pharmacother 43:1084–1095, 2009

Chen Y, Guo JJ, Zhan S, et al: Treatment effects of antidepressants in patients with poststroke depression: a meta-analysis. Ann Pharmacother 40:2115–2122, 2006

Choi-Kwon S, Han SW, Kwon SU, et al: Fluoxetine treatment in poststroke depression, emotional incontinence, and anger proneness: a double-blind, placebo-controlled study. Stroke 37(1):156–161, 2006

Cohen B, Sommer B: Metabolism of thioridazine in the elderly. J Clin Psychopharmacol 8:336–339, 1988

Cohen DJ, Detlor J, Young JG, et al: Clonidine ameliorates Gilles de la Tourette's syndrome. Arch Gen Psychiatry 37:1350–1357, 1980

Cohen LS, Rosenbaum JF: Birth outcomes in pregnant women taking fluoxetine (letter; comment; discussion). N Engl J Med 336:872–873, 1997

Cohen LS, Heller VL, Rosenbaum JF: Treatment guidelines for psychotropic drug use in pregnancy. Psychosomatics 30:25–33, 1989

Cohen LS, Friedman JM, Jefferson JW, et al: A reevaluation of risk of in utero exposure to lithium. JAMA 271:146–150, 1994 [erratum: JAMA 271:1485, 1994; also see comments: 271:1828–1829, 1994]

Cole JO: Research issues, in Anxiety in the Elderly. Edited by Salzman C, Lebowitz BD. New York, Springer, 1990

Cole J, Hardy P, Marcel B, et al: Organic states, in Common Treatment Problems in Depression. Edited by Schatzberg AF. Washington, DC, American Psychiatric Press, 1985, pp 79–100

Colenda CC III: Buspirone in treatment of agitated demented patient (letter). Lancet 1(8595):1169, 1988

Correll CU, Leucht S, Kane JM: Lower risk for tardive dyskinesia associated with second-generation antipsychotics: a systematic review of 1-year studies. Am J Psychiatry 161:414–425, 2004

Courtney DB: Selective serotonin reuptake inhibitor and venlafaxine use in children and adolescents with major depressive disorder: a systematic review of published randomized controlled trials. Can J Psychiatry 49:557–563, 2004

Cumming RG, Le Couteur DG: Benzodiazepines and risk of hip fractures in older people: a review of the evidence. CNS Drugs 17:825–837, 2003

Cuzzell JZ: Paroxetine may increase risk for congenital malformations. Dermatol Nurs 18(1):68, 2006

Dahlin M, Knutsson E, Nergardh A: Treatment of spasticity in children with low dose benzodiazepine. J Neurol Sci 117:54–60, 1993

Dam M, Tonin P, De Boni A, et al: Effects of fluoxetine and maprotiline on functional recovery in poststroke hemiplegic patients undergoing rehabilitation therapy. Stroke 27:1211–1214, 1996

Davis KL, Thal LJ, Gamzu ER, et al: A double-blind multicenter study of tacrine for Alzheimer's disease. Tacrine Study Group. N Engl J Med 327:1253–1259, 1992

Daviss WB, Bentivoglio P, Racusin R, et al: Bupropion sustained release in adolescents with comorbid attention-deficit/hyperactivity disorder and depression. J Am Acad Child Adolesc Psychiatry 40:307–314, 2001

DelBello MP, Kowatch RA, Adler CM, et al: A double-blind randomized pilot study comparing quetiapine and divalproex for adolescent mania. J Am Acad Child Adolesc Psychiatry 45:305–313, 2006

Dennis K, Le Grange D, Bremer J: Olanzapine use in adolescent anorexia nervosa. Eat Weight Disord 11(2):e53–e56, 2006 [Epub]

DeVane CL, Sallee FR: Selective serotonin reuptake inhibitors in child and adolescent psychopharmacology: a review of published experience. J Clin Psychiatry 57:55–56, 1996

Dietrich A, Mortensen ME, Wheller J: Cardiac toxicity in an adolescent following chronic lithium and imipramine therapy. J Adolesc Health 14:394–397, 1993

DiGiacomo J: The hypertensive or cardiac patient, in Common Treatment Problems in Depression. Edited by Schatzberg AF. Washington, DC, American Psychiatric Press, 1985, pp 29–56

Djulus J, Koren G, Einarson TR, et al: Exposure to mirtazapine during pregnancy: a prospective, comparative study of birth outcomes. J Clin Psychiatry 67:1280–1284, 2006

Dodd S, Berk M: The safety of medications for the treatment of bipolar disorder during pregnancy and the puerperium. Curr Drug Saf 1(1):25–33, 2006

Dolovich LR, Addis A, Vaillancourt JM, et al: Benzodiazepine use in pregnancy and major malformations or oral cleft: meta-analysis of cohort and case-control studies. BMJ 317(7162):839–843, 1998

Dopheide JA, Pliszka SR: Attention-deficit-hyperactivity disorder: an update. Pharmacotherapy 29:656–679, 2009

Einarson A, Boskovic R: Use and safety of antipsychotic drugs during pregnancy. J Psychiatr Pract 15:183–192, 2009

Einarson A, Choi J, Einarson TR, et al: Incidence of major malformations in infants following antidepressant exposure in pregnancy: results of a large prospective cohort study. Can J Psychiatry 54:242–246, 2009

Eisendorfer C, Fann WE (eds): Psychopharmacology and Aging. New York, Plenum, 1973

Emslie GJ, Rush AJ, Weinberg WA, et al: A double-blind, randomized, placebo-controlled trial of fluoxetine in children and adolescents with depression. Arch Gen Psychiatry 54:1031–1037, 1997

Emslie GJ, Heiligenstein JH, Wagner KD, et al: Fluoxetine for acute treatment of depression in children and adolescents: a placebo-controlled, randomized clinical trial. J Am Acad Child Adolesc Psychiatry 41:1205–1215, 2002

Emslie GJ, Heiligenstein JH, Hoog SL, et al: Fluoxetine treatment for prevention of relapse of depression in children and adolescents: a double-blind, placebo-controlled study. J Am Acad Child Adolesc Psychiatry 43:1397–1405, 2004

Eros E, Czeizel AE, Rockenbauer M, et al: A population-based case-control teratologic study of nitrazepam, medazepam, tofisopam, alprazolum and clonazepam treatment during pregnancy. Eur J Obstet Gynecol Reprod Biol 101(2):147-154, 2002

Farlow M, Gracon SI, Hershey LA, et al: A controlled trial of tacrine in Alzheimer's disease. Tacrine Study Group. JAMA 268:2523–2529, 1992

Federoff JP, Robinson RG: Tricyclic antidepressants in the treatment of poststroke depression. J Clin Psychiatry 50 (7, suppl):18–23, 1989

Field T: Breastfeeding and antidepressants. Infant Behav Dev 31:481–487, 2008

Findling RL, Aman MG, Eerdekens M, et al: Long-term, open-label study of risperidone in children with severe disruptive behaviors and below-average IQ. Am J Psychiatry 161:677–684, 2004

Findling RL, McNamara NK, Youngstrom EA, et al: Double-blind 18-month trial of lithium versus divalproex maintenance treatment in pediatric bipolar disorder. J Am Acad Child Adolesc Psychiatry 44:409–417, 2005

Findling RL, McNamara NK, Stansbrey R, et al: Combination lithium and divalproex sodium in pediatric bipolar symptom re-stabilization. J Am Acad Child Adolesc Psychiatry 45(2):142–148, 2006

Foster CA, Bafaloukos J: Paroxetine in the treatment of chronic daily headache. Headache 34:587–589, 1994

Frankenburg FR, Kando JC: Sertraline treatment of attention deficit hyperactivity disorder and Tourette's syndrome (letter). J Clin Psychopharmacol 14:359–360, 1994

Friedel R: Pharmacokinetics in the geropsychiatric patient, in Psychopharmacology: A Generation of Progress. Edited by Lipton M, DiMascio A, Killam K. New York, Raven, 1978, pp 1499–1506

Gaete JM, Bogousslavsky J: Post-stroke depression. Expert Rev Neurother 8:75–92, 2008

Geller B, Cooper TB, Sun K, et al: Double-blind and placebo-controlled study of lithium for adolescent bipolar disorders with secondary substance dependency. J Am Acad Child Adolesc Psychiatry 37:171–178, 1998

Geller DA, Hoog SL, Heiligenstein JH, et al: Fluoxetine treatment for obsessive-compulsive disorder in children and adolescents: a placebo-controlled clinical trial. J Am Acad Child Adolesc Psychiatry 40:773–779, 2001

Gentile S: Pregnancy exposure to serotonin reuptake inhibitors and the risk of spontaneous abortions. CNS Spectr 13:960–966, 2008

Gentile S: Antipsychotic therapy during early and late pregnancy: a systematic review. Schizophr Bull September 11, 2008 (Epub ahead of print)

Gentile S, Bellantuono C: Selective serotonin reuptake inhibitor exposure during early pregnancy and the risk of fetal major malformations: focus on paroxetine. J Clin Psychiatry 70:414–422, 2009

Gentile S, Rossi A, Bellantuono C: SSRIs during breastfeeding: spotlight on milk-to-plasma ratio. Arch Womens Ment Health 10:39–51, 2007

Georgotas A, McCue RE, Cooper TB: A placebo-controlled comparison of nortriptyline and phenelzine in maintenance therapy of elderly depressed patients. Arch Gen Psychiatry 46:783–786, 1989

Gibbons RD, Hur K, Bhaumik DK, Mann JJ: The relationship between antidepressant prescription rates and rate of early adolescent suicide. Am J Psychiatry 163:1898–1904, 2006

Gibbons RD, Brown CH, Hur K, et al: Early evidence on the effects of regulators' suicidality warnings on SSRI prescriptions and suicide in children and adolescents. Am J Psychiatry 164:1356–1363, 2007

Glassman A: The newer antidepressant drugs and their cardiovascular effects. Psychopharmacol Bull 20:272–277, 1984

Glassman A, Perel J, Shostak M, et al: Clinical implications of imipramine plasma levels for depressive illness. Arch Gen Psychiatry 34:197–204, 1977

Glassman AH, Bigger JT, Giardino EGV, et al: Clinical effects of imipramine induced orthostatic hypotension. Lancet 1:468–472, 1979

Glassman A, Walsh B, Roose S, et al: Factors related to orthostatic hypotension associated with tricyclic antidepressants. J Clin Psychiatry 43:35–40, 1982

Gleason RP, Schneider LS: Carbamazepine treatment of agitation in Alzheimer's outpatients refractory to neuroleptics. J Clin Psychiatry 51:115–118, 1990 [see comments]

Gold M, Estroff T, Pottash A: Substance-induced organic mental disorders, in Psychiatry Update: The American Psychiatric Association Annual Review, Vol 4. Edited by Hales RE, Frances AJ. Washington, DC, American Psychiatric Press, 1985, pp 227–240

Goldenberg G, Kahaner K, Basavaraju N, et al: Gabapentin for disruptive behaviour in an elderly demented patient (letter). Drugs Aging 13:183–184, 1998

Goldstein DJ, Corbin LA, Sundell KL: Effects of first-trimester fluoxetine exposure on the newborn. Obstet Gynecol 89(5, pt 1):713–718, 1997a

Goldstein DJ, Sundell KL, Corbin LA: Birth outcomes in pregnant women taking fluoxetine (letter; comment; discussion). N Engl J Med 336:872–873, 1997b

Greenberg SM, Tennis MK, Brown LB, et al: Donepezil therapy in clinical practice: a randomized crossover study. Arch Neurol 57:94–99, 2000

Greendyke RM, Kanter DR: Therapeutic effects of pindolol on behavioral disturbances associated with organic brain disease: a double-blind study. J Clin Psychiatry 47:423–426, 1986

Greendyke RM, Berkner JP, Webster JC, et al: Treatment of behavioral problems with pindolol. Psychosomatics 30:161–165, 1989

Greenhill LL, Halperin JM, Abikoff H: Stimulant medications. J Am Acad Child Adolesc Psychiatry 38:503–512, 1999

Greenhill LL, Biederman J, Boellner SW, et al: A randomized, double-blind, placebo-controlled study of modafinil film-coated tablets in children and adolescents with attention-deficit/hyperactivity disorder. J Am Acad Child Adolesc Psychiatry 45:503–511, 2006

Gualtieri CT, Barnhill J, McGimsey J, et al: Tardive dyskinesia and other movement disorders in children treated with psychotropic drugs. J Am Acad Child Psychiatry 19:491–510, 1980

Guerin P, Barthelemy C, Garreau B, et al: The complexity of dopamine receptors and psychopharmacotherapy in children. Acta Paedopsychiatr 56:139–151, 1993

Gupta S, Ghaly N, Dewan M: Augmenting fluoxetine with dextroamphetamine to treat refractory depression. Hosp Community Psychiatry 43:281–283, 1992

Harden CL, Meador KJ, Pennell PB; American Academy of Neurology; American Epilepsy Society: Management issues for women with epilepsy—focus on pregnancy (an evidence-based review), II: teratogenesis and perinatal outcomes. Report of the Quality Standards Subcommittee and Therapeutics and Technology Subcommittee of the American Academy of Neurology and the American Epilepsy Society. Epilepsia 50:1237–1246, 2009

Haw C, Stubbs J: A survey of off-label prescribing for inpatients with mild intellectual disability and mental illness. J Intellect Disabil Res 49 (pt 11):858–864, 2005

Hazell P, O'Connell D, Heathcote D, et al: Efficacy of tricyclic drugs in treating child and adolescent depression: a meta-analysis. BMJ 310:897–901, 1995

Hechtman L: Multimodal treatment plus stimulants vs stimulant treatment alone in ADH: results from a collaborative 2-year comparative treatment study. Presented at the annual meeting of the American Academy of Child and Adolescent Psychiatry, New Orleans, October 1995

Hellings JA, Zarcone JR, Reese RM, et al: A crossover study of risperidone in children, adolescents and adults with mental retardation. J Autism Dev Disord 36:401–411, 2006

Helms PM: Efficacy of antipsychotics in the treatment of the behavioral complications of dementia: a review of the literature. J Am Geriatr Soc 33:206–209, 1985

Hendrick V, Smith LM, Suri R, et al: Birth outcomes after prenatal exposure to antidepressant medication. Am J Obstet Gynecol 188:812–815, 2003

Herrmann N, Mamdani M, Lanctot KL: Atypical antipsychotics and risk of cerebrovascular accidents. Am J Psychiatry 161:1113–1115, 2004

Horrigan JP, Barnhill LJ: Risperidone and explosive aggressive autism. J Autism Dev Disord 27:313–323, 1997

Huessey H, Ruoff P: Towards a rational drug usage in a state institution for retarded individuals. Psychiatr J Univ Ott 9:56–58, 1984

Jacobsen FM, Comas-Diaz L: Donepezil for psychotropic-induced memory loss. J Clin Psychiatry 60:698–704, 1999

Jann MW: Rivastigmine, a new-generation cholinesterase inhibitor for the treatment of Alzheimer's disease. Pharmacotherapy 20:1–12, 2000

Janowsky DS, Barnhill LJ, Shetty M, et al: Minimally effective doses of conventional antipsychotic medications used to treat aggression, self-injurious and destructive behaviors in mentally retarded adults. J Clin Psychopharmacol 25:19–25, 2005

Kafantaris V: Treatment of bipolar disorder in children and adolescents. J Am Acad Child Adolesc Psychiatry 34:732–741, 1995

Källén B, Olausson PO: Maternal use of selective serotonin re-uptake inhibitors and persistent pulmonary hypertension of the newborn. Pharmacoepidemiol Drug Saf 17:801–806, 2008

Kalra S, Born L, Sarkar M, et al: The safety of antidepressant use in pregnancy. Expert Opin Drug Saf 4(2):273–284, 2005

Kaplan CA: Depression in childhood, I: drugs may be useful. BMJ 300:1260–1261, 1990

Keller MB, Ryan ND, Strober M, et al: Efficacy of paroxetine in the treatment of adolescent major depression: a randomized controlled trial. J Am Acad Child Adolesc Psychiatry 40:762–772, 2001

Kelsey DK, Sumner CR, Casat CD, et al: Once-daily atomoxetine treatment for children with attention-deficit/hyperactivity disorder, including an assessment of evening and morning behavior: a double-blind, placebo-controlled trial. Pediatrics e114:1–8, 2004

Kent JD, Blader JC, Koplewicz HS, et al: Effects of late-afternoon methylphenidate administration on behavior and sleep in attention-deficit hyperactivity disorder. Pediatrics 96:320–325, 1995

Killen JD, Robinson TN, Ammerman S, et al: Randomized clinical trial of the efficacy of bupropion combined with nicotine patch in the treatment of adolescent smokers. J Consult Clin Psychol 72:729–735, 2004

Knapp MJ, Knopman DS, Solomon PR, et al: A 30-week randomized controlled trial of high-dose tacrine in patients with Alzheimer's disease. Tacrine Study Group. JAMA 271:985–991, 1994

Koren G, Graham K, Feigenbaum A, et al: Evaluation and counseling of teratogenic risk: the mother-risk approach. J Clin Pharmacol 33:405–411, 1993

Kramer JR, Loney J, Ponto LB, et al: Predictors of adult height and weight in boys treated with methylphenidate for childhood behavior problems. J Am Acad Child Adolesc Psychiatry 39:5617–524, 2000

Kratochvil CJ, Heiligenstein JH, Dittmann R, et al: Atomoxetine and methylphenidate treatment in children with ADHD: a prospective, randomized, open-label trial. J Am Acad Child Adolesc Psychiatry 41:776–784, 2002

Kratochvil CJ, Wilens TE, Greenhill LL, et al: Effects of long-term atomoxetine treatment for young children with attention-deficit/hyperactivity disorder. J Am Acad Child Adolesc Psychiatry 45:919–927, 2006

Kumra S, Frazier JA, Jacobsen LK, et al: Childhood-onset schizophrenia: a double-blind clozapine-haloperidol comparison. Arch Gen Psychiatry 53:1090–1097, 1996

Kumra S, Oberstar JV, Sikich L, et al: Efficacy and tolerability of second-generation antipsychotics in children and adolescents with schizophrenia. Schizophr Bull 34:60–71, 2008

Kunz NR, Goli V, Entsnah AR: Venlafaxine extended release in the treatment of pain associated with diabetic neuropathy. Neurology 54 (suppl 3):A444, 2000

Langemark M, Olesen J: Sulpiride and paroxetine in the treatment of chronic tension-type headache: an explanatory double-blind trial. Headache 34:20–24, 1994

Lavenstein B: Neonatal signs after in utero exposure to selective serotonin reuptake inhibitors. JAMA 294(18):2300 [author reply: 2300–2301], 2005

Lebert F, Pasquier F, Petit H: Behavioral effects of trazodone in Alzheimer's disease. J Clin Psychiatry 55:536–538, 1994

Leonard HL, Swedo SE, Rapoport JL: Treatment of obsessive-compulsive disorder with clomipramine and desipramine in children and adolescents: a double-blind cross-over comparison. Arch Gen Psychiatry 46:1088–1092, 1989

Lipsey J, Robinson R, Pearlsen J, et al: Nortriptyline treatment of post-stroke depression. Lancet 1:297–300, 1984

Lopez-Larson M, Frazier JA: Empirical evidence for the use of lithium and anticonvulsants in children with psychiatric disorders. Harv Rev Psychiatry 14:285–304, 2006

Louik C, Lin AE, Werler MM, et al: First-trimester use of selective serotonin reuptake inhibitors and the risk of birth defects. N Engl J Med 356:2675–2683, 2007

MacMillan CM, Korndorfer SR, Rao S, et al: A comparison of divalproex and oxcarbazepine in aggressive youth with bipolar disorder. J Psychiatr Pract 12(4):214–222, 2006

Madhusoodanan S, Bogunovic OJ: Safety of benzodiazepines in the geriatric population. Expert Opin Drug Saf 3:485–493, 2004

Mandoki MW, Tapia MR, Tapia MA, et al: Venlafaxine in the treatment of children and adolescents with major depression. Psychopharmacol Bull 33:149–154, 1997

March JS, Klee BJ, Kremer CM: Treatment benefit and the risk of suicidality in multi-center, randomized, controlled trials of sertraline in children and adolescents. J Child Adolesc Psychopharmacol 16(1–2):91–102, 2006

Marcus A, Bahro M, Sartoris J, et al: Acute exogenic psychosis following oral ingestion of 2 mg lormetazepam in an eleven-year-old boy. Pharmacopsychiatry 26:102–103, 1993

McClellan J, Werry J: Practice parameters for the assessment and treatment of children and adolescents with schizophrenia. Work Group on Quality Issues. J Am Acad Child Adolesc Psychiatry 33:616–635, 1994

McCracken JT, McGough J, Shah B, et al: Risperidone in children with autism and serious behavioral problems. N Engl J Med 347:314–321, 2002

McDougle CJ, Holmes JP, Carlson DC, et al: A double-blind, placebo-controlled study of risperidone in adults with autistic disorder and other pervasive developmental disorders. Arch Gen Psychiatry 55:633–641, 1998 [see comment: Arch Gen Psychiatry 55:643–644, 1998]

McFarlane A, Kamath MV, Fallen EL, et al: Effect of sertraline on the recovery rate of cardiac autonomic function in depressed patients after acute myocardial infarction. Am Heart J 142:617–623, 2001

McGlashan TH, Zipursky RB, Perkins D, et al: The PRIME North America Randomized Double-Blind Clinical Trial of Olanzapine Versus Placebo in Patients at Risk of Being Prodromally Symptomatic for Psychosis, I: study rationale and design. Schizophr Res 61:7–18, 2003

McKenna K, Koren G, Tetelbaum M, et al: Pregnancy outcome of women using atypical antipsychotic drugs: a prospective comparative study. J Clin Psychiatry 66(4):444–449; quiz 546, 2005

Meador KJ, Baker GA, Browning N, et al; NEAD Study Group: Cognitive function at 3 years of age after fetal exposure to antiepileptic drugs. N Engl J Med 360:1597–1605, 2009

Mellow AM, Solano-Lopez C, Davis S: Sodium valproate in the treatment of behavioral disturbance in dementia. J Geriatr Psychiatry Neurol 6:205–209, 1993

Merlob P, Birk E, Sirota L, et al: Are selective serotonin reuptake inhibitors cardiac teratogens? Echocardiographic screening of newborns with persistent heart murmur. Birth Defects Res A Clin Mol Teratol 85:837–841, 2009

Michelson D, Faries D, Wernicke J, et al: Atomoxetine in the treatment of children and adolescents with attention-deficit/hyperactivity disorder: a randomized, placebo-controlled, dose-response study. Pediatrics 108(5): e83, 2001

Miller LJ: Gabapentin for treatment of behavioral and psychological symptoms of dementia. Ann Pharmacother 35:427–431, 2001

Mondraty N, Birmingham CL, Touyz S, et al: Randomized controlled trial of olanzapine in the treatment of cognitions in anorexia nervosa. Australas Psychiatry 13:72–75, 2005

Morgan MH, Read AE: Antidepressants and liver disease. Gut 13:697–701, 1972

Morrison JL, Riggs KW, Rurak DW: Fluoxetine during pregnancy: impact on fetal development. Reprod Fertil Dev 17:641–650, 2005

Moses-Kolko EL, Bogen D, Perel J, et al: Neonatal signs after late in utero exposure to serotonin reuptake inhibitors: literature review and implications for clinical applications. JAMA 293:2372–2383, 2005

Mosholder AD, Willy M: Suicidal adverse events in pediatric randomized, controlled clinical trials of antidepressant drugs are associated with active drug treatment: a meta-analysis. J Child Adolesc Psychopharmacol 16(1–2):25–32, 2006

Mozes T, Toren P, Chernauzan N, et al: Clozapine treatment in very early onset schizophrenia. J Am Acad Child Adolesc Psychiatry 33:65–70, 1994

Mozes T, Greenberg Y, Spivak B, et al: Olanzapine treatment in chronic drug-resistant childhood-onset schizophrenia: an open-label study. J Child Adolesc Psychopharmacol 13:311–317, 2003

Nelson JC, Kennedy JS, Pollock B, et al.: Treatment of major depression with nortriptyline and paroxetine in patients with ischemic heart disease. Am J Psychiatry 156:1024–1028, 1999

Nemeroff CB, Kalali A, Keller MB, et al: Impact of publicity concerning pediatric suicidality data on physician practice patterns in the United States. Arch Gen Psychiatry 64:466–472, 2007

Nguyen HT, Sharma V, McIntyre RS: Teratogenesis associated with antibipolar agents. Adv Ther 26:281–294, 2009

Nulman I, Koren G: The safety of fluoxetine during pregnancy and lactation. Teratology 53:304–308, 1996

Nulman I, Rovet J, Stewart DE, et al: Neurodevelopment of children exposed in utero to antidepressant drugs. N Engl J Med 336:258–262, 1997

Nulman I, Rovet J, Stewart DE, et al: Child development following exposure to tricyclic antidepressants or fluoxetine throughout fetal life: a prospective, controlled study. Am J Psychiatry 159:1889–1895, 2002

Oslin DW, Ten Have TR, Streim JE, et al: Probing the safety of medications in the frail elderly: evidence from a randomized clinical trial of sertraline and venlafaxine in depressed nursing home residents. J Clin Psychiatry 64:875–882, 2003

Patel NC, DelBello MP, Bryan HS, et al: Open-label lithium for the treatment of adolescents with bipolar depression. J Am Acad Child Adolesc Psychiatry 45:289–297, 2006

Pavuluri MN, Henry DB, Carbray JA, et al: Divalproex sodium for pediatric mixed mania: a 6-month prospective trial. Bipolar Disord 7:266–273, 2005

Paykel E, Fleminger R, Watson J: Psychiatric side effects of antihypertensive drugs. J Clin Psychopharmacol 2:14–33, 1982

Pinner E, Rich CL: Effects of trazodone on aggressive behavior in seven patients with organic mental disorders. Am J Psychiatry 145:1295–1296, 1988

Platt JE, Campbell M, Green WH, et al: Cognitive effects of lithium carbonate and haloperidol in treatment-resistant aggressive children. Arch Gen Psychiatry 41:657–662, 1984

Pliszka SR, Matthews TL, Braslow KJ, et al: Comparative effects of methylphenidate and mixed salts amphetamine on height and weight in children with attention-deficit/hyperactivity disorder. J Am Acad Child Adolesc Psychiatry 45:520–526, 2006

Pomp EF, Gedde-Dahl A: Fluoxetine—safe during pregnancy and breast feeding [in Norwegian]. Tidsskr Nor Laegeforen 121:199–203, 2001

Pool D, Mileke DH, Ronger JJ, et al: A controlled evaluation of Loxitane in 75 schizophrenic adolescents. Curr Res Ther 19:99–104, 1976

Popper CW: Psychopharmacologic treatment of anxiety disorders in adolescents and children. J Clin Psychiatry 54:52–63, 1993

Prien RF: Chemotherapy in chronic organic brain syndrome: a review of the literature. Psychopharmacol Bull 9:5–20, 1973

Profenno LA, Jakimovich L, Holt CJ, et al: A randomized, double-blind, placebo-controlled pilot study of safety and tolerability of two doses of divalproex sodium in outpatients with probable Alzheimer's disease. Curr Alzheimer's Res 2:553–558, 2005

Purdon SE, Lit W, Labelle A, et al: Risperidone in the treatment of pervasive developmental disorder. Can J Psychiatry 39:400–405, 1994

Rahimi R, Nikfar S, Abdollahi M: Pregnancy outcomes following exposure to serotonin reuptake inhibitors: a meta-analysis of clinical trials. Reprod Toxicol 22:571–575, 2006

Raj AB, Sheehan DV: Medical evaluation of the anxious patient. Psychiatr Ann 18:176–181, 1988

Raskin DE: Antipsychotic medications and the elderly. J Clin Psychiatry 46:36–40, 1985

Raskin DE, et al: Presentation at the International College of Geriatric Psychopharmacology, Basel, Switzerland, 2004

Rasmussen A, Lunde M, Paulsen DL, et al: A double-blind, placebo-controlled study of sertraline in the prevention of depression in stroke patients. Psychosomatics 44:216–221, 2003

Ratey JJ, Sovner R, Mikkelsen E, et al: Buspirone therapy for maladaptive behavior and anxiety in developmentally disabled persons. J Clin Psychiatry 50:382–384, 1989

Ray WA, Griffin MR, Schaffner W, et al: Psychotropic drug use and the risk of hip fracture. N Engl J Med 316:363–369, 1987

Ray WA, Griffin MR, Downey W: Benzodiazepines of long and short elimination half-life and the risk of hip fracture. JAMA 262:3303–3307, 1989

Reding MJ, Orto LA, Winter SW, et al: Antidepressant therapy after stroke: a double-blind trial. Arch Neurol 43:763–765, 1986

Reisberg B, Ferris SH, Gershon S: An overview of pharmacologic treatment of cognitive decline in the elderly. Am J Psychiatry 138:593–600, 1981

Reisberg B, Doody R, Stoffler A, et al: Memantine in moderate-to-severe Alzheimer's disease. N Engl J Med 348:1333–1341, 2003

Reiter S, Kutcher S, Gardner D: Anxiety disorders in children and adolescents: clinical and related issues in pharmacological treatment. Can J Psychiatry 37:432–438, 1992

Reyes M, Buitelaar J, Toren P, et al: A randomized, double-blind, placebo-controlled study of risperidone maintenance treatment in children and adolescents with disruptive behavior disorders. Am J Psychiatry 163:402–410, 2006a

Reyes M, Croonenberghs J, Augustyns I, et al: Long-term use of risperidone in children with disruptive behavior disorders and subaverage intelligence: efficacy, safety, and tolerability. J Child Adolesc Psychopharmacol 16:260–272, 2006b

Richardson MA, Haugland G, Craig TJ: Neuroleptic use, parkinsonian symptoms, tardive dyskinesia, and associated factors in child and adolescent psychiatric patients. Am J Psychiatry 148:1322–1328, 1991

Richardson PH, Williams AC: Meta-analysis of antidepressant-induced analgesia in chronic pain: comment (letter). Pain 52:247–249, 1993 [also see comments]

Riddle MA, Geller B, Ryan N: Another sudden death in a child treated with desipramine. J Am Acad Child Adolesc Psychiatry 32:792–797, 1993 [also see comments]

Robinson RG, Schultz SK, Castillo C, et al: Nortriptyline versus fluoxetine in the treatment of depression and in short-term recovery after stroke: a placebo-controlled, double-blind study. Am J Psychiatry 157:351–359, 2000

Roose SP, Glassman AH, Attia E, et al: Selective serotonin reuptake inhibitor efficacy in melancholia and atypical depression. Paper presented at the 147th annual meeting of the American Psychiatric Association, Philadelphia, PA, May 21–26, 1994

Roose SP, Laghrissi-Thode F, Kennedy JS, et al: Comparison of paroxetine and nortriptyline in depressed patients with ischemic heart disease. JAMA 279:287–291, 1998

Roose SP, Sackeim HA, Krishnan KR, et al: Antidepressant pharmacotherapy in the treatment of depression in the very old: a randomized, placebo-controlled trial. Am J Psychiatry 161:2050–2059, 2004

Rosenberg DR, Holttum J, Gershon S: Textbook of Pharmacotherapy for Child and Adolescent Psychiatric Disorders. New York, Brunner/Mazel, 1994

Rugino TA, Copley TC: Effects of modafinil in children with attention-deficit/hyperactivity disorder: an open-label study. J Am Acad Child Adolesc Psychiatry 40:230–235, 2001

Rugino TA, Samsock TC: Modafinil in children with attention-deficit hyperactivity disorder. Pediatr Neurol 29:136–142, 2003

Ryan ND: The pharmacologic treatment of child and adolescent depression. Psychiatr Clin North Am 15:29–40, 1992

Ryan ND: Pharmacological treatment of child and adolescent major depression. Encephale 19:67–70, 1993

Salzman CA: Practical considerations in the pharmacologic treatment of depression and anxiety in the elderly. J Clin Psychiatry 51 (1, suppl):21–26, 1990

Saxena K, Howe M, Simeonova D, et al: Divalproex sodium reduces overall aggression in youth at high risk for bipolar disorder. J Child Adolesc Psychopharmacol 16:252–259, 2006

Schaerf FW, Miller RR, Lipsey JR, et al: ECT for major depression in four patients infected with human immunodeficiency virus. Am J Psychiatry 146:782–784, 1989

Schatzberg AF, Roose S: A double-blind, placebo-controlled study of venlafaxine and fluoxetine in geriatric outpatients with major depression. Am J Geriatr Psychiatry 14:361–370, 2006

Schatzberg AF, DeBattista C: Phenomenology and treatment of agitation. J Clin Psychiatry 60 (suppl 15):17–20, 1999

Schatzberg AF, Kremer C, Rodrigues H, et al: Double-blind, randomized comparison of mirtazapine and paroxetine in elderly depressed patients. Am J Geriatr Psychiatry 10:541–550, 2002

Scheffer RE, Kowatch RA, Carmody T, et al: Randomized, placebo-controlled trial of mixed amphetamine salts for symptoms of comorbid ADHD in pediatric bipolar disorder after mood stabilization with divalproex sodium. Am J Psychiatry 162:58–64, 2005

Schneider LS, Tariot PN, Dagerman KS, et al, CATIE-AD Study Group: Effectiveness of atypical antipsychotic drugs in patients with Alzheimer's disease. N Engl J Med 355(15):1525–1538, 2006

Schreier HA: Risperidone for young children with mood disorders and aggressive behavior. J Child Adolesc Psychopharmacol 8:49–59, 1998

Schvehla TJ, Mandoki MW, Sumner GS: Clonidine therapy for comorbid attention deficit hyperactivity disorder and conduct disorder: preliminary findings in a children's inpatient unit. South Med J 87:692–695, 1994

Shader RI (ed): Psychiatric Complications of Medical Drugs. New York, Raven, 1972

Shapiro AK, Shapiro E, Wayne H: Treatment of Tourette's syndrome. Arch Gen Psychiatry 28:92–97, 1973

Shea S, Turgay A, Carroll A, et al: Risperidone in the treatment of disruptive behavioral symptoms in children with autistic and other pervasive developmental disorders. Pediatrics 114(5):e634–e641, 2004 [Epub]

Shedlack KJ, Hennen J, Magee C, et al: Assessing the utility of atypical antipsychotic medication in adults with mild mental retardation and comorbid psychiatric disorders. J Clin Psychiatry 66:52–62, 2005

Sheehan DV, Raj AB, Sheehan KH, et al: The relative efficacy of buspirone, imipramine and placebo in panic disorder: a preliminary report. Pharmacol Biochem Behav 29:815–817, 1988

Sheikha SH, Wagner KD, Wagner R Jr: Fluoxetine treatment of trichotillomania and depression in a prepubertal child. Cutis 51:50–52, 1993

Shepard TH: The Catalogue of Teratogenic Agents, 4th Edition. Baltimore, MD, Johns Hopkins University Press, 1983

Sikich L, Hamer RM, Bashford RA, et al: A pilot study of risperidone, olanzapine, and haloperidol in psychotic youth: a double-blind, randomized, 8-week trial. Neuropsychopharmacology 29:133–145, 2004

Silver JM, Hales RE, Yudofsky SC: Psychopharmacology of depression in neurologic disorders. J Clin Psychiatry 51 (1, suppl):33–39, 1990

Simeon JG: Use of anxiolytics in children. Encephale 19:71–74, 1993

Simon GE, Cunningham ML, Davis RL: Outcomes of prenatal antidepressant exposure. Am J Psychiatry 159:2055–2061, 2002

Singer HS, Brown J, Quaskey S, et al: The treatment of attention-deficit hyperactivity disorder in Tourette's syndrome: a double-blind placebo-controlled study with clonidine and desipramine. Pediatrics 95:74–81, 1995

Sivojelezova A, Shuhaiber S, Sarkissian L, et al: Citalopram use in pregnancy: prospective comparative evaluation of pregnancy and fetal outcome. Am J Obstet Gynecol 193:2004–2009, 2005

Slone D, Siskind V, Heinonen OP, et al: Antenatal exposure to the phenothiazines in relation to congenital malformations, perinatal mortality rate, birth weight, and intelligence quotient score. Am J Obstet Gynecol 128:486–488, 1977

Solhkhah R, Wilens TE, Daly J, et al: Bupropion SR for the treatment of substance-abusing outpatient adolescents with attention-deficit/hyperactivity disorder and mood disorders. J Child Adolesc Psychopharmacol 15:777–786, 2005

Sovner R: The use of valproate in the treatment of mentally retarded persons with typical and atypical bipolar disorders. J Clin Psychiatry 50 (3, suppl): 40–43, 1989

Sovner R, Hurley A: Do the mentally retarded suffer from affective illness? Arch Gen Psychiatry 40:61–67, 1983

Spencer EK, Kafantaris V, Padron-Gayol MV, et al: Haloperidol in schizophrenic children: early findings from a study in progress. Psychopharmacol Bull 28:183–186, 1992

Spencer TJ, Faraone SV, Biederman J, et al, Concerta Study Group: Does prolonged therapy with a long-acting stimulant suppress growth in children with ADHD? J Am Acad Child Adolesc Psychiatry 45:527–537, 2006

Spiller HA, Ramoska EA, Krenzelok EP, et al: Bupropion overdose: a 3-year multicenter retrospective analysis. Am J Emerg Med 12:43–45, 1994

Steiner H, Petersen ML, Saxena K, et al: Divalproex sodium for the treatment of conduct disorder: a randomized controlled clinical trial. J Clin Psychiatry 64:1183–1191, 2003

Stowe ZN, Kilts C, Ely T, et al: Excretion of sertraline in breast milk. Paper presented at the annual meeting of the Society for Psychosomatic Obstetrics and Gynecology, 1995

Sullivan MJ, Reesor K, Mikail S, et al: The treatment of depression in chronic low back pain: review and recommendations. Pain 50:5–13, 1992 [also see comments]

Sultzer DL, Gray KF, Gunay I, et al: Does behavioral improvement with haloperidol or trazodone treatment depend on psychosis or mood symptoms in patients with dementia? J Am Geriatr Soc 49:1294–1300, 2001

Summers W, Majovski L, Marsh G, et al: Oral tetrahydroaminoacridine in long-term treatment of senile dementia. N Engl J Med 315:1241–1245, 1986

Swanson JM, Lerner M, Williams L: More frequent diagnosis of attention deficit-hyperactivity disorder (letter). N Engl J Med 333:944, 1995

Tariot PN, Erb R, Podgorski CA, et al: Efficacy and tolerability of carbamazepine for agitation and aggression in dementia. Am J Psychiatry 155:54–61, 1998

Tariot PN, Jakimovich LJ, Erb R, et al: Withdrawal from controlled carbamazepine therapy followed by further carbamazepine treatment in patients with dementia. J Clin Psychiatry 60:684–689, 1999

Tariot PN, Farlow MR, Grossberg GT, et al: Memantine treatment in patients with moderate to severe Alzheimer disease already receiving donepezil: a randomized controlled trial. JAMA 291:317–324, 2004

Tariot PN, Raman R, Jakimovich LJ, et al: Divalproex sodium in nursing home residents with possible or probable Alzheimer disease complicated by agitation: a randomized, controlled trial. Am J Geriatr Psychiatry 13:942–949, 2005

Taylor FB, Russo J: Efficacy of modafinil compared to dextroamphetamine for the treatment of attention deficit hyperactivity disorder in adults. J Child Adolesc Psychopharmacol 10:311–320, 2000

Thakur A, Jagadheesan K, Sinha VK: Lamotrigine add-on to valproate therapy for paediatric bipolar affective disorder. Aust N Z J Psychiatry 39(7):639, 2005

Thomas SV, Ajaykumar B, Sindhu K, et al: Motor and mental development of infants exposed to antiepileptic drugs in utero. Epilepsy Behav 13:229–236, 2008

Thompson TL, Moran MG, Nies AS: Psychotropic drug use in the elderly, II. N Engl J Med 308:194–199, 1985

Tinetti ME, Speechley M: Prevention of falls among the elderly. N Engl J Med 320:1055–1059, 1989

Trifirò G, Verhamme KM, Ziere G, et al: All-cause mortality associated with atypical and typical antipsychotics in demented outpatients. Pharmacoepidemiol Drug Saf 16:538–544, 2007

Troost PW, Lahuis BE, Steenhuis MP, et al: Long-term effects of risperidone in children with autism spectrum disorders: a placebo discontinuation study. J Am Acad Child Adolesc Psychiatry 44(11):1137–1144, 2005

Tsuang MM, Lu L, Stotsky BA, et al: Haloperidol vs thioridazine for hospitalized psychogeriatric patients: double-blind study. J Am Geriatr Soc 19:593–600, 1971

Turner DC, Clark L, Dowson J, et al: Modafinil improves cognition and response inhibition in adult attention-deficit/hyperactivity disorder. Biol Psychiatry 55:1031–1040, 2004

Varkukla M, Viguera AC, Gonsalves L: Depression and pregnancy. Compr Ther 35:44–49, 2009

Vetro A, Szentistvanyi I, Pellaj L, et al: Therapeutic experience with lithium in childhood aggressivity. Neuropsychobiology 14:121–127, 1985

Viguera AC, Koukopoulos A, Muzina DJ, et al: Teratogenicity and anticonvulsants: lessons from neurology to psychiatry. J Clin Psychiatry 68 (suppl 9):29–33, 2007 [Erratum in: J Clin Psychiatry 68:1989, 2007]

Vinten J, Adab N, Kini U, et al; Liverpool and Manchester Neurodevelopmental Study Group: Neuropsychological effects of exposure to anticonvulsant medication in utero. Neurology 64:949–954, 2005

Wagner KD, Fershtman M: Potential mechanism of desipramine-related sudden death in children. Psychosomatics 34:80–83, 1993

Wagner KD, Robb AS, Findling R, et al: Citalopram is effective in the treatment of major depressive disorder in children and adolescents: results of a placebo-controlled trial, in Abstracts of the 40th Annual Meeting of the American College of Neuropsychopharmacology, Waikoloa, HI, 2001

Wagner KD, Ambrosini P, Rynn M, et al: Efficacy of sertraline in the treatment of children and adolescents with major depressive disorder: two randomized controlled trials. JAMA 290:1033–1041, 2003

Wagner KD, Kowatch RA, Emslie GJ, et al: A double-blind, randomized, placebo-controlled trial of oxcarbazepine in the treatment of bipolar disorder in children and adolescents. Am J Psychiatry 163:1179–1186, 2006 [erratum: Am J Psychiatry 163(10):1843, 2006]

Weiler PG, Mungas D, Bernick C: Propranolol for the control of disruptive behavior in senile dementia. J Geriatr Psychiatry Neurol 1:226–230, 1988

Weller EB, Weller RA, Fristad MA: Bipolar disorder in children: misdiagnosis, underdiagnosis, and future directions. J Am Acad Child Adolesc Psychiatry 34:709–714, 1995

Whitaker A, Rao U: Neuroleptics in pediatric psychiatry. Psychiatr Clin North Am 15:243–276, 1992

Whittington CJ, Kendall T, Fonagy P, et al: Selective serotonin reuptake inhibitors in childhood depression: systematic review of published versus unpublished data. Lancet 363:1341–1345, 2004

Wilens TE, Biederman J, Mick E, et al: A systematic assessment of tricyclic antidepressants in the treatment of adult attention-deficit hyperactivity disorder. J Nerv Ment Dis 183:48–50, 1995

Wilens TE, Haight BR, Horrigan JP, et al: Bupropion XL in adults with attention-deficit/hyperactivity disorder: a randomized, placebo-controlled study. Biol Psychiatry 57:793–801, 2005

Winn S, Stowe ZN, Landry JC, et al: Sertraline in breast milk and nursing infants, in 1995 New Research Program and Abstracts, American Psychiatric Association 148th Annual Meeting, Miami, FL, May 20–25, 1995. Washington, DC, American Psychiatric Association, 1995, p 73

Winterstein AG, Gerhard T, Shuster J, et al: Utilization of pharmacologic treatment in youths with attention-deficit/hyperactivity disorder in Medicaid database. Ann Pharmacother 42:24–31, 2008

Wragg RE, Jeste DV: Neuroleptics and alternative treatments: management of behavioral symptoms and psychosis in Alzheimer's disease and related conditions. Psychiatr Clin North Am 11:195–213, 1988

Wragg RE, Jeste DV: Overview of depression and psychosis in Alzheimer's disease. Am J Psychiatry 146:577–587, 1989

Yacobi S, Ornoy A: Is lithium a real teratogen? What can we conclude from the prospective versus retrospective studies? A review. Isr J Psychiatry Relat Sci 45:95–106, 2008

Yonkers KA, Wisner KL, Stewart DE, et al: The management of depression during pregnancy: a report from the American Psychiatric Association and the American College of Obstetricians and Gynecologists. Gen Hosp Psychiatry 31:403–413, 2009

Yudofsky SC, Silver JM, Schneider SE: The use of beta blockers in the treatment of aggression. Psychiatry Letters 6:15–23, 1988

Appendix A

Strengths and Costs of Antidepressant and Antipsychotic Drugs

Drug	Strength (mg)	Cost per 100 units, or as specified ($)[a]
Antidepressants		
amitriptyline	25	36
amoxapine	25	62
bupropion (generic)	100	96
bupropion sustained release (generic)	100	169
bupropion extended release (generic)	150	152 (per 30 tablets)
bupropion (Wellbutrin)	100	338
bupropion sustained release (Wellbutrin SR)	100	209 (per 60 tablets)
bupropion extended release (Wellbutrin XL)	150	194 (per 30 tablets)
citalopram (Celexa)	20	372
clomipramine	50	106
desipramine	25	116
desvenlafaxine (Pristiq)	100	129 (per 30 tablets)
duloxetine (Cymbalta)	60	480
doxepin	25	44
escitalopram (Lexapro)	20	338
fluoxetine (Prozac)	20	630

669

Drug	Strength (mg)	Cost per 100 units, or as specified ($)[a]
Antidepressants *(continued)*		
fluoxetine delayed release (Prozac Weekly)	90	130 (per 4 tablets)
fluvoxamine	50	257
imipramine	25	72
mirtazapine (Remeron)	30	126 (per 30 tablets)
nefazodone	100	92 (per 60)
nortriptyline	25	80
paroxetine (generic)	20	81 (per 30 tablets)
paroxetine (Paxil)	20	116 (per 30 tablets)
paroxetine controlled release (Paxil CR)	25	120 (per 30 tablets)
phenelzine (Nardil)	15	53 (per 60 tablets)
protriptyline (generic)	10	307
protriptyline (Vivactil)	10	379
sertraline (generic)	50	285
sertraline (Zoloft)	50	302
tranylcypromine (Parnate)	10	153
trazodone	50	57
trimipramine (Surmontil)	25	226
venlafaxine (generic)	37.5	200 (per 100 tablets)
venlafaxine (Effexor)	37.5	148 (per 60 tablets)
venlafaxine sustained release (Effexor XR)	37.5	382 (per 90 capsules)
Antipsychotics		
aripiprazole (Abilify)	15	485 (per 30 tablets)
aripiprazole ODT (Abilify Oral Disintegrating Tabs)	15	577 (per 30 tablets)
chlorpromazine	100	81
clozapine (generic)	25	136
	100	314
clozapine (Clozaril)	25	261
	100	676
fluphenazine decanoate	25 mg/mL	16 (per 5-mL MDV)

Drug	Strength (mg)	Cost per 100 units, or as specified ($)[a]
Antipsychotics *(continued)*		
haloperidol	5	78
haloperidol decanoate	100 mg/mL	30 (per 5-mL MDV)
loxapine	10	127
olanzapine (Zyprexa)	5	311 (per 30 tablets)
	10	468 (per 30 tablets)
olanzapine (Zydis)	5	346 (per 30 tablets)
	10	503 (per 30 tablets)
perphenazine	8	137
pimozide (Orap)	2	162
quetiapine (Seroquel)	200	949
quetiapine extended release (Seroquel XR)	200	515 (per 60 tablets)
risperidone (generic)	2	456 (per 60 tablets)
	3	536 (per 60 tablets)
risperidone (Risperdal)	2	535 (per 60 tablets)
	3	628 (per 60 tablets)
risperidone (Risperdal M-Tab)	2	279 (per 28 tablets)
risperidone ODT (generic M-Tab)	2	263 (per 28 tablets)
risperidone (Risperdal Consta)	25	296 (per prefilled syringe)
	37.5	445 (per prefilled syringe)
ziprasidone (Geodon)	60	543 (per 60 tablets)
	80	543 (per 60 tablets)
Mood stabilizers		
carbamazepine (Tegretol)	200	34
carbamazepine extended release (Tegretol XR)	200	100
divalproex (generic)	500	325
divalproex (Depakote)	500	385
divalproex extended release (generic)	500	295 (per 100 tablets)
divalproex extended release (Depakote ER)	500	334
gabapentin (generic)	400	160

Drug	Strength (mg)	Cost per 100 units, or as specified ($)[a]
Mood stabilizers *(continued)*		
gabapentin (Neurontin)	400	230
lamotrigine (generic)	100	475 (per 100 tablets)
lamotrigine (Lamictal)	100	582
lamotrigine extended release (Lamictal XR)	100	328 (per 30 tablets)
lithium carbonate	300	19
lithium carbonate ER (generic)	300	47
	450	53 (per 100 tablets)
lithium carbonate ER (Lithobid)	300	218
topiramate (generic)	100	418 (per 60 tablets)
topiramate (Topamax)	100	464 (per 60 tablets)

Note.   MDV = multidose vial.
[a]Cost is reported as the average wholesale price (AWP) based on AmerisourceBergen Drug Distribution, 2009. If a generic drug is available from more than one manufacturer, at least three prices were averaged to obtain an AWP for the drug.

Appendix B

Suggested Readings

For Clinicians

DeBattista C, Glick IR: The Medical Management of Depression, 4th Edition. Dallas, TX, Essential Medical Information Systems, 2003

Brunton LL, Lazo JS, Parker KL (eds): Goodman and Gilman's The Pharmacological Basis of Therapeutics, 11th Edition. New York, Pergamon, 2006

Goodwin FK, Jamison KR: Manic-Depressive Illness, 2nd Edition. New York, Oxford University Press, 2007

Janicak PG, Davis JM, Preskorn SH, et al: Principles and Practice of Psychopharmacotherapy, 2nd Edition. Baltimore, MD, Williams & Wilkins, 1997

Jefferson JW, Greist JH, Ackerman DL, et al: Lithium Encyclopedia for Clinical Practice, 2nd Edition. Washington, DC, American Psychiatric Press, 1987

Ketter TA (ed): Handbook of Diagnosis and Treatment of Bipolar Disorders. Washington, DC, American Psychiatric Publishing, 2009

Koran LM: Obsessive-Compulsive and Related Disorders in Adults. Cambridge, UK, Cambridge University Press, 1999

Nestler EJ, Hyman SE, Malenka RC: Molecular Neuropharmacology: A Foundation for Clinical Neurosciences, 2nd Edition. New York, McGraw-Hill, 2008

Schatzberg AF, Nemeroff CB (eds): The American Psychiatric Publishing Textbook of Psychopharmacology, 4th Edition. Washington, DC, American Psychiatric Publishing, 2009

Schatzberg AF, Nemeroff CB (eds): Essentials of Clinical Psychopharmacology, 2nd Edition. Washington, DC, American Psychiatric Publishing, 2006

Stahl SM: Essential Psychopharmacology: Neuroscientific Basis and Practical Applications, 3rd Edition. New York, MA, Cambridge Press, 2008

For Patients and Families

Allen JG: Coping With Depression: From Catch 22 to Hope. Washington, DC, American Psychiatric Publishing, 2006

Burns D: The Feeling Good Handbook. New York, Plume, 1999

Charney DS, Nemeroff CB: The Peace of Mind Prescription. Boston, MA, Houghton-Mifflin, 2004

Duke P, Hochman G: A Brilliant Madness: Living With Manic-Depressive Illness. New York, Bantam Books, 1992

Fawcett J, Golden B, Rosenfeld N, et al: New Hope for People With Bipolar Disorder. New York, Crown/Random House, 2000

Gilson M, Freeman A: Overcoming Depression: A Cognitive Approach to Taming the Depression Beast. San Antonio, TX, Harcourt Press/Psychological Corporation, 2000

Graves BB: Bulimia: Perspectives on Mental Illness. Mankato, MN, Lifematters Books/Capstone Press, 2000

Hales D, Hales RE: Caring for the Mind. New York, Bantam Press, 1996

Healy D: The Antidepressant Era. Boston, MA, Harvard University Press, 1998

Jamison KR: An Unquiet Mind. New York, Alfred A Knopf, 1995

Jamison KR: Touched With Fire: Manic-Depressive Illness and the Artistic Temperament. New York, Free Press, 1996

Jamison KR: Night Falls Fast: Understanding Suicide. New York, Vintage Books/Random House, 1999

Karp DA: The Burden of Sympathy: How Families Cope With Mental Illness. New York, Oxford University Press, 1999

Kerns LL, Lieberman AB: Helping Your Depressed Child: A Reassuring Guide to the Causes and Treatment of Childhood and Adolescent Depression. Roseville, CA, Prima, 1993

Kramer PD: Listening to Prozac. New York, Viking, 1993

Levenkron S: The Anatomy of Anorexia. New York, WW Norton, 2000

Mondimore FM: Bipolar Disorder: A Guide for Patients and Families. Baltimore, MD, Johns Hopkins University Press, 1999

Rosen LE, Amador XF: When Someone You Love Is Depressed. New York, Free Press, 1996

Rothschild B: The Body Remembers: The Psychophysiology of Trauma and Trauma Treatment. New York, WW Norton, 2000

Shields B: Down Came the Rain: My Journey Through Postpartum Depression. New York, Hyperion, 2006

Solomon A: The Noonday Demon: An Atlas of Depression. New York, Touchstone, 2002

Styron W: Darkness Visible: A Memoir of Madness. New York, Random House, 1990

Torrey EF: Surviving Schizophrenia: A Manual for Families, Consumers, Providers. New York, Harper & Row, 2001

Weiden P: Breakthroughs in Antipsychotic Medications: A Guide for Consumers, Families, and Clinicians. New York, WW Norton, 2000

Weissman M: Mastering Depression Through Interpersonal Psychotherapy. San Antonio, TX, Harcourt Press/Psychological Corporation, 2000

Whybrow P: American Mania: When More Is Not Enough. New York, WW Norton, 2006

Index

*Page numbers printed in **boldface** type refer to tables or figures.*